NEUROLOGICAL AND NEUROSURGICAL NURSING

Barbara A Verran, SRN, SCM, RCNT
Formerly Clinical Teacher, Atkinson Morley's Hospital, London;
Currently Matron, Longdown Nursing Home, Surrey

and

Pamela E Aisbitt, SRN, CMB, RMN
Formerly Sister, Neurological Unit, Atkinson Morley's Hospital,
London; Currently Community Nurse, Kent

Edward Arnold
A division of Hodder & Stoughton
LONDON   BALTIMORE   MELBOURNE   AUCKLAND

© 1988 Barbara Verran and Pamela Aisbitt

First published in Great Britain 1988

British Library Cataloguing Publication Data

Verran, Barbara A.
  Neurological and neurosurgical nursing.
  1. Neurological patients. Nursing
  I. Title   II. Aisbitt, Pamela E.
  610.73'68

    ISBN 0-7131-4521-8

Whilst the advice and information in this book is believed to be true
and accurate at the date of going to press, neither the author nor the
publisher can accept any legal responsibility or liability for any errors
or omissions that may be made.

Typeset in 10/11pt Times by Colset Private Ltd, Singapore
Printed and bound in Great Britain for Edward Arnold, the
educational, academic and medical publishing division of
Hodder & Stoughton Limited, 41 Bedford Square, London WC1B
3DQ by Butler and Tanner Ltd, Frome and London

Contents

Foreword   vi

Preface   vii

Acknowledgements   ix

1   **Neurological Nursing**   1
    Introduction   1

Part I Disorders of the Brain   *3*

2   **Neurological Examination and Investigations**   4
    Anatomy and physiology   4
    Examination of the patient   8
    Investigations   25

3   **Changing Levels of Consciousness and Care of the Unconscious Patient Including Care of the Critically Ill Patient in Intensive Care**   36
    Anatomy as related to unconsciousness   36
    Immediate nursing care   40
    Continuing nursing care and complications of unconsciousness   42
    Rehabilitation   62
    Death   66

4   **Congenital Cranial Disorders**   69
    The ventricular system   70
    Hydrocephalus   71
    Infantile hydrocephalus   72
    Hydrocephalus in later childhood   77
    Congenital tumours   80
    Craniostenosis   81

5   **Head Injury**   82
    Anatomy related to injury   83
    Immediate care of a patient at the scene of the accident   86

    Complications of head injury   89
    Rehabilitation   95
    Birth injuries   96

6   **Intracranial Infection**   97
    Anatomy   97
    Meningitis   99
    Intracranial abscess   103
    Encephalitis   105
    Rabies   107
    Fungal and parasitic infections   110

7   **Intracranial Tumours**   111
    Anatomical and functional localisation   111
    Radiotherapy and cytotoxic chemotherapy   122

8   **Intracranial Vascular Disorders**   124
    Anatomy and physiology   125
    Causes of cerebrovascular accident   127
    Cranial haemorrhage   131
    Cerebral ischaemia   137
    Nursing care following cerebrovascular accident   140
    Routine general nursing care   145
    Mobilisation and rehabilitation   147

9   **Degenerative Disorders of the Brain**   151
    Anatomy and physiology   151
    Dementia   152

Part II Disorders of the Spine   *161*

10   **Disturbances of Sensation and Power**   162
    Anatomy and physiology   162
    Rehabilitation   181

11   **Congenital Spinal Disorders**   185
    Spina bifida and myelo-meningocele   189
    Further care and rehabilitation   196

Syringomyelia 202
Diastematomyelia 205
Spinal angioma 205

12 Spinal Injury **206**
Acute injuries 206
Management of spinal injury 208
Chronic spinal trauma 213

13 Spinal Infection **223**
Myelitis 224
Arachnoiditis 227
Spinal abscess 227
Spinal tuberculosis (Pott's disease) 228
Herpes zoster (shingles) 229

14 Spinal Neoplasm **232**

15 Spinal Vascular Disorders **236**

16 Spinal Degenerative Disorders **238**
Cervical spondylosis 238
Ankylosing spondylitis 241
Spondylolisthesis 242
Paget's disease 242

*Part III Other Disorders of the Nervous
  System* *243*

17 Pain **244**
Anatomy and physiology 245
Headache 245
Migraine 247
Migrainous neuralgia 249
Trigeminal neuralgia (Tic douloureux) 249
Glossopharyngeal neuralgia 252
Atypical facial pain 252
Temporal arteritis 252

18 Demyelinating Diseases **258**
Multiple sclerosis 258
Neuromyelitis optica (Devic's
disease) 263
Rare diffuse demyelinating diseases 263

19 Epilepsy **264**
Generalised epilepsy (involving the
whole brain) 268
Focal epilepsy (involving part of the
brain) 269
Narcolepsy and cataplexy 276

20 Extrapyramidal Disorders **278**
Parkinson's syndrome 279
Heredofamilial or benign tremor 285
Chorea and athetosis 285
Wilson's disease (hepato-lenticular
degeneration) 290
Kernicterus (haemolytic disease of
the newborn) 293

**21 Disorders of the Labyrinth and
Acoustic Nerve** **294**
Anatomy and physiology 294
Meniere's disease 296

22 Motor Neurone Disease **298**

23 Myasthenia Gravis **303**

24 Neurosyphilis **310**
Meningo-vascular syphilis 311
Tabes dorsalis 311
General paralysis of the insane 313
Congenital neurosyphilis 314
Admission to hospital of a patient
with neurosyphilis 314

25 Peripheral Nerve Disorders **318**
Anatomy and physiology 318
Brachial plexus disorders 319
Injuries of the long thoracic nerve 323
The lumbar and sacral plexuses 323
Bell's palsy 325
Polyneuropathy 326

26 Deficiency Disorders **331**
Deficiency of vitamin B_1 332
Vitamin B_{12} (cyanocobalamin)
deficiency 333

27 Poisoning **336**
Poisons 338
Acute poisoning 338
Chronic poisoning 342
Tetanus 345
Botulism 346

28 Muscle Disorders (Myopathy) **347**
Anatomy and physiology 347
Muscular dystrophy 347
Care and management of patients

with muscular dystrophy 349
Polymyositis 352

**29 Inherited and Familial 354
Neuromuscular Disorders**
Friedreich's ataxia 354
Peroneal muscular atrophy
(Charcot-Marie-Tooth disease) 354
Nursing care 355
Dystrophia myotonica 355
Myotonia congenita (Thomsen's
disease) 357
Family periodic paralysis 357

The 'floppy' infant 357

Appendix **358**
The neurological centre 358
The rehabilitation centre 362
Nursing staff 364

Glossary **365**

Bibliography **366**

Index **367**

Foreword

The two experienced nurses who have written this book became friends when each was responsible for a busy ward full of the subjects of diseases of the nervous system. For convenience and from custom the wards were male and female medical and surgical, but really they made one large unit, for neurological physicians and surgeons work together very closely, and it is more true of the neurological surgeon than any other, that he is a physician who operates. These are the specialist wards of St. George's Hospital established at Atkinson Morley's Hospital which is world-famous. The authors had both gained their general nursing experience in St. George's. At Atkinson Morley's Hospital we had the great advantage that the unit was self-contained having all the ancillary services in the same building, the turnover was very rapid, the wards always full and the range of disorders wide – from head injuries to peripheral neuritis. Emergencies were acute and, being on the fringe of South London, patients could be rushed in by ambulance or airlifted in by helicopter.

It was upon all this that the authors gained their experience, and it was upon this experience as well as a recognised formal course of education that their knowledge and wisdom are based. They were always there for the undergraduate teaching rounds and I suspect that they learned more than did many of the students – they certainly saw more. They came to the postgraduate meetings, medical and surgical, and were close friends of technicians, welfare workers and therapists, as well as of the fairly constant senior medical staff and the ever-changing juniors. They must have learned a lot, but I did not then appreciate how much.

As I read each chapter as it was written I wondered whether they told you too much, but then I began to understand the important difference between medicine and nursing. The nurse is constantly concerned for the patient who has the disease, the physician with the disease the patient has. The doctor may sometimes be inclined to forget the patient, the nurse never can. The doctor leavens his science with humanity, the nurse her humanity with science.

So in this excellent treatise there are large and detailed parts of every chapter on how to help the patient, physically, mentally, socially and always as a person, but those sections would not make practical sense if they were not preceded by a fairly detailed account of the anatomy and physiology and the course of the disease. So I changed my mind and I would now say, in these days when there are graduates in nursing, that those of you who want to read to greater depth on a particular topic should refer to one of the specialised texts to be found in any hospital nursing or medical library. I see that this is suggested in the section on aphasia; this is a fascinating subject, the serious study of which is far beyond the scope of a text on neurological nursing, and yet if the nurse is well-informed on the subject she can do just as much as can a speech therapist to encourage hope, and from hope, the first meaningful sounds in the recovery of speech of a patient with a head injury.

This is what the book is all about. It was not written to help you through examinations, though it will. It was compiled after many years of experience in order to pass that experience on, so that you can gain the same degree of intellectual and personal satisfaction in neurological nursing as the authors have enjoyed.

We physicians can do immeasurably more for our patients than I could as a houseman many years ago. Many diseases which were always fatal then, can be reversed in a few days, and yet (if comparison is possible) I still get more satisfaction in helping the patient who has a disorder which I cannot cure, through months or even years of frustration and other distresses, than in the pride of recognition and relief of an amenable disease. This is surely so like the satisfaction of nursing.

Denis Williams

Preface

Our aim in writing this book has been to give a better understanding of injuries, disease and disorders of the nervous system by relating anatomy and physiology, medical, surgical, nursing and community care to a particular disorder. We have suggested principles to improve standards of nursing care in hospital and at home which will lead to more successful rehabilitation and have tried to emphasise that the patient is a unique individual, is one of a family and has his part to play in the community. We hope through our writing to have kindled interest and enthusiasm for the care and happiness of patients who have sometimes been misunderstood owing to mental changes, speech disorders, abnormal movements and other disabling factors. We have openly expressed and tried to discuss impartially ethical matters which we think cause greater anxiety if they remain taboo. The importance of close teamwork and good communication has been repeatedly emphasised and we have attempted to show how anticipation can often prevent anxiety and facilitate the next step in rehabilitation, or in some cases smooth the patient's way through difficult times to a peaceful, painless and dignified death.

Throughout our experience we found certain anatomical and physiological facts difficult to grasp or unexplained, sometimes we tentatively voiced our questions and discovered the answers were still a mystery to medical experts, but other gaps in our understanding have been filled while writing this book through diligent and persistent search. There is constant research into the chemical interactions of the nervous system leading to the possibility of more effective treatment for many neurological disorders, and there have been great advances in the field of genetics.

We hope our readers will find the answers they require in this textbook and will be infected with our enthusiasm for the whole subject. We have tried to discuss each topic in time sequence as the patient experiences his illness from the first development of symptoms, through treatment and rehabilitation to the time when he is totally independent or the illness reaches its fatal outcome. This book has not been written in the nursing process style but any nurse who is practising the nursing process should be able to formulate her plan of care and aims using the information given in this text. Though we appreciate that there are areas of care which can be clearly defined and laid down for all patients, we would emphasise that any plan of care must be flexible as the needs of each patient are unique. As an introduction to the patient's experiences we have tried to make plain the anatomy of the structures involved, relate it to symptoms and describe measures which will help to make a distressing or seemingly impossible situation more bearable for the patient and his relatives. It may not be clear why we have started at the head, proceeded to the spine and ended with those disorders which affect both, or the body generally. A logical system appeared necessary and after a general appraisal of the patient it seemed that one's attention was focused on the head, which contains the central control of the nervous system and is where the doctor's detailed examination usually begins. The head and spinal sections, after an introduction to nursing care, are organised starting with the newborn and young children, through the middle years and ending with disorders which mainly affect the elderly. The third section begins with those disorders which are commonplace and ends with rarer conditions.

Nursing is a repetitive process but in writing we have tried to avoid repetition by gathering all basic nursing care into two chapters (3 and 10) and elsewhere making reference to them, adding in each chapter only that which is specific to the disorder being discussed. We have here and there presumed our readers to have a certain basic nursing knowledge and have for instance deliberately omitted to give details of preoperative preparation and trays and trolleys for nursing procedures partly because hospital procedures vary. We regret that it has not been possible to give detailed description of the invaluable work of physiotherapists, occupational therapists and speech therapists and the many aids designed for the disabled, but nurses would be well advised to consult the specialist therapists and study the individual subjects. (See Bibliography).

We experienced difficulty in the choice of personal pronouns and though we appreciate that doctors, nurses, therapists and patients are of either sex, for clarity we have spoken of the doctor as 'he', the nurse as 'she' and referred to the patient as 'he' unless the condition is more common among women. In addition to the glossary of neurological terms, in the text we have introduced medical terminology in brackets preceded by its explanation, thereafter using the medical term only. There are so many drugs in use at the present time that we have only named those in most common use, deliberately omitting dosage as the prescribing of medication is the province of the doctor; we advise that nurses should use a good pharmacopoeia to keep well informed, up-to-date and know the side effects of drugs. We have tried not to confine our discussion to the Western world, but realise the paucity of our knowledge of the wider aspects of world medicine and would recommend that nurses should read widely to gain a true perspective of the incidence and distribution of neurological disorders, available treatment and resources.

We appreciate that medical science is on the brink of great advance particularly in the fields of electronics, nerve stimulators and drugs. We have witnessed in a few years rapidly changing trends in surgery and medicine; the control of raised intra-cranial pressure has ranged from repeated magnesium sulphate enemas, external ventricular drainage, intravenous urea and intragastric glycerine to intravenous mannitol, steroids and controlled ventilation; stereotaxic thermocoagulation for Parkinson's disease, developed in the 1950s, was twenty years later dismissed in favour of levodopa, which though a miracle in its time is now being revealed to have serious side effects with long-term use. Diagnosis has become more certain since the development of computerised axial tomography, and surgery has benefitted from the use of the microscope. But, what of the patient? He is still frightened of illness and its implications, of entering hospital and being surrounded by experts and space-age machinery. He is the only person experiencing the illness yet because of his lack of knowledge is unable to judge whether a treatment is right or wrong and is forced to accept the decisions of others. In spite of technological advances, nursing has not changed and the most important contribution the nurse can make to the patient's treatment is her ability to see things from the patient's viewpoint; she must listen, understand and be caring and compassionate.

We hope that our logical presentation will help nurses to remember the facts presented, practise the nursing principles suggested and develop further ideas of their own. Nursing as well as medical research is always necessary to improve the patient's comfort, and discussion of knotty problems can be most constructive, no two patients needing identical care.

1988

BV
PA

Acknowledgements

The authors would like to express their gratitude to Dr Denis Williams for his encouragement and help throughout the writing of this book. Also to Mr Alan Richardson of Atkinson Morley's Hospital, Mr Jason Bryce of the Wessex Neurological Centre, Mr Duncan Forrest of Queen Mary's Hospital for Children, Carshalton and Mr Norman Grant of the National Hospital, Queen Square, for their help with the surgical aspects of neurological disease, to the medical staff of the neurological departments of the Royal Free and St. Bartholomew's Hospitals, to Dr James Ambrose, Consultant Neurologist and Dr T Holloway, Consultant Anaesthetist, both of St George's Hospital, London. To Dr E.A. Kauffmann, Rheumatologist, for his help with chronic spinal trauma and to Patricia Collins, Physiotherapist, both from Sevenoaks Hospital. To the staff of Atkinson Morley's Hospital especially Monica Davitt (EEG) and Sister Webber and the staff of the intensive therapy unit; we are particularly indebted to Sheila Bruce, clinical nurse teacher, who responded patiently to all our questions and many phone calls and requests. Our thanks to the staff of the Beckenham Pain Clinic, the nursing staff of Queen Mary's Hospital for Children and the Sydenham Hill Children's Hospital, and to the staff of Lingfield Hospital School for the time freely given to us on our visits. To Mr Duncan Forrest, Mr Rahim Bacchus from Atkinson Morley's Hospital, who painstakingly searched out the required photographs and to Mr Patrick Holme Sellors who gave his permission to print the visual field photographs.

We are indebted to Mr Tom Swinhoe for his encouragement and help in the early days of our writing, and to Nancy Loffler and Ann Corry of Edward Arnold for the preparation of the manuscript for publication and to Teresa Lanigan for converting our rough diagrams into something more meaningful. We are especially grateful to Sue Sinclair and the many friends who looked after our children.

Lastly, but by no means least, we are enormously grateful to our husbands and children, without whose cooperation this book would not have been written, who uncomplainingly accepted and adapted to our 'one week in three' absences from home while we worked alternately in Kent or Surrey.

1

Neurological Nursing

Introduction

In this book we have tried to simplify a subject which many students and trained nurses avoid, thinking it even more complicated than it is in reality. We ourselves found the nervous system a difficult subject for study during our training days. In general medical and surgical wards we met patients suffering from disorders of the nervous system; these were young persons whose outlook for a normal active life appeared hopeless, the aged whose catastrophic 'strokes' led to a fatal outcome within days or weeks, or patients whose behaviour was so disturbed that their transfer to a specialist neurological unit was greeted with a sigh of relief and the thought that those who worked in such units must either be saints or mad! Perhaps partly to allay our curiosity we entered this field of nursing and found it of most absorbing interest and extraordinarily rewarding. It was clear that patients' lives often depended on the nurse's alertness and accurate observations; the will to live and recover powers of speech and movement were also to a large extent dependent on our persistent encouragement, enthusiasm and daily efforts to help the patient regain normality. Relatives turned to us for explanation, reassurance and comfort – it was a great responsibility and we were constantly aware of our lack of knowledge, somewhere we had to find reserves of skill, sensitivity and a new understanding of values; on many occasions we were humbled and filled with admiration for the way our patients faced ordeals with fortitude and even humour and for their relatives who bore years of strain without complaint. There can surely be no greater demand on a nurse's skill than when she is caring for patients who are unable to respond, talk, swallow or move normally and who need mechanical assistance even to breathe; who appreciates a quiet, gentle, thoughtful nurse more than a patient

suffering intense headache, even though he is unable to say so at the time? Patience and good humour are rarely more important than when trying to help those who have suffered years of progressive disability, experienced repeated hospital admission and developed apparently fussy ways and a tendency always to know best how things should be done.

There are occasions when a nurse's knowledge of neurological examination and the significance of certain signs may make the difference between death or complete paralysis, or life with complete recovery. It is essential that early in training all nurses should understand the implication of rising intracranial pressure following head injury, and signs indicative of spinal cord compression; our experience has shown us many pitfalls in nursing patients with disorders of the nervous system when delays and lack of understanding have caused avoidable disability and distress. Someone with severe mental and physical disturbance needs to be in the care of an experienced, sensitive team of people (involving all departments, all grades of hospital and community staff, however brief these encounters) who will have confidence when trying to penetrate semiconsciousness to stir the patient's will to live, and who will not be put off by the patient's sometimes alarming appearance and behaviour, apparent lack of comprehension and inability to converse. The quiet confidence of such staff will allay the fear experienced during confusion and calm tensions which lead to aggressive and disturbed behaviour. Prompt anticipation of physical and psychological needs is essential; we may appear to have overstressed such detail but it is these small details, often brushed off as unimportant, which influence the quality of the patient's recovery and make the difference between his fretful or contented state of mind. A contented patient who has confidence in those caring for him will not be difficult, unco-operative or demanding; he will strive to become independent and not cling to his helplessness, because the caring staff will continue to show their interest and concern for his welfare.

Team effort is necessary for every aspect of the patient's treatment and everyone must put the patient's interests first, understand and communicate aims and objectives of treatment, co-operate with each other without bias or rivalry and never forget to allow the patient and his relatives the freedom to express their viewpoint. Those involved in rehabilitation need to have a hopeful outlook, be prepared to tackle the impossible and enjoy the challenge, remaining undaunted by setbacks and willing to continue their efforts and encouragement even when it is obvious that the patient's condition is deteriorating, but always bearing in mind the quality of the patient's daily life. Rehabilitation should never need to be excessively hearty nor will an inflexible military regime benefit the patient. It should be based on good relationships established from the start of the patient's illness and the introduction of humour whenever this comes naturally. Little will be achieved without tremendous effort, the reward will be the occasional unexpected miracle when all seemed hopeless, the obvious but unspoken look of relief and gratitude in the eyes of a patient who is unable to speak and sometimes just the knowledge that a patient has died peacefully without the discomfort of pressure sores and painful contractures, his relatives spared intense grief through the gentle preparation received in the preceding weeks or months.

There have been many advances recently in methods of investigation, diagnosis and treatment. Unpleasant investigations have been largely superseded and surgical treatment and anaesthesia have improved. The success of treatment is easy to see when a patient is completely cured, much less so in those instances when the patient feels his severe disablement so keenly he would rather have died or his relatives express these feelings. Years of adaptation

may be necessary before the patient finds acceptance, contentment and fulfilment. No effort has been spared to produce devices and aids to improve the quality of life for even the most disabled person. Community services continually attempt to provide for individual needs, and through radio and television programmes the public are encouraged to understand and help the disabled. Treatment must always be considered from many angles by more than one person, and aim to cure or improve. A decision may have to be taken within minutes; a few patients who would otherwise have died are kept alive in a vegetative state – is anyone to blame?

There remains a large number of individuals, children and adults, whose distorted appearance, abnormal speech, helplessness and unavoidable incontinence call for understanding and love, which even in their own families may need to be fostered. The general public are often more willing to help and befriend if they understand the individual's condition. Without explanation and guidance they feel incompetent and fear even to approach him. The disabled person can be fitted with every imaginable device to assist him and still suffer from extreme loneliness, isolation and boredom, something which can happen even in hospital especially when the patient is nursed in a side ward or if there is impairment of consciousness, speech or hearing. The nurse caring for a patient with severe difficulty in communication is often in a position to give him peace of mind merely by putting into words his unexpressed wishes, feelings and thoughts and acting as interpreter, though the patient must always be allowed time to try to express himself. The nurse's role in communication is extremely important; she is responsible for maintaining clear lines of communication between the patient, his relatives and all members of the rehabilitation team. She must ensure that the patient and his relatives are well informed about community services, encourage them to make contact with those which will be helpful and tell them what to do if the patient has a relapse.

Part I
Disorders of the Brain

2

Neurological Examination and Investigations

Anatomy and physiology

Nervous tissue is composed of cells called neurones, which are bound together by connective tissue (glial cells). A typical neurone consists of a nucleated cell with projections called dendrites, one of which is elongated and forms the fibre or axon (Fig. 2.1). These axons vary in length according to the part of the body they supply. Surrounding the axon is a fatty myelin sheath which insulates the fibre enabling it to conduct electrical impulses; these are transmitted from the dendrites of one neurone to those of another across a synapse (Fig. 2.1).

The cell bodies of neurones concerned with movement (upper motor neurones) lie in the motor cortex of the brain. Their axons pass through the brain to synapse with other motor neurones in the brain stem or spinal cord (lower motor neurones), which pass to the muscles where they terminate as the motor end plate (Fig. 2.2); here electrical impulses set up in the motor cortex are discharged to the muscle fibres causing them to contract.

Sensory neurones relay impulses from the sensory receptors in the skin, muscle and joints, along the sensory axon to the cell body. Many cell bodies are grouped together in a ganglion (posterior root ganglion) just outside the spinal cord. Sensory neurones are bipolar, that is a second axon arises from the cell body and passes into the spinal cord to synapse with another neurone carrying sensation to the sensory cortex of the brain (Fig. 2.3; see also Chapter 10). Between the incoming sensory neurones entering the spinal cord and the lower motor neurones leaving it, there is a small linking neurone completing the reflex arc which facilitates reflex activity without conscious control (Fig. 2.4).

The surface of the brain is composed of millions of cell bodies (grey matter); in childhood it is fairly smooth, but the adult brain is highly convoluted, greatly increasing the surface area (Fig. 2.5). The shallower fissures are called sulci and the raised area between two sulci is a gyrus. There are two deep fissures, the fissure of Rolando (between the

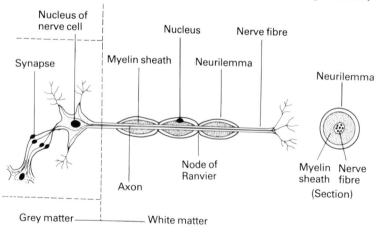

Fig. 2.1 Diagram of a neurone.

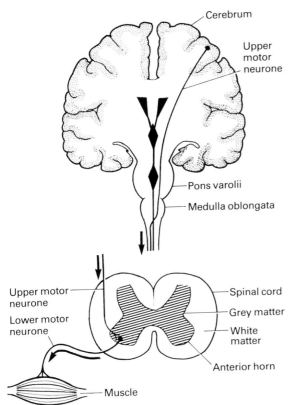

Fig. 2.2   Motor neurone from cortex to muscle.

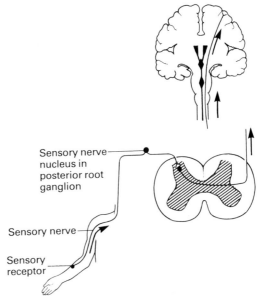

Fig. 2.3   Sensory neurones from receptor to cerebral cortex.

frontal and parietal lobes) and the fissure of Sylvius (separating the temporal from the frontal and parietal lobes). Between the lobes of each hemisphere and adjacent gyri are a multitude of connecting neurones.

The brain is a very soft, delicate organ which is enclosed within and protected by the skull. It is the nerve centre for receiving, interpreting and transmitting messages to and from the entire body and is divided into the cerebrum, cerebellum and brain stem. The cerebrum is divided into two hemispheres, each concerned with motor and sensory functions of the opposite side of the body. Information is passed between the two hemispheres through a broad connecting band of fibres, the corpus callosum (Fig. 2.6). Each hemisphere is divided into lobes, frontal, parietal, occipital and temporal (Fig. 2.5); each lobe is responsible for specific functions although there is considerable overlap of function. Some areas of the cerebrum are called 'silent areas' as their function is not yet determined. The motor cortex lies in the frontal lobe in front of the fissure of Rolando; also in the frontal lobe are inhibitory centres which enable the individual to behave in a socially acceptable manner. The sensory cortex is adjacent to the motor cortex but in the parietal lobe, immediately behind the fissure of Rolando. The occipital lobe contains the visual cortex, visual impulses being transmitted from both eyes to both occipital lobes. In the temporal lobe are the areas of cortex responsible for taste, smell, hearing and memory.

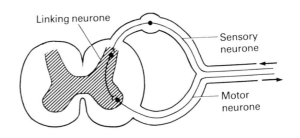

Fig. 2.4   Reflex arc.

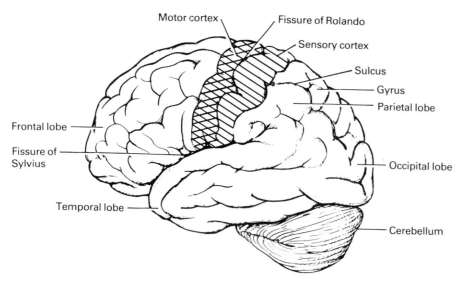

Fig. 2.5 External appearance of the brain showing lobes and convolutions.

1. Tongue
2. Nose
3. Forehead
4. Thumb
5. Fingers
6. Arm
7. Shoulder
8. Trunk
9. Hip
10. Knee
11. Foot
12. Great toe

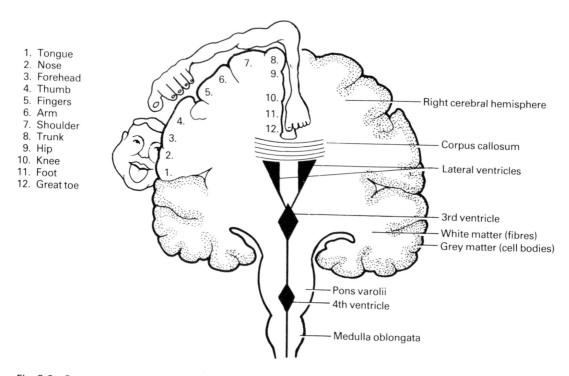

Fig. 2.6 Coronal section showing corpus callosum, grey and white matter and homunculus.

The speech area in a right-handed person is in the left fronto-parieto-temporal region of the cerebrum, the dominant hemisphere (Fig. 2.7), but in the opposite cerebral hemisphere a corresponding area of cortex deals with three-dimensional, non-verbal, spatial recognition; there are connections between these two centres through the corpus callosum. Only a small percentage of people are left-handed; those with an ambidextrous tendency may not fully develop a dominant hemisphere, and speech with its attendant skills, reading and writing, may be shared by both sides of the brain. Incoming information (sensations of vision, hearing, touch, smell and taste) from adjacent areas of cortex and corresponding regions in the other cerebral hemisphere, is passed to the speech area in the posterior part of the temporal lobe and stored in a memory 'bank'. The temporal lobe feeds appropriate words of response to the motor speech area of the frontal lobe which grammatically assembles them into expressive speech which may remain as unexpressed thoughts. All thoughts are emotionally charged as a result of influences from the hypothalamus (Fig. 2.8) and limbic areas of the frontal lobes and are coloured by past experiences stored in the temporal lobes; before they are expressed the brain applies an inhibitory control which, with judgement and intelligence ('higher' centres in the frontal lobes), modify conversation to fit the occasion. The motor cortex in both cerebral hemispheres, which controls the muscles of articulation (the lips, jaw, tongue, palate and pharynx) and phonation (the diaphragm, intercostal muscles, larynx and vocal cords) is very close to the cortex of the speech area in the dominant hemisphere and to the corresponding area on the opposite side. The upper motor neurone pathways of expressive speech pass through the basal ganglia to the brain stem where they link with the nuclei of the cranial nerves (lower motor neurones) supplying the muscles of articulation; they are joined by fibres from the cerebellum.

Clear articulate vocalisation of words 'thought' by the brain is dependent upon:

intact bilateral motor and sensory pathways, including the cranial nerves;

maintenance of muscle tone by the basal ganglia;

co-ordination of muscular movement by the cerebellum; and

healthy muscles of articulation and phonation.

Beneath the superficial layer of grey matter, the greater part of the cerebral hemispheres is composed of axons (motor and sensory white fibres) which come together in a band in the centre of each hemisphere as the internal capsules (Fig. 2.9). Surrounding each internal capsule is a group of nuclei (the basal ganglia), part of the extrapyramidal system which is responsible for maintaining muscle tone through fibres from these structures converging on the internal capsules. The internal capsules unite to form the brain stem (midbrain, pons varolii and medulla oblongata) and are joined by fibres from the cerebellum (the hindbrain) concerned with balance and co-ordination of movement; some of the fibres cross to the opposite side in the lower brain stem and all fibres continue through the foramen magnum, at the base of the skull, as the spinal cord.

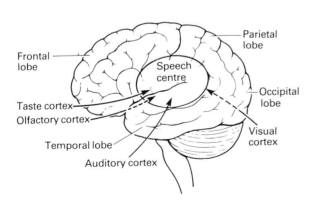

Fig. 2.7 Left cerebral hemisphere showing visual, auditory and olfactory influences on the speech centre.

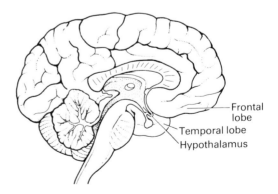

Fig. 2.8 Areas of the brain, in addition to those shown in Fig. 2.7, which influence the speech centre.

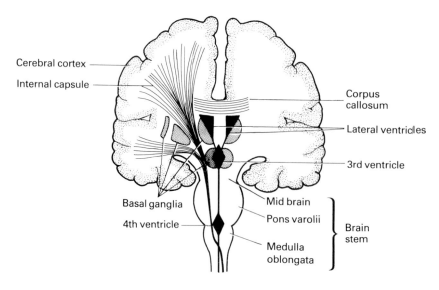

Fig. 2.9   Coronal section showing the internal capsule.

Examination of the patient

The nurse's observations and assessment are described in detail in Chapters 3 and 10, and in each chapter as related to the particular disorders. The doctor's examination of a patient thought to have a disorder of the central nervous system is detailed; its interpretation is interesting and based on logical thought and a detailed knowledge of anatomy and physiology, but if the patient's condition is deteriorating owing to rising intracranial pressure the examination will need to be performed very quickly. The recognition of disease begins when the patient, relative or parent notices mental or physical change; the general practitioner, using broad outlines of knowledge may make a diagnosis and treat the disease; a neurological opinion may be necessary to establish the diagnosis and the patient may be seen as an out-patient or admitted to hospital for observation, investigations and treatment. Sudden events and injuries lead to immediate hospital admission via the casualty department.

Disease of the nervous system leads to:

1   Loss of function through destruction of nervous tissue.
2   Temporary loss of function from transient interference with cell activity.
3   An imbalance of function when disturbance of one part allows overaction of another, e.g. basal ganglia disorders (see Chapter 20).
4   Irritation and excitability of nerve cells, e.g. epilepsy (see Chapter 19).
5   Mental changes affecting comprehension, mood and behaviour.
6   Alteration in the state of consciousness.

Preparation for examination

The nurse will reassuringly explain the nature of the procedure and as the examination is lengthy the patient should be given the opportunity to pass urine, and a specimen should be saved for routine ward testing. Suitable clothing (including briefs) should be worn and the patient helped into a comfortable position in bed. The nurse should ensure that an identity band is fixed to the patient's wrist. A neurological examination tray should be checked and taken to the bedside. While making these preparations the nurse will continue her observations and care of the unconscious or very ill patient (see Chapter 3); she will record and chart the patient's temperature, pulse, respirations and blood pressure. The conscious patient is likely to be apprehensive and the nurse can help to allay his anxiety by her calm approach and explanation. Particular care is necessary if the patient is deaf, has any visual disturbance or is totally blind, and if the patient is a child. A patient who is anxious and agitated will give an inaccurate, muddled history and tremors and disorders of speech will be worse; the patient may have become dependent upon a close relative to interpret for him and will need assurance that the relative will be included later in the interview.

History

This is a most important facet of the examination and may reveal the nature of the patient's illness. The presence of a third person is liable to impose a certain restraint and the nurse is not usually present while the doctor is taking the patient's history, but discussion between the doctor and senior nurse is essential when the examination is completed. Whenever possible the history is taken from the patient; it will however be necessary to question a child's parents or a close relative if the patient has incoherent speech, is deaf, has poor memory, intellectual impairment, change of personality or behaviour, clouding of consciousness, confusion, fits or loss of consciousness. An additional independent history often furnishes details which the patient has unintentionally forgotten to mention.

The doctor will assimilate impressions of the patient from the first moment of meeting: his general appearance, posture, speech, mood, behaviour, personality, intelligence and any obvious neurological abnormality (tremors, titubation, paralysis, hemianopia, etc.). The patient's age may be a pointer to the inclusion or exclusion of certain possible disorders; his occupation may be relevant where there has been injury or exposure to certain toxic substances and will also be a guide to the patient's previous mental and physical abilities. Direct questions will be asked regarding residence in the tropics where infestation and other diseases with neurological sequelae are common.

At an early stage in the interview the patient will be asked to describe his symptoms and the course of his illness. He should be interrupted as little as possible during the account, but may sometimes need guidance to keep to the medically relevant facts. Questions may be necessary to clarify vague or incomplete statements; the patient may use certain words or terms which have ambiguity of meaning, 'giddiness' may describe feelings of faintness, loss of balance or true vertigo; when examining the sensory system the doctor can only rely on the patient's accuracy. A history of particular symptoms will lead the doctor to ask the patient further related questions, for example a right limb weakness will lead to questions about language difficulties (see p. 11). The most important factors in the history are:

1 Exactly when the symptoms were first noticed.
2 How the patient's present condition compares with the start of the illness or other previous episodes. Have the symptoms remained the same, worsened, improved or fluctuated?
3 Any particular factors which influence the symptoms, e.g. does a change of position relieve the 'pins and needles' of nerve compression?

Past medical history In many instances, the past medical history is obviously linked with the present disorder, in others the link may be obscure; it is a well known fact that such diseases as diabetes mellitus and thyrotoxicosis may lead to neurological sequelae, but the relationship between certain personalities and chronic backache is less clear. It is important that the medical history covers the whole of the patient's life. The following points should be included:

Has the patient had any illnesses?

How were the illnesses treated and did they necessitate hospital admission? Previous treatment may be relevant to the present disorder and a report from another hospital is sometimes helpful; results of previous tests and investigations may be especially useful for comparison.

Has the patient had any operations?

Is his general health good?

Is his weight steady?

Has there been any change in sleep rhythm?

What are his smoking and drinking habits?

Is there any change in sexual activity?

Family history Some neurological disorders are genetically determined; have any other members of the family had a similar illness and was the patient's birth abnormal?

General examination

Examination of a patient with disorder of the central nervous system is incomplete unless a thorough general examination is included; facial expression, posture, skin condition and nutrition are all relevant. Each bodily system must be examined; hypertension, cardiovascular disease, anaemia and carcinoma may all be linked with neurological disorder.

Neurological examination

The doctor's assessment of the patient's conscious level, speech and mental state (three faculties which closely overlap) begins when he reaches the bedside and continues during history taking and examination.

Mental state

An accurate assessment of the patient's mental state is difficult when there is clouding of consciousness or difficulty in communication, and ward assessment is always relatively superficial; it is necessary to have formal testing by a psychologist when there is mental retardation, and to differentiate between depression and dementia.

Behaviour   Behaviour is assessed according to age, intelligence, social background and upbringing; disorders of behaviour may be extreme and disruptive or small but significant; an action may be inappropriate to the occasion and contrary to what would be expected from the patient's background, for example a patient ignoring the doctor's presence and continuing to smoke and listen to the radio, or interrupting when the doctor is speaking to another patient. A child's irritability or tantrums may be contrary to his normal behaviour; an adult unusually irritable, aggressive or disinhibited in public. Behaviour may be influenced by false beliefs not amenable to reason (delusions), or by false perceptions in the absence of corresponding external stimuli (hallucinations); hallucinations may be associated with any of the special senses, most commonly they are auditory or visual. A patient with severe dementia sometimes preserves

an excellent façade based on previous social attainments. The patient's response to illness and manner of describing symptoms can be significant, for example an immaculately groomed, healthy looking lady, smilingly complaining is unlikely to have severe pain, but there may be an underlying reason for her complaint.

Mood   The patient's mood or emotional state is revealed in his posture, facial expression and manner. Is the patient:
   Depressed? (Organic disease in the elderly may be heralded by a depressive illness.)
   Anxious?
   Irritable?
   Elated?
   Euphoric? (Euphoria is a false sense of well-being not in keeping with present circumstances.)
   Apathetic?
   Showing bland indifference to his symptoms? (This is characteristic of an hysterical personality and sometimes known as 'la belle indifference'.)
   Withdrawn and inaccessible? (He appears absorbed in his own thoughts, answers in monosyllables, if at all, and lacks facial expression.)

Anxiety and euphoria are often more easily detected than depression. Some conditions give a misleading impression of the patient's emotional state, as does the poverty of facial movement in Parkinson's disease, the presence of bilateral facial weakness or emotional lability.

Orientation in time, place and person   Orientation in time, place and person is dependent upon the patient's alert intelligent perception of all that is happening in his environment and his ability to remember related facts; he will be asked the year, date, day and time and conversation or simple questioning will show whether he knows who he is, where he is and why. It is almost impossible for someone with severe memory impairment or with fluctuation in consciousness to remain orientated and they will behave in a very confused manner.

Memory   Memory is an elaborate process involving attention, retention and recall; only simple testing is possible during a neurological examination; to test recent memory the patient is given a name, address and message or a list of objects to remember for 15 minutes, against the distraction of other activities and conversation, or he is asked to repeat a series of numbers. A patient who is vague and hesitates when giving his history may have memory impairment and this can be confirmed by a comparative history from a relative or friend; the patient may fill in gaps in his memory with imaginary events which sound convincing (confabulation).

Intelligence A general impression of the patient's normal intellectual level will be gained by his conversation and grasp during interview and examination; a psychologist's assessment is sometimes helpful as there are a variety of conditions which cause mental retardation and slowing of cerebration. The patient's school record, employment, social background and opportunities will assist in the assessment. A test called 'serial sevens' tests the patient's agility in calculation, when he takes seven from one hundred and proceeds by subtraction of seven from each result. His general knowledge is tested by discussion of current events, politics, sport or events of recent interest in the news; assessment should always take into account normal interests, for example a housewife may have no interest in politics or sport and therefore little knowledge of these subjects.

Level of consciousness

The doctor will assess the patient's level of consciousness (see Chapter 3).

Speech

Before birth a normal baby will hear the sound of voices; providing his mother, who spends so much time with him, talks to him continually from his earliest days, he will learn to connect sounds with objects and events and there will be normal development of speech through the stages of experimentation, imitation, recognition, use of words and construction of simple sentences to the more complex abstract associations. Reading, writing, mathematics and music are also concerned with recognition and interpretation of symbols and are skills added later. Children who through circumstances in their environment are isolated, deprived of normal conversational stimulation, or are 'spoken' for and never allowed to speak for themselves, will have limited development of speech and conversation; it has been noticed that a child who has not learnt any form of language communication before the age of 5 years will never learn more than elementary speech. A deaf child, though his powers of comprehension, expression and articulation are potentially normal, cannot develop normal speech as he neither hears the spoken word nor his own voice; these children are sometimes wrongly thought to be dumb. There are specific faults in development of the speech area which lead to a lack of comprehension of words; children with these difficulties though they appear mentally retarded have normal intelligence and will benefit from specialist teaching. Any mentally retarded child will be late learning to talk and may not progress beyond very simple words. A child who has not developed a dominant hemisphere by the time he is 5 years of age will have difficulty in recognising the symbols which make up words and, even though he has normal intelligence and a good spoken vocabulary, will find difficulty in learning to read or write (developmental dyslexia). A left-handed child who is forced to write with his right hand is very likely to develop stuttering speech. Any disorder which damages the motor pathways or the structures necessary for articulation causes speech impediments (dysarthria).

Communication disorders
1   Failure in understanding and expression due to language disorder
i   The spoken word
    (a) Aphasia – total loss of language either in expressing or understanding the spoken word, or a combination of both
    (b) Dysphasia – partial loss of language which may be:
        Receptive dysphasia – difficulty in understanding the spoken word
        Expressive dysphasia – difficulty in spoken expression
        Jargon dysphasia – the patient expresses himself in a jumble of unrecognisable sounds, does not notice he is talking gibberish and cannot understand what is said to him
        Nominal dysphasia – difficulty in naming objects
    Tongue apraxia often accompanies aphasia and dysphasia and though the tongue is not paralysed, the patient is unable to will the tongue to move.

ii   The written word
(a) Dyslexia – difficulty in recognising written words (word 'blindness')
(b) Dysgraphia – a difficulty of expression in writing using the symbols that make up words

2   Difficulty in articulation
(a) Anarthria – complete inability to move the muscles of articulation
(b) Dysarthria – difficulty in articulation which causes slurred speech, specific difficulty in the pronunciation of certain sounds and interruption of the normal rhythm and speed of speech; any or all of the structures used when speaking may be weak, clumsy or unco-ordinated. Lesions affecting the upper motor neurones lead to weakness and spasticity and a particular difficulty in the pronunciation of certain consonants made by putting the lips together (labial consonants), e.g. as in pepper, and by putting the tongue behind the top teeth (dental consonants), e.g. as in dirty. When the lesion is in the corpus striatum of the basal ganglia (see Chapter 20), speech is slow, very quiet and monotonous. When the co-ordinating cerebellar control of vocalisation is affected, each syllable is pronounced almost as though it were a separate word (scanning dys-arthria); if the disorder is very severe, speech may also be explosive and accompanied by facial grimacing. Lesions affecting the lower motor neurones cause weakness and wasting of the muscles of articulation beginning in the lips; as the tongue and palate become involved, speech takes on a nasal quality before the patient becomes obviously dysarthric. Early dysarthria can be so slight as to be almost imperceptible, but it is possible to localise the disturbance to a particular area of the brain by recognising the type of dysarthria.

3   Difficulty in phonation
(a) Aphonia – complete loss of voice; lesions in the brain will be differentiated from hysterical aphonia
(b) Dysphonia – the patient can only speak in a whisper

Speech Assessment   When assessing the patient's speech the doctor will take into account variants of the normal, dialects, nervous stutter, badly fitting dentures and such conditions as cleft palate. He will enquire whether the patient is right- or left-handed; dysphasia is a useful localising sign; an attentive experienced ear will detect it during ordinary conversation and will realise that an inappropriate answer may be due to failure of understanding (receptive dysphasia) rather than confusion. A patient who finds difficulty in expres-sion (expressive dysphasia), develops tricks of speech, skirting round a subject to avoid a word which escapes him, characteristically he will des-cribe the function of an item instead of giving its name, for example when shown a clock, he might say 'it tells the time'; to detect nominal dysphasia, the patient will be asked to name familiar objects (naming the parts of a wrist watch is an exacting test). Assessment of a patient with very severe speech disorder needs to be painstaking and detailed. A patient with expressive aphasia will be distressed that he cannot answer the doctor's ques-tions; he may be able to nod and shake his head appropriately, but if he also has receptive aphasia he will be completely bewildered, his smiling greeting changing to a puzzled or blank expression. A patient with jargon dysphasia makes a jumble of sounds, even carrying on a lengthy conversation in this gibberish; he neither understands what is said nor appreciates his own mistakes, becoming very agitated if there is something he particularly wants and failing to understand why his needs are unful-filled. A combination of jargon dysphasia, agnosia (inability to recognise familiar objects) and apraxia (inability to perform simple actions though there is no paralysis), may lead to a complex sequence of events like this: the patient wishing to pass urine fails to communicate his need, attempts to leave the ward fighting with all who restrain him and, when he finally reaches the lavatory, is unable to prepare to pass urine and does not recognise the WC.

Throughout the examination the doctor will listen to the patient's speech and notice whether there is dysarthria; if this is not immediately obvious, certain words or phrases (Royal Irish Constabulary or British Constitution) which are difficult to enunciate will emphasise dysarthria and demonstrate the different types.

Physical examination

Inspection of the face or skull will reveal obvious asymmetry or changes associated with endocrine disturbance. The presence of angiomata or abnormal pigmentation will be noted and the skin and mucous membranes examined for evidence of anaemia, jaundice or cyanosis. Careful examination of the head by palpation may reveal enlargement and increased tension of the fontanelles in infants, separation of the cranial sutures in children up to the age of eight years, congenital abnormality, evidence of haematoma or injury, previous scars or burr holes; an exostosis may suggest the presence of a meningioma. Rare vascular anomalies are sometimes accompanied by a bruit (a swishing noise in a blood vessel synchronising with each heart beat); with a stethoscope the doctor will listen to each carotid artery in the neck, over each orbit, and directly on the vault of the skull. Percussion (tapping with the finger tips) is used to detect raised intracranial pressure in children denoted by a 'cracked pot' sound due to parting of the cranial sutures. The spine is carefully examined throughout its length for evidence of abnormality of bone, posture and mobility (see Chapter 10).

Cranial nerves

The cranial nerves are part of the system of peripheral nerves; there are twelve pairs supplying sensation and motor power to each side of the head and neck (Fig. 2.10). Some nerves are entirely sensory (those of sight, smell and hearing), others are solely motor (those which move the eye and control the muscles of the neck), while the remainder have both sensory and motor pathways. The sensory nerve impulses are relayed to the brain stem and then to the part of the sensory cerebral cortex which interprets each sensation. The motor nerves are lower motor neurones with their nuclei in the brain stem and are controlled by impulses from the cerebral motor cortex.

In his examination, the doctor systematically examines each cranial nerve.

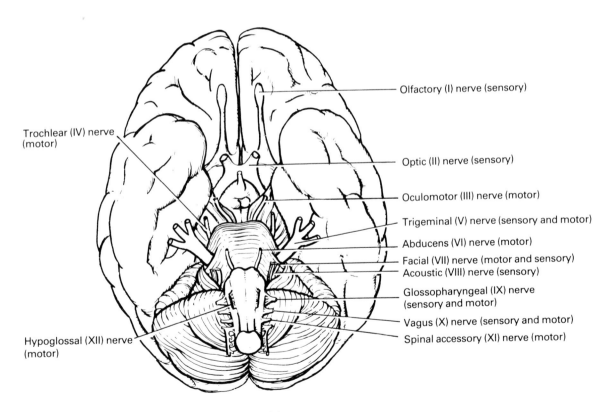

Fig. 2.10   Inferior aspect of the brain showing cranial nerves.

Olfactory or Ist cranial nerve

In the upper part of each nostril are the very fine nerve endings of the olfactory nerves which pass through the cribriform plate of the ethmoid bone above, to the olfactory bulbs which lie close together on either side of the mid-line beneath the frontal lobes. Impulses concerned with the sense of smell are relayed to the uncus of each temporal lobe. The sense of smell is tested by asking the patient to identify the scent of a familiar substance (the name being hidden); each nostril is tested in turn. The test will be of little value if the patient has a cold.

Optic or IInd cranial nerve

This is the nerve of vision. Light falls on the sensory cells of the retina and stimulates impulses in the nerve endings of the optic nerve; the nerve endings converge at the back of the eyeball in the optic disc. Visual impulses are conducted along the optic nerve from each eye; at the optic chiasma (between and behind the eyes and close to the pituitary gland) the two optic nerves unite and the fibres from the nasal side of each retina cross over (Fig. 2.11); nerve fibres from the temporal side of the retina do not cross. On leaving the optic chiasma each optic tract passes through the temporal lobe to a relay station in the thalamus (lateral geniculate body), then the impulses are relayed along the optic radiation through the posterior part of the internal capsule to the visual cortex in the occipital lobe. Nerve fibres which supply the pupillary reflexes leave the optic tracts and establish connections with the third nerve nuclei in the brain stem; the third nerve constricts the pupil and the sympathetic nerve supply

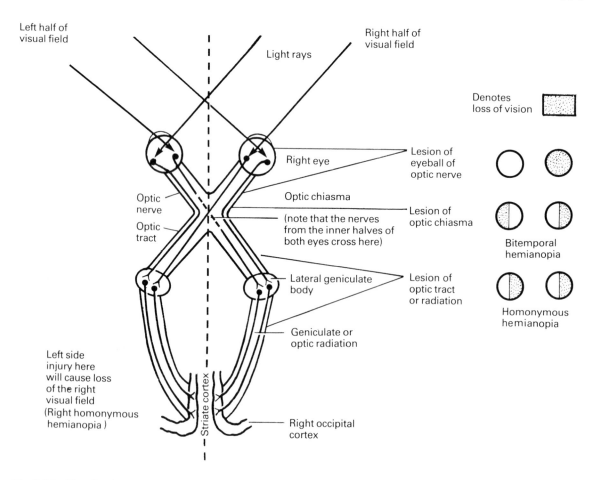

Fig. 2.11   The visual pathways and visual field defects.

dilates the pupil, together controlling the amount of light which falls on the retina.

The general appearance of the eyes will be noted; there may be bilateral exophthalmos associated with thyroid disease, or proptosis resulting from forward displacement of the eye by a space occupying lesion.

Visual acuity

Visual acuity is tested by the use of a graded reading chart. A good light should be provided and if the patient normally wears spectacles or contact lenses, he should do so for the test. A Snellen's chart is used for testing distant vision and Jaeger's types for near vision; more severe defects are tested by asking the patient to count fingers, detect hand movements or distinguish between lightness and darkness. These tests are adapted to suit young children using charts with pictures and other specialised equipment.

Visual fields

The visual field is the whole area which can be seen by the eye when looking straight ahead; to simplify examination each visual field is divided into four quadrants. Confrontation is a method of approximate assessment used in the ward; the patient's visual field is compared with that of the doctor, who sits opposite and about one metre distant. Covering one eye the patient fixes his gaze on the centre of the doctor's forehead; a white-headed pin held midway between the doctor and the patient is used to test each quadrant of the visual field; in testing the peripheral field of vision the object is brought from beyond the periphery towards the centre in each quadrant and the patient is asked to state when he sees it. The central area of the visual field is tested separately by moving the object across the centre from several directions. Each eye is tested and the results charted. Accurate plotting of visual fields (perimetry; Fig. 2.12) is only possible with a mechanical perimeter or Bjerrum's screen. With a young child, unco-operative or semiconscious patient, the presence of field defect can sometimes be suspected when there is no blink response to a menacing flick of the hand from the side towards each eye.

Visual field defects (see Fig. 2.11)

A lesion affecting one optic nerve causes a visual field defect in one eye; complete interruption of the nerve causes blindness in that eye when the pupil will be dilated and unreactive to light or accommodation. An inflammatory condition of the optic nerve (retrobulbar neuritis) gives rise to a central visual field defect (central scotoma). Optic atrophy results in a constricted visual field. Any lesion at the optic chiasma or of the optic tracts or radiations, will result in bilateral visual field defects; compression of the central crossing fibres at the optic chiasma (often due to a pituitary tumour) causes bitemporal hemianopia, a bilateral defect involving the temporal halves of each visual field; the defect is often asymmetrical at first, affecting only the upper quadrant. Lesions involving the optic tract or the optic radiation cause an homonymous hemianopia, an obscuration of half the visual field on the same side in each eye; a lesion in one cerebral hemisphere results in a homonymous hemianopia on the opposite side. The patient will ignore anyone who approaches or stands on his blind side.

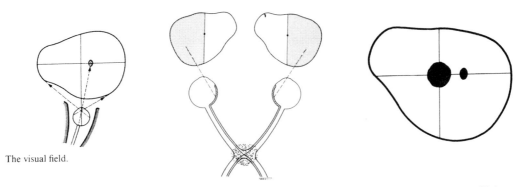

The visual field.

Fig. 2.12 Normal and abnormal visual field charts. *Left:* the usual field. *Centre:* bitemporal hemianopia. *Right:* central scotoma in optic hemitis. From Coakes, R.L. and Holmes Sellors, P.J. *An Outline of Ophthalmology* (1985), John Wright & Sons, Bristol.

Ophthalmoscopy

With an ophthalmoscope it is possible to see the head of the optic nerve as it emerges at the back of the eye (optic disc) and the blood vessels which enter the eye with the optic nerve and radiate into the retina; the normal optic disc is circular, pale pink, slightly raised on its margin and dipped in the centre (physiological cup); it lies towards the nasal side of the eye (Fig. 2.13). Important abnormalities may be seen in the optic disc and blood vessels. Papilloedema, an important sign of raised intracranial pressure, is caused by increased pressure of cerebrospinal fluid in the sheath of the optic nerve. This obstructs the venous return from the retina and the disc becomes pinker, blurred at the edges, the central depression fills up, the blood vessels become congested and tortuous and there may be haemorrhages and exudates. Papilloedema is usually bilateral (see p. 118) and without relief the constant pressure on the optic nerve and blood vessels will result in secondary optic atrophy and blindness. Unilateral papilloedema occurs in association with optic neuritis and thrombosis of the central retinal vein. Primary optic atrophy may be the result of direct pressure on the optic nerve, inflammation, vascular disease or exposure to toxic substances; the disc becomes paler, the margins clear-cut, the physiological cup becomes deeper and the blood vessels shrink. Evidence of hypertensive changes may be seen in the blood vessels of the retina; the signs are similar to and can be confused with papilloedema.

Oculomotor or IIIrd cranial nerve (see page 37)

The nuclei of the third cranial nerves are in the upper part of the midbrain; each nerve leaves the brain stem at the level of the tentorial hiatus, it passes forward along the floor of the skull to the lateral wall of the cavernous sinus, where it lies close to the fourth and sixth cranial nerves, and then enters the orbit; fibres from the oculomotor nerves connect with the optic nerves. The oculomotor nerve innervates the muscles of the iris, the upper eyelid and the muscles which turn the eyeball downwards towards the nose. The size of the pupils is controlled by sympathetic and parasympathetic nerves which normally work in harmony; the sympathetic nerves dilate the pupils and the parasympathetic nerves constrict them. The oculomotor nerve is the parasympathetic nerve supply and when this nerve is damaged, either at its nucleus or

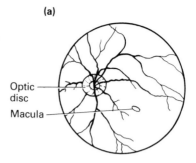

(a)

Optic disc
Macula

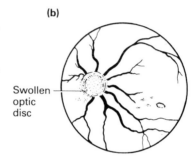

(b)

Swollen optic disc

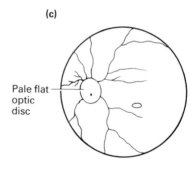

(c)

Pale flat optic disc

Fig. 2.13 The fundus of the eye. (a) Normal optic disc and blood vessels (arteries and veins). (b) Papilloedema and congested tortuous blood vessels. (c) Optic atrophy and threadlike blood vessels.

along its pathway, the pupil becomes dilated and sluggish or unreactive to light and accommodation, due to the unopposed action of the sympathetic nerve supply; **this is an important sign of rising intracranial pressure.** A third nerve palsy also affects the movement of the upper eyelid; when there is complete paralysis (ptosis) the patient will be unable to open his eye on the affected side; slight ptosis is difficult to detect unless there is careful comparison of the palpebral fissure of both eyes with the eyes open (Fig. 2.14).

Observation of the pupils (see p. 46):

Are they circular in outline?

Are they equal in size?

Are they normal in size considering light conditions and the patient's age? (In childhood the pupils are normally larger.)

Do they react briskly to light and is this reaction equal in both eyes?

Do they react to accommodation, i.e. get smaller when looking at near objects?

Do they react consensually, i.e. when light is directed at one pupil does the other also react?

Pupil abnormalities

Argyll Robertson pupil is almost always due to neurosyphilis; the pupil is small, irregular in outline and reacts to accommodation, but not to light.

Holmes Adie syndrome (myotonic pupil) is a benign, symptomless condition usually found in females in which the abnormal pupil may be slightly dilated, shows no reaction to light, but slowly constricts and dilates to accommodation. There may be an associated abnormality of tendon reflexes with absence of ankle and knee reflexes.

Horner's syndrome suggests damage to the sympathetic nerves in the neck; on the affected side the pupil is constricted but reacts to light, there is a slight degree of ptosis and absence of sweating on the face and neck.

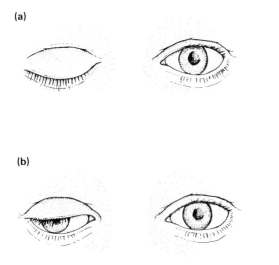

(a)

(b)

Fig. 2.14 Ptosis. **(a)** Complete right ptosis. **(b)** Partial right ptosis.

Trochlear or IVth cranial nerve

The nuclei of the fourth cranial nerves are in the midbrain in front of the aqueduct of Sylvius. Each nerve passes forwards and after entering the cavernous sinus crosses the oculomotor nerve and reaches the eye through an opening in the orbit; it innervates the superior oblique muscle which rotates the eyeball outwards and downwards.

Abducens or VIth cranial nerve

The nuclei of the sixth cranial nerves are in the pons varolii. The nerve reaches the eye after passing through the cavernous sinus, innervates the lateral rectus muscle and is responsible for turning the eye outward.

Eye movements

The eyes normally move together in parallel fashion (conjugate movement) except on convergence; most eye movements are reflex. Co-ordinated movements are controlled by an area in the frontal lobe, by centres in the brain stem and by the third, fourth and sixth cranial nerves which innervate the ocular muscles. Eye movements are tested by asking the patient to follow a moving object with his eyes without moving his head; the object is held about 60 cm from the patient and moved to right and left, upwards and downwards and brought in from a distance towards the nose to test convergence.

Squint (strabismus), convergent or divergent, occurs when a lesion affects the nerve pathways in the brain, brain stem, cranial nerve nuclei or cranial nerves; paralysis of eye movements causes double vision (diplopia). Concomitant squint is not caused by disease of the nervous system, but by defective balance of the eye muscles; it is not associated with diplopia and the affected eye has full range of movement.

Diplopia is a common symptom following paralysis of eye movement because images of a single object fall at different points on each retina and cannot be brought into focus. By careful examination the doctor is able to detect the affected eye and determine which muscle is paralysed; plastic goggles with one green and one red lens help the patient to give a clear account of the images. Specialised tests by an ophthalmologist will be necessary for a patient with transient or slight diplopia.

Nystagmus

While examining the patient's eyes the doctor may notice a rhythmic jerking of the eyeball (nystagmus), which is an inco-ordination of gaze seen in horizontal, vertical or rotatory plane. Nystagmus is caused by:

1 Impairment of fixation; a blind or very short-sighted (myopic) person will be unable to find an object on which to fix his gaze.
2 Disorder of the labyrinth when it is usually associated with vertigo and deafness.
3 Brain stem and cerebellar disorders.
4 Congenital or familial factors; there is a constant fine pendular oscillation of the eyes which is increased by eye movement.

Trigeminal or Vth cranial nerve (see Fig. 17.3)

This nerve is mainly sensory with a small motor root. The nucleus is in the pons varolii; shortly after leaving the brain stem, at the apex of the petrous bone and beneath the temporal lobe is an expansion of the sensory root, the Gasserian ganglion; from this ganglion arise the three divisions of the trigeminal nerve:

i the ophthalmic branch which includes the corneal reflex;
ii the maxillary branch; and
iii the mandibular branch.

The cutaneous distribution of the three divisions is suggested by their names. The trigeminal nerve also supplies sensation to the nasal mucosa, hard and soft palates, teeth, anterior two-thirds of the tongue (not taste) and buccal mucosa. The motor root supplies the muscles of mastication.
The nerve is examined by testing:

1 Each sensory division for appreciation of light touch, pain and thermal sensibility.
2 The corneal reflex – the cornea is lightly touched with a wisp of cotton wool; if the corneal sensation is diminished or absent the blink response is also reduced or absent.
3 The jaw jerk – the patient is asked to let his mouth hang open loosely; the doctor then places his finger across the patient's chin and taps it gently with a patella hammer. An exaggerated jaw jerk indicates a lesion between the cerebral cortex and the nucleus in the pons varolii.

4 The power of the muscles of mastication; the patient is asked to clench his teeth, and the doctor palpates the temporalis and masseter muscles on each side, comparing their strength and equality. He then asks the patient to open his mouth; if there is weakness the jaw will deviate towards the paralysed side. The jaw will hang open if there is bilateral paralysis.

Facial or VIIth cranial nerve

The facial nerve has a mainly motor function, supplying the muscles of facial expression and the scalp; its motor nucleus is in the pons varolii. A small sensory pathway relays sensation of taste from the anterior two-thirds of the tongue, sensation from the soft palate and excites salivary secretion.
The pathway of the nerve is complex and devious; the important factors are:

i Its close proximity to the auditory nerve as it leaves the pons varolii and crosses the posterior fossa.
ii Its passage through the internal auditory meatus.
iii Its situation in the facial canal and emergence from the skull at the stylo-mastoid process.
iv The location of the geniculate ganglion (the nerve cells of the taste fibres) in the facial canal.
v The passage of the nerve through the parotid gland on its final pathway to the facial muscles.

Disease of the structures through which the facial nerve passes may affect its function. The motor functions of the facial nerve are tested as follows:

1 The face is observed for symmetry.
2 The patient is asked to screw up his eyes tightly; the eyelashes will be less well buried on the side of the facial weakness.
3 The patient is asked to raise his eyebrows and frown; furrowing of the brow is less noticeable on the side of the weakness.
4 The patient is asked to smile (a request to whistle is often effective); is he able to smile normally, purse the lips, blow out the cheeks and whistle? Poverty of movement will be observed on the weak side.

The part of the facial nerve supplying the forehead receives its upper motor neurone stimulation from the cortex of both cerebral hemispheres whereas the part of the facial nerve supplying the lower part of the face receives its cortical stimulation from the opposite hemisphere only. An upper motor neurone facial weakness caused by a lesion in one cerebral hemisphere affects the lower half of the face more severely because the forehead has this bilateral nerve supply. A lower motor neurone facial weakness in contrast affects the upper and lower part of the face equally as it is produced by a lesion affecting the final pathway of the nerve (Fig. 2.15). Facial weakness due to muscle disorders is usually bilateral and affects all the facial muscles.

(a)

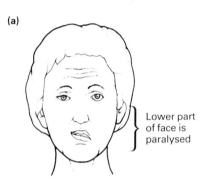

Lower part
of face is
paralysed

(b)

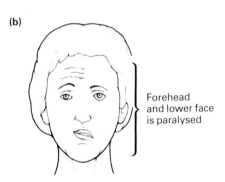

Forehead
and lower face
is paralysed

Fig. 2.15 Facial weakness. **(a)** Upper motor neurone facial weakness. **(b)** Lower motor neurone facial weakness.

The sense of taste
The sensation of taste is transmitted from the tongue by the facial and glossopharyngeal nerves; the cortical area for appreciation of taste lies in the region of the uncinate gyrus of the temporal lobe. The facial nerve supplies the anterior two-thirds of the tongue and the glossopharyngeal nerve supplies the posterior one-third. For the purposes of testing, the tongue is divided into areas. There are only four tastes, sweet, salt, bitter and sour; other 'flavours' are olfactory sensations. The sense of taste is tested by the use of weak solutions of sugar, salt, quinine and vinegar. The patient is asked to put out his tongue, the tongue is dried and with a pipette, a drop of the required substance is placed on the test area; the procedure is repeated for each substance and each area of the tongue.

Acoustic or VIIIth cranial nerve (see Chapter 21)

This nerve has two functions, hearing and equilibrium. The cochlear part of the nerve is concerned with hearing which it relays to the auditory cortex of the temporal lobe; the vestibular part relays information, regarding the position of the head, to the cerebellum. The two parts of the nerve pass from the inner ear, through the internal auditory meatus to the pons varolii; the nerve lies in the cerebello–pontine angle close to the facial nerve (see p. 114 and Fig. 2.10). When there is disturbance of the acoustic nerve the patient's complaints are of deafness, vertigo or tinnitus (an abnormal high or low pitched hissing, whistling or swishing noise, sometimes in time with the pulse).

A rudimentary test of hearing is performed in the ward using a whispered voice, ticking watch and tuning fork. The hearing in each ear is tested separately and a comparison made. An audiometer will be used for more detailed testing of pitch and sound. Nerve conduction deafness causes loss of high tones, and middle ear disease, loss of low tones. The doctor will try to locate the cause of deafness by using one of the following tests.

Weber's test (a test of bone conduction of sound) In this test a vibrating tuning fork is placed on the forehead or vertex in the mid-line. When both ears are normal the sound is 'heard' in the mid-line; in nerve deafness the sound is referred to the normal ear, and in middle ear deafness to the affected ear; this is because in nerve conduction deafness the diseased nerve is incapable of transmitting any sound impulses to the auditory cortex, and in middle ear deafness bone conduction is enhanced on the affected side.

Rinne's test (a comparative test of air and bone conduction) A vibrating tuning fork is placed on the mastoid process while the external auditory meatus is occluded. When the sound is no longer heard through the head, the tuning fork is held near the meatus. Sound through the other ear is effectively blocked by rubbing the fingers together at the meatus. As air conduction is normally better than bone conduction, in normal persons or when there is some degree of nerve deafness, the sound can be heard by air conduction after bone conduction has ceased; in middle ear deafness the sound cannot be heard once bone conduction of sound has ceased.

Vestibular function
A complicated mechanism exists to maintain the body in its appropriate position in space and for the individual to be aware of that position. Sensory impulses are received by the brain from many parts of the body, from the soles of the feet as the person stands, the joints, the muscles of the neck which give the relationship of the head to the body, the eyes and the labyrinths in the ears (semicircular canals, utricle and saccule). All this information is relayed to the cerebellum which reflexly corrects balance. In order to bring this to conscious awareness there are connections with an area of cortex in the posterior part of the temporal lobe. Similarly this sensory network connects with the spinal motor pathways (see p. 168) enabling corrections of posture to be made.

The vestibular branch of the acoustic nerve innervates the labyrinth. Disordered function of this nerve will result in vertigo, an unpleasant symptom in which the patient experiences a feeling of rotation, either of his body or his surroundings which he may describe as 'giddiness'. The doctor will test the patient's balance and caloric tests (specific tests for vestibular function) may be necessary (see p. 35 and Chapter 21).

Glossopharyngeal or IXth cranial nerve

The glossopharyngeal nerve arises in the medulla; it supplies sensation and taste to the posterior third of the tongue and sensation to the tonsils and pharynx; it is responsible for the secretion of saliva from the parotid gland. The motor portion of the nerve supplies power to the muscles of the pharynx. The nerve is seldom damaged in isolation, but usually in association with the vagus and spinal accessory nerves.

The posterior one-third of the tongue is tested for appreciation of taste (see p. 19).

Gag reflex
This is a normal protective reflex elicited when the walls of the pharynx are touched; if the gag reflex is brisk it is a clear indication that the pharynx has normal sensation.

Mechanism of swallowing
This involves the normal function of several cranial nerves (glossopharyngeal, vagus and hypoglossal). Food and fluid are channelled into the pharynx by the tongue, the soft palate rises to close off the nasal passages, the epiglottis closes the trachea to prevent inhalation into the lungs, the larynx rises and food or fluid passes into the oesophagus.

Vagus or Xth cranial nerve

This nerve is widely distributed and has sensory and motor fibres. It emerges from the medulla, lies close to the glossopharyngeal and spinal accessory nerves and, as one large trunk, leaves the skull through the jugular foramen; it supplies sensation to the pharynx, trachea and external ear, then travels downward in the neck where it gives off the laryngeal nerves supplying sensory and motor nerve fibres to the larynx and vocal cords; it continues into the thorax and through the diaphragm to the abdomen supplying the thoracic viscera and the gastrointestinal tract.

The motor functions of the vagus nerve are tested by observing the appearance of the soft palate and pharynx and noting whether the soft palate rises freely in the mid-line when the patient says 'ah' and responds when each side is touched (palatal reflex); the gag reflex is tested as already described. These reflexes have their motor component from the vagus nerve, but their sensory components from the trigeminal and glossopharyngeal nerves. Should the tone of the voice suggest an abnormality in the vocal cords it may be necessary to examine them at rest, during inspiration and phonation.

Bilateral palatal paralysis gives the voice a nasal tone and causes regurgitation of food and fluids into the nose as the palate fails to shut off the nasopharynx during swallowing. Unilateral paralysis of the larynx causes hoarseness and difficulty in coughing, and bilateral paralysis causes complete loss of voice and cough, and stridor on deep inspiration. Bilateral pharyngeal paralysis causes difficulty in swallowing (dysphagia).

Spinal accessory or XIth cranial nerve

This is a motor nerve which arises partly in the medulla and partly in the spinal cord. At the foramen magnum the two parts join to form a single trunk leaving the skull through the jugular foramen with the vagus nerve; at this point the accessory fibres join the vagus nerve. The spinal accessory nerve supplies the sternocleidomastoid and the trapezius muscles.

Weakness of the sternocleidomastoid muscles will be demonstrated by asking the patient to turn his head to each side in turn against the resistance of the doctor's hand; the muscle will also be inspected and palpated for signs of wasting. The patient will be asked to flex his neck and if there is muscle paralysis on one side his head will tilt and his chin turn towards the paralysed side. The trapezius muscles are observed and palpated and the patient is asked to shrug his shoulders against resistance; on the affected side, there may be an abnormal position of the scapula, the shoulder will be lower and its movement weaker.

Hypoglossal or XIIth cranial nerve

This is the motor nerve of the tongue, its nucleus is in the medulla. Paralysis of this nerve causes the tongue to deviate to the weak side. The protruded tongue is examined for deviation, wasting, fasciculation (flickering of the muscle bundles), tremor and involuntary movement; the patient will then be asked to waggle his tongue rapidly from side to side; it will move very sluggishly if there is weakness or spasticity. When tongue movement is limited or there is deep furrowing due to wasting and atrophy the affected area often becomes furred due to lack of friction. Sometimes the patient experiences difficulty in protruding his tongue even though it is not paralysed (apraxia).

Hypoglossal paralysis leads to dysarthria and dysphagia.

The motor system

This is composed of three closely inter-related systems which together produce controlled purposeful movement, the pyramidal, extrapyramidal and cerebellar systems.

The pyramidal system (see Fig. 2.9 and Chapter 10)

The body is represented upside down in the motor cortex (see Fig. 2.6) and the areas which have the greatest skills (the fingers and the face) have the largest cortical representation. One side of the brain controls the opposite side of the body. Impulses from these cells pass along the nerve fibres through the cerebrum, the internal capsule and the brain stem to the level in the medulla where they cross to the opposite side. The impulses then travel down the nerve fibres in the lateral columns of the spinal cord. The nerve fibres of the upper motor neurones throughout the entire length of the brain stem and spinal cord, synapse with the cell bodies of the lower motor neurones (anterior horn cells). The lower motor neurones (including those of the cranial nerves) then leave the brain stem and spinal cord, become part of the peripheral nerves and terminate in the motor end plates of the muscles they supply.

The extrapyramidal system

This is concerned with muscle tone, posture and initiation of movement. The basal ganglia lie deep within each cerebral hemisphere (see Fig. 2.9), the structures on one side controlling functions on the opposite side of the body through extrapyramidal nerve fibres in the spinal cord which synapse with the lower motor neurones. The basal ganglia communicate with each other and also with the cerebrum, cerebellum and brain stem; they have a suppressant action on each other and if one ganglion is damaged, the others overact giving rise to the various syndromes associated with extrapyramidal disorders (see Chapter 20).

The cerebellar system

The cerebellum is concerned with balance and co-ordination of movement; it lies in the posterior fossa beneath the tentorium and behind the brain stem and has two hemispheres connected by a central portion, the vermis (Fig. 2.16). The surface of the cerebellum is closely and deeply convoluted and is composed of cell bodies; the fibres pass through the centre of each cerebellar hemisphere to the brain stem and spino-cerebellar tracts in the spinal cord, where they synapse with the lower motor neurones. The fibres of the cerebellar system do not cross, but supply structures on the same side of the body.

Balance is maintained by impulses from the semicircular canals in the inner ear which are relayed to the cerebellum by the vestibular portion

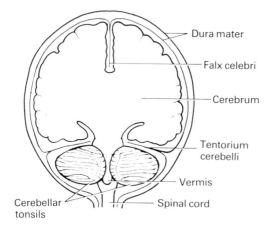

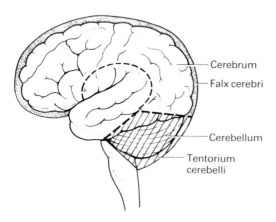

Fig. 2.16 The cerebellum.

of the eighth cranial nerve and sensory impulses from all parts of the body (including those of sight), which provide an image of the body in space and its relation to its surroundings.

Examination of the motor system

The examination is performed with the patient reclining comfortably in bed. Tone, power, posture and co-ordination of all muscle groups are tested and the size of the limbs, and wasting or fasciculation of the muscles is noted.

Muscle tone
The limbs are moved passively; resistance to movement indicates an increase in tone (spasticity, hypertonia) and a floppy limb, decrease in tone (flaccidity, hypotonia). Lesions involving the

upper motor neurone produce increased tone and those involving the lower motor neurone, decreased tone. Disorders of the extrapyramidal system may produce either increased or decreased tone. Cerebellar disorders lead to decreased tone.

Power
The patient is asked to move his limbs against resistance exerted by the doctor; each group of muscles is tested in turn and comparison is made between both sides of the body. Unless contraindicated, the patient will be asked to sit up, stand and walk a short distance, if necessary with help. A hemiparesis (weakness on one side) will cause difficulty in rising from the recumbent position, standing unaided, and a characteristic gait, the weak arm either hanging limply at the patient's side or held in a stiff partially flexed position, the leg and foot dragging with an outward swinging movement. A co-operative patient may be able to move an apparently paralysed limb if the pull of gravity is counteracted by the observer supporting the weight of the limb.

Posture
Throughout the examination the patient's posture is observed; how does he sit or stand, is he stooped or does he lean backwards and in what position are his limbs in use and at rest?

Co-ordination
Ataxia indicates a disturbance of cerebellar function; mild inco-ordination may be due to weakness, but cerebellar ataxia is confirmed when, on testing, the power is found to be greater than would be expected from the degree of disability displayed. Severe ataxia is obvious when the patient walks or attempts to move from wheelchair to chair or bed when he will veer towards the affected side. Tests for co-ordination will be performed as follows:

1   Finger/nose test   The patient is asked to touch his nose and the doctor's finger alternately as rapidly and accurately as possible. This test will be performed with the patient's eyes open and then closed; inco-ordination due to cerebellar lesions is demonstrated in each instance, but when due to loss of joint position sense (loss of proprioception), is only present when the patient's eyes are closed.

2   Tests for ability to perform repetitive movements
i   Tapping one hand rapidly on the back of the other, or tapping with the foot.

ii Rapidly alternating supination and pronation of the wrist and hand.

3 Heel/shin test The patient is asked to place the heel of one foot on the knee of the other leg and run the heel smoothly down the shin to the ankle.

4 Rebound phenomenon The patient holds his arms outstretched and the doctor attempts to press them downwards while the patient puts up resistance; on sudden release, on the affected side, there will be excessive rebound due to disturbance of cerebellar control of the compensating muscle tone relationships.

5 Romberg's test The patient, standing with feet together, is asked to close his eyes. Cerebellar dysfunction or loss of position sense, or both, cause the patient to sway; he may suddenly fall over unless protected.

Limb size
Examination of the size of the limbs may reveal a smaller limb on one side; the difference may be so small that it can only be confirmed by comparing the size of the great toe or thumb nails; this may be a congenital defect or associated with a disorder which occurred during the developing years (e.g. poliomyelitis).

Wasting
Muscle bulk is inspected; mild discrepancies may only be revealed when the limb girth is measured and compared.

Fasciculation
Individual muscle bundles contracting and relaxing rapidly will be seen as ripples of movement beneath the skin; momentary fasciculation may be induced by tapping the muscles. Fasciculation only occurs in motor disorders involving anterior horn cells.

Reflexes
These are inborn responses to certain stimuli. For reflex actions to take place the reflex arc (see Fig. 2.4) must be intact. It consists of:

i the receptor – a special sense organ in skin, muscle or tendon;
ii the sensory neurone which forms part of the peripheral nerve; in the posterior horn this synapses with another small neurone which relays the impulse to

iii the lower motor neurone; and
iv the effector – the muscle or gland which produces the response.

There is no conscious control of reflex actions, though the conscious person will be aware of the reactions as impulses are also relayed to the cortex.

The doctor systematically examines the reflexes:

1 Tendon reflexes of the limbs (elbows, wrists, fingers, knees and ankles) are elicited by tapping individual muscle tendons to cause sudden stretching of the muscle body; in response there is reflex contraction of the muscle causing the limb to jerk. To obtain this response, the patient must be relaxed and the limbs correctly positioned and supported; a distracting activity may be necessary to prevent the patient tensing the limbs. When the muscles are suddenly stretched, intermittent muscular contraction and relaxation will be seen, causing a rhythmic jerking at the joint (clonus); this may be elicited at the wrist, ankle or knee and is an indication of increased muscle tone and upper motor neurone disorder.

2 Cutaneous reflexes
(a) Corneal reflex ⎫ these are tested during
(b) Gag reflex ⎬ examination of the
(c) Jaw reflex ⎭ cranial nerves
(d) Abdominal reflexes – the skin of the abdomen is lightly scratched from the umbilicus in the direction of each quadrant of the abdomen; if the reflex is present, the umbilicus is drawn towards the quadrant stimulated. Absence of abdominal reflexes may be of no pathological significance in obese patients, following several pregnancies, after abdominal operations or in old age.
(e) Peri-anal reflex – a light stroke with a pin causes anal contraction.
(f) Plantar reflex (Babinski response) – when the sole of the foot is gently scraped along its outer border in the direction of the great toe, the normal plantar response is flexor, the toes curling downwards. In children under the age of one year, the normal response is extensor, the great toe turning upwards with outward fanning of the other toes, but over this age this extensor response is abnormal and is a sign of upper motor neurone disorder.

Lesions of the motor neurones

Upper motor neurone	*Lower motor neurone*
1 Weakness or paralysis	1 Weakness or paralysis
2 Spasticity	2 Flaccidity
3 Muscle wasting – developing at a later stage	3 Muscle wasting – developing at an early stage
4 Increased reflexes	4 Diminished or absent reflexes
5 Abdominal reflexes diminished or absent	5 Abdominal reflexes present
6 Plantar response extensor	6 Plantar response flexor or absent

Sudden development of lesions in the brain and spinal cord affecting the upper motor neurones result in flaccidity of the affected muscles for the first few days (cerebral or spinal shock), then the tone increases rapidly and the limb becomes spastic due to the unopposed action of the extrapyramidal system.

Sensory system (see also Chapter 10)

Impulses of sensation are relayed to the parietal lobes; one side of the brain interprets the sensation from the opposite side of the body. The pathways of sensation divide when they reach the spinal cord (see chapter 10 and Figs 10.11–16).

Pain and temperature sensation   The nerve fibres cross immediately to the opposite side of the spinal cord and then pass upwards in the lateral spinothalamic tract to the thalamus; sensation is then relayed to the cerebral cortex.

Light touch   These nerve pathways, on entering the cord travel upward for a few segments before crossing to the opposite side; they then continue in the ventral spinothalamic tract.

Joint position, vibration and pressure sensation   Impulses are transmitted in the dorsal columns of the cord to the medulla where they cross to the opposite side and are relayed to the cerebral cortex; joint position sense (proprioception) is also relayed to the cerebellum.

Examination of the sensory system

The patient's full co-operation is necessary for an accurate assessment. The doctor first asks questions relating to any abnormal sensation (paraesthesia) experienced by the patient; those described may include numbness, tingling, 'pins and needles' or crawling feelings.

Discriminative sensations

Pain and temperature sensations   These will be affected simultaneously. A patient who has lost these sensations may have many scars and make light of the injuries. The doctor maps out the exact area where the sensation is abnormal, by pricking lightly with a pin and holding test-tubes of hot and cold water against the skin.

Light touch   To demonstrate an area of defective sensation the skin is lightly touched with a wisp of cotton wool.

Sensory inattention   The patient recognises individual stimuli but when both sides of the body are touched simultaneously, one stimulus is repeatedly ignored; a sign of a lesion in the opposite cerebral hemisphere.

Joint position sense   The patient is asked to close his eyes; the doctor may then:
> *(a)* move the patient's toes or fingers up or down and ask the patient to state the direction, or
> *(b)* place the patient's hand and fingers in a certain posture and ask the patient to place the other hand in the same position.

Romberg's sign (see p. 23) will be positive if there is diminution of joint position sense.

Vibration sense   A vibrating tuning fork is placed on a joint and the patient is asked to describe the sensation; normally there is a 'buzzing' feeling.

Two point discrimination   A pair of pronged calipers is used to find and measure the closest distance at which two simultaneously applied stimuli can separately be felt. The power to discriminate sensation is particularly highly developed in the finger tips, the normal distance is 3–6 mm whereas on the palms of the hands and soles of the feet it is 15–20 mm.

Pressure sensation This modality is tested by pressing a blunt object against the skin.

Stereognosis This is tested by asking the patient to close his eyes and identify familiar objects (key, coin, etc.) placed in his hand.

Investigations

The patient's medical history and doctor's clinical examination are always of prime importance; they may be the only basis for treatment in remote parts of the world, but in specialist units with up-to-date equipment investigations can be selected to assist a speedy, accurate diagnosis and prompt successful treatment.

Routine ward urine test

Blood tests

Routine blood tests are always performed, i.e.

i   haemoglobin estimation
ii full blood count
iii blood sedimentation rate
iv Wassermann and Kahn reaction

For other specific tests see chapters relating to specific disorders.

Chest X-rays

Chest X-rays are performed routinely to obtain information about the patient's general health and to reveal abnormalities which may be associated with disorders of the central nervous system, for example carcinoma and tuberculosis.

Skull X-rays

Hair pins, dentures, spectacles, earrings and bandage pins must first be removed. Plain X-rays of the skull are performed whenever cranial disorder is suspected. The X-rays will reveal:

1   Fractures (Fig. 2.17)
2   Areas of calcification
i   The pineal gland, calcified in a certain number of adults, lies in the mid-line; when this gland is shifted to one side an intracranial space-occupying lesion is indicated
ii   Certain tumours become calcified
3   Raised intracranial pressure
i   Widening of the sutures in children up to the age of eight years
ii   Thinning of the dorsum sellae of the sella turcica of the sphenoid bone and erosion of the posterior clinoid processes
iii Markings resembling those of beaten copper on the vault of the skull
4   Areas of infection
i   Osteomyelitis
ii   Pus and fluid levels in the sinuses
5   Changes in bone density in association with a tumour
6   Enlargement of foramina and dilatation of venous channels within the bone in the presence of certain tumours
7   Congenital abnormalities, e.g. dermoid cyst (see p. 80)
8   Foreign bodies
9   Previous burr holes
10 Aeroceles (see p. 93)

Simple linear

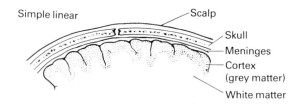

Comminuted

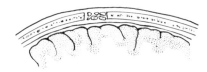

Compound

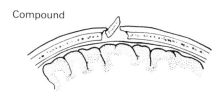

Depressed

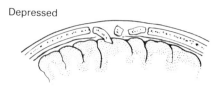

Fig. 2.17   Skull fractures.

dure is simple, the patient is potentially ill and may collapse, have a fit, feel overcome by anxiety and be worried about the outcome of the test; a nurse must always accompany a patient and stay with him throughout the test. The scan takes only ten minutes; it has no side-effects and the total exposure to radiation is no more than from a single ordinary X-ray.

Preparation
The procedure is explained to the patient who must understand the need to lie still during the examination; though the patient's face is not enclosed, his head is confined in the scanning machine's close-fitting cuff and a few patients will experience feelings of claustrophobia. Restless confused patients or children may require sedation or a light general anaesthetic; it is wise for all patients to fast before the examination.

Procedure
The X-ray department must be informed in advance if the patient's head is unduly large or small. When the patient is satisfactorily positioned, X-ray photons are passed through the skull and picked up by crystal detectors; the pictures are built up by the differential absorption of X-rays by the tissues. The results are calculated mathematically by computer, simultaneously translated on to a small screen and reproduced in a series of sectional photographs throughout all levels of the brain, including the cerebellum and structures at the base of the skull.

Computerised axial tomogram (CAT scan)

The CAT scanner produces clear pictures (Fig. 2.18) of sections through the brain and skull and enables the doctor to locate the site of a space-occupying lesion and in some instances to suspect its composition by detecting differences in the density of brain tissue. It is particularly useful in detecting tumours, in revealing the extent of cerebral oedema, as a repeat comparative investigation and in the diagnosis of postoperative complications, for example haematoma.

The CAT scanner is a very expensive piece of equipment and some patients travel a distance to have a scan as an out-patient. Though this proce-

Magnetic resonance imaging (MRI)

Magnetic resonance imaging (Nuclear Magnetic Resonance) is an investigation which gives clear pictures of the tissues of the nervous system without the need to introduce radioactive or other substances into the body. The patient's head or entire body is placed inside the machine which is a large electromagnet. This causes the nuclei of the cells to align themselves with the magnetic field. A burst of radiofrequency is then applied to these cells which causes them to resonate, the radiofrequency which these cells emit is recorded and analysed and transformed by a computer into cross-sectional pictures of the central nervous system.

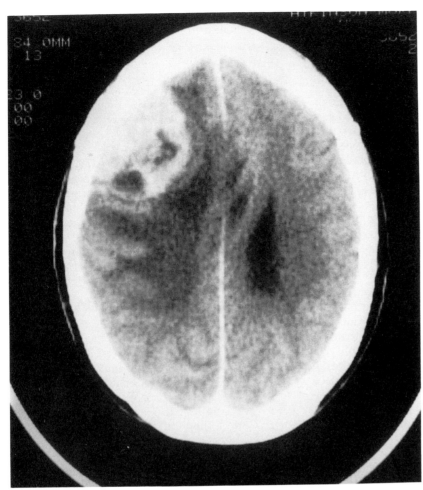

Fig. 2.18　Computerised axial tomogram, showing space occupying lesion.

This investigation is reserved for those disorders which cannot clearly be defined by other investigations as the machinery is very expensive and, in Great Britain, is only available in a few centres throughout the country.

Echoencephalogram (ultrasound)

For intracranial lesions in adults this investigation has largely been superseded by the CAT scan, but it remains useful for the diagnosis of intracranial disorders in children. It is a simple painless procedure which shows displacement of the mid-line structures within the brain, the size of the ventricles, the position of the tentorium cerebelli and the presence of extracerebral lesions. Glycerine is used to make contact with the scalp; the 'probe' sends high frequency sound waves through the brain which are deflected from the solid structures (meninges and the walls of ventricles) as an echo, are picked up by the machine and relayed to a viewing screen, on which distances can be measured and the presence of abnormal echoes seen. The patient's hair needs a shampoo after the procedure.

Ultrasonic studies are useful in the investigation of occlusion within the carotid arteries.

Electroencephalogram (EEG)

An electroencephalogram is a record of electrical potentials in the brain (Fig. 2.19). It is a useful aid to diagnosis and localisation of many neurological disorders. The procedure is in no way unpleasant and a simple explanation will allay fears and gain the patient's co-operation. It is usual and desirable for the test to be performed in the specially equipped EEG department where the presence of only the patient and a technician prevents distraction. An electroencephalogram can be performed in the ward if the patient is too seriously ill to be moved. The patient's head should be clean, hair oil should not be used before the recording is made and hairpins and metal clips removed.

Procedure

The record is made by attaching small electrodes to the scalp in relation to the lobes of the brain beneath. A variety of adhesives or electrode jelly can be used to make contact. Wires from the electrodes convey electrical activity to an amplifying machine which operates pens to draw lines in graph form. Small dermal needles may be used to speed up the recording. Special needles, inserted through the cheek, obtain a recording from the under surface of the anterior part of the temporal lobe. Electrocorticography is occasionally performed during operation by inserting needles into the brain.

The sequence of wave forms of the EEG record is fed into a computer for analysis and interpreted by an experienced neurologist. The normal rhythm is recognised as an alpha rhythm with a frequency of 10 cycles per second. There are normal variations in accordance with the person's age, state of consciousness and mental activity. Muscular activity such as blinking or frowning interrupts the normal alpha rhythm with irregularities in the wave pattern known as artefacts. Abnormal records are found in about 10% of clinically normal subjects. Generalised or focal abnormalities may be seen on some records in association with epilepsy, organic brain disease and mental disorder. Characteristic dysrhythmias are found in certain types of epilepsy, for example the spike and wave record of alternating fast and slow waves at 3 cycles per second which is associated with petit mal. Local slow or delta waves may suggest the presence of a tumour. A series of EEG records taken at intervals are sometimes useful for comparison.

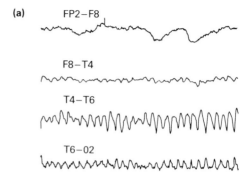

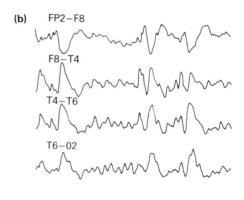

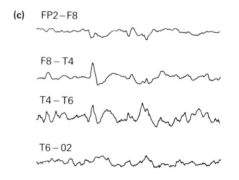

Fig. 2.19 Electroencephalographic **(a)** Normal tracing from right cerebral hemisphere. **(b)** Idiopathic epilepsy with spike and wave. Grand Mal. **(c)** Lateralised discharges from right hemisphere in presence of cerebral tumour. F = frontal; P = Parietal; T = Temporal; O = Occipital.

During the procedure the patient is required to sit or lie quietly with his eyes open for part of the time and then closed while the record is received from the visual cortex in the occipital lobes; restless patients and children may need sedation or a general anaesthetic. Abnormal electrical discharges may be provoked by asking the patient to breathe deeply and rapidly (hyperventilate) for a short period or look at a flashing light, by giving certain stimulant drugs or by withholding the patient's normal drugs.

Consent for radiological procedures

The following special investigations require either the written consent of the patient, or if they are incapable of giving it, the consent of their next-of-kin. In case of emergency, verbal consent is accepted by telephone; if no relative is available the investigation of a seriously ill or unconscious patient is permitted to proceed without consent to avoid delay. The nature of each procedure is explained to the patient and to the next-of-kin.

Angiography

This is a radiological investigation which demonstrates the cerebral circulation (see Chapter 8), primarily to reveal abnormalities in the structure and position of blood vessels (Fig. 2.20). When there has been subarachnoid haemorrhage it is necessary to discover the source of bleeding. The doctor's clinical examination may localise the lesion and suggest the diagnosis; a CAT scan will give further information, for example the site of a haematoma or angioma, or suggest the side on which the haemorrhage originated, but it is necessary to perform angiography to give a clear picture of the cerebral circulation and to determine which aneurysm has bled when multiple aneurysms are present. The procedure will be performed under a local or general anaesthetic. Depending on the patient's condition and awareness, a suitable explanation should be given and enquiry made as to whether he has any allergies; the patient should be

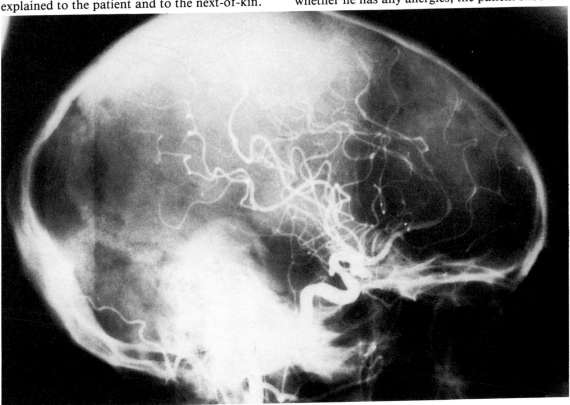

Fig. 2.20 Carotid angiography showing circulation to the anterior part of the brain.

assured that a nurse will stay with him throughout the investigation and the only discomfort he will experience is a momentary harmless sensation of heat suffusing his head as the dye is injected.

Procedure

A suitable premedication will be prescribed and administered between half an hour and an hour before the angiogram. In the X-ray department a radio-opaque dye is injected into a selected artery; access to the artery is either by direct puncture or by passing a catheter from the femoral artery to the origins of the carotid and vertebral arteries (Fig. 2.21). Four vessel angiography (i.e. simultaneous injections of dye into the carotid and subclavian arteries) may be performed only if the patient is young and in good general health; an arch aortogram will show occlusive lesions low in the carotid or vertebral arteries. When the dye is injected a series of films is taken in quick succession; once the needle is removed the artery is compressed for several minutes to prevent the development of haematoma. Very occasionally a patient may react adversely to the contrast medium.

After-care

1 Level of consciousness – the procedure should cause no deterioration in conscious level and a normal rapid recovery from anaesthesia should be expected. Neurological assessments should be made and recorded at half-hourly intervals. Arterial spasm is a serious complication particularly associated with angiography following sub-arachnoid haemorrhage (see p. 132); it is usually avoided by allowing several days to elapse after the haemorrhage, to allow the cerebral circulation to settle down.

2 Vital functions – a half-hourly record of pulse and respirations, and 2-hourly blood pressure should be made unless the patient is very ill, when a more frequent record is necessary; when he has regained his previous level of consciousness the frequency of records depends upon the patient's condition; from the beginning it should be made clear to the patient that these frequent assessments

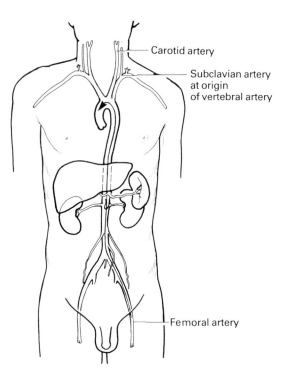

Carotid artery

Subclavian artery at origin of vertebral artery

Femoral artery

Fig. 2.21 Sites for angiographic injections.

are routine otherwise he may fear something has gone wrong.

3 Inspection of the injection site for oozing and haematoma formation.

4 Dyspnoea or complaint of chest pain following a subclavian angiogram should never be ignored (see iii below).

Complications of angiography

i Deterioration in conscious level The patient's condition may continue to deteriorate while he is anaesthetised and undergoing angiography; he may fail to regain his previous level of consciousness and any deterioration – however slight – must be reported immediately.

ii Haematoma at the site of the injection Haemorrhage into the tissues should be arrested by direct pressure and the doctor must be informed immediately as severe haemorrhage in the neck would displace and compress the trachea and cause asphyxiation; an emergency tracheostomy may be necessary.

iii Pneumothorax The subclavian artery lies close to the apex of the lung and the pleura may be unintentionally punctured. The patient will be breathless, cyanosed and complain of chest pain. A chest X-ray will reveal the severity of the resulting pulmonary collapse; if severe, a chest drain will be necessary. Intensive physiotherapy will be required to assist re-expansion of the lung.

Ventriculography

(for the anatomy and physiology of CSF production, circulation and re-absorption, see p. 70)

This investigation is fortunately now rarely performed as it has been superseded by CAT scan. The investigation involves replacing some of the ventricular CSF by a contrast medium, air or radio-opaque dye which will show the size, shape and displacement of the ventricles (Fig. 2.22).

Preparation
The patient will need a simple explanation of this rather unpleasant investigation and constant reassurance during the procedure. A 4-hour period of fast is necessary to prevent vomiting and in case major surgery is urgently needed. The posterior

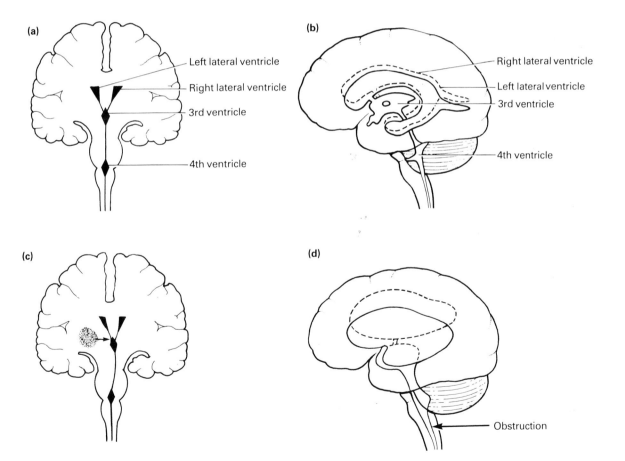

Fig. 2.22 The ventricular system. **(a)**, **(b)** Normal position of the ventricles. **(c)** Ventricles displaced by lesion in left cerebral hemisphere. **(d)** Dilated ventricles caused by obstructive lesion at exits to 4th ventricle.

parietal region is shaved for a burr hole. A general anaesthetic is necessary for children or very restless confused patients; otherwise a local anaesthetic is preferred to allow careful neurological observation.

Procedure

The surgeon first makes a small incision in the scalp and using a drill makes a burr hole in the skull before opening the dura; he passes a cannula through the brain into one lateral ventricle and by alternately withdrawing a few drops of CSF and instilling the same amount of the contrast medium (replacing in all 10 ml), he avoids sudden change of intraventricular pressure. The dura and scalp are then sutured. As air is lighter than CSF it will rise to the uppermost part of the ventricle; to obtain a sectional outline of lateral, third and fourth ventricles the patient's head is tilted in various positions as a series of films is taken. A second burr hole is only necessary if the air cannot be induced into the other lateral ventricle; failure of the air to enter one of the ventricles may be due to a blockage in the ventricular system.

After-care

1 Conscious level – half-hourly neurological assessment will be made and any deterioration must be reported immediately. Rising intracranial pressure may be caused by changing the intraventricular pressure (especially if there is a lesion blocking the ventricular system) or when accidental rupture of a vein has caused intracranial haemorrhage.

2 Vital functions – half-hourly pulse, respirations and blood pressure will be recorded and observations made for signs of rising intracranial pressure.

3 Scalp wounds will be inspected for haemorrhage.

Lumbar puncture

Indications for lumbar puncture:
i   To obtain a specimen of CSF for laboratory analysis and to estimate CSF pressure.
ii   To establish a diagnosis, relieve pressure and remove inflammatory or irritative substances, e.g. in subarachnoid haemorrhage and meningitis.

iii To introduce therapeutic drugs or epidural anaesthetic.
iv   To introduce radio-opaque substances (see p. 34).

Contraindications to lumbar puncture:
i   A lumbar puncture is dangerous when there is raised intracranial pressure due to suspected intracranial space-occupying lesions, especially if these are in the posterior fossa, because the withdrawal of CSF from the lumbar region will encourage descent of the brain and impaction of the cerebellar tonsils in the foramen magnum, compression of the vital centres and sudden respiratory arrest (cerebellar 'coning').
ii   The presence of cutaneous infection in the lumbar region.
iii Spinal deformity makes lumbar puncture difficult or impossible.

The patient's co-operation is necessary; he will naturally feel apprehensive and the way he reacts to lumbar puncture may be coloured by past experience or tales he has heard. Confused patients may be alarmed at the mere sight of doctor and nurse approaching with a trolley and may resist the whole procedure through fear and misunderstanding.

Parents should always be interviewed when a lumbar puncture is planned for their child and should receive an explanation and a reason for the procedure. The child also needs an explanation adapted to suit his age and understanding. A restless child may need sedation or a light general anaesthetic to prevent the experience being unpleasant and the child developing a dread of lumbar puncture, a procedure which, in certain diseases, is life saving and may need to be repeated daily.

The patient is positioned on his left side, with only one pillow under his head, his neck flexed so that his chin touches his chest, his knees drawn up to his chin and his back close to the edge of the bed. This is an uncomfortable position to maintain and some patients, particularly the elderly, may find it difficult and painful to flex stiff joints and be fearful of falling off the bed. Any patient with meningeal irritation will resent interference and because of severe headache and painful neck rigidity will be reluctant to curl up.

The nurse will face the patient and with one hand behind his knees and the other behind his head will give reassurance throughout the procedure and encourage him to keep absolutely still until he is told he may move. She will be prepared to forcibly maintain the patient in this position should he move suddenly or be unco-operative and restless, when she will kneel on the bed and hook her arms round his knees and neck; the assistance of another nurse will be necessary.

The puncture is usually performed between the 3rd and 4th or alternatively between the 4th and 5th lumbar vertebrae (Fig. 2.23); this enables the doctor to penetrate the subarachnoid space surrounding the cauda equina and avoids damaging the spinal cord which usually ends at the level of the 1st lumber vertebra (see p. 165). Strict asepsis is essential to prevent infection of the meninges; a cleansing agent is used to prepare the skin prior to the injection of local anaesthetic. When the anaesthetic has taken effect the lumbar puncture needle is introduced between the vertebrae passing through the intervertebral ligaments until it reaches the dura mater; the needle is then advanced slowly, the doctor withdrawing the stylet after each movement; a resistance is felt before the needle finally penetrates the meninges and CSF drips out. The patient should not feel any pain as the lumbar puncture needle is inserted, but he will feel pressure

against his back. Sometimes pain radiates down one leg, into the buttocks or genital area due to the needle touching one of the nerve roots of the cauda equina; it should disappear when the doctor withdraws and redirects the needle. The CSF pressure is measured by attaching a manometer to the needle; the rapid oscillation of fluid in the manometer synchronises with the pulse beat, the slower oscillation with the respirations. As muscular tension increases the CSF pressure, the patient is asked to relax his position, to straighten his legs a little and breathe quietly; tests are then performed to determine free communication within the CSF system.

Queckenstedt's test

The nurse, warning the patient that she is going to press his neck, will in turn compress each jugular vein at the angle of the jaw; the normal reaction is an immediate rapid rise of the CSF in the manometer of at least 100 mm, and almost as rapid a fall when pressure is released; this 'free rise and fall' indicates free communication between the ventricular system, CSF channels, venous sinuses (where the CSF is absorbed) and the venous circulation; no rise and fall indicates a blockage somewhere in the system. Other tests for increasing CSF pressure include applying pressure to the abdomen and asking the patient to cough or strain. When the tests have been completed one or more specimens of CSF will be collected and carefully labelled for laboratory analysis. The needle will then be removed, pressure applied to the puncture site to prevent leakage of CSF and a small adhesive dressing applied; this can be removed within a few hours. The ambulant patient should be advised to rest in bed for the remainder of the day and headache will be treated with a mild analgesic.

Cerebrospinal fluid (CSF)

Total volume – 130 ml which is constantly being secreted by the choroid plexus of the ventricular system and re-absorbed into the superior sagittal sinus (see Figs 4.3 and 4.4).

Normal pressure when the body is in the horizontal position is 90–120 mm/water.

The normal appearance of CSF is crystal clear and colourless.

Normal constituents

protein	15–40 mg%
sugar	50–80 mg%
chlorides	725–750 mg%
cells	0–5 lymphocytes/cubic mm.

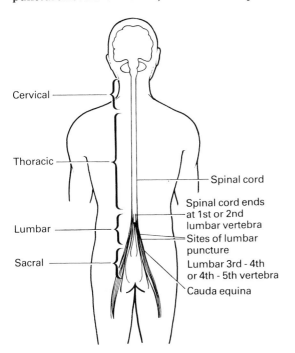

Cervical

Thoracic

Spinal cord

Spinal cord ends at 1st or 2nd lumbar vertebra

Lumbar

Sites of lumbar puncture

Sacral

Lumbar 3rd - 4th or 4th - 5th vertebra

Cauda equina

Fig. 2.23 Sites for lumbar puncture.

Myelography

Lumbar myelogram

This is a radiological investigation in which a contrast medium, metrizamide, is injected into the subarachnoid space through a lumbar puncture needle to outline the spinal cord and nerve roots. The procedure must be explained to the patient beforehand; a meal is unwise before myelography as anxiety and the tilting X-ray table are liable to induce nausea and if the investigation is expected to be followed by surgery the patient will be fasted for four hours. A tranquillising or anticonvulsant preparation (diazepam or phenobarbitone) may be given as a premedication because metrizamide can cause an epileptic fit in susceptible individuals.

A lumbar puncture is performed, pressure recorded, a specimen of CSF is obtained for laboratory analysis and then the contrast medium is injected. The patient, lying prone, is strapped to a tilting X-ray table; as the contrast medium moves within the subarachnoid space it is viewed on a screen and a series of films is taken which will reveal space-occupying and other compressing lesions (Fig. 2.24).

Cisternal myelogram

When a lumbar injection is not possible or is contraindicated by a suspected lesion in the lumbar region (spinal deformity or abscess), the contrast medium can be injected into the cisterna magna. The sub-occipital region is shaved before the procedure. As the cisternal needle is close to the medulla and sudden movement would be dangerous, it is most important that the patient is reassured and remains calm throughout the procedure; the investigation is performed with the patient in a sitting position, his neck flexed. The skin is cleaned, infiltrated with local anaesthetic and a special cisternal puncture needle is used to introduce the contrast medium into the subarachnoid space (Fig. 2.25); a series of X-rays is then taken.

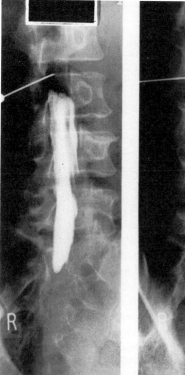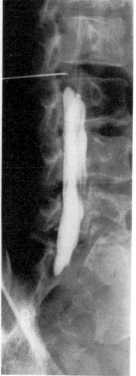

Fig. 2.24   Lumbar myelogram, showing compressing lesion at lumbar 4/5 level.

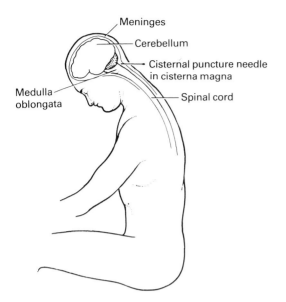

Fig. 2.25 Site for cisternal myelogram.

Radiculography

This procedure is as for myelography but with the specific intention of outlining the nerve roots; metrizamide is used and is confined to a localised area by tilting the table only slightly. This investigation can proceed to myelography if the need arises.

After care following myelography
It is advisable for the patient to rest in bed for 24 hours; when metrizamide has been used the patient must sit upright in bed for the first 6 hours and for the next 16 hours he should have no less than 4 pillows; these measures are to prevent metrizamide causing irritation of the cervical cord and brain. Myelography may aggravate the patient's symptoms and regular analgesics are often necessary.

Caloric tests
(Tests of labyrinthine function; see Chapter 21)

Caloric tests are helpful in determining the nature and site of lesions which affect labyrinthine function. The tests are not conclusive, but in conjunction with the history, examination and other tests, are helpful in diagnosis and treatment. The test are performed by an ear, nose and throat specialist after he has studied the patient's medical history. It is advisable for the patient to fast for a few hours beforehand as the test may cause nausea and vomiting. Romberg's and finger/nose tests and examination for nystagmus will be performed before caloric testing, as a comparative record. The test equipment is prepared and a second person should be available to keep records. Before commencing, the doctor will examine the patient's ears to exclude a perforated ear drum, which would contraindicate the use of water in this test though air could be used. The patient should be given a clear explanation of the test, and if he is deaf this will include a written explanation to ensure that he understands the procedure and the importance of telling the doctor immediately any symptoms are experienced.

The patient lies on a couch with his head raised at an angle of 30°; with the head in this position the labyrinths are more sensitive to changes of temperatures. He will then be asked to gaze straight ahead and 250 ml of tap water at 30°C (cold test) is used to irrigate the ear taking 40 seconds. The doctor watches the patient for the first appearance of nystagmus and notes its direction and duration; the procedure is timed from the beginning of the irrigation to the time when nystagmus ceases. The other ear is tested in the same way and the whole procedure is repeated using water at 44°C (hot test). Records are compared with the normal.

Abnormal responses

1   The response may be diminished or absent in one ear (canal paresis); this abnormal response is on the same side as the lesion and accompanies the condition of Menière's disease and tumours of the acoustic (VIIIth cranial) nerve.
2   There may also be directional preponderance – whichever labyrinth is stimulated, nystagmus in one direction lasts longer than in the other; this is found in lesions affecting the vestibular areas in the cerebral hemispheres and the brain stem.

The patient may be very distressed by these tests which cause intense giddiness, nausea and sometimes vomiting; he should be encouraged to bear this temporary unpleasantness for the sake of a possible diagnosis and cure. A period of rest for an hour or two is necessary after the tests.

3

Changing Levels of Consciousness and Care of the Unconscious Patient

Including Care of the Critically Ill Patient in Intensive Care

The care of an unconscious or semiconscious patient presents many special problems in nursing technique and understanding, and the quality of nursing care is of crucial importance to the patient's recovery. Stresses imposed on the nursing staff are considerable and it is essential that they have a sound understanding of the physical and psychological problems involved. Any patient who is not fully conscious runs the same risks to a lesser or greater extent as a totally unconscious patient. The authors' reference to 'unconscious patient' therefore includes all patients who have any degree of clouding of consciousness.

There is an unfortunate lack of knowledge of many simple things which may influence the survival of an unconscious person. The life of the unconscious road accident victim may rest with the casual passer-by who may or may not have a first aid knowledge of how to prevent choking. The victim of 'stroke' may be found by a relative or friend who has no medical knowledge. In hospital an inexperienced junior nurse may find her patient collapsed in the lavatory.

Medical advances mean that a greater number of very seriously ill patients are being kept alive; the use of pacemakers and respirators is increasing. The tensions of this age lead to psychiatric disorders which are treated with drugs; many of those attempting suicide take an overdose and are found unconscious. On the road there is a high toll, and a large proportion of these accident victims sustain head injury.

Whatever the cause of unconsciousness, whether it is trivial or serious, wherever the event occurs (in the home, on the street or in hospital), the patient's life depends on the knowledge and presence of mind of those who find him and the care he receives until he regains normal health. He should not die as the result of ignorance or poor nursing standards or be unnecessarily maimed for life.

Anatomy as related to unconsciousness

The skull, encasing the brain, is composed of many bones intricately linked together by sutures. In an adult it forms a rigid, unyielding box whereas, in a child under the age of 8 years before the sutures have united, it will yield to an internal pressure and the bones will part. The base of the skull is divided into fossae or recesses and in these lie different parts of the brain (Fig. 3.1). The cerebrum occupies the whole of the vault, anterior and middle fossae; the cerebellum and brain stem lie in the posterior fossa (Fig. 3.2). There are many openings in the skull, most of them small, allowing entry and exit of cranial nerves and blood vessels; one large outlet, the foramen magnum, allows the passage of the nerve fibres from the brain to the spinal cord.

The brain is covered by three membranes (meninges); the pia mater is closely applied to the surface of the brain and is separated from the arachnoid mater by a protective shock-absorbing cushion of fluid (cerebrospinal fluid); the dura mater, a very tough inelastic double membrane, surrounds the whole brain (Fig. 3.3). The outer layer of the dura mater is attached to the inner surface of the skull and the inner layer dips into the brain dividing the cranial cavity into compartments. A sickle-shaped sheet of dura mater (the falx cerebri) separates the two cerebral hemispheres and runs in the mid-line from the frontal bone to the occipital bone where it becomes continuous with a tent-like sheet of dura mater (the tentorium cerebelli) which separates the cerebrum from the cerebellum and forms the roof of the posterior fossa (Fig. 3.4). The brain stem passes through an opening in the tentorium cerebelli (the tentorial hiatus).

The brain stem consists of the nerve fibres passing to and from the brain and the nuclei of the cranial nerves. The third cranial nerves (oculomotor) are very important, their nuclei are in the midbrain at the level of the tentorial hiatus (see p. 16 and Fig. 3.5). The nerves (one to each eye) leave the midbrain, pass through the hiatus to supply movement to the upper eyelids and the pupils; they are the parasympathetic nerve supply and cause the pupils to constrict in reaction to light and accommodation. Located in a central core of the brain stem is a network of cells and fibres called the reticular formation which in the midbrain is concerned with consciousness and in the medulla oblongata, with respiration, cardiovascular control, swallowing and vomiting.

From this simple anatomy it can be deduced that an increase in pressure in the cranial cavity above the tentorial hiatus will force the soft brain tissue through any available outlet (Fig. 3.5). It will at first plug the small foramina of the skull close to the expanding lesion affecting local cranial nerve function and blood supply, and then force the free lower edge of the falx cerebri to one side and squeeze under it. Finally the medial part of the temporal lobe (the uncus) is forced through the only remaining outlet, the tentorial hiatus (uncal or

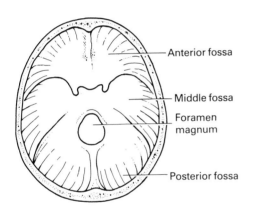

Fig. 3.1 Interior base of the skull showing fossae.

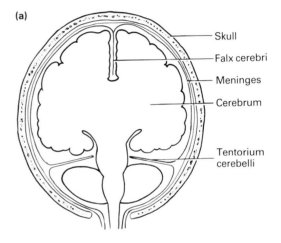

(a)

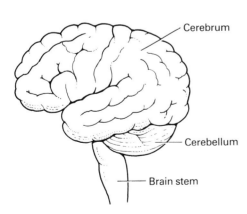

Fig. 3.2 The brain.

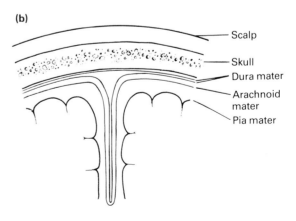

(b)

Fig. 3.3 Coronal section showing (a) meninges, falx cerebri and tentorium cerebelli; (b) layers of the meninges.

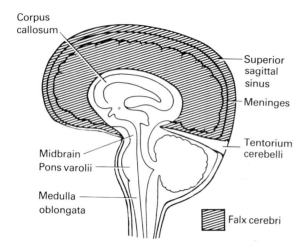

Fig. 3.4 Sagittal section showing the falx cerebri and tentorium cerebelli.

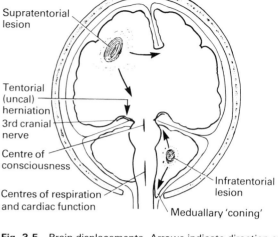

Fig. 3.5 Brain displacements. Arrows indicate direction of displacement.

tentorial herniation), where it will nip the third cranial nerve against the edge of the tentorium cerebelli on the same side as the lesion causing a third nerve palsy. It will compress the midbrain affecting the function of the limbs on the opposite side of the body, and the conscious centre causing lowering of consciousness and will proceed to compress the contents of the posterior fossa.

An increase in pressure in the posterior fossa will affect the functions of the cerebellum, the sympathetic (autonomic – see p. 169) nerve supply to the pupil, constricting the pupil often to pinpoint size (as the IIIrd cranial nerve is functioning unopposed), and will compress the brain stem as the contents of the posterior fossa are squeezed out. Cerebellar displacement through the foramen magnum affects the vital functions of the medulla oblongata (medullary 'coning'); upward displacement through the tentorial hiatus compresses the midbrain.

Causes of unconsciousness

Whatever the cause of unconsciousness (Table 3.1), the principles of nursing care are the same. The normal reflexes which protect the conscious patient have been lost and their function of protection must be taken over by diligent and watchful nurses. **Reflexes act promptly and so must the**

nurse. The patient must be kept free of the many complications which can beset him while diagnosis is made, treatment given and nature uses her restorative powers. Time is necessary, and during that time the patient may die of bronchopneumonia caused by lack of suction, inhalation of vomit or cross infection. Recovery may be prolonged or marred if poor nursing care allows such disabilities as corneal ulceration, joint contractures, foot drop or pressure sores.

It cannot be overemphasised that the care of an unconscious patient must follow certain principles, from the onset of unconsciousness and thereafter for twenty-four hours each day, with the utmost conscientiousness on the part of all staff who come in contact with the patient. This requires, in the first place, enlightenment of the general public, then careful instruction of ambulance attendants, all grades of nursing staff, theatre and X-ray porters. In particular each one should know how to maintain a clear airway and the positions which facilitate this to prevent additional complications. Any routine must have an obvious purpose which is communicated to the staff as, if they are ill-informed and do not understand priorities, they will become casual and negligent in carrying out routine nursing procedures. Each individual is important and every quarter of an hour vital, as negligence in changing the position of an unconscious patient, which begins in a small way by being just half an hour beyond the appointed time,

Table 3.1 Causes of unconsciousness

1 Poisons and drugs
Alcohol
General anaesthetics
Overdose of drugs, e.g. barbiturates or opiates
Gases, e.g. carbon monoxide and phosgene
Heavy metals, e.g. lead or mercury

2 Vascular causes
Ischaemia – acute ischaemia (syncope), e.g. following
      haemorrhage or coronary
      thrombosis
    – chronic ischaemia, e.g. resulting from
      cerebral thrombosis or cerebral embolus
Hypertensive encephalopathy
Haemorrhage – subarachnoid or cerebral haemorrhage

3 Infections
Septicaemia
Organisms – encephalitis (viral)
      – meningitis (bacterial)
      – protozoon, e.g. malaria and sleeping
        sickness
      – metazoon, e.g. hyatid and cysticercus
      – fungal, e.g. actinomycosis and torulosis
Abscess

4 Endocrine causes
Myxoedema
Addison's disease

5 Fits
Epilepsy
Eclampsia

6 Metabolic causes
Diabetes – insulin overdose – hypoglycaemia
       – ketoacidosis
Uraemia
Hepatic coma

7 'Mechanical' causes
Trauma
Hypothermia
Hyperthermia
Dehydration

8 Tumours

9 Hysteria – sometimes mimics coma

can be as serious in its consequences as to ignore the signs of internal haemorrhage. This may seem an exaggeration, but emphasis is necessary, for all those responsible for an unconscious patient should be constantly urged to maintain a high standard of exactitude in all matters relating to the patient who is unable to complain himself and may be in this condition for a very long period, the very length of which may naturally cause a decline in the staff's interest as they turn, wash and feed this unresponsive body, day in and day out.

Emergency equipment

The special equipment described in Table 3.2 must be available for immediate use. For ward design, staff and equipment see Appendix A.

Table 3.2 Emergency equipment to be available for immediate use

1 Post-anaesthetic instruments in a receiver
2 Suction apparatus
3 Resuscitation trolley containing
  i Resuscitation tray holding drugs
    (a) cardiac stimulants
    (b) various sizes of syringes and needles
    (c) intracardiac needle
    (d) swabs and cleaning agent
  ii Emergency ventilation equipment
    (a) a Brook airway
    (b) an Ambu resuscitator
  iii Intubation tray
4 A mechanical ventilator
5 Electric clippers for preparing a head shave if this should be necessary
6 Shaving tray
7 Apparatus for the passage of an oesophageal tube to aspirate the stomach contents, or wash out the stomach if overdose of·drugs is suspected
8 Neurological examination tray
9 Charts and routine admission forms

Immediate nursing care

The unconscious patient will arrive in the ward or intensive care unit on a stretcher trolley and may be accompanied by several relatives, hospital porters and ambulance attendants. To ensure that the patient receives necessary care swiftly, responsibilities should be delegated to members of the nursing staff according to the staff situation. One nurse or the ward hostess should meet the relatives and take them to the visitors' room or other suitable interview accommodation. She will impart any information required concerning visiting times, telephone enquiries, hospital procedure and canteen facilities, and will arrange for an interview between the relatives and the ward doctor. A nurse from the transferring hospital may be present and able to furnish useful details concerning the patient's condition and previous history.

When nursing an unconscious patient it is most important that at no time does any member of the staff talk about the patient, his condition, illness and prognosis at the bedside. The sense of hearing may remain intact and it is always kinder to regard the patient as being able to hear and to treat him as though he were conscious. An experienced nurse of the ward staff should accompany the stretcher-borne patient to help and supervise as he is lifted on to the bed, making sure that his head and neck are always supported; **the possibility of neck injury must always be considered when the patient has sustained a head injury**. The nurse will ensure that the patient is placed in the lateral or semi-prone position with his neck slightly extended to improve his airway (Fig. 3.6). These positions are used as they prevent the tongue obstructing the airway, inhalation of foreign bodies (a small denture plate with a single tooth or a broken tooth) and allow drainage of secretions from the nose and mouth. **At no time should an unconscious patient lie flat on his back.** An identity name band must be attached to the patient's wrist or ankle.

Maintenance of a clear airway

The nurse must take immediate steps to see that the airway is clear by:

1 removing any obvious obstructions; and

2 using suction to remove excess secretions, vomitus or sputum. Nasal suction is contra-indicated if the patient has sustained a head injury or has CSF rhinorrhoea.

As soon as the patient reaches the ward it is likely that he will require suction as facilities during an ambulance journey may be inadequate; an artificial airway will improve the patient's respira-

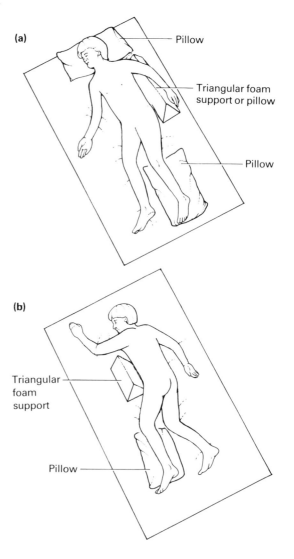

Fig. 3.6 Positioning of the unconscious patient. (a) Lateral position. (b) Semiprone position.

tions. It is naturally unwise and unnecessary to introduce suction catheters into the air passages if the patient's respirations appear quiet and regular and his colour is good; the passages are lined with delicate mucous membrane and are very easily damaged. Oxygen may be prescribed if the patient has respiratory difficulties even though he may not be cyanosed as the brain suffers from anoxia before peripheral cyanosis is evident.

Suction technique

This procedure is extremely important and the correct technique must be used on each occasion and by every nurse. Any carelessness in this matter is a potential source of infection to the patient; incorrect methods will cause abrasion of the mucous membrane with resulting haemorrhage and oedema, introduce infection which will increase the swelling and obstruction of the air passages, and cause anoxia which has such serious effects upon the brain. Cross-infection will endanger other patients and the nursing staff.

Types of suction apparatus

A small portable apparatus, though rarely used in a ward, is useful when an unconscious patient is being moved from one place to another. In the ward the most effective system is piped suction. Equipment at the bedside must be well maintained and neatly arranged so that, in an emergency, the nurse can practise the correct technique without hindrance.

Procedure

1 The patient's neck should be slightly extended and an artificial airway inserted into the mouth to facilitate the passage of suction catheters into the trachea.
2 The suction apparatus is turned to a pressure of 10 cm of mercury.
3 The catheter is connected to the Y-connection on the suction apparatus exposing only the connecting end of the catheter while leaving the other end in the sterile packet.
4 The nurse puts on clean disposable polythene gloves to protect herself from painful infection of the fingers; the gloves are not sterile, but every attempt is made to keep the procedure as clean as possible.

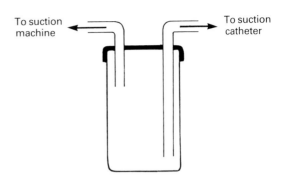

To suction machine   To suction catheter

Fig. 3.7 Sterile sputum trap.

5 The catheter is carefully withdrawn from the sterile packet (avoiding contact with the bed, locker or nurse's clothes), introduced into the mouth or nasal passages and gently passed until it reaches the excess secretions. At this point, the nurse covers the open end of the Y-connection and, slowly withdrawing the catheter, applies suction. Once suction has begun the catheter should never remain stationary as, if it does, it will adhere to the mucous membrane and cause an abrasion. Sometimes suction stimulates the patient to cough which produces more sputum, an indication that the procedure should be repeated.

The nurse should observe the character of secretions and sputum and note whether it is simple mucoid, purulent or bloodstained and frothy. It may be necessary to collect a specimen for laboratory examination in the special sputum trap suitable for this purpose (Fig. 3.7). The aim of suction is gently and speedily to remove secretions which are embarrassing the patient's respirations. Suction should not be prolonged and the nurse should pause at intervals and listen to the patient's breathing.

Indications to stop suction
1 When the lungs and air passages appear clear and the respirations are quiet.
2 If, in spite of prolonged attempts at suction, the lungs sound moist, an interval of 10 to 15 minutes should be allowed before further suction is given.
3 Should laryngeal stridor develop suction should cease and medical aid should be sought.

Suction completed

The catheter is disconnected from the suction apparatus and, held coiled in the palm of the hand, is enclosed within the glove by turning the glove inside out starting at the wrist. With the first glove held in her second hand the nurse removes her second glove in the same way and the dirty catheter is thus enfolded in two layers of polythene; it is then placed in the disposal bag.

Artificial airways should be changed at regular hourly intervals as they may become blocked with sputum and obstruct breathing. Suction apparatus must be replaced with sterile equipment twice daily.

Continuing nursing care and complications of unconsciousness

General assessment

The nurse responsible for the admission of an unconscious patient will be making pertinent observations from the moment he is brought into the ward and these observations must be written down before they are forgotten. Under the supervision of the nurse the patient is lifted from stretcher to bed by the ambulance attendants and placed in the correct position; suction is used to remove excess oral secretions and the nurse will be considering and relating the observations she makes to the possible causes of coma, using her well-trained senses and making a rapid mental note of the following points:

1   Listen
    Do the respirations sound 'bubbly', laboured or stertorous?
    Are the respirations slow or rapid?
    Are the respirations irregular or of the Cheyne–Stokes type?
    Is there stridor?

2   Look
    Is there any obvious injury, are there abrasions, lacerations, bruising, oedema or deformity caused by fractures of the skull or facial bones?
    Is there any obvious cranial nerve palsy, e.g. facial weakness or deviation of the eyes?
    Is the tongue coated, clean, dry or moist?
    Is there any discharge from the ears or nasal passages? (If there is bleeding, blood from these orifices may disguise a leak of cerebrospinal fluid).
    Is the patient pallid, florid, jaundiced or cyanosed?
    Is the patient obese, well-nourished or emaciated?
    Is the patient dehydrated? (If so, the patient will appear drowsy and ill, will have a dirty mouth, dry cracked tongue, sunken eyes and dry inelastic skin.
    Does the patient's hair condition suggest endocrine disturbance?
    Is there a rash, pigmentation or any form of skin eruption?
    Are there pressure sores?
    Is there any abnormality of posture, e.g. head retraction as in opisthotonos?
    Is the patient moving spontaneously, and if so is this movement equal in all four limbs?
    Is there evidence of limb fractures?
    Are there any abnormal movements, e.g. twitching of a part as in focal epilepsy?
    Is the chest expanding well and equally or is there evidence of a fracture of the clavicle or ribs?
    Is the abdomen distended?
    Is the patient pregnant?
    Is the patient menstruating?

3   Smell
    Is the patient ketotic?
    Does the patient smell of alcohol?
    Is there a sickly-sweet smell indicative of hepatic disturbance?
    If the patient has been incontinent, is the urine offensive in odour?
    Is there faecal incontinence?

4   Touch
    Are the extremities cold?
    Is the skin cold and clammy or hot and dry?
    Is there surgical emphysema?

Levels of consciousness

In discussing levels of the consciousness, it is first necessary to define 'full consciousness'. The fully conscious patient is mentally alert, rational, orientated in time, place and person, and able to react to sensory stimuli in an appropriate way. It is not possible to describe here every small degree of alteration in consciousness, but six levels of consciousness which are convenient for assessment purposes are set out below. The patient may be:

1 Fully conscious (see above).

2 Drowsy but easily roused. The patient who is drowsy may be rational but more commonly there is some degree of disorientation and confusion.

3 Very drowsy, but can be roused with difficulty. This patient is often confused and disorientated in time and place; if he is also disorientated in person he may not recognise his relations and friends, or the status of medical and nursing staff.

4 Stuperose. The patient is virtually unconscious, but with stimulation, either by the loudly spoken word or by pain, he may respond by opening his eyes, by grunting or by moving his limbs spontaneously, but soon lapses into unconsciousness. Some patients who are stuporose become extremely restless and even aggressive when disturbed, especially if they are suffering from headache or have a full bladder.

5 Unconscious. None of the above-mentioned methods of stimulation will rouse the patient, but it may be possible to elicit some form of reflex movement in response to painful stimuli. Occasional spontaneous movement may be seen.

6 Deeply unconscious. The patient is completely unrousable by any method of stimulation. His pupils may react sluggishly to light or may be fixed, i.e. non-reactive to light. There may be no response to painful stimulus in any limb or there may be extension to pain or spontaneous extension of all four limbs (decerebrate response).

Neurological assessment

When assessing the neurological state of a patient the nurse must gain his full co-operation. A patient who is not fully awakened from sleep before an assessment is made may be recorded as drowsy; later, when his neurological condition deteriorates and he becomes truly drowsy, it may be thought that there has been no change in his conscious state and early detection of deterioration will have been missed. This becomes more important when dealing with very drowsy, stuporose and unconscious patients, when even a slight deterioration will render the patient deeply unconscious; by then irreversible damage may have been sustained by the midbrain and medulla. It is important, too, that the nurse writes down the assessment of each patient (see Neurological Assessment Charts, Fig. 3.8) when working in a ward with unconscious and drowsy patients; it is extremely difficult for the inexperienced person to remember all the relevant details of each patient. When relieved by another nurse a careful and detailed report must be given before relinquishing her duties.

To rouse the patient, light stimulation such as calling his name, touching his hand or a gentle shake of his shoulder, may be sufficient. The drowsy patient may require repeated instructions before obeying requests to open his eyes or move his limbs. Should this be ineffective then greater stimulation will be necessary, the nurse using a louder voice, perhaps kneading the trapezius muscle with her knuckles or even inflicting pain in order to get the greatest response from the patient. It is always a matter of regret to the nursing and medical staff that they are forced to use painful stimuli to assess a patient's condition, but when it is necessary there are methods which cause the least possible damage to the tissues, and others which are not recommended. Painful stimulation by supra-orbital pressure, pinching or pummelling limbs or trunk will cause extensive bruising and swelling and should be avoided. The maximum response from a stuporose or unconscious patient will be obtained by pressing the thumb nail into the base of the patient's finger or toe nail, taking care to avoid the cuticle; should the cuticle be damaged it

Fig. 3.8   Neurological assessment charts. Below: **(a)** In association with simultaneous TPR and BP chart. Right: **(b)** Glasgow chart.

TIME	LEVEL OF CONSCIOUS- NESS AND SPEECH	PUPILS	LIMB MOVEMENTS	GENERAL REMARKS
8.30 a.m.	Conscious but drowsy. Fairly easily roused. Mumbled intelligible verbal response.	R slightly larger than L. Normal size. React briskly to light.	Moving all limbs spontaneously and to command. Grips strong L slightly weaker than R.	Observe meantime and report any changes. ½ hourly chart.
9.00 a.m.	Conscious but drowsy. Some difficulty in rousing patient. Verbal response mumbled, brief, but intelligible.	R slightly larger than L. Normal size. R pupil more sluggish to react than L.	Moving R limbs spontaneously and all limbs to command. Obvious L hemiparesis. Withdraws L limbs briskly from painful stimulation.	Dr notified ¼ hourly record to be kept I.V. set up.
9.15 a.m.	Very drowsy and difficult to rouse. Brief monosyllabic verbal response. Irritable – resents interference.	R larger than L. More dilated. R pupil reacting sluggishly. L briskly to light.	Moving R limbs to command. Occasionally spontaneously. L hemiparesis more marked. Arm worse than leg. Withdraws limbs briskly from pain.	I.V. mannitol set up. To run in in 20 minutes.
9.30 a.m.	Very drowsy. Difficult to rouse. Brief verbal response. Still irritable.	Smaller. R slightly larger than L. R reacting more briskly.	Moving R limbs spontaneously and to command. L hemiparesis unchanged. Withdraws limbs briskly from pain.	
9.45 a.m.	More easily roused. Verbal response mumbled, brief but intelligible.	R slightly larger than L. Normal size. Reacting briskly.	Moving R limbs spontaneously and to command. Occasional slight spontaneous movement L leg. Withdraws both L limbs briskly from pain.	Good diuresis

may lead to paronychia; this method does not cause significant bruising.

When she has done her utmost to rouse the patient by some form of external stimulation, for example either vocal or painful, the nurse should continue her assessment as follows:

1   Conscious level. What is the patient's best conscious level?

2   Speech. Is it:
   (a)   clear and intelligible
   (b)   muttered or incoherent
   (c)   dysphasic or aphasic
   (d)   dysarthric or anarthric

3   Mental state (see p. 10). Is the patient:
   (a)   confused
   (b)   disorientated
   (c)   hallucinated
   (d)   behaving abnormally

4   Observations relating to the patient's eyes. Can the patient voluntarily open his eyes? If not it will be necessary to open them gently and make the following observations:
   i   General observations
   (a)   Can the patient see?
   (b)   Has there been any eye injury?
   (c)   Is there chemosis, proptosis, ptosis or obvious squint?

NEUROLOGICAL OBSERVATION CHART

AFFIX PATIENT IDENTIFICATION LABEL

Surname: SMITH

Date of birth: 6.5.70

Unit number: 12345

First Names: JOHN

Sex: M

Consultant/s:

....

Frequency of Recordings ½ HOURLY

DATE

TIME

				30 6	7	30 7	8	30 8	9	30 9	10	30 10	11	30 11	12										

COMA SCALE

			Eyes closed by swelling = C
Eyes open	Spontaneously		
	To speech	✓ ✓ ✓ ✓ ✓	
	To pain	✓ ✓	
	None		
Best verbal response	Orientated		Endotracheal tube or tracheostomy = T
	Confused	✓ ✓	
	Inappropriate words	✓ ✓ ✓	
	Incomprehensible sounds	✓ ✓	
	None		
Best motor response	Obey commands	✓ ✓ ✓ ✓	Usually record the best arm record
	Localise pain	✓	
	Flexion to pain	✓ ✓	
	Extension to pain		
	None		

Written comments – See Over

Pupil scale (m.m): 1, 2, 3, 4, 5, 6, 7, 8

Blood pressure and Pulse rate

240 230 220 210 200 190 180 170 160 150 140 130 120 110 100 90 80 70 60 50 40 30 Respiration 20 10

Temperature C: 41 40 39 38 37 36 35 34 33 32 31

PUPILS

right	Size	3	3	4	4	5	5	6			+ reacts – no reaction c. eye closed by swelling
	Reaction	+	+	+	+	–	–	–			
left	Size	3	3	3	3	3	3	3			
	Reaction	+	+	+	+	+	+	+			

LIMB MOVEMENTS

ARMS	Normal power	✓ ✓	R	R	R		Record right (R) and left (L) separately
	Mild weakness		L	L		R	
	Severe weakness			L			
	Spastic flexion						
	Extension				L	L	
	No response						
LEGS	Normal power	✓ ✓ ✓ ✓	R	R		If there is a difference between the two sides
	Mild weakness		L		R	
	Severe weakness			L		
	Extension				L	
	No response					

(d) Is the patient able to focus?

(e) Is there nystagmus?

ii   Pupillary observations

(a) What is their size, are they pinpoint, normal, moderately or fully dilated?

(b) Are the pupils equal in size? If not, which is the larger?

(c) Is there irregularity in the outline of the pupils?

(d) What is the pupil reaction to light and does each react in the same way? Reaction may be described as brisk, sluggish or fixed. The normal pupil reacts briskly to light, but also constricts when confronted by near objects (reaction to accommodation); to ensure a true response to light only, the nurse should direct light obliquely into the eye. If the reaction is very sluggish and the pupil small it may be necessary to test it by a sudden direct flash of light.

5   Limb movements and tone

i   Observe for spontaneous movement; are the limbs moved as often and as vigorously on each side?

ii   Is there any abnormal involuntary movement?

(a) twitchings

(b) tremors

(c) choreiform or athetoid movements

iii   Is the patient able to move his limbs to command, and if so, is there any apparent weakness? Receptive dysphasia, deafness or other difficulty in comprehension may cause misunderstanding of the commands given; gesture may convey the idea where spoken word fails. The patient should be asked to grip the nurse's hand and then release his grip; in some instances a grasp reflex is present, when the nurse places her fingers in the palm of the patient's hand, he will continue to grip firmly even when asked to let go – attempts to withdraw her hand forcibly further intensify the patient's grasp. Slight weakness of the upper limbs may only be detected if the patient, with eyes closed, is asked to hold out his arms with fingers outstretched; a slight lowering of one arm (fall-away) may be due to weakness or loss of the appreciation of position sense; if the patient is able to co-operate, when he is asked 'are your arms in the same position?', if the fall-away is due to weakness he will correct it, but not if it is due to sensory loss.

iv   When the limb is paralysed what is its response to painful stimulation? Is the response purposeful, does the patient reach out to the painful focus with his unaffected hand (localise to pain), is there reflex withdrawal from pain or a completely abnormal decerebrate response in which the patient extends the limb to pain?

v   When there is no movement from painful stimulation is this due to sensory loss?

vi   Is the muscle tone normal, increased or decreased?

Vital functions

Following immediate care to obtain a clear airway, careful positioning of the patient, general appraisal and neurological assessment, a record of temperature, pulse, respiration and blood pressure will be made and charted. It is important that these records are taken on admission, as they provide a baseline for comparison when future variations occur; subsequently these recordings and neurological assessment will be performed frequently, as often as half-hourly if the patient is unconscious or his condition is deteriorating. Frequent regular observation of vital functions over a period of time, will demonstrate the bodily reaction to the insult which has caused unconsciousness, indicate recovery and be an early pointer to the onset of complications. The patient's temperature will be recorded in the axilla or rectum, NEVER by placing a thermometer in the mouth. Mild pyrexia may be due to many causes, such as respiratory and urinary infections, blood in the cerebrospinal fluid or deep vein thrombosis. Hyperpyrexia and hypopyrexia are sometimes due to hypothalamic disturbance though the latter may be caused by prolonged exposure to cold; urgent measures will be necessary to correct extremes of temperature (see p. 88). According to the patient's condition and the cause of unconsciousness there may be abnormality in the rate and character of the pulse; it may be very slow in association with raised intracranial pressure or a Stokes–Adams attack, increased when there is infection, or rapid and thready in the presence of haemorrhage. The rate and character of the unconscious patient's respirations are extremely significant and the rate should be recorded carefully for a full minute; many variations occur (see p. 121). Blood pressure recordings range from normal to extreme hypertension or hypotension; the blood pressure rises with rising intracranial pressure.

Routine admission forms will be completed and a continuing record of neurological assessment and vital functions will be maintained; a history of epilepsy or an observed epileptiform attack will necessitate the commencement of a 'fit' chart, recording each attack in detail (see Chapter 19).

Consent for operation and investigations, and a telephone number for contacting the next-of-kin, will be obtained before the relatives leave.

There are other factors related to the cause of unconsciousness which must be discussed.

1 When coma is thought to be due to diabetes mellitus or uraemia, the urine should be tested as soon as possible.

2 When subarachnoid haemorrhage and meningitis are suspected, a lumbar puncture will be performed for diagnostic and therapeutic purposes.

3 Wounds may need surgical debridement.

4 Other injuries may need urgent treatment and a replacement blood transfusion may be necessary.

5 When coma is thought to be due to an overdose of drugs there are some additional nursing responsibilities and considerations (see Chapter 27). The incidence of acute poisoning has increased and the possibility of 'overdose' is always considered when the cause of unconsciousness is not immediately obvious. The patient, admitted with head injury, fits or 'stroke', may be addicted to alcohol or drugs, or suffer from depression or other mental disorder.

Deterioration in conscious level

The most serious complication is a deterioration of the conscious· level due to rising intracranial pressure.

Signs of raised intracranial pressure

Raised supratentorial pressure
When a supratentorial lesion expands very rapidly the signs of deteriorating conscious level from full

consciousness to deep coma also develop very rapidly; on the other hand a large slow-growing supratentorial lesion which may have existed for several years, although it causes marked brain displacement, will not have any effect on consciousness for a very long time. Increased supratentorial pressure causes tentorial (uncal) herniation (see p. 37) leading to:

1 Increasing drowsiness
2 Deterioration in mental state and verbal response
3 Inequality of the pupils with sluggish reaction to light
4 Development of a hemiparesis which may rapidly become a hemiplegia
5 Incontinence in a previously continent patient
6 The patient may complain of headache and this may be associated with nausea and vomiting
7 The pulse rate becomes slower
8 The blood pressure rises

The onset of increasing restlessness and irritability, possibly due to a headache, is an indication that the patient's condition is deteriorating; these signs are especially significant if accompanied by increasing drowsiness, localising signs of pupillary changes and limb weakness.

When the patient is already unconscious the following signs indicate rising intracranial pressure.

i Spontaneous movements will cease
ii One pupil will become more sluggish in its reaction to light, enlarges and then becomes non-reactive to light
iii The response of the limbs to painful stimulation changes, where there had been withdrawal there may be no response or extension, or the patient may spontaneously extend his limbs
iv The rate, depth and rhythm of respirations change when the vital centres of the medulla are compressed

Unless this state can be rapidly reversed the patient will die; even with treatment there may be irreversible brain damage.

Raised infratentorial pressure
(medullary 'coning' – see p. 38)

1 Intense headache and vomiting
2 Increasing drowsiness

3   The pupils become small, then pinpoint and unreactive to light

4   The patient may become mute and akinetic

5   Hemiparesis or quadriparesis develop which rapidly result in total paralysis

6   The respirations become irregular with periods of apnoea, they may be Cheyne–Stokes or suddenly cease

7   The blood pressure can suddenly change and become very high or very low

Any of these signs (which must be reported immediately to the doctor) suggest impending medullary 'coning' which may lead to respiratory arrest; the nurse must stay with the patient and be ready to give emergency resuscitation.

Methods of reducing raised intracranial pressure

The cerebral oedema which accompanies injury, intracranial space-occupying lesions, generalised cerebral inflammation or anoxia is sometimes extensive, and treatment must be given to relieve pressure on the brain and tide the patient over until such time as surgical or medical treatment have been effective or natural recovery has occurred. Intracranial pressure can be monitored by the use of a transducer inserted beneath the dura mater or into a lateral ventricle.

Mannitol

Mannitol is a hygroscopic intravenous solution which rapidly reduces intracranial oedema by drawing excess fluid from the brain into the blood vessels by osmosis and is used when oedema is life-threatening; it is supplied as 500 ml of a 20% solution and should be stored in a warm draught-free place to prevent crystallisation. Care must be taken during administration to prevent rapid cooling and crystal formation, by excluding draughts from open windows and doors and from electric fans; should accidental crystallisation occur the infusion must be discontinued immediately and the doctor informed. The mannitol infusion is administered rapidly, taking 10–20 minutes; this results in an increase in blood volume and a temporary rise in the blood pressure level. The kidneys rapidly excrete this excess fluid from the bloodstream resulting in a marked diuresis and lowering of blood pressure. The patient is usually incontinent of a vast amount of urine and for this reason some authorities recommend catheterisation for accu-

rate measurement of urinary output. If the patient is not catheterised it is essential that the nurse observes carefully for a good diuresis; urine should be passed within about half an hour of the commencement of the infusion by which time the patient's neurological condition should also be showing some improvement. If diuresis is delayed it may be due to urinary retention and this will make the patient restless. On the other hand restlessness may mean that the patient, being more aware, is controlling the urge to pass urine and needs to be offered a urinal or bedpan and told to pass urine. The improvement brought about by mannitol is short-lasting and needs to be reinforced by a substance which has a longer-lasting effect upon cerebral oedema.

The use of a mechanical ventilator

Poor oxygenation of the brain increases intracranial pressure. The use of a mechanical ventilator is necessary when the patient's respirations are inadequate or the exchange of oxygen and carbon dioxide in the lungs is unsatisfactory. A build-up of carbon dioxide in the blood causes dilatation of the cerebral blood vessels; this in turn increases the total bulk of the brain and leads to an increase in intracranial pressure causing a worsening of any pre-existing condition. The brain must have oxygen; brain cells can die from lack of oxygen long before the patient shows any sign of peripheral cyanosis. Oxygen is given through the ventilator, the amount being determined by regular estimation of blood gases.

Ventilation is necessary for several days. Frequent injections of tubocurarine are given to paralyse the respiratory muscles and overcome resistance from the patient's spontaneous attempts to breathe.

Dexamethasone

Dexamethasone is a steroid used to relieve intracranial oedema; its effect is more gradual and longer-lasting than that of mannitol. Initially it is given intravenously and continued intramuscularly or orally depending on the patient's condition. A high dosage is given for about a week or until the patient's neurological condition begins to settle down; then it is gradually reduced over several days to avoid a serious fall in blood pressure or deterioration in conscious level, before being finally discontinued.

External ventricular drainage
See Chapter 4.

Lumbar puncture
A lumbar puncture (see p. 32) is only permitted in the presence of raised intracranial pressure when there is known to be free communication between the ventricular system and the spinal theca, for example following subarachnoid haemorrhage and in meningitis. The history, signs and symptoms of these disorders are usually conclusive. In any condition when a suspected obstructive lesion is the cause of raised intracranial pressure the removal of cerebrospinal fluid from the lumbar theca is an extremely dangerous procedure, as fluid from the high pressure zone in the skull will attempt to flow to the low pressure zone in the spinal theca forcing the cerebellar tonsils through the foramen magnum. 'Coning' in this instance, may be immediate, but can occur up to 24 hours after lumbar puncture.

Maintenance of a clear airway

The unconscious patient must never be allowed to lie on his back as he is likely to asphyxiate; alternate semiprone and lateral positions (see Fig. 3.6) are favoured as they are the most natural positions for maintaining a clear airway and they provide the best postural drainage for the posterior basal region of each lung, the area most likely to become consolidated. Most unconscious patients are nursed with their head slightly higher than their feet as this helps to reduce intracranial pressure; seldom is the patient nursed with his head down, even for postural drainage of the lungs; the position of the patient and the tilt of the bed is in accordance with medical instructions.

The patient's position should be changed at least 2-hourly, day and night in order to:

1   Prevent chest complications by
    (a) postural drainage
    (b) allowing each side of the chest to expand fully, free from the compression of body weight and bedding
    (c) stimulating the cough reflex
2   Prevent pressure sores and give an opportunity for frequent skin inspection
3   Provide an opportunity for passive movements to be given to all the patient's limbs to prevent contractures

These occasions provide an additional opportunity for observations, inspection, communication with the patient and neurological assessment.

Immediately it is noticed that the patient has signs of a moist chest, has been incontinent or the undersheet is rucked he must receive further attention even though he has been attended to only minutes before.

Respiratory complications (bronchopneumonia)

Drowsy, ill, elderly and unconscious patients are particularly susceptible to infection of the respiratory tract because they lie in bed inert, lose their cough reflex, may have difficulty swallowing (dysphagia) and therefore inhale their own secretions; habitual smokers are at greater risk. The risk of respiratory complications is significantly reduced if these patients are well nursed, their position is changed regularly, excess secretions are removed by correct suction technique and attention is paid to oral hygiene; early signs of infection should receive immediate attention. Bronchopneumonia is an especially serious complication for an unconscious patient, as it increases cerebral anoxia and brain oedema, causing further deterioration in conscious level; it may be suspected if there is an increase in the pulse and respiratory rates, pyrexia and moist sounding respirations.

Any one of these signs should alert the nurse to the possibility of respiratory infection and the doctor should be informed immediately so that percussion, auscultation and chest X-ray may be performed, and a sputum specimen collected to determine the infecting organism and sensitivity to antibiotics.

Nursing care for respiratory complications

Prevention of respiratory complications is always of first consideration, but infection may occur despite every precaution; the patient's survival is then even more dependent on the skill and co-operation of nurses and physiotherapists in the treatment regime; the ratio of physiotherapists to patients is often impossibly low and nurses must be able to practise effective 'clapping', shaking and suction. Though antibiotics are effective against organisms, unless the patient is vigorously roused and insistently urged to co-operate in regular deep breathing exercises and coughing, he may drown in his own purulent secretions. There must never be any hesitation about using oral and tracheal suction just because the patient will be aware of the unpleasantness of the procedure, but every care must be taken to explain to the patient how vital it is because he is unable to clear his lungs himself. Ideally a physiotherapist will visit the patient three times daily to assist in chest care by 'clapping', shaking and suction; these procedures should not be performed immediately after an intragastric feed as this may induce vomiting.

'Clapping'   The physiotherapy procedure 'clapping' is a method of loosening sputum within the lungs by externally 'beating' the chest wall; it is performed by using cupped hands alternately in a gentle, relaxed, rhythmic manner. 'Clapping' is performed over the whole chest wall, starting at the base and working towards the bronchi and is following by shaking the chest to dislodge sputum and stimulate coughing.

Methods of improving air entry   The simplest method of improving air entry is to insert an artificial airway into the mouth which also allows easier passage of suction catheters. Endotracheal intubation, bronchoscopy or tracheostomy may be necessary if a severe respiratory infection develops, when there is imminent or sudden respiratory failure or when obstruction is due to inhalation of a foreign body. Though tracheostomy is not usually an emergency measure, the nurse should know when to summon medical aid, the emergency call system, and where the equipment for this procedure is kept.

Oxygen and humidity   A great many patients admitted to hospital unconscious, are middle-aged or elderly and already suffer from hypertension, heart and lung disease. The long term effects of smoking can be an additional hazard especially if the patient needs an anaesthetic, and may very rapidly lead to bronchopneumonia. In spite of the nurses' efforts to maintain a clear airway, breathing may still be laboured and though there are no signs of cyanosis, administration of oxygen may be prescribed to protect viable brain tissue; this will be given by a ventimask through which the patient will receive the correct percentage of oxygen, air and moisture. A mask is not without its problems; it is particularly difficult to keep in position when the patient is semiprone, the mask and

elastic can ride up into the patient's eyes or cause pressure marks on his face, the semiconscious and confused patient may repeatedly take the mask off and, not understanding the danger, the confused patient may light a cigarette while the oxygen is flowing; **cigarettes and matches should be taken from all confused patients**, and other patients should be persuaded not to smoke in the ward. The use of a mechanical ventilator may be considered if oxygen therapy is needed over a long period; a child may be nursed in an oxygen tent.

Respiratory obstruction and failure

Every nurse should know the factors which can lead to respiratory obstruction and failure and how to prevent them; she should also know how very simple it is for breathing to be obstructed when the tongue of the unconscious patient falls into the back of the throat, how to prevent inhalation of vomitus, how important it is to prevent respiratory infection, recognise the situation which requires prompt attention and be able to perform suction competently.

Respiratory obstruction

Signs
1   Respirations are noisy (stertorous).
2   Extremities are cyanosed (seen most clearly in the nail beds, tongue and inside of the lips).
3   Chest and diaphragmatic movements are laboured; the patient's lower ribs and sternum are drawn in on inspiration.
4   The accessory muscles of respiration are being used; the nostrils are splayed at each attempted inspiration and the sternomastoid muscles are prominent.
5   It is difficult to squeeze the patient's chest when attempting artificial respiration and impossible to use a mechanical ventilator.

Maintenance of a clear airway is always of prime importance and every member of the nursing staff should be aware at all times of the possibility of respiratory distress. Nurses must always be alert for any sound indicative of respiratory embarrassment. No matter what other task may be on hand, **if any patient in the ward is heard to be breathing noisily the nurse must investigate the cause immediately**. Should she find that a patient's airway is obstructed, she must send for medical aid and, in the meantime, do everything possible to relieve the obstruction. She must:

i Position the patient well over on his side.
ii Ensure the tongue has not fallen into the back of the throat.
iii Insert an artificial airway into the mouth.
iv Remove secretions, sputum or vomitus by suction.
v Pull the angle of the jaw forward to prevent the tongue falling back.
vi Clap and shake the chest wall to loosen plugs of sputum.

When these measures fail to relieve obstruction, the doctor will pass an endotracheal tube and the equipment for this procedure should be immediately available. When the doctor arrives, the nurse having screened the bed, pulled it out from the wall and removed the bedhead, will help to position the patient on his back with a pillow under his shoulders and his neck slightly extended over the end of the bed. She will have suction apparatus ready and a mechanical ventilator at hand.

Respiratory failure
Respiratory failure is caused by unrelieved respiratory obstruction, disturbance of the respiratory centre in the medulla oblongata or paralysis of the muscles of respiration.

Signs
1 Respirations quietly fade out.
2 Chest movement is poor or absent.
3 The patient becomes rapidly cyanosed.
4 The chest wall compresses easily when artificial respiration is given.

All nurses should know which patients might develop respiratory failure and should record the neurological assessment and vital functions at frequent intervals, noticing the character of respirations and counting their rate for a full minute; periods of apnoea and Cheyne–Stokes respirations indicate impending respiratory failure. These patients should be kept under constant surveillance; experienced nurses are tuned-in to every sound in the ward and will immediately notice the silence of failing respirations.

When a nurse discovers a patient has failing respirations or has stopped breathing she must immediately give artificial respiration and send for medical help; she may have to send a patient to enlist help if no other member of staff is present. As soon as the doctor arrives the patient will be intubated and attached to a mechanical ventilator.

Care of the patient using a ventilator
The principles of care for a patient using a ventilator remain the same although the type of machine will vary from hospital to hospital. A nurse must be in attendance at all times in case there is mechanical failure or other emergency: she should know the basic principles of how the machine works and how to operate it manually in the event of a power failure. The following half-hourly observations and records must be made.

1 Chest movement
The nurse should watch the chest wall and if it is not rising and falling in time with the ventilator's action she should check the machine for leaks and observe whether the patient is trying to breathe spontaneously. The doctor must be notified if the nurse has not been able to establish respirations satisfactorily or if the patient continues to fight the respirator. He may be given a trial period without it, or if it is still considered necessary to use the ventilator to reduce raised intracranial pressure the patient will be given a muscle paralysing agent, e.g. tubocurarine, to allow the ventilator to take over.

2 Colour of extremities
Oxygen is given through the machine according to the estimations of blood gases

3 Vital functions

4 Total volume of air given at each inspiration

5 Volume of expired air

6 Positive and negative pressures of the machine
A rising pressure indicates obstruction which may be anywhere along the pipeline from the machine to the patient's lungs and the nurse must:
(a) Check whether the tubing is kinked
(b) Empty water which collects in the loops of tubing
(c) Use suction to remove sputum from the trachea
(d) Note whether the patient is attempting to breathe spontaneously

(e) Notify medical staff immediately if positive pressure continues to rise

A falling positive pressure is due to leakage of air from the tubing; the nurse must check all tubing and connections and listen for air leaks, especially around the cuff of the endotracheal or tracheostomy tube.

7 Check the mechanical humidifier

Normally the air drawn into the lungs is moistened and warmed as it passes through the nose; if the patient has an endotracheal or tracheostomy tube the air is dry unless a humidifier is used. This is filled with sterile distilled water heated to a temperature of 40°C which allows for a drop to body temperature by the time the air reaches the patient. It is necessary to regularly check the temperature and water level in the humidifier.

8 Administer and record prescribed drugs at the appointed time.

9 Give chest physiotherapy and suction hourly, more often if obvious infection is present. The nurse must ensure that the stopper on the connection to the endotracheal tube is firmly replaced on each occasion.

10 Make a frequent and accurate neurological assessment. When muscle relaxant drugs are being administered, the only guide to change in the patient's neurological condition is the size and reaction of the pupils (tubocurarine does not affect pupil reaction) and changes in the intracranial pressure, and the pulse and blood pressure.

General nursing care must be maintained and it must be remembered that the patient can hear conversation. He must be turned hourly or 2-hourly for chest and pressure area care and receive regular eye and oral toilet. An intravenous infusion will be maintained and an accurate up-to-the-minute record kept of fluids given and urine excreted. Passive movements should be given to all joints (whenever there is a spare moment) at least three or four times daily.

Tracheostomy

Skilful nursing of unconscious patients will usually avoid the need for tracheostomy, but occasionally it will be of real benefit and will be performed

without delay to avoid irreparable brain damage from anoxia.

Indications for tracheostomy:

1 Laryngeal obstruction due to
(a) Oedema – overvigorous introduction of suction catheters can be a contributory cause
(b) Severe respiratory infection
(c) The presence of a foreign body and associated oedema
2 Laryngeal trauma
3 Thoracic injuries
4 Facio–maxillary injuries, especially if the patient is unconscious or unco-operative
5 When mechanical ventilation is necessary for longer than 48 hours to prevent the prolonged use of an endotracheal tube and the formation of ulcers and sores in the mouth and throat

Care of the patient who has a tracheostomy

Respiratory distress, even of mild degree, is terrifying for the conscious patient and no-one can be sure how the struggle to breathe affects an unconscious patient. Tracheostomy is usually performed under local anaesthesia, and even though the patient is unconscious he must be given explanation and reassurance. This will also be necessary whenever the tracheostomy receives attention as it must be a nightmare suddenly to be stimulated by a nurse or physiotherapist inducing a fit of painful coughing as she introduces a suction catheter into the tracheostomy tube.

A cuffed tracheostomy tube which prevents inhalation of· saliva and vomitus is used for an unconscious patient or one who cannot swallow. The incision will be protected by a gauze dressing. The nurse receiving a patient from the operating theatre must have with her a pair of sterile tracheal dilators and a spare tracheostomy tube of the same size and type as the patient's. These will remain beside the patient at all times as he may in his confusion or restlessness remove his tube or it may become blocked and need to be changed hurriedly. A trained nurse must supervise the care of the tracheostomy and must comply with the instructions given to her by the surgeon or anaesthetist in charge of the patient, relating to humidification, deflation of the cuff and changing the tracheostomy tube.

On return from the operating theatre the patient may be nursed in the lateral or supine position, but the semiprone position should never be used as he may lie on his tracheostomy tube and suffocate. Humidification is necessary for the first few days otherwise the inhaled air is cold, dry and dust-laden and will encourage the formation of plugs of sputum which can cause pulmonary collapse, anoxia and possible death. There are many mechanical humidifiers, some more effective than others. In the absence of a humidifier or to compensate for any deficiency the nurse may be instructed to instil 1–2 ml normal saline into the tracheostomy tube at hourly intervals to loosen the sputum. Unless the patient coughs immediately a few moments should be allowed for the sputum to soften before suction is used. The patient should be warned that this procedure may make him cough, but if coughing is not spontaneous it should be encouraged. The bloodstained dressing will be changed as necessary using a sterile dressing and a non-touch technique. Blood oozing should only be slight and once it has ceased, twice-daily dressings are usually adequate. The tracheostomy cuff must remain correctly inflated (Fig. 3.9). Underinflation will allow secretions to trickle into the lungs; overinflation causes pressure necrosis of the trachea. The cuff will be periodically deflated according to the doctor's or anaesthetist's instructions. To reinflate the cuff, the nurse occludes the tube with a gloved finger while instilling air into the cuff. At the point when the patient gasps for breath the exact pressure has been achieved, for the patient can no longer breathe around the tube. If the patient is using a ventilator a gurgling sound will be heard at each inspiration when the cuff is underinflated.

A strict regime of chest care is essential during the days immediately following tracheostomy. Half-hourly or hourly suction will be necessary at first to remove bloodstained secretions and sputum. Sterile catheters and a non-touch technique are always necessary when suction is used. The chest requires clapping and shaking hourly to loosen the secretions and the patient's position must be changed 2-hourly to prevent collections of sputum gathering in the lungs causing pneumonia. The patient with a tracheostomy should be encouraged to breathe deeply, cough and expectorate. A sputum specimen will be required for culture and sensitivity to antibiotics, and further specimens are needed twice weekly.

As the patient's general and respiratory condition improves removal of the tracheostomy tube will be considered. The first step is to replace the cuffed tube with an uncuffed tube to accustom the patient to swallowing his saliva; after a few days when the patient is swallowing satisfactorily, preparations can be made to remove the tube. It is then spigotted for increasing periods to make certain that the patient can manage without it before it is finally removed and the stoma is allowed to heal.

The principles of tracheostomy care also apply for the period when a patient has an endotracheal tube *in situ*.

General hygiene and care of the skin

Every time the nurse approaches the patient, even though he seems to be unconscious, she should try to rouse him and explain exactly what she is going

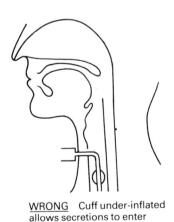

WRONG Cuff under-inflated allows secretions to enter trachea

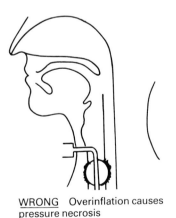

WRONG Overinflation causes pressure necrosis

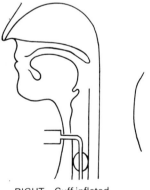

RIGHT Cuff inflated just sufficient to prevent secretions from entering lungs

Fig. 3.9 Tracheostomy cuff.

to do. The daily persistent repetition of instructions by different voices with the stimulus of physical care may finally rouse the patient to make a supreme effort to raise himself one rung up the ladder towards full consciousness; this may be noticed in such a simple action as holding up his own arm while it is washed.

A daily blanket or hoist bath should be given to keep the patient's skin clean, cool, dry and supple; great care should be taken to prevent soap getting into the patient's eyes; eye care (see p. 57) is a separate procedure. The bath ensures that every area receives careful inspection and any crack or sore is immediately noticed, reported, and treated. Nurses should carefully wash and dry any area where two folds of skin meet, between the buttocks and groins and beneath the breasts. On every occasion when the patient is incontinent he should be washed thoroughly, especially in the crevices, using warm soapy water and a soft disposable 'flannel', rinsed, then pat-dried carefully. Talcum powder should be used sparingly and then only when the skin has been thoroughly dried. Plastic drawsheets and the plastic edges of incontinence sheets should not come into contact with the patient's skin or they will stick and may peel away the skin; drawsheets should not be used at all with restless patients. The patient's fingernails should be trimmed regularly and hair (hair brushes and combs) washed at least once weekly.

The type and texture of the patient's skin dictates the use of ointments and oils; a healthy skin requires no application; a dry skin benefits from frequent application of arachis oil. Should soreness occur between the buttocks (likely when a patient has loose stools), zinc and castor oil cream or petroleum jelly protects the area. Spots which occur when a patient's skin is greasy, may be dabbed with methylated spirit. Silicone barrier creams which are thought to protect the skin from the effects of incontinence may have a drying effect upon the skin, are difficult to apply without friction and are best avoided.

The care of every patient's skin should be decided by the nurse-in-charge (in consultation with the doctor if there are any problems); she should make certain that all her staff (day and night) are informed of the proposed plan of treatment, to which they should adhere unless the nurse-in-charge gives further instructions. Exact specifications should be given for each patient including applications, turning regime and position, special beds, dressings, etc.

Pressure and friction sores

Sores are caused by many factors, and can be avoided if the patient's position is changed at least 2-hourly, attention is paid to cleanliness and the condition of the skin, the bed linen changed as soon as it becomes wet or soiled with faeces, and sheepskins, foam channels, ripple and water beds used from the beginning for patients whose skin is vulnerable. Skin surfaces must be separated to prevent sweat rash, friction or pressure. The following patients are at risk (Fig. 3.10), i.e. those who are:

Fig. 3.10   The Norton Scale. Devised by Doreen Norton, the scale helps to anticipate which patients are most likely to develop pressure sores. Simply choose one description from each column which nearest resembles the patient's condition. *Lower the score, higher the risk*. Score of below 14 will require a detailed *Nursing Care Plan* to prevent wounds forming.

Physical Condition	Mental Condition	Activity	Mobility	Incontinent
Good 4	Alert 4	Ambulant 4	Full 4	Not 4
Fair 3	Apathetic 3	Walk/Help 3	Slightly Limited 3	Occasionally 3
Poor 2	Confused 2	Chairbound 2	Very Limited 2	Usually/Urine 2
Very Bad 1	Stuporous 1	Bedfast 1	Immobile 1	Doubly 1

1 Unconscious
2 Incontinent and immobile
3 Restless
4 Thin or elderly with prominent bones and poor circulation
5 Fair-skinned
6 Heavy, paralysed and with sensory impairment
7 Ill-nourished and dehydrated
8 Suffering from barbiturate overdosage
9 Whose limbs are encased in plaster of Paris

Friction sores which result from friction against bedding or the patient's own body start superficially, but can result in ulcerated sores if not treated immediately. When the patient's position is changed he should be lifted clear of the bed to prevent scuffing the skin. The undersheet should always be taut, free of rucks, and items of equipment should be well clear of the patient, for example catheter and tubing.

The very restless hyperactive patient, who may be aggressive and resent interference and for whom sedation would be unwise, may completely rub an area of skin off his body in a very short time; a full-length sheepskin which is soft and less easily rucked is essential. The patient's skin should be given frequent liberal applications of soothing zinc and castor oil cream. Occasionally when this state persists for several days, it is necessary to protect the sore areas with soft pads firmly held in position.

Sores which can develop in a few days may take weeks or even months to heal; however arduous the task of prevention, the nurse has a duty to protect the patient from unnecessary pain and keep his stay in hospital as short as possible.

Suggested principles of treatment for pressure sores

1 Prompt action to relieve pressure from a sore area immediately it is discovered.

2 Even the smallest area of broken skin should be covered with a sterile dressing; a semipermeable adhesive film or non-adherent gauze dressing secured by a non-allergenic adhesive will prevent further damage to the tissue and skin reaction and excoriation. The dressing should be inspected daily.

3 Infected pressure sores require cleansing with a desloughing agent such as Eusol and paraffin, or aserbine lotion or cream; usually daily dressings are all that are necessary. It should be protected from contamination by urine and faeces; soiled dressings must be changed promptly. A penile sheath attached to a urinary drainage bag will keep the male patient dry; catheterisation may be necessary.

4 There must be insistence that there is no deviation from the line of treatment prescribed; good communication between all staff will ensure continuity. It is necessary to persist with a treatment for at least a week even though at first the sore seems to get worse as the slough softens prior to separation as all infected matter must be removed before the sore is allowed to heal by granulation; if there is any depth to the sore, ribbon gauze packing will prevent a sore from healing on the surface too soon leaving an infected sinus.

Positioning of limbs and physiotherapy

The aim of the nursing staff and all members of the rehabilitation team is to help the patient to become fully independent without complications, but the necessary simple care to prevent contractures may be overlooked when everyone is so busy fighting for the patient's life or the prognosis is thought to be so hopeless that the idea of physiotherapy is overlooked; when the patient's condition begins to improve contractures may already be quite severe and very difficult to remedy. There is considerable ignorance among nurses as to the ease and speed with which contractures can develop; early neglect may considerably lengthen the patient's stay in hospital, cause him pain, prevent him resuming his previous occupational and social activities, make him depressed and, when he returns home, place an additional burden on his family.

The care of every unconscious and paralysed patient must include careful support of every joint when a limb is moved and regular passive movements must be given from the first day of the illness. At rest limbs should be supported on pillows to prevent unnecessary strain on joints and muscles, and should be only slightly flexed at elbow or knee, never curled up tightly; fingers should be outstretched, wrists slightly extended to prevent wrist drop and ankles supported to prevent internal rotation. Sand-bags may be useful to keep the ankle flexed at an angle of 90° to prevent foot drop; care should be taken to avoid pressure on calf muscles which can cause deep vein thrombosis.

Exercises are designed to keep joints mobile and prevent shortening of muscles by fibrosis; the reflex tone and power of the strong flexor muscles in a weak or paralysed limb cause contractures unless the muscles are regularly and gently stretched; for the patient who has little or no voluntary movement, passive exercises will help to re-establish the pattern of normal movement.

A trained physiotherapist will give a full range of passive movements twice each day; the nursing staff should observe the physiotherapist's technique and give the patient skilled physiotherapy whenever she changes his position. The limb should always be supported and knees and elbows never over-extended.

Every approach to the bedside of an unconscious or drowsy patient is an opportunity to rouse and recall him to awareness, effort and normality. Hearing his own name and attempting to attend to instructions is a mental exercise of almost as much importance as the physical treatment; if he is handled without first being roused he will probably resist treatment and may develop severe muscle spasms.

In certain brain stem disorders when severe flexor spasms are uncontrollable it is very difficult, if not impossible, even to straighten the limb. Spasms may be spontaneous or triggered by the merest touch; the only physiotherapy possible in these circumstances may be slowly and gently to ease the limb straight and hold it still until the spasm wears off; the application of ice-packs to the contracted muscles will help to relax the spasm. One might suppose that splints would be useful in maintaining the position of weak and paralysed limbs affected by spasms, but splints become wet and soiled, cause friction to the skin, increase spasm in a spastic limb and deter nurses from giving passive movements and are therefore best avoided.

Active movements should be encouraged as soon as power, however slight, returns to a limb. During the recovery period the drowsy, apathetic patient, whose brain is still suffering from the insults of trauma, anoxia, infection, ischaemia or other factors, will need constant firm encouragement to move the limbs he has begun to accept as useless, disowns (see p. 117) or is reluctant to move because of pain. If the patient fails to understand or remember continual explanations for the necessity of treatment or acts childishly or abusively, it may be the effect of brain damage (see p. 62).

The occupational therapist should be informed of the patient's admission, know his medical history and background, follow his progress and assess his disability even though at this stage she may be unable to participate in his treatment.

Contractures and deformities

Physiotherapy for these conditions is very painful, mainly ineffective and surgical transplantation of tendons does little to improve the deformity. What a tragedy that a man who recovers from a cerebrovascular accident, is unnecessarily deformed and disabled.

Oral hygiene

Regular 3-hourly oral hygiene is an extremely important feature in the care of an unconscious patient. Extra care will be necessary when an artificial airway is in use as secretions adhering to the inside of the airway can obstruct the patient's breathing; the airway may need changing hourly or more often. The following factors contribute to a dry and dirty mouth.

1   Dehydration
2   Mouth breathing. The insertion of an artificial airway to some extent prevents the mouth itself becoming dry, as the air passes through the airway and does not come into contact with the mucous membrane of the mouth.
3   Feeding by intragastric tube or intravenous infusion will not stimulate the salivary glands.
4   Absence of mouth and tongue movements.
5   Collection of muco–purulent secretions in the mouth.

Method   It is not uncommon for a junior nurse to be given the responsibility for the patient's oral hygiene without adequate instruction and reassurance; she thinks if she removes an airway the patient will stop breathing, does not understand how to gain access to the mouth through tightly clenched teeth and in many instances gives up after cleaning only the outer surface of the teeth. The result of this inadequate oral hygiene is very unpleasant to see – the hard and soft palate, inner surface of the teeth and gums encrusted with blood-stained secretions and the tongue a dirty yellow–brown colour.

The nurse, explaining the procedure to the

patient, puts on protective polythene gloves, gives suction to remove excess secretions and removes the airway if one is being used. She opens the patient's mouth carefully and inspects it using a torch. Difficulty is sometimes experienced when the jaws are tightly clenched, but the use of a mouth gag can usually be avoided; gags cause trauma to soft mucous membranes when the patient is edentulous, teeth may be loosened or dislodged and the protective covering from the gag may be pulled off and inhaled. The patient may open his mouth if a soft toothbrush is used (do not use toothpaste); if this fails a satisfactory manoeuvre is to insert one forefinger inside the cheek and prise open the jaws by pushing the finger in behind the last molars; this opens the teeth sufficiently for the nurse to insert her mouth-cleansing forceps which are covered with a firmly secured gauze swab soaked with sodium bicarbonate solution. Every part of the mouth, particularly the hard and soft palates, should be cleaned carefully. Liquid paraffin is a suitable lubricant for a dry tongue and a thin application of petroleum jelly to the lips on each occasion will prevent soreness, cracking and bleeding.

Parotitis
Infection of the parotid gland may be caused by lack of oral hygiene and should respond to regular thorough mouth toilet and a suitable antibiotic; should an abscess develop it will require drainage.

Stomatitis
Stomatitis (inflammation of the mucous membrane of the mouth) will respond to regular and frequent cleansing with a mild antiseptic mouthwash. Only in the very severe form when ulceration occurs is antibiotic therapy indicated. Thrush infection requires specific treatment.

Eye care

The eyelids and blink reflex prevent foreign matter entering the eye and spread moistening and cleansing tears over its whole surface; the highly sensitive corneal reflex responds instantly when any particle, however small, enters the eye, by stimulating the increased production of tears and rapid blinking to wash the eye clean. This is the body's natural protection of a very delicate organ. The protection will be lost if:

1   the eyes do not or cannot close and the blink reflex is absent
(a) in the unconscious patient
(b) when there is facial weakness
(c) if there is severe proptosis; or
2   the corneal reflex is absent.

The nurse has extra responsibilities while nature's normal protective mechanisms are disturbed. A patient who has lost his corneal reflex and is drowsy, confused or has a poor memory will need frequent clear explanations and reminders to prevent him rubbing or touching his insensitive eye.

The utmost care must be taken in positioning an unconscious patient so that his eyes are never buried in the pillow; this is more likely in the semi-prone position, but a small firm pad which lifts the side of the head, will keep the eye clear of the bed. Electric fans, used to reduce pyrexia, should never be directed on to the patient's face. Frequent neurological assessment includes examination of the pupils and nurses must always make sure that the patient's eyes are left completely closed. Even so, the eyes may slowly reopen; to protect them in this circumstance, the outer part of the upper eyelids should be taped obliquely on to the cheeks (Fig. 3.11) using a transparent non-allergenic tape; the reason for this procedure should be explained to the relatives. It should be possible to inspect the pupil safely without removing the tape if it is correctly applied.

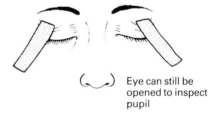

Eye can still be opened to inspect pupil

Fig. 3.11 Taping eyelids closed using non-allergenic tape. Note that the eye can still be opened to inspect the pupil.

Eye care should be performed 4-hourly unless the eyes are 'sticky', then it would be unreasonable to wait for the routine hours of treatment. Should there be the least hint of infection (reddening of the conjuctiva or purulent discharge) the doctor should be informed, a swab taken for culture and eye care including irrigation should be given more often; local antibiotic treatment will be prescribed. Correct procedure is essential to avoid inflammation of the cornea (keratitis), corneal abrasion and ulceration and great care should be taken to prevent cross-infection to the other eye or to other patients.

Bathing the eyelids

Though the patient may appear unresponsive the nurse must always explain what she intends to do as eyelids are very sensitive; she should have adequate light, position the patient's head comfortably and protect the bedclothes with a polythene sheet and paper towel, then wash and dry her hands. Care should be taken to prevent any contact with the eyeball while the eyelids are being bathed. Each eye should be swabbed separately and each dampened swab used only once, swabbing from the inner canthus outwards, to remove matter and secretions without risking the spread of infection; swabbing should be continued until the lid margins and eyelashes are clean. After inspecting the eye, the eyelids should be gently dried with medical wipes.

Irrigation of the eye

Irrigation is necessary if the cornea is insensitive, the eyelids are swollen and bruised, there are excessive serous secretions, or there is infection. The patient should be prepared; the nurse, having washed and dried her hands, should swab the eyelids, check the temperature of the lotion is 36°C before filling the undine and then, standing a little behind the patient with the receiver held against the patient's face, she should gently draw down the lower eyelid to expose the lower conjunctival sac; with the undine held about 5 cm from the eye the fluid is directed into the sac at the inner canthus; the upper eyelid is then gently drawn against the orbital ridge to expose the upper conjunctival sac which can then be irrigated. Finally the eyelids are dried carefully with medical wipes. Before leaving the patient the nurse should make sure that the patient's eyes are closed, his airway is clear and position is satisfactory; however busy the nurse, this routine must always follow any treatment.

Tarsorrhaphy

Tarsorrhaphy is a surgical procedure designed to protect the eye when facial weakness and loss of corneal reflex are likely to persist for a long period. A sliver of skin is removed, laterally or in the midline, from the inside of the upper and lower eyelids before they are sutured together; to prevent the suture cutting into the eyelids it is passed through

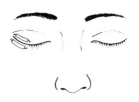

Fig. 3.12 Tarsorraphy.

two small pieces of tubing before it is tied (Fig. 3.12). Antibiotic eye ointment will be applied along the lid margins to prevent or counteract infection. No-one should attempt to open the eye. After 10–14 days when the eyelids have united the suture is removed.

Corneal abrasion and keratitis

Every attempt must be made to protect the cornea from injury and infection, as either may lead to corneal ulceration, scarring and blindness. Keratitis is treated with antibiotic eye drops or ointment containing hydrocortisone, given promptly and regularly as prescribed for a lengthy period; the decision to stop treatment must rest with the doctor as, though the eye may appear to have recovered, insufficient treatment may lead to recurrence of the infection.

Feeding the unconscious patient

The nutritional and fluid requirements of an unconscious patient will depend upon the following factors:

1   The cause of unconsciousness
2   The patient's age, weight and previous health
3   The blood electrolyte balance

The aims of nutrition are:

i   To provide an adequate fluid intake of at least 2½ litres per day (previous medical history must be taken into account as, for example, patients with heart and renal disease may be unable to tolerate this amount)
ii   To provide protein, carbohydrate and fat in the correct proportions
iii   To maintain a balance of essential chemicals
iv   To provide essential vitamins and minerals
v   To provide roughage

It must be remembered that the unconscious patient's metabolism is inevitably abnormal whatever the cause of unconsciousness.

It is usual for the medical officer to discuss each patient's metabolic requirements with the nursing staff and dietitian; the senior nurse-in-charge should supervise the patient's fluid intake and output throughout the 24-hour period; a daily adjustment of nutritional requirements may be necessary depending upon the patient's condition, his need for intravenous fluids, whether he is absorbing intragastric feeds and the results of blood electrolyte estimation. The electrolyte balance is a very critical factor in the recovery of consciousness; severe imbalance may delay recovery of consciousness or in the critically ill, tip the balance unfavourably between life and death. At first, a daily electrolyte estimation may be essential and the nutritional requirements will be prescribed accordingly. As the patient's condition improves, less frequent estimations are needed and the dietary requirements will stabilise.

Some patients with cerebrovascular disease or raised blood urea need a low protein diet; a patient with diabetes mellitus needs care in balancing his carbohydrate intake, and for the patient who is unconscious for a long period, iron and vitamin additives, and increased protein may be recommended. Though much is known about the part metabolism plays during and following illness and injury, considerable research is still necessary.

An intravenous infusion is essential if the patient is very ill or deeply unconscious and unable to absorb intragastric fluids; intravenous fluids will be prescribed according to the patient's electrolyte levels and blood volume; should intravenous fluids be needed for a considerable time, a soluble protein or fat solution will be necessary to avoid muscle wasting. As soon as possible after admission an intragastric tube will be passed to empty the stomach, prevent vomiting and reduce the risk of inhalation of vomitus; sometimes a large amount of fluid is withdrawn (½ litre or more) which may contain undigested food, large quantities of beer or altered blood. Coffee ground aspirate is not always such an alarming sign as when associated with gastric ulcer; it occurs when the body has sustained a severe shock or when blood has been swallowed, but it also occurs in the terminal stages of deep coma. Intragastric feeding would be inadvisable in this instance and the stomach should be aspirated hourly until the aspirate becomes negligible. Small quantities of water (30 ml) should then be given hourly via the intragastric tube; if this is absorbed the quantity will be gradually increased until the patient is absorbing 120 ml of water; then fluid can be given 3-hourly. It is advisable to build up the quantity and strength of the feed mixture gradually before introducing the standard intragastric feeding regime. The stomach should always be aspirated before intragastric feeds are given to check that the previous feed has been absorbed. Intravenous fluids should be carefully calculated during this transitional period to avoid over-hydration.

A suggested method of introducing intragastric feeding is shown in Table 3.3. Continuous intragastric 'drip' feeding is an alternative method used when a patient has problems of absorption.

Administration of intragastric feeds
First the nurse should check the treatment card regarding type and quantity of feed to be given. A paper towel will be placed over the patient's chest to protect the bedclothes. When the oesophageal tube is to be passed nasally the nostrils should be gently cleaned; **the nasal route is contraindicated if the patient has sustained head injuries or has a CSF rhinorrhoea** (see p. 93), when the oral route should be used; in this instance the tube should be removed after each feed. The oesophageal tube, lubricated with liquid paraffin, should be inserted into the nostril and passed gently along the floor of the nose; if the patient's neck is then flexed slightly the tube is more likely to enter the oesophagus than the

Table 3.3 A suggested method of introducing intragastric feeding

Feed 1	120 ml of water
Feed 2	120 ml of half-strength milk followed by 60 ml of water to wash the tube through
Feed 3	240 ml of half-strength milk followed by 60 ml water to wash the tube through

If at any stage of this introductory scheme a feed is not fully absorbed it will be necessary to remain at that quantity and strength for longer.

Feed 4	240 ml milk followed by 60 ml water.

If feed 4 is satisfactorily absorbed, standard intragastric feeds may be commenced using Clinifeed to supply an intake of 8000 kJ (2000 calories) each 24-hour period; a liquidised normal diet is preferred in some centres.

trachea; occasional inspection to ensure that the tube is not coiling in the mouth is advisable. When it is thought that sufficient length of tube has been passed to have reached the stomach, the position is checked by listening with a stethoscope over the hypogastric region as a small amount of air is injected down the tube; a loud rumbling will be heard at the time the air is injected. It is important that the sound exactly synchronises with the injection of air and is not the result of normal bowel sounds; if the patient belches the tube is in the oesophagus. Should there be any doubt about the position of the tube it must be withdrawn and repassed. Two nurses (one of them fully qualified) should always check the position of the tube before each feed is given. A syringe is used to aspirate gastric secretions, which are measured and recorded, and then to give the feed. The syringe funnel should be held 15–30 cm above stomach level; all prescribed medicines should be given first and then the feed, at the correct temperature, is poured in slowly and continuously; the tube is cleared with 60 ml water, spigotted and taped to the side of the face. Before leaving the patient, the nurse should check that his bed-linen is dry, position satisfactory and airway clear; she should record the aspirate, medicines, feed, and urinary output on the appropriate charts.

The oesophageal tube can remain in position in the nostril for one week; there may be indication for the tube to be changed more frequently, but unnecessary changing should be avoided to lessen the chance of damaging the nasal mucosa, throat or oesophagus. Fluids should be introduced by mouth as soon as the patient regains consciousness and is able to swallow satisfactorily.

Dehydration

Inadequate fluid intake will cause dehydration. The signs and symptoms are:

1   Deterioration in the patient's level of consciousness
2   Dirty crusted mouth with dry tongue and cracked lips
3   Inelasticity of the skin
4   Low urinary output

The maintenance of an adequate fluid intake is the responsibility of the nursing staff and at times it is an onerous task. Except where there is malabsorption or loss of fluid, the unconscious patient, on a settled regime of intragastric feeds, is less likely to become dehydrated than the confused, drowsy, dysphasic or nauseated patient who refuses to drink. In this instance, time and patience are required to persuade the patient to take small amounts of fluid at very frequent intervals during the daytime and when awake at night. The patient may drink if he is offered a fluid he likes, out of a drinking vessel he recognises and finds acceptable; enquiries may need to be made about the patient's preferences. Despite every effort the fluid intake may still be inadequate; intragastric fluids will be necessary or the doctor will set up an intravenous infusion. Febrile patients need a greater fluid intake and an anti-emetic is required if the patient is nauseated or vomiting. When hypertonic solutions are given to relieve cerebral oedema, normal fluid intake must be maintained to prevent bodily dehydration.

Overhydration

Although dehydration is more common, overhydration can occur, especially when an intravenous infusion is supplementing intragastric feeding; overhydration overloads the heart and leads to venous congestion in the lungs. Respiratory distress develops when the lungs become waterlogged (pulmonary oedema) producing copious amounts of frothy sputum. Exchange of gases will be impaired, intracranial pressure will rise and the level of consciousness will deteriorate. It is most important that all intravenous, intragastric and oral fluids are recorded at the time the fluid is given and the daily totals reviewed.

Loss of weight

Maintenance of nutritional requirements is important during any period of unconsciousness, however brief. Irritability, restlessness, general metabolic disturbance and prolonged unconsciousness, lead to weight loss despite a high calorie intake; anabolic steroids are sometimes given.

Care of the bladder

The bladder of an unconscious patient usually empties spontaneously. Each time the patient is incontinent the genital area must be thoroughly washed with plenty of warm, soapy water to protect the skin and prevent urinary tract infection. The nurse should:

i record the incontinence on the fluid balance chart;

ii estimate by a recognised system of signs the amount of urine passed; this is inevitably an inexact method, as a small quantity of urine dampens sheets out of proportion to the amount and there may have been an accumulation of dribbling incontinence since the last change of linen;

iii notice any offensive odour suggesting infection;

iv inspect the abdomen for distension;

v percuss and palpate to assess bladder distension and if the nurse is in any doubt about her findings she should consult the doctor;

vi observe for haematuria.

Urinary retention and infection

An unconscious patient cannot complain of abdominal discomfort or difficulty in passing urine; restlessness is a very important sign suggesting a full bladder. Though the patient has been incontinent of urine, inspection of the abdomen may reveal gross distension; slight manual pressure just above the symphysis pubis may be sufficient to empty the bladder. Manual pressure should never be used when an elderly man has retention of urine as he may have an enlarged prostate gland; a doctor should be consulted without delay. Constipation and impaction of faeces sometimes causes retention of urine which will resolve if suppositories or an enema are given.

Catheterisation
Catheterisation should only be performed when there is a specific reason as it leads to urinary infection. Indications for catheterisation are:

1 Retention of urine
2 The need for accurate measurement of urine, e.g. following administration of mannitol or in renal failure
3 To obtain regular specimens of urine for testing, e.g. in diabetes mellitus
4 To prevent pressure sores becoming saturated with urine
5 When 24–hourly collections of urine are required for laboratory analysis

A catheter should never be left in for longer than necessary. A patient who has had retention of urine must be carefully observed for recurrence.

Care of the bowels

Normal evacuation of the bowel is always the aim, but the ideal is rarely achieved as the unconscious patient is immobile and some fluid diets do not provide normal bulk. Constipation is common and aggravates raised intracranial pressure, but it is a mistake to administer aperients in haste and two to three days may safely elapse before a mild aperient is given. A mild liquid aperient may be given by intragastric tube each day, but should this be ineffective, suppositories will be necessary. When a regular bowel habit has been re-established medications can be gradually withdrawn, but it is important that the bowels are evacuated at least once every three days.

Diarrhoea may be caused by:

1 Impacted faeces – this is frequently misunderstood by the nursing staff
2 An idiosyncratic reaction to a particular food substance
3 Infection or other medical reason

Menstruation and pregnancy

Menstrual periods must be recorded; there may be amenorrhoea during a serious illness. Tampons should be used during menstruation as they are more hygienic; a record should be made when tampons are inserted to ensure they are changed at least twice daily and are not forgotten. Dysmenorrhoea may be a reason for restlessness and should be treated with a mild analgesic. There is the possibility of pregnancy in a woman of child-bearing age; relatives will often furnish information or the pregnancy may be obvious. Vaginal bleeding must be reported, as a serious illness may cause abortion. A patient in the later stages of pregnancy will be seen by an obstetrician who will advise management; an emergency Caesarian section will be performed if the mother's condition deteriorates; the infant will be transferred to a premature baby unit.

Management of a confused patient

When a patient is regaining consciousness, he rarely wakes up saying drowsily 'hello' and 'where am I?' as is often shown on stage and screen. A senior nurse, understanding the process of recovery, its possible slowness, periods of confusion and non-recognition, can prepare relatives in advance and save them much distress. There is usually a period of clouding of consciousness with confusion and disorientation which, with restlessness, noisiness, irritability, inability to communicate, aggression and unco-operative behaviour, sometimes presents extreme difficulty for the nursing staff and great anxiety for the relatives. It is no wonder that a patient appears disturbed when he first regains consciousness in hospital; he may have no recollection of events leading to his admission and on 'coming to' finds his head is throbbing, there is a tube in his nose, tracheostomy tube in his throat, his hands are restrained, bedsides obscure his view and he is in an unfamiliar noisy environment. Unless restraint is removed and clear explanation given, he will fight continously to escape; explanations may need to be repeated many times before the details sink in and the nurse must be watchful to prevent the patient injuring himself.

No two patients are the same. Confusion and disturbed behaviour may last for minutes or extend to hours, days or months. The length of time and degree of confusion depend upon many factors, the cause of unconsciousness, the part of the brain involved, the patient's age and difficulty in communication if he is deaf or dysphasic. Visual perception may be poor and distortion of ordinary objects, especially at night, increase frightening illusions.

The nurse must always be quiet and gentle in manner, but should convey confident firmness, obviously expecting the patient to follow her suggestions and requests; it may be necessary to try many different tactics to pacify and settle the patient. Sensible management of his physical needs will often avoid the necessity for treatment with drugs. Is the patient cool and comfortable, is he hungry or thirsty, has he a full bladder or does he want to have his bowels open? The use of normal lavatory facilities instead of unfamiliar urinal or bedpan, is often helpful. Bedsides are sometimes a useful deterrent to the patient getting out of bed, but may on the other hand, increase the height from which the patient can fall. Restraint is often resented and sometimes unnecessary, though shortage of staff makes 'freedom under supervision' a difficult principle for a patient who wanders round the ward, interfering with other patients' belongings and endangering himself as he stumbles along unsteadily. The very disturbed patient who constantly strips to the skin, climbs out of bed and is abusive and noisy, is upsetting to other patients and visitors; their co-operation and tolerance can often be gained by explanation that this is a transitory stage of recovery. Nurses should be on their guard for unpredictable behaviour and avoid personal injuries; it is unwise to argue with an aggressive, deluded or hallucinated patient.

Rehabilitation (see also pages 181 and 362)

The nurse's responsibility in the care of the patient with brain damage is particularly concerned with the protection of viable brain tissue and avoidance of complications. Rehabilitation begins when the patient is first taken ill and continues until he is as well as possible and has readjusted satisfactorily to daily living. The nurse should always engender in her patient, his relatives and all members of the hospital staff involved in his care, an attitude of optimism and she should keep an open mind to the future outlook for even the most seriously ill. There must be no relaxation or lack of perseverance in day to day rehabilitation in spite of difficulties and slowness of recovery which can take several years.

The conscious patient must always be encouraged to be as independent as possible in spite of

confusion, dysphasia, slowing of cerebration and other factors. The semiconscious or drowsy patient needs frequent intermittent stimulation or he will not bother to rouse himself. A baby who is merely fed and changed regularly will not progress as quickly as one whose mother also talks, smiles and bestows other encouragement upon him; the same applies to nursing a patient recovering consciousness.

During the recovery period there may be times when, owing to intellectual deficit and personality change, the patient may not be very likeable, he may resist rehabilitation and be facetious or abusive; patience and understanding are very necessary. The patient often shows a great lack of self-confidence and if a spirit of optimism reaches him he will be encouraged to pursue his rehabilitation to the limit; all his achievements, however small, should be noticed and praised. He should not be pushed too hard or too fast at any point during the recovery period because repeated failure will cause loss of confidence and will retard progress; on the other hand, harm can be done by recommending too much rest.

Physical and mental abilities do not always improve simultaneously; impairment of memory, powers of concentration, apathy and fatiguability further influence progress. It is wise not to ask too frequently whether the patient has a headache, pain or feels sick as the patient is often very suggestible regarding symptoms, and hypochondriasis will be encouraged. Whether in hospital, convalescent home, rehabilitation centre or in the patient's own home, rehabilitation programmes need to be thoughtfully planned to suit each individual; personality and home background are various. Relatives are usually over-protective until they understand that this is not in the patient's best interests, and must be guided in the part they have to play.

The nurse should adapt her manner of conversation to suit each particular patient taking into account the degree of recovery, understanding, personality, interests and intellect; this is something learned only by experience and sensitivity to each situation. Habit retraining may be necessary, but derogatory and humiliating phrases like 'potty training' should never be used; a disturbed patient may regress to incontinence solely because he does not know where the lavatory is or is unable to express his needs. At all stages of illness the nurse must avoid 'talking down' to the patient or falling in with his confused ideas; she should gently and repeatedly attempt to put the patient in touch with his surroundings and with events, and gradually guide and upgrade his conversation and behaviour to as near normal as possible. Her example in these matters will probably be copied by other patients in the ward, relatives and friends, as well as staff of all grades; in this way she can contribute very greatly to the patient's rehabilitation. The patient's mental state and powers of communication should be explained to his relatives and friends.

Each individual will react differently to neurological deficit and the problems facing him; it is not always appreciated that a school child, student or person in a responsible position, trying to maintain his previous standard of performance with a brain made inefficient as the result of a disorder of the nervous system, may develop a severe neurosis. The patient should not return to work too soon nor to a job which is beyond his capabilities; sometimes a change of career or occupation is necessary and assessment by a clinical psychologist may be helpful.

Personality changes are common; patients may be antisocial, unpredictable and extremely difficult to live with. This may lead to the saddest situation of all – causing distress to families and children, wrecking marriages and breaking up previously happy homes. Relatives will need the help of the social services, their general practitioner, local counselling services and/or their local church community.

Nurse–relative support

A good relationship should be established between the nurse and the patient's relatives from their first meeting; this will help the nurse to obtain an accurate history of the illness and will be a good basis for future co-operation and understanding during the course of the patient's illness and rehabilitation. Sometimes relatives have to bear with the considerable inconvenience of the patient being moved to a special unit far away for investigation and treatment.

It should be remembered that before the patient entered hospital the relatives have suffered varying periods of stress perhaps of many months' duration; both patient and relatives may have become anxious about the symptoms, their cause and significance. The patient may have become irritable, depressed, unable to pursue his normal activities, strange in behaviour, asocial and, as personality changes and confusion have developed, there may have been an unwillingness to seek medical advice. The nurse will sometimes meet criticism of the patient's previous treatment and it is as well for her to realise and to mention how common is the symptom of headache and how rare are some of the disorders encountered in neurological and neurosurgical units. When the patient has collapsed suddenly, the relatives will be in a state of intense shock. The nurse who appreciates this background of stress and distress when talking to relatives will not be irritated by lack of clarity in the history given, the relatives' inability to grasp explanations unless they are repeated many times over, and will understand the critical, almost aggressive response which is frequently met in these circumstances. Relatives are anxious, bewildered, agitated, overtired and may have many other worrying responsibilities.

Interviews (see p. 9)

The doctor will see the patient's relatives, but a quiet talk between the nurse and relatives is helpful as there are times when distressed relatives will talk more freely to a nurse. The interview should be uninterrupted, unhurried and informal; a friendly manner, a smile and an appearance of calm confidence and competence are reassuring. Relatives should be guided with suitably phrased questions; time taken in obtaining an accurate history is never wasted, dates and events should be written down. The nurse should enquire into the patient's social background as an early contact with the medical social worker may be helpful; the patient may have lost his job or had long periods off work owing to ill health. Is he receiving National Health benefit and when is his next certificate due?

Some relatives are pleased to know that there is a chapel in the hospital and that visiting ministers and representatives of different religious denominations and faiths can be called upon at any time.

Future outlook

The nurse-in-charge should know what the doctor has told relatives concerning the patient's illness and should impart this knowledge to all members of the nursing staff. Though it is necessary to show an attitude of confidence in investigation and diagnosis, and optimism regarding the success of operation or treatment, the nurse should be careful not to paint an over-optimistic picture, only to find it necessary to retract it shortly afterwards; relatives who have had their hopes falsely raised are more distressed than those who expect the worst. Though complete recovery is always the goal, there may be a residue of mental or physical handicap; there may be sudden death. Fluctuations in the patient's condition are likely to occur and if relatives are prepared they will be more resilient when facing a crisis. They should be introduced to the idea that when damage is sustained by the central nervous system, recovery is a very slow process, and may take several years.

Visiting

Normal hospital visiting times must be clearly specified for these are planned to fit in with the patient's nursing care, doctors' examinations, X-rays, investigations, physiotherapy and occupational therapy. On their first visit relatives should be accompanied to the patient's bedside and forewarned about the patient's appearance and any apparatus in use; when there has been a rearrangement of beds in the ward visitors should again be met and accompanied to the bedside to prevent the shock of finding an empty bed and wrongly fearing the worst.

Relatives will usually be pleased to adapt their visiting times if the patient's programme for the day is explained, but occasionally it should be possible to make exceptions and allow visiting out of hours. Even an interruption during a visit for the patient to receive nursing care is a good thing; if no nurse comes near the patient during visiting, the relatives may leave thinking and often saying, 'they don't seem to do much for him'. While the relatives are visiting they may be pleased to help in a practical way especially if the patient is unresponsive or unable to talk, by performing some simple task like feeding the patient, arranging his flowers or washing his hairbrush or comb. As visiting hours in many hospitals are flexible and spread over a long period of the day, relatives may need advice about the best times to visit; because the visiting times are long, relatives should not feel compelled to stay for the full time nor arrange for other visitors to fill up the time, for patients can be exhausted by a constant stream of visitors. The burden of daily visiting for the next-of-kin can sometimes be shared with other relatives and close friends. Short but frequent visits by family and close friends may help the confused patient to regain his orientation and put less strain on the relatives. The visits may be unsettling to the patient and make him restless, agitated and distressed, but in the long run may be beneficial in hastening his return to normality. The parents of sick children and relatives of the critically ill should be given the opportunity to visit at any time of day and may need accommodation in or near the hospital. Is there any point in visiting the unconscious patient or staying with the unconscious patient who is dying? The final decision must be made by the relatives who must decide whether they wish to stay near the patient or whether family commitments are the first priority.

Visiting ministers of all denominations and

faiths should feel welcome and in order to be at ease with the patient it may be necessary for them to know something of the patient's background, illness and future prospects. The nurse, by her attitude and general conversation when she introduces the minister, can sometimes help the patient to overcome embarrassment caused by his appearance (shaven head, facial weakness, etc.) and difficulty in conversing. Sometimes relatives need more help than the patient and it is a pity that hospital chaplains have so few opportunities to meet and talk to them. It is helpful if there is good liaison between chaplain, patient, relatives and the patient's local church community.

Telephone enquiries

There will be fewer telephone enquiries if relatives are seen regularly by the nurse-in-charge during visiting times. Only one member of the family should be in regular contact with the hospital and he should act as an 'information bureau' for the rest of the family. The nurse-in-charge should always be consulted about telephone enquiries as it is she who knows how up-to-date the relatives are with changes in the patient's condition and treatment and may wish to give them some particular information or ask a question. The official hospital bulletin, 'as well as can be expected', is a most unsatisfactory reply for relatives who cannot visit; a more personal touch should be added, for example 'his breathing is a little easier', 'he was able to take some lunch', 'he is absorbing his tube feeds today', or some other factual statement. This means a great deal to relatives; if information is given honestly stage by stage, most relatives will even accept deterioration in the patient's condition with greater equanimity.

Caution should be exercised if an enquiry is received from anyone other than the next-of-kin; no information should be given to employers or other parties involved in an accident, and enquiries from the press should be referred to the hospital administrator.

Consent for investigations, anaesthetic and operation

Explanation should be given by the doctor to the patient about the nature of investigations and operations and the patient should sign his consent. When a patient is unconscious, confused, dysphasic or paralysed he will be unable to sign his own consent and it will be necessary for the doctor to discuss the nature of proposed treatment with the patient's next-of-kin and gain their consent. Investigations and surgical treatment may be urgent and verbal consent may be obtained over the telephone to avoid delay, but a written consent should still be obtained at the earliest opportunity. A life-saving measure, e.g. the operation of burr hole for removal of extradural haematoma, may proceed without consent if no relative can be contacted.

Property

The task of caring for the patient's property can be a tedious one for nurse or ward hostess but they will be careful and conscientious on every occasion if they are aware of the expense, time wasted and trouble caused by a search for one lost article.

A patient entering hospital should be advised to ask their relatives to take home any valuable property (except wedding ring), excess cash and unnecessary clothing. Should the patient be unable to make decisions for himself or be unaccompanied, valuable property and cash should be listed and deposited with the hospital administrator for safe keeping; it is unwise to hand cash to the patient's relatives without his permission. Valuable property retained by the patient should be listed and the signatures of two witnesses obtained.

All clothing should be marked with the patient's name otherwise it will get lost. The clothing of incontinent patients can so easily reach the hospital laundry in error; pyjamas and nightgowns are expensive items on a family's limited budget, a point which nurses sometimes forget, used as they are to handling large quantities of hospital-supplied stock.

A careful list of all the patient's belongings including spectacles and dentures (specify top and/or bottom set) should be compiled when the patient is admitted to hospital; the list should be kept up to date. Care with this list and in marking things with the patient's name is important as the patient, admitted to hospital fully alert and responsible may become confused or lapse into coma. Confused patients do not necessarily keep their dentures in the obvious place and they can all too easily be thrown out with the rubbish or sent to the laundry. It is always necessary to mention to relatives that, though every care will be taken, the hospital does not accept liability for any loss that may occur.

Opportunities for discussion

Daily contact between relatives and nursing or medical staff, with good communication of information, prevents misunderstandings. First, there must be good communication between all members of the medical and nursing team. Results of any tests or investigations should be available as soon as possible and relatives informed in a simple way that a layman can understand. Every member of the nursing staff should be aware of the general situation so that they can talk intelligently to relatives should the occasion arise. The nurse should refer matters to a senior member of the nursing staff or the doctor in charge if confronted with questions which she feels unable to answer either through lack of knowledge or because the answer requires a special experience in its psychological approach. Any 'caginess' on the part of members of the staff is often misinterpreted by relatives as lack of competence – 'they don't seem to know what is the matter with him'; this may be true, but if the diagnosis is uncertain an honest, 'we don't know yet, but we are trying to find out' and discussion of further tests planned, will give the relatives greater confidence in the hospital staff.

Relatives must be regarded as part of the team who are interested in the patient's welfare; they are closely concerned, but usually lack understanding of the changes which occur as the result of an illness affecting the central nervous system; it is so much easier for them to understand a gastric ulcer or heart attack than incoherent speech, fits, confusion and unconsciousness. The nursing staff, by simple explanation and example, can show relatives how to approach someone who is dysphasic, whose appearance has been grossly altered by a 'stroke' or whose personality has changed.

Relatives learn from the nurse; can she learn anything from them? The nursing staff should always be receptive to suggestions, comment and even criticism. The patient can no longer speak and act for himself or fight for his rights, others must do it for him. Relatives are under stress, unfamiliar with hospital routine and may appear to speak out of turn, but the nurse should listen quietly, explain methods misunderstood and benefit by what she is told. It is most useful, for example, to learn the personal preferences of a dysphasic patient; it has been known for a patient to reply 'yes' meaning 'no' when asked if he took sugar in his tea. This may sound a trivial irrelevant detail, but might lead to a situation in which the fighting, distressed patient refuses oral fluids and has such a low fluid intake that intragastric feeding becomes necessary.

A critically ill unconscious patient will present a horrifying picture to the inexperienced; bandaged head, eyes taped closed, endotracheal tube attached to mechanical ventilator, oesophageal tube in the nose, intravenous infusion in the arm, the unnatural quiet of the ward only disturbed by the sounds of machinery, ventilator, suction apparatus, electric fans. How can the nursing staff help the relatives? Firstly by giving preparatory explanation in anticipation of the distress which will be experienced by relatives when they first see the patient; secondly by accompanying relatives to the bedside. When the relatives have been closely involved in discussion and the patient's treatment they will be less likely to harbour discontent, even if the illness has a fatal outcome for they feel that everything possible was done.

Death

In the past death was seldom sudden, but was more usually a gradual process whereby the major organs failed successively, culminating in cessation of respiration and heart beat. In the late 1950's came heart massage which brought a person 'back from death', and the widespread use of mechanical ventilators which kept 'alive' deeply comatose and unresponsive patients indefinitely. With this came the dilemma of when to switch off the ventilator, sometimes patients being kept alive for years without hope of recovery, the anguished relatives clinging on to the thought of 'while there's life there's hope'.

There has always been fear amongst the general population that they may be wrongly proclaimed dead and be buried alive; when organ transplants became commonplace these people feared that unscrupulous doctors might hasten death to acquire organs they needed. Amongst the medical profession there was also concern about their responsibility in diagnosing death and it was helpful once it was established that a situation of brain death could be defined, from which there was no chance of recovery. Laws have had to be passed which protect both the doctors and the patients, and strict guidelines laid down and criteria set for establishing brain death.

In neurosurgical wards young people with otherwise healthy bodies will die as the result of head injury, cerebral haemorrhage or other acute disorder of the central nervous system. Nurses in intensive care units are in close contact with the relatives of critically ill, brain-damaged patients being maintained by a mechanical ventilator, and will be sensitive to how the relatives feel about death and organ donation for transplant; the ward sister/charge nurse may be in the position to have preliminary discussion with the relatives and she will be aware of those who, because they cannot accept the prospect of death, would react unfavourably to the idea of organ donation. This information she will convey to the medical staff.

All treatment given to the patient is always solely aimed towards his survival, never because his organs might be taken for transplant.

Diagnosis of brain death

Two doctors, jointly or independently, are required to diagnose brain death, one must be a consultant or experienced doctor in charge of the patient and the second a consultant or doctor who is not of the same clinical team; neither doctor should be connected with the transplant team. Death can only be confirmed when the criteria for brain death have been met on each of two separate occasions.

The doctors must first satisfy themselves that the conditions for consideration of the diagnosis of brain death have been met.

1 The patient is deeply comatose.
  (a) There should be no suspicion that this state is due to depressant drugs. Some drugs have a prolonged or cumulative action particularly some used as anticonvulsants or used to assist synchronisation with mechanical ventilators. Adequate intervals are allowed for the effects of drugs to be excluded.
  (b) Primary hypothermia must be excluded –

hypothermia will also prolong the effects of drugs.
  (c) Metabolic and endocrine disturbances which can be responsible for or can contribute to coma should be excluded. Tests for serum electrolytes, acid-base balance, and blood glucose will be performed.

2 The patient is being maintained on a ventilator because spontaneous respiration had previously become inadequate or had ceased altogether. Neuromuscular blocking agents, hypnotics and narcotics must be excluded as the cause of respiratory failure.

3 There should be no doubt that the patient's condition is due to irremediable structural brain damage. The diagnosis of a disorder which can lead to brain death must be fully established. This diagnosis may be straightforward when the patient has suffered a severe head injury, but may be considerably delayed when an indefinite period of cerebral anoxia has been caused by cardiac arrest or other circulatory disturbance.

Diagnostic tests for the confirmation of brain death

All brain-stem reflexes are absent.

1 The pupils do not react to light.

2 The corneal reflex is absent.

3 The vestibulo–ocular reflexes are absent. They are tested by the slow injection of 20 ml of ice–cold water into each external auditory meatus in turn; the reflexes are absent when no eye movements occur.

4 No motor responses within the cranial nerve distribution can be elicited by adequate stimulation.

5 The gag reflex is absent and there is no reflex response to a suction catheter passed into the bronchus.

6 No respiratory movements occur when the patient is disconnected from the mechanical ventilator for long enough to ensure that the arterial carbon dioxide tension rises above the threshold

for stimulation of respiration. The administration of 5% CO_2 in oxygen through the ventilator will bring the patient's blood CO_2 level to as near as possible the threshold for stimulation of respiration before the ventilator is disconnected. This is determined by measuring the blood gases. Hypoxia during the period of apnoea when the machine is disconnected is prevented by giving oxygen at 6 litres/minute through a catheter into the trachea; this will safeguard the patient should he not be at the point of brain death, and his organs should they be for transplant.

The possibility of a rapidly fatal outcome within 24–48 hours should always be borne in mind and every opportunity must be taken to communicate with the relatives and establish a relationship; when there has been sudden collapse or accident the relatives will be bewildered and repeatedly go over the scene and conversation when they last saw the patient fit and well; sometimes there will be unresolved conflicts and difficulty in accepting the possibility that they may never be able to talk to the patient again. They will be in a state of extreme shock and must be given time to talk and ask questions. It is inevitable that the nurses and doctors will be saddened at the death of the patient and feel a sense of failure, especially if he is young and they have fought hard to save his life; these feelings will be intensified if the staff have come to know the patient's family well. When a good rapport has had time to be established between the nurses, doctors and the relatives there will be mutual understanding, often unexpressed, when the patient dies. The knowledge that organs are to be donated will help the relatives and the nurses to feel that at least something good has come from a tragic event.

4

Congenital Cranial Disorders

(This chapter should be read in conjunction with Chapter 11 as the two subjects closely overlap.)

Nervous tissue begins to develop very early in embryonic life; a length of ectoderm on the back of the embryo sinks inwards to become completely enfolded within the embryo (Fig. 4.1a), sealing off at each end into a closed tube (the neural tube) (Fig. 4.1b). At one end cells rapidly multiply to become the forebrain, midbrain and hindbrain (Fig. 4.1c), while in the remainder of the tube the cells form the spinal cord. The cerebral hemispheres develop from the forebrain, becoming the largest portion of the brain, while the hindbrain develops into the cerebellar hemispheres, and the midbrain into the brain stem which connects brain and spinal cord (Fig. 4.1d). The cavity formed initially as the neural tube persists in the centre of the brain as the ventricular system and in the centre of the spinal cord as the neural canal; the two cavities are continuous.

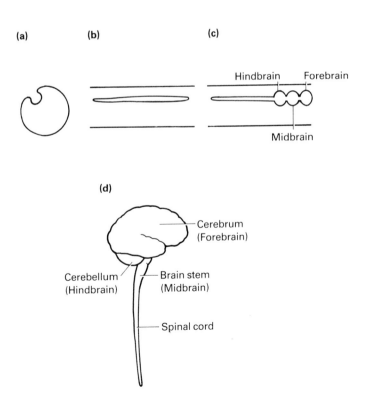

Fig. 4.1 Embryological development of brain and spinal cord. **(a)** Enfolding of ectoderm; **(b)** development of the neural tube; **(c)** formation of forebrain, midbrain and hindbrain; **(d)** developed brain and spinal cord.

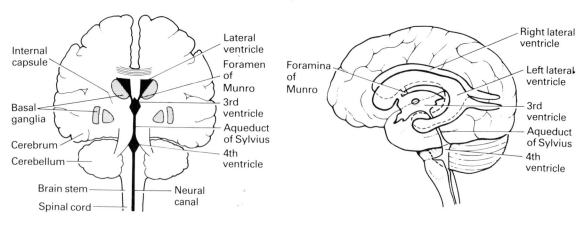

Fig. 4.2   The ventricular system.

The ventricular system

The ventricular system is shown in Fig. 4.2. There are two lateral ventricles, one in each cerebral hemisphere lying beneath the corpus callosum and immediately above the basal ganglia; they project into the frontal lobe (anterior horn), the occipital lobe (posterior horn) and laterally into the temporal lobe (inferior horn). Each lateral ventricle connects with the third ventricle through the foramina of Munro; the third ventricle lies in the mid-line beneath the lateral ventricles, at its anterior end is the optic chiasma and posteriorly is a recess for the pineal gland. The thalami (part of the basal ganglia) lie on either side of the third ventricle. From the third ventricle a very narrow tube, the aqueduct of Sylvius, passes downward through the midbrain to the fourth ventricle which lies between the cerebellum and the brain stem (pons varolii and medulla oblongata); the lower portion of the fourth ventricle is continuous with the neural canal of the spinal cord. There are three openings from the fourth ventricle into the subarachnoid cisterns at the base of the brain, in the mid-line posteriorly is the foramen of Magendie, and laterally the two foramina of Luschka.

The ventricles are lined with ependymal cells and in each ventricle, a collection of small blood vessels, the choroid plexus, is responsible for the production of cerebrospinal fluid (CSF); this cir-

culates from the lateral ventricles to the third, then fourth ventricle and out into the subarachnoid space surrounding the brain and spinal cord (Fig. 4.3). The CSF returns to the circulation when, by a simple process of osmosis, it passes from the subarachnoid space, through the arachnoid villi (small balloon-like projections) into the superior sagittal sinus (Fig. 4.4); this reabsorption is dependent upon the anatomical structures being normal and the CSF pressure being slightly higher than the venous pressure.

Faulty development in early embryological life may affect any system or part of the body, resulting in more than one congenital abnormality. In the brain the defects involve:

1   Faulty closure of the neural tube (encephalocele).
2   Failure of development of brain tissue (anencephaly and microencephaly).
3   Faulty communication within the ventricular system due to narrowing (stenosis) of the aqueduct of Sylvius or absence (atresia) of the foramina of Munro, Luschka or Magendie.
4   Abnormal enlargement of the cerebellum (Arnold Chiari malformation – see Fig. 4.10) when the elongated cerebellar tonsils descend through the foramen magnum obstructing the flow of CSF from the fourth ventricle.

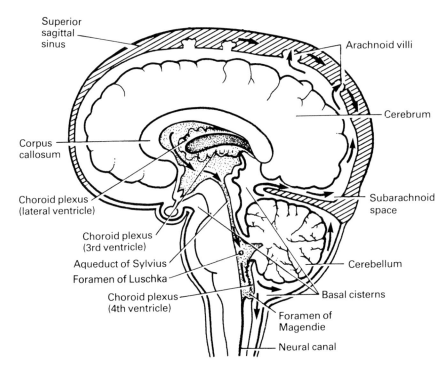

Superior sagittal sinus

Arachnoid villi

Cerebrum

Corpus callosum

Choroid plexus (lateral ventricle)

Choroid plexus (3rd ventricle)

Aqueduct of Sylvius

Foramen of Luschka

Choroid plexus (4th ventricle)

Subarachnoid space

Cerebellum

Basal cisterns

Foramen of Magendie

Neural canal

Fig. 4.3 Cerebrospinal (CSF) fluid pathways. CSF is produced in the ventricles and reabsorbed into the circulation in the superior sagittal sinus.

These abnormalities are often associated with spina bifida and myelo-meningocele and other congenital abnormalities in other parts of the body (see p. 188). With adequate antenatal care many of these abnormalities are detected before birth.

Hydrocephalus may occur as the result of injury at birth or infantile meningeal infection (see pp. 188 and 99) which cause adhesions in the subarachnoid space at the base of the brain preventing CSF from reaching the superior sagittal sinus to be reabsorbed; it may also be caused by rare intraventricular tumours which obstruct the ventricular system or cause excessive production of CSF (choroid plexus papilloma).

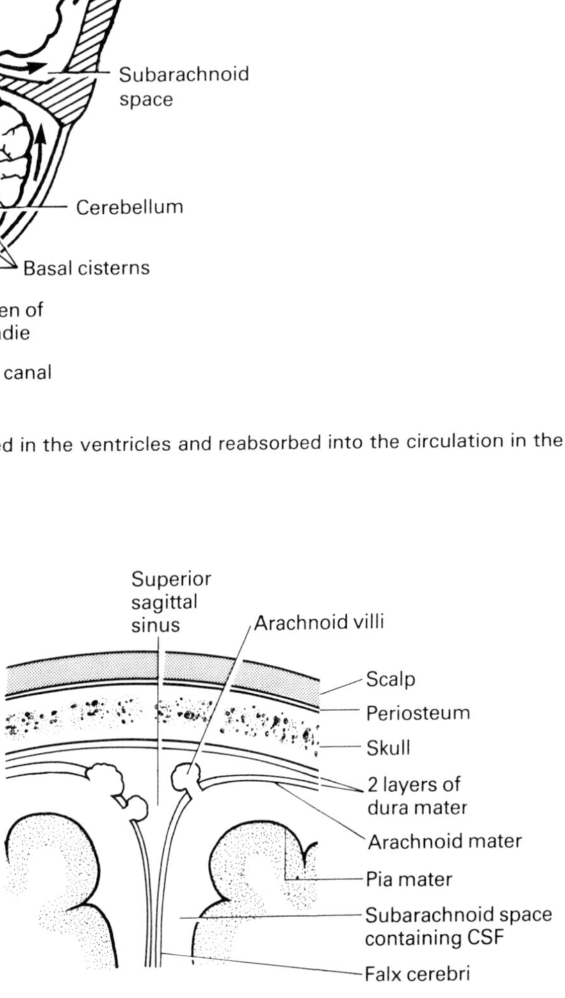

Hydrocephalus

Hydrocephalus, a condition recognised for centuries and described by lay persons as 'water on the brain', is caused by faulty development, ventri-

Superior sagittal sinus

Arachnoid villi

Scalp

Periosteum

Skull

2 layers of dura mater

Arachnoid mater

Pia mater

Subarachnoid space containing CSF

Falx cerebri

Fig. 4.4 CSF reabsorption from the subarachnoid space into the superior sagittal sinus.

cular obstruction, excessive secretion of CSF, inadequate reabsorption or a combination of these factors.

Infantile hydrocephalus

Hydrocephalus may be diagnosed before a baby is born when, on palpation, the head is felt to be abnormally large, a fact confirmed by abdominal scanning; the baby is delivered by Caesarean section if the head is exceptionally large.

At birth a baby's head is always inspected for abnormality and its size, shape, presence of naevi, facial or palatal abnormality are noted. The anterior and posterior fontanelles are palpated and should be soft and slightly depressed; the head circumference is measured and is normally about 37 cm in diameter though there is a limited variation according to birth weight and inherited characteristics. All babies should be seen by a paediatrician soon after birth. Those who have suffered foetal distress or whose birth has been complicated will be followed up by the paediatrician in the outpatients' department. Any baby whose head circumference is definitely larger than normal, all babies who have spina bifida abnormality and babies that suffered intracranial haemorrhage from premature or precipitate delivery will be kept under close observation for signs of hydrocephalus.

All babies, after discharge from the maternity unit, should be seen regularly at the Health Visitor's clinic where they are weighed and any feeding problems are discussed. Some normal babies suck poorly and are slow to feed for the first few days after birth, but should this persist for a longer period and the baby continue to be lethargic and fail to gain weight, hydrocephalus may be suspected; similarly it may be suspected when a baby is irritable, hungry and sucks eagerly but vomits immediately after feeds and fails to thrive. A baby with feeding problems will be seen by the doctor at the Health clinic who will refer him to a paediatrician for examination, and arrangements will be made for his admission to hospital for investigations; the parents will naturally be very anxious but should hydrocephalus be suspected they should never be given an over-optimistic outlook.

History and examination

A careful history of the mother's pregnancy and delivery, the baby's birth weight and progress, and details of the family history will be obtained from the baby's parents; the baby may already have been a patient in the neurosurgical unit for surgery for spina bifida.

A baby who has hydrocephalus has a characteristic appearance (Fig. 4.5); the head is large in proportion to the body and the forehead prominent causing the face to appear small. The skin of the skull and forehead is shiny and stretched and the veins easily seen. The eyes gradually take on the so-called 'setting sun' appearance, being displaced downwards, and the upper eyelids are retracted showing the whites of the eyes above the iris. A full general and neurological examination will be performed. When the doctor palpates the baby's head he will notice, even when the baby is held upright and is quiet, that the anterior fontanelle is enlarged, bulging and tense, that the sutures have parted and on percussion there is a fluid thrill because the enlarged ventricles are filled with fluid and the brain is like a thin rind (Fig. 4.6).

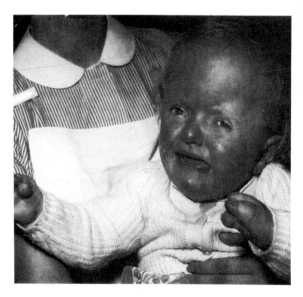

Fig. 4.5 Baby with hydrocephalus.

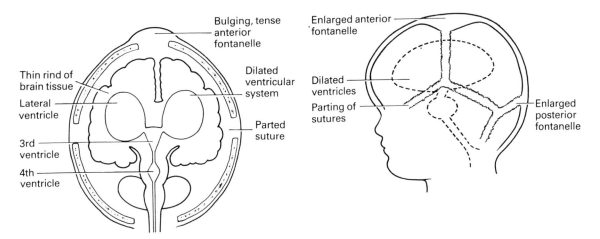

Fig. 4.6 (a) Coronal section showing infantile hydrocephalus. (b) Parting of sutures and dilatation of the ventricles in the presence of raised intracranial pressure in infants.

Nursing care
(see also Chapter 11)

When the baby is received into the ward the nurse should be sensitive to the mother's acute anxiety and aware that during this post-natal period she is likely to be emotional and may even be physiologically depressed. The baby's relationship with his mother must be maintained and the mother should be encouraged to help with all his care, staying in the hospital if her home commitments permit. The nurse needs information about the baby's feeding regime (brand of milk, quantity and frequency of feeds) and the difficulties that have been experienced.

The baby is given all routine care and love to keep him well nourished, contented and his skin in good condition. He may be fretful, slow taking feeds and vomit because he is suffering from raised intracranial pressure. Patience will be necessary to ensure that sufficient feed is taken; tube feeding will become necessary if the baby is too drowsy and lethargic to suck. He should be weighed regularly and feeds increased and adjusted as for the normal infant, but at a slower rate. The head circumference is measured at regular intervals and recorded on a chart, and the fontanelles are palpated when the infant is quiet and nursed sitting upright; any variation from the normal is reported. It must be remembered that dehydration caused by poor feeding or vomiting will cause slackening or depression of a fontanelle which would otherwise be tense and bulging due to raised intracranial pressure. The baby will be observed for fits. A routine record will be kept of temperature, pulse and respirations.

Investigations
(see Chapter 2)

Investigations will be performed to try to discover the cause of hydrocephalus and to determine which treatment will best alleviate the condition. The parents must be informed of any proposed tests and their consent obtained.

Echoencephalogram (ultrasound)

This investigation will demonstrate the midline and the size of the ventricles.

Computerised axial tomography (CAT scan)

A CAT scan may be performed to show the size of the ventricles.

Ventricular tap

This investigation excludes or proves subdural haematoma, measures and relieves raised intracranial pressure and obtains a specimen of CSF for analysis. The baby's scalp will be shaved and thoroughly cleaned; encrustations must be removed with either soap or similar substance. This very necessary preparation which may take up to 24 hours will lessen the serious risk of introducing infection into the ventricles. An irritable baby may need sedation. The nurse helping with the procedure is responsible for keeping the baby warm, steadying his head to prevent the needle moving and accidentally injuring the brain, and keeping the baby quiet so that accurate measurements of the intracranial pressure can be obtained. Using a short lumbar puncture needle, the doctor first taps the subdural space by inserting the needle through the anterior fontanelle; if there is no haematoma he will pass the needle into a lateral ventricle and gain an impression of the thinness of brain tissue. The pressure of CSF in the ventricles is recorded with a manometer while the baby is lying level and quiet. A specimen of CSF will be collected for laboratory analysis, there may be red cells present or the CSF may be yellow (xanthochromic) due to previous haemorrhage, there may be a raised protein indicating inflammation, old haemorrhage or blockage in the ventricular system or reduced sugar when pus cells are present. The CSF will be cultured for organisms.

Treatment

When the cerebrospinal fluid pathways have been radiologically visualised a course of treatment will be selected. A very small number of babies with mild hydrocephalus may benefit from administration of isosorbide which is though.   ılay some part in controlling the formation o.   · without seriously disturbing the blood chemi. ʼ y; in some instances babies can be tided over for a few weeks with isosorbide ultimately avoiding the necessity of a ventriculo-peritoneal shunt.

Most babies with hydrocephalus need one of the surgical manoeuvres designed to provide continuous drainage of excess CSF from the ventricular system to another cavity in the body, where it is absorbed and returned to the cardiovascular system. In the past CSF has been shunted from the ventricles to the pleural or peritoneal cavities or the right atrium of the heart; at present the ventriculo-peritoneal shunt is favoured using the valveless unishunt (Fig. 4.7), the pressure at which the CSF drains is determined by the bore of the tubing.

Earlier shunts incorporated a one-way valve which operated at a predetermined pressure and could be used to pump the CSF from the lateral ventricle. Several types of valve have been used:

(a) Spitz-Holter valve (Fig. 4.8)
(b) Till's valve
(c) Pudenz valve
(d) Hakim's valve

For many years ventriculo-atrial shunts were in vogue, but problems were experienced; the catheters could be blocked by a high CSF protein and infection could block and colonise the valve and lead to septicaemia. In recent years the trend has reversed in favour of a ventriculo-peritoneal shunt using the unishunt.

Choroid plexus coagulation, performed with the aid of a microscope, is a treatment for hydrocephalus caused by choroid plexus papilloma.

Ventriculo-peritoneal shunt

A doctor will fully explain the shunt procedure to the parents and obtain their consent. Though such

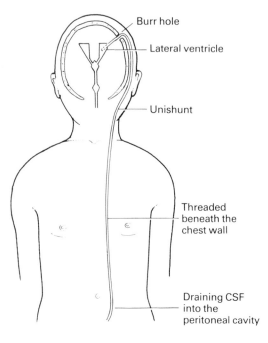

Fig. 4.7 Unishunt (ventriculo-peritoneal).

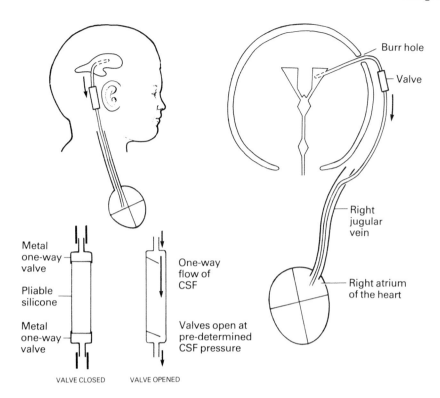

Fig. **4**.8 Spitz-Holter valve.

artificial devices are commonplace, there are still some parents who dislike the whole idea of the baby's head being shaved and of tubes being passed into his brain. A simple factual explanation and advice about after care will help to dispel their fears.

The unishunt is a piece of silicone tubing approximately 1 mm in diameter; its perforated end is inserted through a parietal burr hole into the lateral ventricle, the distal end of the tube is threaded under the scalp, neck and the chest wall through a series of small incisions to the abdomen where it terminates in the peritoneal cavity; when a valve is used this is sited beneath the scalp behind the ear. The position of the tube is checked by X-ray.

There are many people with ventriculo-atrial shunts and some surgeons still use this method incorporating the Spitz-Holter valve. This shunt is usually performed on the right side of the head (unless there is local skin infection) and the tube is passed into the right external jugular vein which gives a more direct route to the heart.

Postoperative care

On return to the ward the baby will be nursed flat and kept under close observation; pulse, respiration and temperature will be monitored and any abnormality reported. The baby needs 'mothering', to hear comforting sounds and feel physical contact. The wounds will be watched for haemorrhage, haematoma formation and the head wound for leakage of CSF. Extra fluids will be given to correct dehydration; if the anterior fontanelle appears sunken it may be necessary to lower the head of the bed for about 48 hours or until the fontanelle returns to normal; then the baby should gradually return to normal positions spending regular periods propped up in an adjustable infant chair. Once the shunt is working normally the baby will be more alert and feed more eagerly. A suitable feeding regime will be planned to meet individual requirements; frequent small feeds are best. In all the baby's care it is important to prevent cross-infection.

Complications following ventriculo-peritoneal shunt using the unishunt

1 The fine catheter is easily blocked by debris in the CSF or by stickiness of CSF if it becomes infected. Should symptoms of raised intracranial pressure occur, it suggests the shunt is not functioning.

2 There may be a CSF leak from the wound; barrier nursing then becomes essential to prevent the introduction of infection into the ventricles.

Complications following ventriculo-atrial shunt using a Spitz-Holter valve

1 The proximal or distal catheters can become blocked; the medical officer may request that the valve is pumped (by pressing with the thumb on the centre of the valve); the valve will feel hard and is resistant to pumping if the distal section of the tubing (from valve to heart) is blocked, or will not refill if the proximal tubing (from lateral ventricle to valve) is blocked. Should the valve not clear with pumping, the blocked section of tubing will need to be replaced.

2 A low grade infection may occur when organisms colonise the valve; this leads to persistent pyrexia, progressive anaemia, enlargement of the spleen and positive blood culture. Infection in the valve is unamenable to treatment with antibiotics and the valve will be removed. Antibiotics will, however, be given to treat septicaemia, and ventricular taps will be performed when necessary to reduce raised intracranial pressure. When infection has resolved a further ventriculo-atrial shunt will be performed using the opposite lateral ventricle; there is a limit to the number of times the ventriculo-atrial shunt can be renewed as the veins already used lose their patency; however, ventriculo-peritoneal shunt is still possible and is a procedure which needs fewer revision operations as the child grows; infective colonisation of the valve is less serious, but unfortunately the peritoneal end of the tubing blocks more easily.

3 A CSF leak (see 2 in previous list).

4 The valve occasionally ulcerates through the skin resulting in infection; to prevent this complica-

tion the baby should not lie on the valve.

5 A few youngsters, who have reached teenage years with satisfactory control of hydrocephalus by a ventriculo-atrial shunt, have developed narrowed ventricles which block the ventricular catheter (slit ventricle syndrome) and cause repeated episodes of raised intracranial pressure; treatment consists of inserting an anti-siphon device into the shunt system, or for the patient to have a subtemporal decompression on the side of the catheter which allows the lateral ventricle to expand slightly and avoid blockage.

Discharge from hospital

As the mother has participated in the baby's care during his stay in hospital she will not be afraid of handling him, but when the time comes to take her baby home she may be apprehensive of the full responsibility and especially worried about the shunt. She should be aware of the importance of the fontanelle tension and be given many opportunities to feel it for herself so that she knows when it is abnormal; she should know the symptoms of rising intracranial pressure (increased fontanelle tension, fretfulness, poor feeding and vomiting) and the importance of seeking skilled advice quickly; relief of hydrocephalus should always be undertaken as soon as possible to prevent permanent brain damage.

Apart from these observations the mother should be encouraged to treat her baby as though he were normal and try to put the valve 'in the back of her mind'. A neurological outpatient appointment will be made and the mother and baby should resume normal attendance at the Health Visitors's clinic where the baby's progress will be assessed and recorded. The mother should be warned that her baby's normal milestones are likely to be a little delayed.

Reasons for readmission to hospital

i Shunt failure with raised intracranial pressure.
ii Revision of the shunt; longer tubing will be necessary as the baby grows; this small opera-

tion usually takes place between the ages of 9 months and three years.

iii Other illnesses and treatment of other congenital conditions.

Prognosis

Without treatment, infants with hydrocephalus rarely live more than five years; occasionally the condition arrests spontaneously, but by then there is usually mental deficiency, epilepsy and blindness. Infants treated by the operative procedures previously mentioned have a variable prognosis; less than one-fifth are free from any kind of handicap, one-third have normal intelligence but are physically handicapped, a third have no physical abnormality but are mentally handicapped, and a small percentage have both mental and physical handicap.

Hydrocephalus in later childhood
(Nine months onwards, Fig. 4.9)

This is caused by
1   Arnold Chiari malformation (Fig. 4.10) – this is a congenital abnormality which may remain asymptomatic for many years; symptoms can occur at any age, even in adulthood.
2   Stenosis of the aqueduct of Sylvius.
3   Tumours of the 3rd and 4th ventricles and cerebellum.
4   Basal meningitis.

Symptoms and signs in young children before the cranial sutures have fused

i   Slow development – the infant is late to sit up, crawl, walk and become independent.
ii Poor co-ordination – he is unable to feed himself
iii Lethargy – the infant is disinclined to play or explore
iv Mental retardation – development of speech is delayed
v   Minor epilepsy – there is head sagging, eye rolling and twitching of the face or limbs

These children may have other congenital abnormalities, are snuffly as babies and are prone to infection.

The child may be admitted to hospital for investigation of mental retardation, slow development, epilepsy or head injury. The parents will be asked about the child's birth, his development and whether he has had any fits or falls; head injury can cause a subdural haematoma and the symptoms are similar to those of hydrocephalus (see p. 96). A full general and neurological examination will reveal the severity of the disability; the child may be almost blind due to optic atrophy, he may be deaf which affects his speech and understanding, and his limbs may be spastic, undeveloped and weak. There may be cerebellar inco-ordination and signs of cranial nerve palsy, particularly affecting movement of the eyes.

Nursing care and observations

The child's behaviour and activity will be closely observed and the occurrence of fits recorded (see Chapter 19); he must be protected against injury. The sick child with very large head may have poor head control and should have his head supported, without using pillows which might cause suffocation; his position should be changed frequently to prevent pressure sores developing on his head and ears. The child with hydrocephalus may find it difficult to lift his head, sit up, maintain his balance and move in bed; a pillow under the mattress will raise the head slightly and an adjustable infant chair is a useful support when the baby is sitting up.

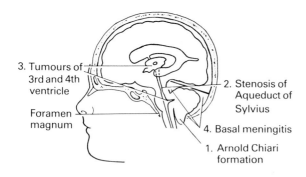

Fig. 4.9 Hydrocephalus in later childhood – sites of ventricular obstruction.

Investigations

i   Plain skull X-rays
ii   Echoencephalogram
iii A CAT scan will be performed to demonstrate the size of the ventricles (see Fig. 4.11)
iv An electroencephalogram (EEG). This record will show the frequency and nature of abnormal electrical discharges
v   Ventriculography is sometimes helpful in locating obstructive lesions

Treatment

Surgery will be decided according to the site and nature of the lesion. Arnold Chiari malformation is treated by a posterior fossa craniectomy which enlarges the foramen magnum and relieves the pressure exerted by the cerebellum upon the foramina of the 4th ventricle. When there is aqueduct stenosis a by-pass operation (Torkildsen's) will be performed, a silicone tube is inserted beneath the scalp with one end passed through a burr hole into a lateral ventricle and the other end into the cisterna magna through a posterior fossa craniectomy; this procedure may be used to by-pass obstructions caused by 3rd and 4th ventricle tumours which can be only partially removed or are inaccessible to surgery; these tumours are always treated with radiotherapy. Cerebellar tumours also obstruct the ventricular system and will be surgically removed. When there are adhesions caused by meningitis a

ventriculo-peritoneal drain will by-pass the obstruction.

All children with congenital abnormalities will be seen regularly by a paediatrician to follow their development and suggest corrective measures as the needs arise. Education may be a problem and an assessment by an educational psychologist will help place the child in the right educational environment. For further details of education, employment and social factors see pages 201 and 350.

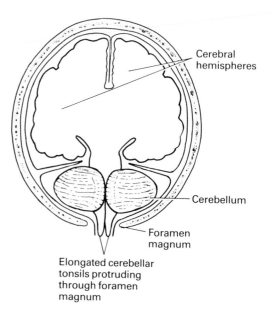

Fig. 4.10 Arnold Chiari malformation.

Symptoms and signs in the older child

The older child's skull is less able to yield to internal pressure because the sutures have fused, and blockage of the CSF circulation will produce symptoms of raised intracranial pressure.

1 Headache – especially on waking in the morning, but as pressure increases this may be at any time of day; it is increased by stooping, coughing and straining and may radiate into the neck.
2 Effortless morning vomiting which immediately relieves headache.
3 Marked neck retraction – this is associated with pain in the neck.
4 Drowsiness and lethargy.
5 Sudden loss of consciousness (drop attacks) – without warning the patient falls to the ground but rapidly recovers. These attacks may be associated with tumours temporarily plugging a ventricular foramen (see p. 113).
6 Papilloedema.
7 Sudden obscuration of vision – vision suddenly goes black and then quickly recovers.
8 Cranial nerve palsies.

Apart from signs of raised intracranial pressure the child may have other congenital abnormalities or show signs of endocrine disorder (obesity, hypogonadism, diabetes insipidus and premature puberty) due to pressure on the hypothalamus (see Fig. 7.7).

A child is amazingly tolerant of unpleasant symptoms; if he feels unwell he may not complain of severe headache but be found lying quietly on his bed. Once he has vomited and his headache disappears he may get up and behave quite normally for the rest of the day. Headaches may be falsely attributed to anxiety about school work, eye strain or sinusitis.

Hydrocephalus may have been developing slowly for several months, but when it reaches a certain level the symptoms develop very rapidly and the child is rushed into hospital. On admission a history will be taken from the parents and an examination will be performed without delay. The parents' consent will be obtained for the child to have investigations under anaesthetic:

i plain skull X-rays
ii CAT scan (Fig. 4.11)

There may not be time for these investigations if the child has raised intracranial pressure and is on the point of 'coning' (see p. 38), instead:

iii bilateral posterior parietal burr holes will be performed under general anaesthetic, the ventricles will be tapped to relieve pressure and external ventricular drainage is set up.

External ventricular drainage

External ventricular drainage is set up only as a temporary measure to drain excess CSF and reduce raised intracranial pressure, until a shunt operation, decompressive surgery or excision of tumour can be performed. A tube is inserted into a lateral

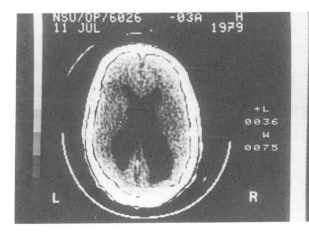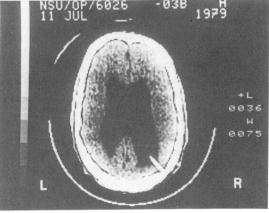

Fig. 4.11 CAT scan showing hydrocephalus.

ventricle, stitched to the scalp, connected to a sterile disposable drainage bag and set on a level with the ventricle or 10 cm above, as specified by the surgeon (Fig. 4.12). The drainage bag should never be below the level of the ventricles or the CSF will be siphoned out and a serious low pressure state will be created. When the child regains consciousness many of his symptoms will have resolved; he must be warned not to tamper with the drainage nor sit up suddenly. Whenever the child is moved the nurse should ensure that his head is kept at the same level in relation to the drainage apparatus and when he is to be transferred to a trolley or is allowed up in a chair, the tubing must be clamped off until the apparatus can be resited.

Observations relating to the ventricular drainage:
  (a) the fluid should be clear – cloudiness indicates infection;
  (b) the quantity should be measured daily;

(c) the drainage bag should be changed only when necessary; a sterile technique is essential.

The parents must be seen again by the doctor who will explain the results of investigations and discuss further treatment; the gravity of the child's condition will be emphasised.

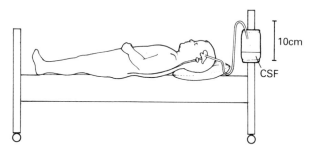

Fig. 4.12   External ventricular drainage.

Congenital tumours

Congenital tumours are rare and slow-growing, they will cause symptoms and signs according to their situation. The tumours are benign, if suitably situated will be amenable to surgery and are usually treated by radiotherapy. They cause no symptoms until late childhood or early adult life, but are discussed here as they are congenital in origin.

Teratoma   A teratoma may contain any kind of human tissue foreign to the area in which it is situated. It often develops in the pineal region and is large in size before detection; the bilateral supratentorial mass often compresses the midbrain and causes hydrocephalus.

Cholesteatoma (epidermoid)   A cholesteatoma has a pearly appearance and consists of epithelial debris inside a thin capsule. Although it is benign, it penetrates deep structures in such a way that complete removal is sometimes impossible. The most common situation is near the basal subarachnoid cisterns although sometimes a tumour arises within a ventricle.

Dermoid cysts   These cysts are the result of defective closure of the ectoderm and contain hair, sebaceous material and fluid. Dermoid cysts may be:

  (a) pericranial (of the periosteum) and erode through the bone near the anterior fontanelle;
  (b) orbital; or
  (c) in the posterior fossa – some entirely extradural dermoid cysts have a skin sinus leading to a dimple above the occipital protuberance which may give rise to recurrent meningitis or a posterior fossa abscess. The sinus may be revealed when the head is carefully inspected or the cyst and sinus are seen on plain skull X-rays as a circular defect on the inner table of the bone and a fine channel penetrating the overlying bone.

A dermoid cyst may cause hydrocephalus and signs of cerebellar disturbance.

Chordoma   This tumour arises from an embryonic remnant at the base of the skull and extends upwards in the mid-line; its slow-growing, hard invasive nature causes extensive bone destruction; there is dense calcification which can be seen on X-ray, and surgical removal is difficult as the tumour encircles cranial nerves and blood vessels.

Craniopharyngioma (tumour of Rathke's pouch)
This tumour develops from an embryonic remnant of the craniopharyngeal pouch which contains the pituitary gland. During embryonic development two sacs of tissue form the gland, one extending upwards from the pharynx (Rathke's pouch) forming the anterior lobe and the other descending from the brain to form the posterior lobe. The tumour lies above the sella turcica and expands upwards towards the hypothalamus and third ventricle where it may obstruct the foramen of Munro causing hydrocephalus; it is usually cystic and is liable to become partially calcified; its rate of growth is variable, sometimes the tumour remains quiescent for years.

Symptoms usually occur in childhood or adolescence, but may be delayed until middle-age. In children craniopharyngioma causes raised intracranial pressure; the skull enlarges, sutures separate and there is headache, vomiting and papilloedema. In adults, the symptoms are usually caused by compression of the optic nerves, chiasma or tracts (see Fig. 8.5); visual field defects are common and without treatment the patient will ultimately lose his sight; the frontal lobes, temporal lobes or the cerebral peduncles may also be compressed. Almost any type of endocrine disturbance may be seen; a child often shows signs of underdevelopment, growth is stunted, the child is fat and late developing secondary sexual characteristics; at any stage of life there may be very marked features of pituitary dysfunction (polyuria or oliguria, dwarfism, sexual infantilism or premature physical senility).

Angioma (see p. 134) Angioma (arteriovenous malformation), a vascular anomaly, is a tangle of dilated, tortuous, fragile-walled, disorganised blood vessels which may be superficial or deep-seated and is commonly found in the territory of the middle cerebral artery. In time, the angioma expands to become an intracranial space occupying lesion, or the fragility of its blood vessels leads to rupture and a subarachnoid haemorrhage. The abnormal angiomatous circulation may steal blood from large areas of the brain causing ischaemia or the angioma acting as a space-occupying lesion may cause epilepsy. Angiomata can arise in the posterior fossa, affecting the cerebellum or brain stem, and in the spinal cord.

Sturge Weber syndrome

This is a rare condition in which a facial naevus is associated with an intracranial angioma.

Craniostenosis

Craniostenosis is a condition in which there is early closure of the fontanelles and premature fusion of one or more of the skull sutures; compression of the growing brain within a rigid box will cause rising intracranial pressure, which pushes the eyes forward. When the condition affects some sutures more than others the head becomes lop-sided; fused sutures are felt as a hard ridge. Craniostenosis may be accompanied by other congenital abnormalities such as webbed fingers, bronchiectasis and congenital heart disease. These unfortunate children may also be mentally retarded and suffer from epilepsy. Skull X-rays will reveal fusion of the sutures and signs of raised intracranial pressure. Surgical intervention involves separation of the sutures, and to prevent fusion, the edges of the bones are kept apart by enclosing them in strips of nylon sheeting.

5

Head Injury

Hardly anyone escapes head injury during their lifetime. The skull is tough and takes much abuse; a large lump the size of an apple may appear on the forehead or crown of the head within minutes of a blow, but may have no significance beyond immediate pain, shock and possible scalp laceration. The brain is well protected by bone and cushioned by CSF, but is vulnerable in the very young and the aged when the bones and blood vessels are fragile; in these age groups comparatively minor injuries may cause haemorrhage and brain damage. During peacetime most head injuries are sustained in road traffic accidents, but in warring parts of the world more are the result of bomb blast and gunshot.

There are many causes of head injury, depending on age, environment and activity; it would be impossible to enumerate the many unique and extraordinary circumstances leading to some injuries; they may be purely accidental, self-inflicted, due to lack of supervision, the result of deliberately taking risks or of violence. When admitting the patient to hospital, nurses need to consider all the social circumstances, which may not be straightforward – for example 'Did he fall or was he pushed?'. Babies may be injured at birth or when they fall from cot or pram, but a baby with extensive bruising or repeatedly admitted with head injury may be the victim of parental battering. Toddlers and young children in their inquisitive and exploratory years may fall from a height or find and play with potentially dangerous objects which can penetrate the skull, e.g. knitting needles or an umbrella. Swings may strike a severe blow to a passing child; many youngsters are cycling on the roads; horse riding is very popular and a child may easily be thrown and kicked on the head. Young teenagers are exposed to head injury when playing football and cricket, skating or when violence erupts within a group; young adults because of their inexperience of road conditions and tendency to travel at speed, may be injured in motor cycling or car accidents; only after their first accident do they become more cautious, if they get a second chance. Boxing causes brain damage through repeated minor head injuries causing 'punch drunkenness' and dementia (see Chapter 9). The middle-aged are exposed to occupational hazards or road traffic accidents due to fatigue or to the effects of alcohol. The elderly, whose blood pressure drops as they get out of bed in the early hours of the morning, may totter and fall or lose their balance on the stairs. Liking to remain independent they also continue their spring cleaning and home decorating activities; at their age, climbing ladders is risky and they may temporarily interrupt the vertebral blood flow to the brain stem, by reaching upwards with neck extended, causing them to 'black out' and fall ('drop attack'). The elderly are also more likely to be the victims of mugging. Many general conditions cause loss of consciousness (see Chapter 3) when, if the patient falls, he may sustain a head injury.

National awareness of accident prevention at home, on the road, at work and in recreation, and the serious consequences of head injury with its possible life-long problems, is vital. More publicity is necessary on radio, television, in the press and on eye-catching posters to emphasise the need for safety measures and the responsibility of all road users.

Parents must teach their children road safety and supervise them until they are of an age to safeguard themselves; throughout the school curriculum there should be repeated instruction. This is especially necessary for teenagers who should understand their responsibilities as motor-cyclists and motorists, respect weather conditions and never treat the road as a race track. Many accidents can also be prevented by:

i   the use of crash helmets and seat belts and careful, regular maintenance of vehicles and highways;

ii   better safety standards in the home, shops,

public buildings and institutions:
(a) steps and stairs should be well lit;
(b) floors should be non-slip and mats and rugs used cautiously;
(c) the use of appropriate safety equipment which meets national safety standards is advisable, e.g. gates on stairs, catches on windows, infant's car seats and pram and high chair harnesses;

(d) supervision of young children and the elderly (especially those taking sedative and antidepressant drugs);
iii enforcement of safety standards in industry;
iv supervision of recreational pursuits; equipment should be well maintained and correct clothing and safety apparel worn; riding hats must be well-fitting and of the correct design.

Anatomy related to injury
(See also Chapter 3)

Injury may be superficial involving only the scalp, or deep involving skull, meninges and brain tissue; there may be other injuries, to the chest, abdomen, limbs or spine (see Chapter 12). Injuries may be caused by a blow from a blunt object which may or may not fracture the skull and tear the dura. A penetrating injury will always cause a fracture and dural laceration (Fig. 5.1); a blow on the head with an axe will cause localised damage at the site of the blow whereas a bullet will leave a track of damage from the point of entry to its exit; occasionally a bullet may lodge in the brain. Parts of the brain and skull may be completely torn away by bomb blast. Some patients sustain very severe brain damage yet there is little evidence of external injury, no

fracture of the skull or dural tear (closed head injury). There is always cerebral oedema when the brain is damaged and if there is no escape for the swollen brain it can only herniate through the tentorium cerebelli or foramen magnum (see p. 37); when brain damage is associated with a fractured skull (especially if there is a dural tear with CSF leak), the expanding brain has an outlet and raised intracranial pressure will be less severe; the patient with a 'closed' head injury may be deeply unconscious and unresponsive and one with brain oozing out of his skull, alert and co-operative.

The scalp is highly vascular, receiving its blood supply from the external carotid arteries; if lacerated it bleeds profusely, but heals quickly. The

(a)   (b)

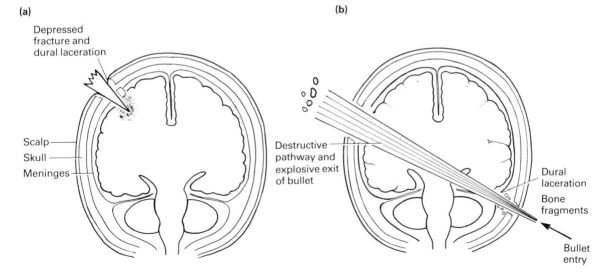

Fig. 5.1 Penetrating injuries. (a) Localised penetrating stab injury. (b) Injury caused by high velocity bullet.

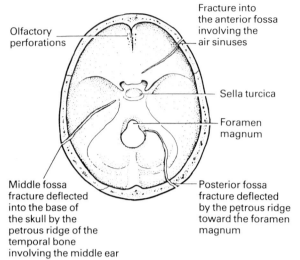

Olfactory perforations

Fracture into the anterior fossa involving the air sinuses

Sella turcica

Foramen magnum

Middle fossa fracture deflected into the base of the skull by the petrous ridge of the temporal bone involving the middle ear

Posterior fossa fracture deflected by the petrous ridge toward the foramen magnum

Fig. 5.2   Fractures of the base of the skull.

skull bones are of varying thickness and some parts are more liable to fracture than others. Thick, strong internal ridges tend to deflect fractures into the base of the skull (Fig. 5.2). The many air sinuses in the frontal and ethmoidal regions are fragile, and fractures with underlying dural tears allow easy access for infection from the nasal passages. Fractures of the base of the skull where the dura mater is most firmly attached to the bone almost always cause dural tears whereas over the vault, tears are less common. The skull receives its blood supply bilaterally from the meningeal arteries, branches of the external carotid arteries; the middle meningeal artery lies in a groove in the temporal bone and is easily ruptured by a blow in the temporal region (see p. 89 and Fig. 5.3).

The living brain is a very soft, semi-fluid organ cushioned by CSF in the subarachnoid space, protected from infection by the impermeability of the dura mater and securely contained and protected in compartments formed by the dura mater and the skull. Any blow on the head causes movement of the brain within these compartments which is damaged as it strikes the free edges of the meninges and the irregular inner surface of the skull; small arterioles are stretched and torn and blood haemorrhages into the brain substance.

Contre-coup injury

When the body hurtles through the air and the head strikes a stationary object the rigid skull is stopped instantly, but the softer brain continues its progress forward, rebounds and continues to oscillate back and forth within the skull; there will be contusion of the brain not only at the point of impact, but also of an area directly opposite, for example an injury to the vault of the skull causes damage not only to the sagittal sinus and upper surfaces of the cerebral hemispheres, but also to the under surfaces of the frontal and temporal lobes, even damaging the hypothalamus; in addition the corpus callosum may be damaged when it strikes the free edge of the falx cerebri (Fig. 5.4).

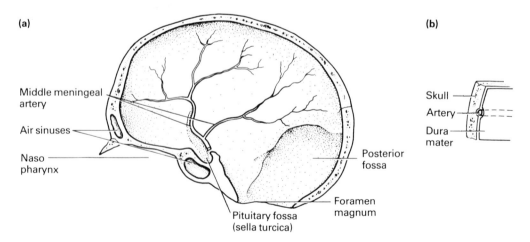

(a)

Middle meningeal artery

Air sinuses

Naso pharynx

Pituitary fossa (sella turcica)

Foramen magnum

Posterior fossa

(b)

Skull

Artery

Dura mater

Fig. 5.3   The blood supply of the skull: **(a)** Interior of skull showing distribution of middle meningeal artery. **(b)** Section showing artery in groove of the skull, outside of the dura mater.

Shearing lacerations

Shearing strains tear axons from their cell bodies and these neurones will not regenerate; when there has been severe head injury there will be shearing lacerations throughout the brain. The living brain has a jelly-like consistency and the effect of this type of injury can be likened to the splits and loss of shape which occur when a jelly is vigorously shaken. Tearing of small cortical capillaries causes widespread petechial haemorrhages, amalgamation of several of these form a haematoma; veins entering the superior sagittal sinus may similarly be torn, causing subdural haematoma.

Brain stem injury

A glancing blow to the side of the head will twist the skull rapidly sideways; the brain, which always moves more slowly than the skull, will screw round on its axis the brain stem (Fig. 5.5) causing injury, oedema and even haemorrhage. Brain stem injury will render the patient deeply unconscious, with marked head retraction, stertorous Cheyne–Stokes respirations and spontaneous extension of all limbs. Recovery is possible, but it is a very slow process.

Cranial nerve damage

The cranial nerves may be damaged at the time of injury or compressed when intracranial pressure

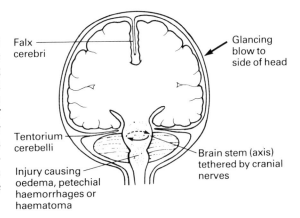

Fig. 5.5 Brain stem injury.

rises. The olfactory nerves are often involved when the face and forehead are injured, their nerve endings which pass through the cribriform plate of the ethmoid bone being severed from the olfactory bulbs; when there is bilateral nerve severance there will be permanent complete loss of the sense of smell (anosmia). The eye may be irreparably damaged by penetrating glass and the optic nerve severed by fractures of the orbit; when the eye is unscathed but the optic nerve is severed, though the pupil does not react to direct light, it will constrict when light is shone into the other eye (consensual reaction). Damage to the abducens nerve which moves the eye outwards causes a convergent squint with diplopia. It is extremely rare for the oculomotor nerve to the pupil to be damaged by direct injury, but this is the nerve which is so important in the early detection of raised intracranial pressure (see p. 38). The glosso-pharyngeal and vagus nerves are damaged by brain stem injury, causing dysphagia and loss of cough reflex.

Other injuries

Approximately 30% of patients who have sustained head injury also have injuries to other parts of the body, which may have even more serious consequences than the head injury itself and may be overlooked unless the patient is examined carefully. When two or more urgent conditions are present at the same time, teams of surgeons may need to operate simultaneously, for example when there is an extradural haematoma and a ruptured spleen.

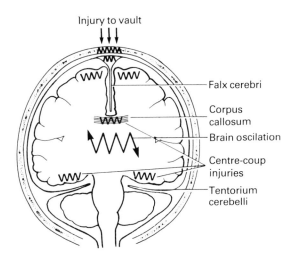

Fig. 5.4 Contre-coup injury.

Other injuries include:

1   Chest injuries
   (a) 'Stove in' chest
   (b) Pneumothorax or haemothorax

2   Fractured cervical spine
3   Abdominal injuries – ruptured spleen, liver or kidneys
4   Fractures of facial bones, limbs or pelvis
5   Severe lacerations and burns

Immediate care of a patient at the scene of the accident

(See also Chapter 3)

Everyone should be well-informed in first aid care, as speed in obtaining skilled help and careful observation may be life-saving. Is the patient breathing? It is vital to prevent respiratory obstruction through the tongue falling back into the throat, dentures becoming dislodged or inhalation of vomitus; profuse vomiting often occurs when the patient has had a heavy meal or has drunk large quantities of beer before an accident. To prevent obstruction of the airway the victim should be turned into the semi-prone position, his dentures removed and he should not be given anything to drink. Is the patient bleeding profusely? There should be no hesitation in removing the patient's clothing to locate the source of haemorrhage and stop its flow. An ambulance must be summoned urgently. Accurate observations of the patient's conscious level, pupillary size and reaction, and limb movements, should be noted immediately after the injury and communicated to those receiving the patient at the hospital. A doctor may give an injection of pethidine when peripheral injuries are intensely painful, but analgesics such as morphine are contraindicated, as they depress respirations. Before the ambulance arrives, the patient should be moved only if this is essential for his safety, and then with the utmost care as he may have sustained a fracture of the cervical spine (see Chapter 12).

Admission to hospital

Admission to hospital will depend upon the nature, severity and site of the injury; any patient who has been concussed, unconscious – however briefly, has a skull fracture, is vomiting or has multiple injuries, must be admitted to hospital for observa-tion and treatment; only a few patients need neuro-surgical intervention.

The aims of every nurse and those responsible for the care of someone who has suffered a head injury are to keep him alive, protect viable brain tissue and prevent complications. It must always be remembered that a patient with a head injury might also have a cervical fracture. No one should presume that a deeply unconscious patient has sus-tained irreparable brain damage, for powers of recovery are great; every effort must be made to resuscitate the patient who has stopped breathing or who has cardiac arrest; a young person with quite severe head injury may make a remarkably good recovery even after several respiratory or car-diac arrests.

In the casualty department, depending on urgent priorities, the following observations and care are necessary.

1   Neurological assessment and record of vital functions will be made by the nurse immediately she sees the patient.

2   A general and neurological examination. The casualty officer will examine the patient for exter-nal signs of injury; a boggy swelling over the tem-poral region will alert him to the possibility of an extradural haematoma (see p. 89), and bruising over the mastoid process (Battle's sign) will suggest a fractured base of skull. The eyes will be examined for proptosis, indicating bony displacement or hae-morrhage into the orbit. The doctor will not be able to examine the patient's neck movements until X-rays of the spine have been taken, but will look for external signs of injury and notice the posture of head and neck. A rapid scrutiny of the chest, abdomen and limbs will reveal any other injuries and there will be urgent discussion about the need for immediate surgery.

3 An intravenous blood transfusion will be set up; it is essential that blood lost through haemorrhage is replaced as soon as possible and many litres will be required if there has been profuse haemorrhage.

4 Skull, chest, cervical spine and limb X-rays. The use of a multi-purpose trolley and special stretcher canvas enable X-rays to be taken without lifting the patient unnecessarily.

5 Wound toilet – an area of 3–5 cm will be closely shaved around all small scalp lacerations before they are cleaned and sutured; larger head wounds will be treated in the operating theatre.

6 Setting fractured limbs in plaster of Paris or putting up traction.

7 Tetanus prophylaxis.

When a patient is admitted with severe open head injury and possibly many other injuries, he will be taken straight to the operating theatre where he will be anaesthetised, his respirations controlled by a positive pressure ventilator and a blood transfusion will be commenced while teams of specialist surgeons attend to his injuries. Head wounds will be thoroughly cleaned, all damaged tissue and fragments of bone removed, bleeding points sought and haemorrhage stopped. Limbs may need extensive debridement, surgical repair or amputation; all minor grazes and lacerations must be thoroughly scrubbed before they are sutured to prevent gas gangrene; chest and abdominal injuries will be treated and fractured jaws wired. Postoperatively the patient's respirations will be maintained by the ventilator for a few days, as early control of respirations improves cerebral oxygenation, reduces cerebral oedema and leads to a better recovery.

Examination and investigations

A full neurological and general examination (see Chapter 2) will be performed by the medical officer as soon as immediate treatment and emergency surgery have been completed. Regular laboratory examination of blood will be needed to find the levels of haemoglobin, white cell count, blood urea and electrolyte balance. A CAT scan is a useful aid to discover shift of mid-line structures, developing haematomata or oedema. Electroencephalography is rarely useful in the immediate investigation of head injury, but it is a useful guide to recovery when a patient is being maintained by a ventilator and is valuable to demonstrate a focus of epilepsy.

Nursing care
(See Chapters 3 and 10)

All patients with head injuries require

i frequent careful observation and neurological assessment; and
ii maintenance of general health by diligent nursing care to:
  (a) prevent complications;
  (b) provide adequate nutrition and ensure satisfactory excretion; and
  (c) encourage full rehabilitation and gain the helpful participation of the patient's relatives.

On admission to hospital it is important that a clear description is obtained from eye witnesses, relatives or ambulance attendants, of the circumstances of the accident, the condition of the patient immediately following injury and during the journey to hospital. Was the patient conscious? A lucid interval has very important significance and urgent treatment will be required (see p. 90). It is also important to discover preceding events or illnesses which may have caused the incident and influence treatment, for example a 'stroke' may cause an accident. The patient may be unable to give his own history if he is drowsy, confused or has amnesia. When an unconscious patient is unaccompanied by relatives and the nursing staff cannot contact the next-of-kin until they have been traced by the police, urgent surgical measures may have to be performed without obtaining consent. Enquiries should be answered with discretion as in some circumstances there are legal implications.

Observations

Whenever there has been a head injury a clear, concise and accurate description of the patient's conscious state and neurological assessment must be made immediately after the accident and then at regular frequent intervals. The patient is likely to be irritable, irrational and resent interference especially if he has been taking alcohol or drugs, and at night when he expects to be asleep. He may lie in bed curled up with bed clothes over his head, or being confused and amnesic, constantly clamber out of bed half-naked and try to leave the ward; he will probably be unsteady on his feet and will reel around endangering himself and others. The nurse must not be deterred from making her regular thorough and accurate assessments and if the patient is exceptionally abusive and aggressive she must seek assistance each time before she examines the patient.

During the first 24–36 hours following injury a neurological assessment, pulse, respiratory rate and blood pressure should be recorded half- to 1-hourly, and temperature hourly; if the patient's condition is critical he will be kept under constant observation and his vital signs will be monitored. Urine should be tested for blood. Any deterioration should be promptly reported to the doctor as it may indicate the development of an extradural haematoma or other complicating condition requiring treatment; a conscious patient may complain of increasing headache, a semiconscious patient may become extremely restless; the patient may have an epileptic fit (see Chapter 19); all details should be accurately recorded. Hourly measurement of abdominal girth will detect internal haemorrhage, particularly from the spleen. Tachycardia and a fall in blood pressure may indicate internal haemorrhage. A slow pulse and rising blood pressure are late indicators of increasing intracranial pressure, but in the terminal stages of raised intracranial pressure, the pulse rate will rise and the blood pressure will fall. Respirations are often stertorous and there may be periods of apnoea.

Pyrexia and hyperpyrexia

After a severe head injury the patient's axillary or rectal temperature should be recorded hourly; any rise above 38°C is serious as it may indicate hypothalamic damage, when the temperature can rise to a dangerous level in a very short time. Methods of temperature reduction should be discussed with the doctor.

1   The ward should be well ventilated with a room temperature not exceeding 18°C.

2   The patient should be nursed naked between linen sheets only, to avoid the rucks of draw sheets, gowns or pyjamas as pyrexia increases the skin's susceptibility to pressure sores.

3   The use of an electric fan is especially effective in conjunction with a wet sheet placed over the patient; the unconscious patient's eyes must be kept closed with a non-allergenic adhesive (see Fig. 3.12) to avoid corneal abrasion which can be caused by the drying effect of the fan.

4   When hyperpyrexia does not respond to the above measures, ice bags can be placed over the heart and major arteries, and vigorous rubbing with sponges soaked in iced water will cause peripheral vasodilatation in the patient's trunk and limbs and bring more rapid temperature reduction.

A very high temperature caused by hypothalamic damage must be reduced quickly with careful monitoring of the rectal temperature to prevent over-reduction to subnormal temperatures. Shivering, one of the body's natural mechanisms for raising the temperature, should be reported to the doctor as soon as it is noticed as it counteracts the nurse's efforts to reduce pyrexia; promazine may be prescribed if the patient's blood pressure is above 110 mm Hg and ice and fanning treatment may need to be withheld for a while; shivering may recur when the effect of promazine is wearing off.

Hypopyrexia

Subnormal temperatures may occur after head injury especially in the elderly, and warming measures including the use of an electric heat pad or foil space blanket, will restore a near normal body temperature.

Care of the eyes (see p. 57)

Care of the eyes should be carefully supervised as their appearance may frighten an inexperienced nurse. The patient often has extensive bruising and oedema of the eyelids, severe chemosis and sometimes proptosis; it may be impossible to open the eyelids to look at the pupils; iced compresses will help to reduce the swelling.

Care of associated injuries

In all instances of associated injuries the neurosurgeon, neurologist and the nurse will work in close cooperation with consultants in orthopaedic, general ENT or plastic surgery. Positioning the patient is often a problem when there are one or more fractures, but whenever possible the lateral or semiprone positions should be used if the patient is unconscious. Care of the patient's skin may be hampered by plaster of Paris splinting. The upper end of a full-length leg plaster is liable to cause pressure and friction especially when it is damp due to incontinence; the skin must be relieved of pressure by using a piece of foam, broken skin protected by a dressing and a urinary catheter will be necessary.

Sedation and relief of pain

Though sedatives are contraindicated during the first 36 hours as they will mask the true level of consciousness, the patient should not be allowed to suffer unnecessarily. Intramuscular codeine phosphate will relieve headache, and stronger analgesics may be prescribed if there are other painful injuries. Sometimes the patient's behaviour is so disturbed despite skilful management (see p. 61) that sedation becomes necessary.

Recovery of consciousness (see p. 61)

The pattern of recovery following loss of consciousness is variable, according to the severity of brain damage, the area involved and the length of time the patient has been unconscious; there is usually confusion, disorientation and amnesia and the patient may be completely unco-operative, irritable and aggressive. There is sometimes a period of automatism when the patient appears to behave normally, but on regaining full consciousness has no recollection of events during this period. A patient who has been unconscious for a prolonged period will regain consciousness and awareness more gradually.

Complications of head injury

Most patients make an uneventful recovery from head injury, only a few will suffer from serious complications.

Cerebral oedema (see p. 48)

When the brain is damaged it always swells, causing raised intracranial pressure and lowered level of consciousness; oedema is worsened by respiratory complications. It is impossible to predict those patients with head injury who will develop severe cerebral oedema. Oedema can be demonstrated by CAT scan and the treatment is to withdraw fluid from the brain by using a hypertonic solution (mannitol), high doses of steroids (dexamethazone) or by controlling the exchange of gases in the lungs through the use of an intermittent positive pressure respirator.

Haematomata

Only a small number of those who sustain head injury will develop an intracranial haematoma; when this occurs it may develop outside the dura (extradural), beneath the dura but outside the brain (subdural) or in the brain substance (intracerebral);

there may be bilateral haematomata or more than one type present at the same time. Some small haematomata need no treatment and will be reabsorbed naturally, but when there are localising neurological signs and the patient's condition is deteriorating, further investigations become necessary and the patient may require surgical treatment.

Extradural haematoma

Extradural haematoma (Fig. 5.6) is a most important complication requiring emergency surgery. The haematoma is usually the result of injury in the temporal region causing rupture of the middle meningeal artery; an injury in this region should always be regarded seriously as a comparatively minor blow can fracture the temporal bone or damage the artery, and the injured person must be examined by a doctor. However well the patient may seem, if he has had loss of consciousness however brief, a period of amnesia, headache and vomiting, a boggy swelling is found above the ear or skull X-rays show a fracture of the temporal bone, he must be admitted to hospital for 24-hour observation; a longer period is necessary should

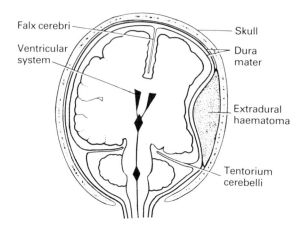

Fig. 5.6 Extradural haematoma.

symptoms persist, as extradural haematoma sometimes takes longer to develop. There is often a lucid
interval of up to 12 hours following injury when the
patient appears normal, vehemently claims he is
'quite all right' and may refuse to see a doctor; this
can be an entirely misleading and dangerous situation as there may be sudden deterioration and
death. Someone who sustains an injury while under
the influence of alcohol is at even greater risk as he
may be allowed to 'sleep it off' and 'sober up', and
even stertorous respirations may be wrongly interpreted as noisy snoring.

When a patient is in hospital for observation
following a head injury the nurse must continue her
frequent assessments of his conscious level, pulse
and blood pressure, even at night, as the patient can
deteriorate extremely rapidly to death within the
hour; if there is prompt treatment unnecessary loss
of life can be avoided and complete recovery
expected. The doctor must be notified immediately
the nurse notices any change, however slight, in the
patient's neurological assessment; signs for
concern are drowsiness, incontinence, dilatation of
one pupil and weakness of the limbs on one side. As
most patients following head injury are admitted to
general hospital wards, an urgent decision will be
taken as to whether there is time to transfer the
patient to a neurosurgical unit, for within minutes
the patient's condition will markedly deteriorate,
the other pupil becomes unreactive and begins to
dilate, a rapidly progressive contralateral hemiplegia will develop and before long all limbs will
extend spontaneously or in response to painful
stimuli; the respirations become rapid and

stertorous, then Cheyne–Stokes. Successful early
treatment means miraculous complete recovery
from coma in a very short time. The delays entailed
in organising and transferring a patient would
threaten his life or, perhaps even worse, would
make the expected full recovery impossible; occasionally a general surgeon will need to make the
life-saving burr hole to let out the blood and relieve
the raised intracranial pressure. The patient will
then be transferred to a neurosurgical unit where,
following a temporal craniotomy, the bleeding
artery will be located and coagulated and the haematoma fully aspirated; a blood transfusion will be
necessary when considerable blood has been lost.

Less characteristically extradural haemorrhage
follows a severe injury; the patient is unconscious
from the outset and his condition unrelentingly
deteriorates. Extradural haematoma may also be
caused by bleeding from the diploeic vessels (small
venous channels) in the skull or from the venous
sinuses when it will not be found in the classical
temporal region, but over the vault of the skull or in
the posterior fossa.

Subdural haematoma

Acute subdural haematoma
Acute subdural haematoma (Fig. 5.7) occurs
within a few hours of a severe head injury, rarely
does it result from trivial injury; the patient is
usually unconscious from the beginning and the
underlying brain damage is severe. The haematomata are often bilateral and vary in size and
speed of development depending on the severity of
the injury; they cause downward displacement of
the cerebral hemispheres and tentorial herniation
with rapid deterioration in conscious level. When
there is time a CAT scan is performed, to confirm
and localise the haematoma, but the urgency of the
situation frequently calls for immediate craniotomy to aspirate the haematoma and control
haemorrhage. The outlook is unpredictable as it is
impossible to assess underlying brain damage;
the patient's failure to recover may be due to other
haematomata (extradural or intracerebral), to
severe oedema, injury to vital structures or
haemorrhage into the brain stem.

Subacute subdural haematoma
Subacute subdural haematoma occurs within 14
days of the injury and should be suspected if the
patient fails to recover or begins to deteriorate a

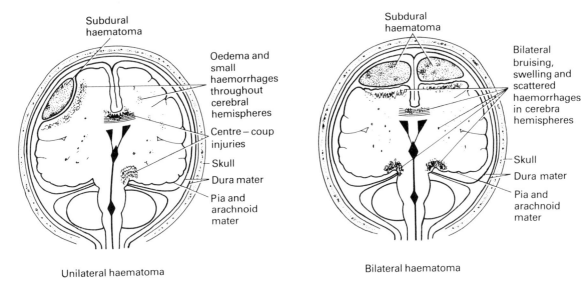

Fig. 5.7 Acute subdural haematoma.

few days after the injury; a CAT scan will usually reveal and localise the haematoma which can then be aspirated through suitably placed burr holes.

Chronic subdural haematoma
(for infantile subdural haematoma see page 96)
Chronic subdural haematoma may be the result of a minor head injury often so trivial it was immediately forgotten. The haematomata are usually bilateral, build up very slowly over a period of weeks or months and are more common in the elderly whose poor eyesight and unsteadiness lead to bumps and falls and whose cerebral blood vessels are fragile. The gradual development of the haematomata allows the brain to compensate and the patient may remain conscious with very slight symptoms in spite of large bilateral haematomata (up to 100 ml in each, see Fig. 5.8). The symptoms develop slowly and are so like the normal features of old age (a tendency to sit around and doze, forgetfulness, slight confusion at night and occasional incontinence) that they may be overlooked. A fluctuating level of consciousness, from being unrousable to fully conscious, and fleeting mild hemiparesis of either or both sides are suggestive of chronic subdural haematomata. Other helpful signs are partial or complete inability to look upwards and mild ptosis due to the downward compression of both oculomotor nerves. Those caring for the elderly, especially in nursing homes and

institutions, need to be aware of the serious consequences of minor knocks on the head, and common illnesses which cause dehydration, lower the blood pressure, diminish cerebral circulation and may even rupture blood vessels (see Chapter 8); it has been known for chronic subdural haematoma to develop following a bout of diarrhoea and vomiting when dehydration has caused the shrunken brain to drag upon and rupture fragile blood vessels. Any elderly person who regularly complains of severe headache, whose mental state

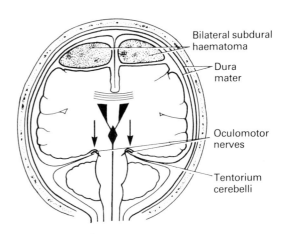

Fig. 5.8 Bilateral chronic subdural haematoma.

and memory appear to be deteriorating more rapidly and who is lethargic and increasingly drowsy should be thoroughly examined and undergo investigations. When there are no localising signs, a mistaken diagnosis of frontal lobe tumour may be made or the patient may be admitted to a psychiatric hospital with dementia.

Investigations will include skull X-rays and a CAT scan and treatment is by aspiration of the haematomata through bilateral parietal burr holes; the dark, partly broken-down stale blood is easily aspirated, but repeated aspirations of the subdural space will be necessary at intervals of 2–3 days as fluid reaccumulates, though usually in decreasing amounts and changing to a xanthochromic fluid; a graph record is kept of the appearance and amount of aspirate from each burr hole. Very occasionally if fluid continues to collect (subdural hygroma), the subdural membrane will need to be removed.

A contributory cause of subdural haematoma in the elderly may have been low intracranial pressure caused by ill health, low blood pressure, or poor hydration. As the haematomata have been present for a long time, the brain does not quickly re-expand to fill the space. To help re-expansion the patient is nursed with his head lower than his feet and given a high fluid intake. Recovery is generally good, but as these elderly patients have to remain in bed for several days, every effort must be made to prevent complications, especially respiratory infection and pressure sores, and once they are allowed to sit up and get out of bed they must be encouraged and stimulated to become active, independent and to take a renewed interest in life.

Intracerebral haematoma

Intracerebral haematoma usually occurs at the time of injury but occasionally develops after several days have elapsed; the haemorrhage is sometimes sudden and catastrophic, even rupturing into the ventricular system. Neurological signs will depend upon the size of the haematoma and the area of the brain involved, the patient is usually unconscious with signs of raised intracranial pressure, with localising signs of pupillary change and dense hemiplegia. A CAT scan will help to locate the haematoma which can then be removed through a craniotomy. The outlook is unpredictable as the brain may have already sustained extensive damage.

Respiratory complications (see page 49)

Additional factors which make the nursing care of a patient with head injury difficult are:

(a) Maxillo–facial injuries
Blood and serous fluid from these injuries will collect in the nasal passages and throat, obstructing the air entry to the lungs, and when the fractured jaws are also wired together, suction is difficult, but small suction catheters may be passed through any gap in the teeth; suction through the nose is contraindicated. The conscious patient may be taught to perform his own suction, the unconscious patient may require a tracheostomy.
(b) CSF rhinorrhoea
The unconscious patient must be nursed in the semiprone position to prevent CSF draining to the back of the pharynx and being inhaled.
(c) Cervical fractures – see Chapter 12
High cervical fractures are likely to paralyse the muscles of respiration
(d) Thoracic injuries
When thoracic injury accompanies head injury it is very serious as the already injured brain is subjected to increasing anoxia, which also increases cerebral oedema.

Fractures of the skull and CSF leak

When a fracture of the skull is seen on X-ray the patient is admitted to hospital for observation. Linear fractures require no surgical treatment, but are important when they cross underlying structures such as blood vessels and where they may tear the dura mater; this is especially likely in the base of the skull because the dura mater is more adherent to the bone than it is over the vault.

Simple depressed fractures, without dural tear, need to be elevated as they may be a focus for epilepsy, but surgery is usually delayed for 24–48 hours to allow the patient to recover from shock. Fractures involving the venous sinuses are dangerous as, when the fragments of bone are lifted from the sinus, haemorrhage may be profuse and difficult to control and transfusion of several litres of blood will be required. Compound comminuted depressed fractures, fractures of the base of skull and those which involve the air sinuses, all open a pathway for the entry of infection (meningitis and cerebral abscess – see Chapter 6

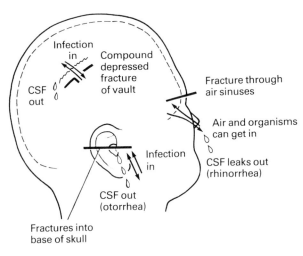

Fig. 5.9 CSF leak.

and Fig. 5.9). Surgical excision of ragged necrotic tissue and removal of fragments of bone and foreign bodies will be necessary, the dura mater will be repaired and antibiotics instilled into the wound before it is closed; head wounds must always be covered with a sterile dressing and bandaged securely into place, and when there is a leakage of CSF from wound, nose (rhinorrhoea) or ear (otorrhoea) the patient must be barrier nursed; systemic antibiotics will be given. A CSF leak may not be apparent at first as the oedematous brain plugs the dural defect; alert nursing staff will watch all patients with head injury for a CSF leak especially when it is known that a patient has a compound or basal fracture. After a day or two a thin watery fluid leaks from wound, ear or nose or it may be noticed that the patient is constantly sniffing. It may not be obvious whether a nasal discharge is serous or CSF; a specimen should be collected for analysis. Should there be difficulty in obtaining a specimen, clinistix can be used for a ward test as CSF contains sugar. The patient with CSF rhinorrhoea must not smoke and he must be told not to sniff, sneeze or blow his nose, as this will cause the entry of infecting organisms, and air which forms an aerocele (a pocket of air usually in the frontal region). **The passage of oesophageal tubes and suction catheters through the nose is contraindicated as they will introduce infection.** When there is CSF otorrhoea the patient should be told not to

poke his finger into his ear and the ear should be covered with a sterile dressing firmly bandaged into placed. The patient will find a CSF leak very uncomfortable and it may be difficult for him to keep to the nurse's instructions; a confused, dysphasic or very drowsy patient will not be able to co-operate. The patient will be nursed in an upright position and the leakage will usually cease spontaneously within 7–10 days, but if it does not, the dural defect must be surgically repaired. It is very difficult for the surgeon to locate a minute puncture hole in the dura mater, but when found it is plugged with a small piece of fascia taken from the thigh, or artificial dura. When rhinorrhoea develops weeks or months after the injury there will be no spontaneous healing and surgical repair is the only option.

When parts of the scalp and skull are destroyed as in bomb blast or other mutilating injuries, cranioplasty using a moulded sheet of plastic will be an emergency measure and plastic surgery will be necessary to recreate the lost scalp. In all other instances of large cranial defect where scalp is not lost and can be repaired the cranioplasty can be left until a later date, but during the waiting period the patient should wear a protective helmet to prevent damage to the brain.

Meningitis and cerebral abscess
(See Chapter 6)

Meningitis and cerebral abscess may complicate compound fractures and should be suspected when headache, neck stiffness, photophobia, positive Kernig's sign and pyrexia develop. A lumbar puncture is necessary to confirm the diagnosis by obtaining a specimen of CSF for culture and sensitivities; the appropriate antibiotics can then be given systemically and intrathecally. It may be extremely difficult to recognise meningitis when the patient is unconscious and if treatment is delayed the patient may develop a cerebral abscess or die. When the signs of meningitis are accompanied by deterioration in the level of consciousness with focal neurological signs (dysphasia, hemiparesis and the onset of generalised or Jacksonian epilepsy fits) the cause may be a cerebral abscess. Recurrent bouts of meningitis following head injury indicate a dural defect even though a CSF leak is not apparent.

Subarachnoid haemorrhage

When the arachnoid mater is torn blood escapes into the subarachnoid space, explaining the severe headache, photophobia, neck stiffness and irritability experienced by so many patients with head injury; blood in the subarachnoid space will gradually be absorbed and the symptoms will recede. The patient should rest in bed until the symptoms subside but should they recur when he gets up, a further period of rest is necessary. It has been found that if patients with these symptoms are urged to resume normal activities too soon, they frequently develop a postconcussional syndrome or accident neurosis (see p. 95). Headache may persist intermittently for several weeks and simple analgesics should be administered regularly (see p. 137). There is a small chance that the head injury occurred as the result of a spontaneous subarachnoid haemorrhage (see Chapter 8).

Fat emboli

Fat emboli are a risk for any patient who has a fracture of a marrow bone, for example the femur. Globules of fat enter the circulation at the site of the fracture and are carried to the lungs, kidneys and brain. Very occasionally cerebral fat emboli are the cause of unconsciousness following head injury. Cerebral and pulmonary signs and symptoms usually occur simultaneously within 24 hours of injury:

i   restlessness
ii lowering of consciousness
iii irritability
iv epileptic fits
v   increasing respiratory and pulse rates
vi pyrexia
vii petechial haemorrhages, mainly on the trunk and neck, appear on the second or third day and confirm the diagnosis; there may also be haemorrhages into the kidneys causing haematuria.

Epilepsy
(See Chapter 19)

There is a high risk of epilepsy following head injury if the patient has sustained a depressed fracture, dural tear, penetrating injury or had an intracranial haematoma. Should the patient have a fit during the first week following injury the risk of further fits is greatly increased, but if he does not, it does not preclude his having a fit later. Epilepsy developing in a child under 5 years of age is much more serious as he may rapidly develop status epilepticus and could die. When a fit is noticed it should be promptly reported to the doctor; the attack may only be the brief twitch of a finger or corner of the mouth, but it may be grand mal or progress to status epilepticus within a very short time; anticonvulsant therapy will be prescribed and all attacks and medication should be carefully recorded. Some doctors recommend prophylactic use of anticonvulsant drugs from the beginning for all patients who are at risk, for a period of between eighteen months and two years or more. The disadvantage of these drugs is that they mask the level of consciousness in the early days following injury and cause lethargy during rehabilitation. Sudden cessation of anticonvulsant therapy can provoke a grand mal fit or status epilepticus if the patient has a potential epileptic focus. True post–traumatic epilepsy begins several months or years after a head injury, is persistent and must be treated with anticonvulsant therapy for the rest of the patient's life. Even a single fit following head injury may have serious consequences as the patient may have to forfeit his driving licence and experience difficulty in obtaining employment or be forced to abandon career plans.

Cortical atrophy
(See Chapter 9)

Large areas of cortex are destroyed by severe head injury, either at the time of the injury or when local vascular damage with thrombosis leads to gliosis and atrophy. The patients will either show personality changes and intellectual impairment from the beginning, or slow slight improvement during the first days and weeks will suddenly come to a halt, or deterioration occurs much later with signs of dementia and there may be epilepsy. Investigations will be performed to exclude chronic subdural haematoma and to demonstrate enlarged ventricles and cortical atrophy. Treatment for this condition is not very satisfactory; the insertion of a ventriculo–peritoneal shunt may help slightly if the enlarged ventricles are due to obstruction by adhesions in the CSF pathways.

Metabolic disorders

Severe head injury is a shock to the patient's system and causes disturbance of metabolism. The administration of intravenous fluids in the early days following injury must be carefully controlled to avoid overhydration and in accordance with the patient's electrolyte levels, blood urea and blood volume which are checked daily. There may be damage to the pituitary gland and hypothalamus causing diabetes insipidus with electrolyte imbalance and dehydration; if the patient is unconscious he will be unable to ask for extra fluid, his increased excretion may pass unnoticed because of incontinence and he will become severely dehydrated, losing vital salts. The conscious patient constantly demands fluid to satisfy his excessive thirst and in desperation will drink water from the flower vase or his own urine. An accurate fluid balance chart must be kept and when diabetes insipidus is suspected the urinary specific gravity should be tested; if the condition is present the specific gravity will be low, 1002 or less. Treatment is to replace pitressin by administering an intranasal solution of desmopressin or pitressin by injection.

Brain death
(See p. 66)

Rehabilitation
(See also Chapter 3)

Although head injury affects any age group a large proportion of those injured are children and young adults whose lives are before them; the sudden catastrophic incident affects previously healthy young people and robs them of their hopes and plans for the future. It is all very well if the patient completely recovers and is able to pick up the threads of life where he left off, but so often there is mental and physical disability and the patient and his relatives have to completely readapt their lives; there can be every shade of disability from something so slight that it is only noticed by the patient or those who know him well, to such severe disablement that the patient needs permanent institutional care. It is heart-breaking when a previously bright, intelligent young man or woman loses their potential and becomes totally dependent, excessively demonstrative and mentally subnormal. The relatives are so delighted that the patient has survived and regained consciousness and are ever hopeful that there will be complete recovery that they do not see the snags, are eager to take him home and think that if they devote themselves to his care 'everything will be all right'; only later comes the realisation of the burden they have taken on.

Many families learn to accept their lot and cheerfully soldier on; they must of course be given every possible support from relatives, friends, social services, community clubs and day centres. Others never come to terms with the problems, cannot accept changed personality, dementia and restrictions to social life, and inevitably there is family disruption and break-up; only then do the authorities find a place for this young chronic sick person, but often it is too late to save a marriage. Husbands and wives may find that the changed personality of their spouse following head injury makes them totally incompatible, leading to separation or divorce.

Besides the head injury, which may have been quite mild, there are other disfiguring and disabling injuries to come to terms with; severe facial injuries cause embarrassment, loss of confidence, possible employment difficulties, may even ruin a young person's marriage prospects and will mean repeated hospital admission for reconstructive surgery; blindness demands total readjustment and loss of limbs seriously curtails activities.

Compensation neurosis

It has been noticed that some patients who have postconcussional headache, dizziness, poor concentration and impaired memory, lose their persistent and prolonged symptoms when legal processes are completed and financial settlement has been made. There is no doubt that those who are comfortably well off and can afford paid help when they need it, being less dependent on the goodwill of others, will not feel guilty about asking for help and will therefore have greater freedom and suffer less strain. Financial anxieties sap the energy and goodwill of even the most willing relative; the delay of 2–3 years for compensation settlement can cause great hardship.

Birth injuries

Prevention of birth injuries is the concern of midwives and obstetricians, whose duty it is to recognise disproportion between the maternal pelvis and the foetal head, foetal deformity and to ensure safe delivery.

Minor injuries, caput succedaneum and cephalhaematoma need no treatment. Depressed fractures are rare and may be due to maternal pelvic deformity or badly applied forceps; the fracture may right itself as the infant grows, but occasionally surgical elevation of the depressed bone is necessary. Dural tears and intracranial haemorrhage occur when there is excessive and rapid compression of the foetal skull during delivery, the falx cerebri or tentorium cerebelli may be torn, damaging nearby blood vessels; haemorrhage is usually into the subdural space. The baby will be shocked and ill, with shallow breathing, his body may be rigid with muscular twitching or generalised convulsions, he will not suck well and often vomits. He should be carefully observed, handled as little as possible and nursed in an incubator in a quiet darkened room; feeds should be withheld for 24 hours, then he should be 'cot' or tube-fed. Intramuscular injections of vitamin K are given to prevent further haemorrhage and a sedative will be prescribed. Should the baby be cyanosed or have a convulsion, he should be turned on his side to maintain a clear airway and secretions from the nose and mouth should be removed, the doctor must be notified and his instructions for the administration of oxygen and prescribed medication must be followed carefully.

Infantile subdural haematoma

Subdural haematoma may either be due to injury at birth or to a later blow on the baby's head. Evidence of haematoma (usually bilateral) may not at first be apparent, but develops gradually within a few months; the skull enlarges, the sutures part and the fontanelles become wide, bulging and tense. The infant becomes drowsy, irritable, refuses feeds, vomits or may have convulsions. The diagnosis is confirmed when blood is aspirated from the subdural space by inserting a needle through the fontanelle; only a small amount of blood is removed at first to avoid precipitating further haemorrhage. The subdural haematomata are aspirated daily until there is negligible aspirate; when repeated subdural taps reveal consistently large amounts of stale blood, bilateral temporal burr holes may be necessary to aspirate other parts of the subdural space; if large amounts still continue to collect the surgeon may perform a craniotomy to remove the dense unyielding subdural membrane which, until it is removed, prevents re-expansion of the brain.

A subdural hygroma will develop after several months if a subdural haematoma is untreated, serous fluid being osmotically drawn into the cavity previously occupied by blood.

6

Intracranial Infection

(Read also Chapter 13 on spinal infection.)

Intracranial infection was once very common and many people died or were severely disabled, but in recent years many factors occurred almost simultaneously to reduce the incidence and improve the outlook for those who contracted infection, the most important being the discovery of antibiotics. Other important factors have been less crowded living conditions, better general health and hygiene including careful preparation of food, pasteurisation of milk and an unpolluted water supply, prompt treatment of ear and sinus infections and awareness of the serious complications which

follow their neglect. Publicity campaigns draw attention to the danger of diseases such as tuberculosis, the availability of mass X-ray facilities and vaccination, and the notification of certain infectious diseases enables them to be monitored and controlled. Laboratory equipment and techniques have improved and organisms can be more easily and speedily identified and their sensitivity to antibiotics established. A greater variety of antibiotics are available, but sometimes antibiotic-resistant bacteria occur. The introduction of anti-viral agents has improved the outlook for patients with viral infection of the nervous system.

Anatomy

(See Chapters 2 and 3)

The brain is protected from many harmful chemicals and infective substances by an efficient blood–brain barrier; it is a complex system which is partly concerned with the permeability of the meninges and blood vessels. Most people have, from birth, efficient immune mechanisms and also inherit or develop resistance to most harmful organisms.

Infecting organisms

Intracranial infection is caused by:

1 Bacteria
i Organisms causing pyogenic meningitis are the meningococcus (affecting children and young adults), pneumococcus, streptococcus, escherichia coli and haemophilus influenzae (the most common cause of meningitis in infants).

ii Tubercle bacillus may cause tuberculous meningitis in children and young adults; the infection is mainly from the human tubercle bacillus, but in some instances is from the bovine variety.

iii Spirochaete organisms cause neurosyphilis (see Chapter 24) and Weil's disease – caused by the leptospira icterohaemorrhagica which is found in the urine of infected rats and contracted through bathing in contaminated water or working in an infected environment, e.g. in sewers, mines or on farms.

iv Brucella abortus causes brucellosis (undulant fever or Malta fever) – a notifiable disease contracted by drinking infected cow's or goat's milk.

2 Viruses
Viral infections cause an acute non-pyogenic (aseptic) meningitis; viruses known to cause intracranial infection include:

i   Coxsackie virus
ii   Echo (enteric cytopathogenic human orphan) virus
iii Mumps, measles, chickenpox and whooping cough viruses
iv   The virus of glandular fever (infectious mononucleosis)
v   Influenza virus
vi   Herpes simplex virus
vii Herpes zoster virus (see Chapter 13)
viii Poliomyelitis virus (see Chapter 13)
ix   The viruses of encephalitis lethargica and inclusion body encephalitis
x   Rabies virus

Occasionally the virus is not identified.

3   Fungi
i   Torula histolitica causes torulosis – a fatal disorder, widespread throughout the body, which affects the brain, spinal cord and meninges
ii   Other rare fungal infections

4   Parasites
i   Protozoa which include
       Malarial parasites (*Plasmodium falciparum, P. vivax, P. ovale* and *P. malariae*)
       Trypanosomes, which cause trypanosomiasis ('sleeping sickness') – transmitted to man by the bite of an infected tsetse fly and which involves the central nervous system, lymph glands and spleen.
       Toxoplasma gondii which cause toxoplasmosis – a congenital or acquired disorder, probably transmitted from household pets, which is widespread in the body and causes encephalomyelitis
ii   Metazoal infestations which include:
       Cysticercosis
       Toxocara canis
iii Helminths (worms) – human beings can become infested by the eggs or larvae of worms which are commonly harboured by animals. Larval infestation of round worms from dogs or cats mainly affects children who can also ingest the larvae from eating dirt. Pets should be healthy and free from worms and children should be instructed to wash their hands after handling animals. The eggs of tapeworms may be ingested through eating undercooked pork or beef. The larval stage of these infestations may occur in the brain causing cerebral irritation and epilepsy.

Routes of entry for infection

Many general systemic infections occasionally affect the brain and even the drowsiness and loss of concentration experienced with a common cold is probably a mild cerebral reaction. Organisms either invade the nervous tissue or their toxins act as an irritant causing inflammation, oedema, tiny scattered haemorrhages, gliosis, degeneration or the formation of cysts.

There are four main routes by which infection can reach the brain (Fig. 6.1):

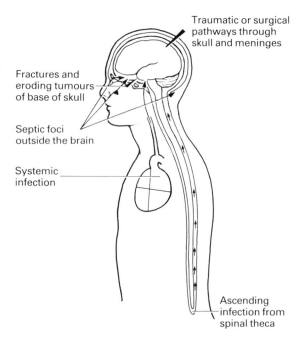

Fig. 6.1   Routes for infection to the brain.

1   A pathway through the skull caused by
(a)   Head injuries. Penetrating injuries of the skull will carry organisms into the brain from the scalp; a fracture of the base of the skull with dural tear may lead to infection reaching the CSF from the nasopharynx, middle ear or mastoid process (CSF rhinorrhoea and otorrhoea see p. 93).

(b)   Abnormal sinuses and dural faults associated with congenital tumours (dermoid cyst), eroding tumours in the region of the air sinuses and the base of the skull (osteoma and cholesteatoma) and destruction of bone by irradiation.

(c)   Following neurological investigations or surgical procedures. Certain operations carry a high risk of infection either because they involve the dura and may leave a defect, use an approach which is potentially infectious, e.g. the naso–pharynx, or are extremely lengthy surgical procedures.

2 Ascending infection through the spinal theca, e.g. ruptured meningocele.

3 Spread from a septic focus in the head or face. Most commonly the infection, which may be acute or chronic, spreads from the nasal sinuses, middle ear or mastoid process; uncommonly infection may spread from a boil on the face to cause an infected cerebral venous sinus thrombosis. These centres of infection, in particular chronic otitis media, are sometimes associated with intracranial abscess.

4 Carried in the bloodstream.

Secondary infection in the brain may result from systemic viral, bacterial, fungal and parasitic infections (e.g. infectious mononucleosis, tuberculosis, torulosis and trypanosomiasis).

Meningitis

Meningitis is an infection of the meninges, the coverings of the brain and spinal cord. The infection is of any of the three layers, pia mater, arachnoid mater and dura mater, and also involves the subarachnoid space and the CSF; there may be associated encephalitis (inflammation of brain tissue) or encephalomyelitis (inflammation of the brain and spinal cord).

Pyogenic meningitis

Many different bacteria cause pyogenic meningitis, in which the whole surface of the brain and spinal cord is coated with a greenish-yellow pus (Fig. 6.2a); the meninges are very inflamed, the blood vessels are congested and the brain is swollen.

The onset of the illness is rapid with severe frontal or diffuse headache building up in a few hours and associated with photophobia, vomiting and fever; a child may have an unexpected convulsion. As the illness worsens, signs of meningeal irritation develop, pain in the nape of the neck radiates down the back to the legs, the patient becomes irritable, resents interference and is often seen curled up in bed with his head under the bedclothes. When disturbed, babies and children emit a high-pitched cry and adults sometimes cry out with the severity of the pain. Deterioration is rapid and the patient, within a few hours, passes from irritability and delirium to drowsiness, stupor and coma.

Meningococcal meningitis (cerebrospinal fever) – now very rare, is a secondary infection which spreads from the nasopharynx into the blood stream causing septicaemia, and enters the CSF through the choroid plexus; the brain and spinal

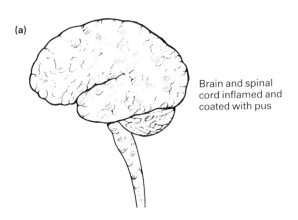

(a)

Brain and spinal cord inflamed and coated with pus

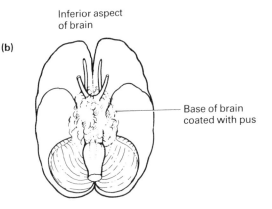

Inferior aspect of brain

(b)

Base of brain coated with pus

Fig. 6.2 **(a)** Pyogenic meningitis. **(b)** Tuberculous meningitis.

cord may also be affected (encephalomyelitis). It is a highly infectious notifiable disease and the patient should be nursed in isolation. The organism is spread by droplet infection from a carrier or other infected person. The disease is most common in infants and young adults, especially where there are overcrowded conditions, though it is not contracted by all those exposed to the infection; outbreaks usually occur in the winter or early spring. The illness starts with a high fever (up to 40°C) and acute septicaemia which may, within a few hours, cause the patient's death before there are any signs of meningitis. When meningitis develops there will be signs of meningeal irritation; a child may have convulsions and an adult rigors. Nearly half the patients develop a purpuric rash after approximately 48 hours which gives the illness the name 'spotted fever'. The rash occurs mainly in those areas of the skin subjected to pressure and improves when the general infection is controlled. Herpes simplex on the lips is common at the end of the first week. The illness may be very severe (acute fulminating type) with positive blood culture, severe septicaemia and haemorrhage into mucous and serous membranes, and into the adrenal medulla leading to collapse and death. Infants develop marked head retraction and opisthotonos during the course of the illness and vomiting and dehydration are common. Sometimes, following meningococcal meningitis, infants develop hydrocephalus, progressive dementia and blindness and death usually occurs within 3 months.

History and examination

To avoid disturbing the patient unnecessarily as much information as possible should be obtained from a close relative. Particular care will be taken to elicit any information relating to a possible source or focus of infection; there may be a history of sinusitis, ear or respiratory infection, or contact with another infected person. A thorough general and neurological examination will then be made. The doctor will notice signs of meningeal irritation; neck stiffness which occurs early in the illness causes pain and limitation of movement when an attempt is made to flex the neck, the pain being caused by stretched inflamed meninges. Kernigs sign (pain in the hamstring muscles caused by an attempt to straighten a flexed knee with the hip fully flexed) is often present in association with meningeal irritation, but is less common than neck stiffness. Head retraction may develop as the

disease progresses due to spasm of the posterior neck muscles; opisthotonos (Fig. 6.3), an extreme degree of neck and spine extension, occurs most commonly in children. There may be other abnormal clinical signs and symptoms, papilloedema, unequal pupils with abnormal reaction to light, ocular palsies and diplopia. The limbs are limp, tremulous and poorly co-ordinated without definite weakness. Reflexes are usually sluggish or absent; plantar responses which are at first flexor, become extensor as the illness progresses. Incontinence of urine occurs with lowering of consciousness.

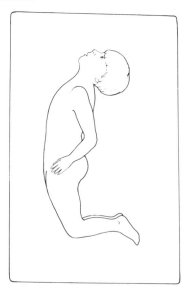

Fig. 6.3 Opisthotonus.

Investigations

i   Haemoglobin, full blood count and blood sedimentation rate.

ii   Blood culture – in meningococcal meningitis it is usually positive.

iii Throat swab.

iv   Skull X-rays to reveal fractures.

v   Chest X-ray.

vi   Lumbar puncture (see p. 32). The CSF pressure is raised, the fluid is turbid and xanthochromic, there is an abundance of polymorphonuclear cells which invade the CSF in great numbers to ingest the bacteria, there is an increase in the protein content, the chlorides are reduced and the sugar content is very low or absent. Organisms will be cultured from the CSF and sensitivities obtained.

Treatment

As soon as the doctor has completed his examination a lumbar puncture will be performed; CSF (10 ml) will be required to determine the organism and its sensitivity to antibiotics.

Intrathecal antibiotics will be given with the first lumbar puncture before the CSF has been examined and the sensitivities determined when meningitis is severe or if the patient is a child. Systemic chemotherapy (oral, intramuscular or intravenous) is usually effective, but if the infection is exceptionally severe, the patient is not responding well to treatment or the antibiotic is one which poorly penetrates the blood-brain barrier, an additional intrathecal antibiotic is necessary. Regular anticonvulsant therapy will be commenced if an epileptic fit occurs at any time during the illness.

Tuberculous meningitis

Tuberculous meningitis is a comparatively rare condition which before the advent of the specific anti-tuberculous drugs was invariably fatal; it is still a dangerous illness having a high mortality rate. Early diagnosis is most important, but often difficult owing to the insidious onset of the disease which resembles other conditions. Prompt, adequate and prolonged treatment can be very successful, but even so there may be residual mental deficiency, paralysis, optic atrophy and deafness.

The primary tubercular focus is often in the mediastinal or mesenteric lymph nodes, but may be in the bones, joints, lungs or genito-urinary tract. The infection spreads to the brain in the blood stream and infects the meninges. The pia and arachnoid meninges, particularly at the base of the skull become matted together with a yellow gelatinous exudate (Fig. 6.2b).

The patient, usually a child or young adult, becomes generally unwell, apathetic, fretful or irritable, restless in sleep with night sweating, anorexic and loses weight; an adult may have marked mental changes. There is a low grade evening pyrexia and frequent headaches which continue for some weeks before an obvious and rapid deterioration occurs with increasing drowsiness.

The history and examination of the patient is often singularly unhelpful as the symptoms are rather vague; the diagnosis may only be suspected by the exclusion of other conditions. There may be slight neck stiffness and sometimes there are cranial nerve palsies especially affecting eye movement. During ophthalmoscopy tubercular lesions may be seen in the ocular fundi. The doctor will need to know whether the patient has had BCG vaccination and whether any member of the family has tuberculosis.

Investigations

A wide range of investigations is usually necessary to find the primary infection and to diagnose tuberculous meningitis.

i　A full blood count and sedimentation rate.

ii　Chest X-rays and tomography. There may be a primary focus or miliary tuberculosis in the lungs.

iii　Plain skull X-rays help to exclude space-occupying lesions and may show evidence of raised intracranial pressure.

iv　Laboratory examination for tubercle bacillus – specimens of sputum, throat and intra-gastric washings, and urine are required.

v　Electroencephalogram.

vi　Mantoux test.

vii　Computerised axial tomogram.

viii　Lumbar puncture. This is the most important investigation and will be repeated on many occasions, to diagnose the condition, introduce intrathecal drugs, measure CSF pressure, determine the free flow of CSF in the subarachnoid channels (Queckenstedt's test) and obtain CSF at regular intervals for laboratory analysis. The CSF is clear and colourless unless the cell content is much increased when it appears hazy; it may be under normal or increased pressure. When left to cool, a white web-like clot is sometimes seen which is formed by fibrin in the fluid. The cell count, mainly lymphocytes, may be increased from 10–350 per cu. mm, sugar is diminished and the chloride level is low. A special staining technique is necessary to demonstrate the tubercle and even when the patient is thought to have tuberculous meningitis, repeated laboratory examination may not at first reveal tubercle in the CSF.

Treatment

Treatment with systemic and intrathecal anti-tuberculous drugs will be commenced as soon as tuberculous meningitis is suspected, even before the tubercle has been isolated from the CSF, for delay may jeopardize complete recovery or cost the patient his life; the search for the tubercle often takes some time. Intrathecal drugs are administered for up to three weeks and systemic chemotherapy for 6 months to 1 year until all risk of re-infection is past, or otherwise the tubercle may lie dormant for a while and flare up months or years later.

Complications of pyogenic and tubercular meningitis

1   Adhesions sometimes form between the inflamed pia and arachnoid meninges, at the base of the brain, impeding the free circulation of CSF in the subarachnoid space and preventing intrathecal antibiotics from reaching the entire area of inflammation. Intrathecal hydrocortisone is given to prevent adhesions obstructing the outlets of the 4th ventricle causing hydrocephalus, a complication especially likely in children and when meningitis is severe. Signs of impending obstruction are a low CSF pressure, an increase in the CSF protein and a poor rise and fall on Queckenstedt's test, and can be confirmed by brain scan.

2   Development of intracranial space-occupying lesions.
 (a)   Multiple intracerebral abscesses (see p. 103) sometimes complicate pyogenic meningitis.
 (b)   Tuberculoma. This is a rare complication of tubercular infection in children, but may not be accompanied by tuberculous meningitis. It is a space-occupying granulomatous lesion mainly found in the posterior fossa, causing raised intracranial pressure. The tumour must be excised and a full course of anti-tuberculous treatment given.

3   Cranial nerve palsies. Deafness and blindness sometimes complicate tuberculous meningitis.

4   Corticothrombophlebitis. The cerebral veins sometimes become infected and inflamed causing thrombosis and infarction. This is a very serious complication; babies and children are particularly susceptible. The patient's condition deteriorates with increasing drowsiness, severe pyrexia, rigors, epileptic fits and weakness of the limbs on the opposite side. Lumbar puncture will show a high CSF pressure; the CSF may be xanthochromic and laboratory examination will reveal excess leucocytes and red cells, and a high protein content.

Acute aseptic meningitis

When there is an outbreak of viral infection in a community it is likely that a patient who shows signs of meningeal irritation is suffering from viral meningitis. Generally the patient is nursed at home unless he is a child, exceptionally ill or there is some doubt about the diagnosis. Relatives should be advised to keep the patient in bed, encourage a high fluid intake and notify their doctor should any new symptom develop or the patient become very drowsy. The doctor will prescribe antipyretics, analgesics for headache and will visit regularly until the patient has recovered. Should the patient be admitted to hospital a lumbar puncture will be performed; the CSF pressure will be raised, the fluid is usually clear, but many lymphocytes will be found, the protein content will be increased, but the chloride and sugar levels will be normal; organisms can only be demonstrated by special virological techniques. Blood will be tested for virus antibody titres.

Nursing care of a patient with meningitis

The patient should be nursed in quiet surroundings, if possible in a single room, and protected from the glare of bright light as he will have photophobia. Strict barrier nursing precautions are necessary for patients with meningococcal meningitis and those with active pulmonary tuberculosis, and precautions must be observed by everyone who enters the patient's room. The nurse's approach should be quiet and gentle, taking particular care to avoid jerking the patient unexpectedly and bumping his bed. Careful observation is essential especially for a patient nursed in isolation; frequent neurological assessments and a record of the vital functions must be made at regular intervals throughout the 24 hours and combined with other nursing care to avoid repeatedly disturbing the patient. Deterioration in his level of consciousness must be reported immediately as he may be developing one of the previously described complications (see p. 102). Pyrexia fluctuates and the temperature must be recorded at hourly intervals when the patient is very ill; if he becomes hyperpyrexic, cooling measures (see p. 88) must be commenced immediately. Antibiotics should be administered and recorded promptly at the hour they are due, and analgesics and anticonvulsants given as prescribed.

Although antibiotics have revolutionised the treatment of meningitis, a very high standard of nursing care (see Chapter 3) is still essential for the patient's survival without complications, and to keep him even moderately comfortable. The patient feels awful, he has a thumping headache, burning hot skin and does not want to be disturbed; he is only half aware of what is going on, to open his eyes hurts and he may be unable to see clearly. His tongue is furred, he may be vomiting and everything tastes foul, oral antibiotics may make his mouth sore and give him indigestion, heartburn and diarrhoea especially if he is not eating much. Children and some adults fear injections; during the course of this illness there will be repeated blood tests, painful intramuscular injections and sometimes daily lumbar puncture which the patient begins to dread. Just getting into the correct position for the procedure causes pain and as the procedure becomes more and more difficult for the doctor each time a lumbar puncture is performed, the patient may need to stay in this uncomfortable position for some time.

The patient may be reluctant to drink if he is drowsy, irritable and nauseated, but a high fluid intake is essential as in any pyrexial illness and should he refuse to drink or become dysphagic, fluids will be given by intravenous infusion. An accurate measurement of the patient's urinary output is necessary as there is sometimes retention of urine; the abdomen should be palpated daily to ensure that the bladder is not distended. Constipation is frequently a problem which requires treatment with suppositories. During the acute phase of the illness, the patient will not want to eat and nourishing fluids must be given; when this time has passed and the patient has regained his appetite, a high calorie diet must be encouraged. Tuberculous meningitis is a long, debilitating illness and every effort must be made to tempt the patient's palate and build up his strength and resistance to infection; additional nourishing milk drinks are necessary.

Intracranial abscess

An intracranial abscess is a collection of pus which is either:
  (a) intracerebral;
  (b) subdural; or
  (c) extradural.
The source of infection (Fig. 6.4) may be directly through a wound or from nearby structures or distant organs (secondary infection). There may be one or more abscesses:

1   A single abscess
i   Sinusitis – particularly frontal and ethmoidal sinusitis which leads to an abscess in the frontal lobe or subdural space
ii   Otitis media – the abscess usually develops in the temporal lobe, but sometimes in the cerebellum

iii   Mastoiditis – the abscess is in the temporal lobe or cerebellum
iv   Compound fractures and penetrating injuries of the skull – an abscess develops at the site of the injury

2   Multiple abscesses
i   Thoracic infections – infected emboli lodge in the brain, causative conditions are
    (a) bronchiectasis
    (b) lung abscess
    (c) congenital cyanotic heart disease
ii   Meningitis
iii   Suppurative encephalitis

The patient with cerebral abscess looks pale and very ill, his eyes sunken with dehydration, his

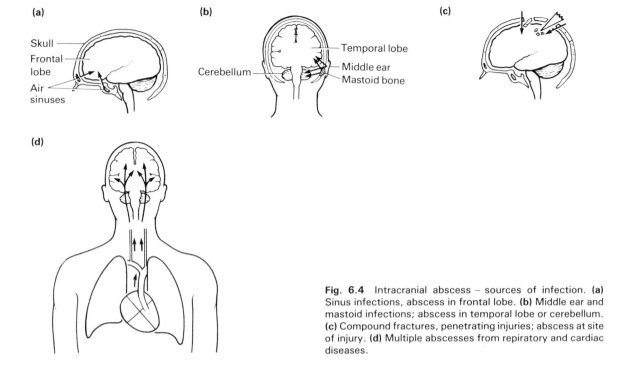

(a)

Skull
Frontal lobe
Air sinuses

(b)

Cerebellum
Temporal lobe
Middle ear
Mastoid bone

(c)

(d)

Fig. 6.4 Intracranial abscess – sources of infection. **(a)** Sinus infections, abscess in frontal lobe. **(b)** Middle ear and mastoid infections; abscess in temporal lobe or cerebellum. **(c)** Compound fractures, penetrating injuries; abscess at site of injury. **(d)** Multiple abscesses from repiratory and cardiac diseases.

mouth very dirty, and with septic spots on his face and shoulders. The patient has a high temperature, signs of raised intracranial pressure (see p. 47) localising neurological signs and focal or generalised epilepsy, depending upon the situation of the abscess.

Investigations and treatment

1 Intracerebral abscess
A history and clinical examination often reveal a focus of infection and localised brain disturbance. Skull X-rays may show a brain shift (see p. 25), infected air sinuses or compound fractures, and a CAT scan will localise the abscess. An EEG will demonstrate an area of slow wave delta activity in the region of the abscess.

The abscess is located and aspirated as quickly as possible to prevent its rupture into the ventricular system, as this is usually fatal. The abscess is aspirated through a burr hole and the pus sent to the laboratory to be cultured. Antibiotics and a radio-opaque substance are instilled into the cavity; the exact size, location and pocketting of the abscess cavity will then be seen on X-ray. Systemic antibiotics must be given in large doses until the pus is sterile, but as many patients have already received antibiotics for treatment of the primary infection the organisms may have already been destroyed; on the other hand the organisms may have become resistant to many antibiotics. The abscess will be tapped two or three times at intervals of a few days according to the patient's condition, the amount of pus aspirated and the radiological appearance of the shrinking abscess. During this time the patient will be observed carefully and if he is more alert, his hemiparesis improving and pyrexia subsiding this is an indication that the abscess is resolving; should the abscess capsule fail to shrink or cause epilepsy, surgical excision will be necessary.

2 Subdural abscess
The pus floats in the subdural space over a wide area of the brain. The cortical blood vessels become infected and when they thrombose, cause widespread brain ischaemia. This frequently leads to

epilepsy, starting as a focal attack, rapidly becoming generalised and possibly leading to status epilepticus; prompt anticonvulsant treatment is essential. Should the patient have a fit, other localising signs, for example hemiplegia, may be noticed for the first time.

Several burr holes will be made for the insertion of catheters into the subdural space (Fig. 6.5) to allow frequent aspiration of pus and instillation of antibiotics; systemic antibiotics (intramuscular or intravenous) are also given.

Subdural abscess is difficult to treat, prognosis is very poor, and residual hemiparesis and dysphasia are common.

3 Cerebellar abscess
Cerebellar abscess is a rare occurrence and follows

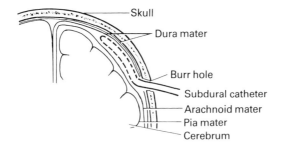

Fig. 6.5 Catheter draining a subdural abscess.

an ear or mastoid infection; the signs are ataxia, nystagmus and raised intracranial pressure. Once the abscess is located it is removed through a posterior fossa craniectomy; antibiotic therapy will be given.

4 Extradural abscess
Extradural abscess is associated with osteomyelitis of the skull and may follow head injury or cranial surgery; when the dura is intact infection will not spread to the other meninges or the brain. A discharging sinus is sometimes seen on the scalp and skull X-rays show erosion of the skull bone. This is a chronic condition which persists for many months and often fails to respond to treatment with systemic antibiotics. A course of antibiotics will be given and the infected bone and pus will be removed. When the infection has completely resolved a cranioplasty will be performed.

Nursing care

Nursing care is as for a patient with meningitis. Delay in observing and reporting deterioration in the patient's level of consciousness, focal neurological signs or epilepsy will be detrimental to recovery.

Encephalitis

Encephalitis (inflammation of the brain) is a rare condition, occurring mainly in the young and is usually the result of a viral infection; the areas most often affected are the cortex, basal ganglia, nuclei of the brain stem and the hypothalamus; the meninges and spinal cord may also be affected (meningoencephalitis and encephalomyelitis). Viruses may be transmitted by human contacts, animal, bird or insect carriers.

Encephalitis is a serious illness which causes almost any of the signs and symptoms associated with disorder of the nervous system. When these closely follow a recognised viral infection it is likely that there is a connection between the two conditions; otherwise the diagnosis is made by excluding

other disorders, the progress of the illness and changes in the CSF. The cause of encephalitis often remains a mystery and the virus is rarely identified, though a rising antibody titre in the blood serum is significant and is the most reliable method of identification. The virus is occasionally found in the stools during the acute illness.

The illness usually starts with a mild fever and headache, followed by increasing drowsiness, stupor and even coma. Epileptic fits are common especially in children. There is often disorientation, irritability, minimal neck stiffness, mild papilloedema and pupillary changes. The brain stem and cerebellum are frequently affected, leading to cranial nerve palsies, nystagmus and ataxia.

Abnormal sensory symptoms are less common, though there may be areas of hyperaesthesia. Tendon reflexes are usually diminished and plantar responses flexor or extensor; Kernig's sign is sometimes positive. Hemiparesis is unusual, if it occurs it is transitory.

Investigations

1 Those needed to establish the diagnosis
i A full blood count will show an increase in white cells and the blood sedimentation rate will be raised
ii An EEG will show a characteristic diffusely abnormal record
iii Lumbar puncture will be necessary to:
(a) measure the CSF pressure which is likely to be increased
(b) obtain CSF for laboratory analysis. There is usually an increase in the lymphocyte count (10–50), a rise in protein, but sugar and chloride levels are normal
iv Viral studies. Specimens of blood, stools and CSF are obtained

2 Investigations which may be necessary from time to time during the illness
i A CAT scan to exclude space-occupying lesions, e.g. intracerebral abscess
ii Blood for electrolyte levels, urea estimation and haemoglobin
iii Chest X-ray
iv Sputum culture

Treatment

An antiviral agent (acyclovir) is given intravenously for 7 days and this will limit the infection and improve the chances of recovery. The use of steroids is thought to limit inflammation and diminish reactive gliosis. Anticonvulsants may be necessary, analgesics will be needed for headache and sedatives given if there is extreme restlessness and behaviour disorder. Sedatives are used with caution as they mask deterioration in the patient's conscious level and further irritate the already disturbed nerve cells.

Nursing care

Care of a patient with encephalitis is a real challenge to the nursing staff as the patient invariably gets worse almost to the point of death, before his condition begins to improve; he is very ill for a very long time and runs the risk of any one of the many complications which beset the unconscious patient (see Chapter 3). All resuscitative equipment should always be available as, even for the most critically ill patient, hope should never be abandoned. Complete recovery has been known to occur after many weeks' coma and several episodes of respiratory arrest, providing that every effort is made to protect viable brain tissue by preventing hyperpyrexia, and episodes of cyanosis due to respiratory obstruction. A patient may be akinetic rather than unconscious and well able to understand what is said in his presence – a point always to be remembered. A suitable environment must be created for the acutely disturbed, restless, confused and irritable patient. Rehabilitation must aim to restore the patient to full mental and physical health; rest is an important factor during the illness and physiotherapy and other measures of rehabilitation should not be pursued to the point of fatigue, as this may lead to relapse, delay in recovery and possible to neurosis when the patient finds his inefficient brain unable to cope with daily activities.

Recovery may be a very slow process, powers of concentration are affected and a long period of adjustment is particularly necessary for those with responsible jobs or engaged in academic studies; some patients never fully regain their potential.

Other forms of encephalitis

There are a few other forms of encephalitis which though acute in onset have special characteristics or are progressive, and have long-term effects or are fatal within 6 months to 10 years. These include the following.

1 Herpes simplex encephalitis, which affects the cerebral blood vessels and causes necrotic lesions which give rise to localising signs and suggest intracranial abscess.

2 Encephalitis lethargica (see Chapter 20) is a form which occurred in epidemics between 1916

and 1926 and is now rarely encountered. It is characterised by a reversed sleep pattern and its effects on the basal ganglia. Parkinsonian symptoms occur as early as the acute stage of the illness, but are frequently a later manifestation.

3 Inclusion body encephalitis is a form which affects children and is characterised by three distinct phases during the 2–6 months' fatal illness:

i   intellectual impairment;
ii akinetic mutism; and
iii involuntary movements and grimacing.

4 Rabies

Rabies

Rabies is a virus infection which causes an acute fulminating fatal encephalomyelitis and invades every organ of the body. It is transmitted to man by the infected saliva of a diseased animal, most commonly the domestic dog and sometimes the cat, affecting the male of the species more than the female. The incubation period varies, from as little as 10 days to one year, the average being 4–6 weeks. Wounds of the face and head, as would be sustained by children due to their small stature, give a shorter incubation period than those of the extremities, as they are nearer the brain. The virus, having entered through a wound, invades the local muscles, enters the peripheral nerve axons and tracks into the spinal cord and brain; it leaves the brain along all voluntary and involuntary nerve pathways to infiltrate the entire body.

Rabies is a world-wide, much feared disease; it has been in existence for centuries, can affect all warm-blooded animals and is rarely contracted by man. In those countries where rabies is common, outbreaks of the disease come and go in the same way as other virus infections and pass across a continent like a wave from east to west. In many countries dogs are very popular pets and because they are so numerous, dog bites are extremely common, ranging from the very minor playful bite to the isolated occasion when a child is fatally savaged. As the dog is chiefly responsible for transmitting the virus to man it would be reasonable to expect the incidence of rabies to be dramatically reduced if the dog population were healthy and controlled, and this has proved to be correct. In Great Britain and Australia which are free of the disease there are stringent controls at all sea and air ports and a compulsory period of 6 months' quarantine for all dogs entering the country; import licences are required for all animals whether for private ownership, zoos or research institutions. The police have the power to seize and confine stray dogs, which are destroyed if they are not claimed within 7 days, and law breakers are heavily fined if caught smuggling an animal into the country. In some countries all dogs must be vaccinated against rabies and in others they must be muzzled.

The question of wild animals and rabies must be kept in proportion; it would be ecologically unwise to destroy completely a particular group of animals even though they are likely to transmit the disease. There has recently been much anxiety about the increasing fox population and the spread of rabies; the fox may travel many miles in a day, will kill indiscriminately, even attacking domestic animals, and often visits or inhabits urban areas; a rabid fox may therefore be the link between wild and domestic animals over a wide area and bring the disease one stage nearer to man. It has been proved that reducing the fox population controls the spread of rabies.

There is no way that rabies can be totally eradicated from the animal population; where a country is free of the disease, as in Great Britain, every effort must be made to prevent its entry by gaining the co-operation of the general public, by informing them of the horror of the disease and the implications of one rabid animal entering the country. All who work in ports and harbours in Great Britain must be diligently watchful to prevent anyone contravening the law and the disease crossing the natural sea barrier. The developing countries of Asia have a particularly high incidence of rabies infection because there are no regulations to control the dog population and stray dogs abound. Preventive and prophylactic treatments are not generally available and facilities for investigation and vaccination are prohibited by cost.

Veterinarians, the police, animal handlers and dog owners need to know the symptoms of animal rabies so that a suspect is immediately isolated. The early symptoms of change in temperament when a dog slinks away and hides, becomes restless and has bursts of affection when he licks his owner's hands and face (which could transmit the disease through a break in the skin or through a mucous membrane), may not at first be attributed to rabies. The dog then becomes feverish, his appetite changes, he may chew unnatural things and develop an abnormal bark. He takes on a characteristic wild mad-dog look, eyes glinting, pupils dilated and saliva dribbling from the mouth; he may be seen biting at an old wound, becomes excessively thirsty (but not hydrophobic), rushes around madly making unprovoked attacks, snapping wildly at man or other animals, and disappears from home. He may later return, weak and emaciated, develop paralysis of the hind quarters and die within a short while.

When a person is bitten by a mad dog the amount of infected saliva reaching the wound will be greatly reduced and the wound less severe if the animal bites through clothing. The wound must be thoroughly cleaned as soon as possible to wash away infected saliva; it is not sutured immediately to reduce the risk of trapping the virus in the wound.

When a person has been bitten by a rabid or suspected rabid animal he must receive prompt treatment; the further the bite is from the brain, the longer the period that the patient has to develop his own antibodies (an unknown number of people have natural immunity), or antibodies in response to vaccination, but when the injuries are extensive or on the face or head, the patient must be given an immediate injection of a serum containing rabies antibodies. The only disadvantages to this injection are that it may cause serum sickness or cancel some of the effect of a vaccine given to stimulate the production of the patient's own antibodies.

There are several vaccine preparations, some safer and more effective than others. In Britain, vaccine prepared by growing the virus in duck embryo is favoured and is given as a 14-day course of subcutaneous injections; these injections are usually given into the abdomen as there is a large area and the injections can be widely spaced. There is often localised reaction at the injection site and there will be severe general and local reactions in patients who are allergic to egg protein. Most individuals, including those at high risk of contracting the disease, laboratory workers preparing vaccines, workers in quarantine kennels or the team of hospital workers who will be caring for patients who have rabies, will be given this type of vaccine. It will also be given when a bite is thought to be infected by rabies virus (and this may be after every animal bite in countries where rabies exists).

As rabies encephalitis is a fatal condition it is imperative that the patient is given a full course of vaccination without delay in spite of the unpleasant side effects, but when the dog has been checked by the vet and if it is found not to have rabies, the hospital must be notified and anti-rabies vaccination can cease. A tissue culture vaccine prepared from animal or human cells is more effective in fewer doses than the duck embryo vaccine; it has been accepted by some countries, has only minor reactions, but is very costly to prepare and research continues to find an effective, but cheaper vaccine. Human serum antibodies can be acquired from vaccinated subjects and stored in a serum bank for future use with rabies victims.

During the incubation period patients who know of the threat of rabies are extremely anxious, feeling as though under sentence of death, they may even understandably develop hysterical symptoms of the disease. The vaccination programme will to some extent alleviate their anxiety.

The signs and symptoms which develop when the brain is attacked by the rabies virus are due to damage in the regions of the hypothalamus, limbic areas of the frontal lobes and the brain stem, and their connections with the pituitary gland and autonomic nervous system (Fig. 6.6). The functions and inter-relations of these areas are complex and concerned with emotional reactions, arousal, sexual arousal, temperature regulation, glandular activity, urine concentration, sweating, salivation and lacrimation. A much less common form of rabies is sometimes seen which appears as an ascending myelitis with progressive paralysis and respiratory failure.

Human rabies starts with a generalised 'flu-like illness when the patient feels unwell, has a fever, headache, loss of appetite, and aches and pains in his limbs; he may also develop nausea, vomiting, diarrhoea, stomach pain, sore throat and a cough. Abnormal sensations (paraesthesiae) at the site of a healed bite wound and increasing weakness and tremor of the affected limb follow or precede these symptoms and are grave early signs of the virus irritating the nervous system. After a day or two the patient becomes very tense and progressively more restless, apprehensive, agitated and hyperactive with insomnia or nightmares. He then shows all the characteristic features of rabies, hydrophobia (dread of water), excessive salivation, sudden choking spasm at each attempt to drink and violent retching, extreme agitation, expression of terror

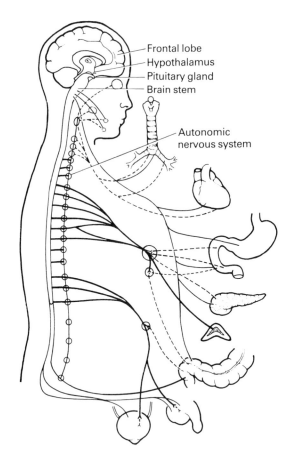

Frontal lobe
Hypothalamus
Pituitary gland
Brain stem

Autonomic
nervous system

Fig. 6.6 Parts of the nervous system affected by the rabies virus.

diaphragm and pharynx or viral destruction of the respiratory centres in the brain stem will ultimately cause respiratory arrest. Cardiac arrest will follow respiratory failure or result from damage to the vasomotor centres in the brain stem. This whole sequence of events takes from 7–10 days.

Once the virus has reached the central nervous system it passes into the bodily secretions and for about 7 days the patient is infectious. Though it is practically unknown for the rabies virus to be transmitted from person to person, none the less, because there is such horror attached to this fatal disease, it is wise for all members of the medical, nursing and ancillary team to be vaccinated. The effects of vaccination should be checked by assessment of the blood antibody level; unless this is satisfactory the individual cannot be accepted for the team. Ideally there should be a special centre where the staff are already protected by vaccination and there are facilities for intensive care and effective barrier nursing. It is possible that a patient with undiagnosed early rabies may be admitted to a general hospital ward or to a psychiatric unit. As soon as rabies is suspected arrangements should be made to isolate the patient and implement barrier nursing procedures; the patient may be transferred to a specialist unit. Immediately preparations should be made to brief all personnel who will come into contact with the patient, the ambulance crew, the porter who disposes of infected material, the nursing, medical and ancillary staff.

The importance of diagnosis is to confirm that the patient has rabies so that all known contacts can be vaccinated, and to differentiate from other forms of encephalitis which have very similar symptoms, but carry a much better prognosis.

and the whole body distorted by violent spasms which throw the arms into the air and arch the head and back into extreme opisthotonos. The patient is so gripped by terror that he feels compelled to escape and struggles furiously with anyone who tries to restrain him; these wild spasms last for a few minutes and occur many times a day. After a spasm the patient becomes calm and is often able to discuss his unpleasant experience. As the condition worsens the spasms become more frequent and severe and are brought on even by the thought of water, by a draught of cool air on the face or finally, without any obvious provocation. The patient becomes increasingly confused as the disease advances, has dramatic swings of excessively high or low temperatures, may have very marked diuresis or oliguria, becomes paralysed and loses consciousness. The intense spasms of the

Investigations

1   Samples are taken from those parts of the body where rabies virus may be found.
    (a)   Corneal smear – most commonly the virus can be isolated from the corneal cells.
    (b)   Specimens of saliva and sputum.
2   Blood samples are tested for rabies antibodies.
3   Lumbar puncture – the CSF is normal in many instances, but sometimes shows an increase in cells, mainly lymphocytes, and a slightly raised protein.

Nursing care

The aims should be to prevent infection being transmitted to any other person, to keep the patient comfortable by alleviating painful and distressing symptoms and, though the condition is said to be invariably fatal, to keep the patient alive by the use of all available life support systems, for as long as possible in the hope of recovery and in case the diagnosis of rabies is incorrèct.

Barrier nursing is essential. Nursing and medical staff must be completely in control of the situation from the beginning, to give the patient and his relatives confidence. The patient's awareness varies considerably and between periods of apparent unconsciousness he may have intervals when alert and lucid. Apart from sedatives, the greatest comfort to the patient will be knowing and having confidence in the team of nurses and doctors caring for him. Patients are very alert to every passing remark and will quickly sense staff anxiety, though the nurse's face is masked; the whole barrier nursing procedure adds to the patient's nightmare experience, for all who approach the bedside must wear operating theatre head-covering, gown, gloves, overshoes, mask and a complete perspex face shield which protects the nurse's eyes from droplet infection. Sedation will be necessary to alleviate the patient's hydrophobic spasms which, apart from distressing the patient, are very disturbing to witness especially if a nurse or relative realises they have been responsible for inducing the spasm by the slightest touch, thoughtless noise or reference to water. In the later stages of the illness heavy sedation may fail to control the spasms which occur even when the patient is unconscious. A quiet atmosphere is helpful and working surfaces should be covered with a cloth to reduce noise. Nursing care should be performed soon after sedation has been given. To reduce disturbance monitoring aids (electrocardiogram, central venous pressure line and electrical thermometer) should be used; intravenous fluids should be given and urine collected by an indwelling catheter and urinary drainage bag. Persistent excessive salivation and the necessity for frequent suction cannot be avoided though administration of atropine is helpful.

Relatives will need every consideration and explanation; they have a very short time to understand and accept the patient's condition, his distress and alarming behaviour, the mechanical apparatus needed in his care and his death within the week. They should have an opportunity to speak to the doctor and nurse in charge whenever they wish; the advisability of visiting the patient must be discussed. Relatives and all other contacts must have rabies vaccination.

Fungal and parasitic infections

Fungal and parasitic infections are so rare in the Western world that they will be mentioned here only briefly. The interval from primary infection to involvement of the central nervous system is variable. Diagnosis is often very difficult and the patient will undergo many investigations in an effort to trace the infecting organism which invades many organs of the body. Many of the conditions have a fatal outcome; specific treatments are available for some fungal and parasitic diseases, they are toxic and not necessarily curative. Steroid therapy may be given to reduce inflammation and oedema and should epilepsy develop, which is very common in some of the disorders, anticonvulsant therapy is essential to prevent status epilepticus.

7

Intracranial Tumours

The brain may be the site of primary or secondary tumours; primary brain tumours affect any age group and either sex, some are peculiar to childhood and others usually occur in middle age. They are single tumours, do not metastasise and are as various as the different structures of the brain. Primary brain tumours are classified as benign if they are encapsulated and slow-growing and such tumours develop in the meninges, cranial nerves, ventricular system, blood vessel walls and in the cranial endocrine glands. Primary brain tumours are described as malignant when they rapidly infiltrate the brain substance. These invasive brain tumours are due to abnormal proliferation of the neuroglia and arise in the cerebrum and cerebellum; curiously enough, tumours of the neurones themselves are extremely rare. Secondary brain tumours are multiple, malignant, metastasise from other organs and occur in the fifth and sixth decades of life.

Anatomical and functional localisation

Any expanding intracranial tumour disrupts local brain function, displaces intracranial structures, interferes with blood circulation and finally causes raised intracranial pressure. The signs and symptoms it produces are very varied as they depend upon the site of the tumour and the speed of its growth. Perhaps the simplest way to understand brain tumours is to consider them anatomically, from the scalp and skull through to the innermost structures of the brain.

Tumours of the scalp and skull

The scalp is always inspected carefully during any examination for evidence of neoplasia; simple lesions such as sebaceous cysts will be distinguished from the more important tumours of the skull, or the exostosis of a meningioma. Tumours of the skull, for example benign osteoma, and primary and secondary carcinoma, may not be apparent unless they produce an exostosis, involve other structures such as the orbit or nasopharynx, or become large enough to cause pressure on the brain and affect its function. The lesion will be visible on skull X-rays, but a CAT scan may be necessary to demonstrate the extent and involvement of deeper structures.

Tumours of the meninges

A **meningioma** is a benign slow-growing tumour of the meninges, which arises from the arachnoid mater and may invade the overlying dura mater and skull, forming an exostosis; it is very vascular, does not usually invade the brain, but takes up valuable space within the skull compressing cerebral tissue (Fig. 7.1). Meningiomas form only a small percentage of intracranial tumours, occurring in women more than men and occasionally found in children. They are mainly found in the frontal region, most commonly beneath the frontal lobes where they grow from the meninges covering the sphenoid bone and may surround cranial nerves, arteries and venous sinuses; frontal parasagittal meningiomas growing from the falx cerebri displace both cerebral hemispheres (Fig. 7.1). A few meningiomas grow over the vault, in the posterior fossa or in the ventricular system. Meningiomas may calcify and can then be seen on X-ray, they can be detected by a CAT scan and have a slow circulation which can be demonstrated by angiography. The use of a microscope during surgery enables the surgeon to operate with great accuracy, reducing the risk of nerve damage and postoperative haemorrhage. Such an operation may take many hours, but with improved anaesthesia this should not be an additional risk to the patient; closed circuit television allows other members of the operative team to watch the lengthy procedure. Radiotherapy is often necessary following surgery to ensure the destruction of any remaining tumour cells; the prognosis for meningioma is good.

Carcinomatous meningitis is a very rare untreatable condition in which a film of secondary deposits coats the meninges.

Tumours of brain tissue

The hemispheres of the cerebrum and cerebellum are composed of neurones and neuroglia (connective tissue). Tumours of the neuroglia (gliomas) develop from two types of glial cells (Fig. 7.2a) astrocytes and oligodendrocytes, forming **astrocytomas** and **oligodendrogliomas**, the former being the more common. As these are tumours of connective tissue they infiltrate the brain substance leaving no clear demarcation between tumour and normal brain tissue (Fig. 7.2b). Astrocytomas are graded according to the degree of malignancy. Grade I is a slow-growing, usually cystic cerebellar tumour, most commonly found in children, which has a favourable prognosis if totally removed. Grades II, III and IV (the latter sometimes referred to as **glio-**

blastoma) are more malignant and are found in the cerebral hemispheres; corpus callosum gliomas may involve both hemispheres. Infiltration into a large part of the cerebrum may have taken place before the patient shows any symptoms; complete surgical removal is impossible and the prognosis is poor. Oligodendrogliomas are slow-growing, localised, often calcified tumours which though apparently totally excised may recur several years later. Radiotherapy is given following excision of any type of glioma to try to achieve complete destruction of all remaining tumour cells, but unfortunately the tumour often recurs.

Carcinomatous metastases in the brain (Fig. 7.3) are composed of cells foreign to the brain, which have most commonly spread from malignant

(a)

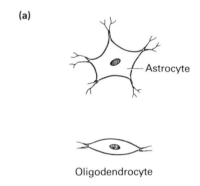

Astrocyte

Oligodendrocyte

(b)

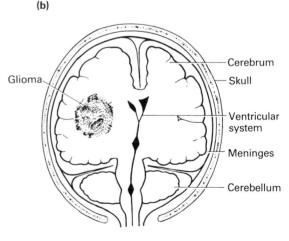

Fig. 7.2 **(a)** Neuroglial cells forming connective tissue. **(b)** Infiltrating glial tumour. Note there is no clear demarcation between the glioma and the healthy brain tissue.

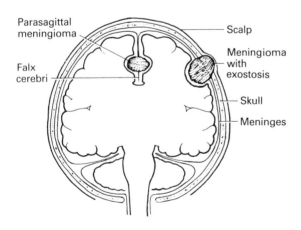

Fig. 7.1 Meningioma.

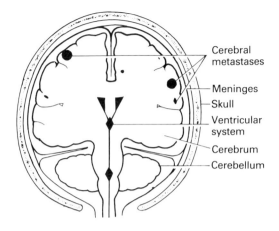

Fig. 7.3 Carcinomatous metastases.

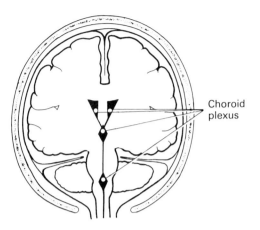

Fig. 7.4 Sites for choroid plexus papilloma.

tumours of the bronchi and breast, or less commonly from the stomach, prostate gland, thyroid gland and nasopharynx; metastases are suspected if a patient with neurological symptoms is known to have had primary carcinoma, but symptoms sometimes arise while the primary growth is asymptomatic and if a metastasis is examined histologically, the evidence will indicate the site of the primary growth, as the cells from the primary and secondary tumour are similar. Neurological evidence of more than one cranial lesion suggests metastatic tumours. Metastases are firm, well circumscribed tumours which usually form in the cerebral cortex or subcortical region, less commonly in the cerebellum. A CAT scan is helpful in confirming the presence of small lesions undetectable by other radiological investigations. Surgical treatment is unsatisfactory as it is impossible to excise several tumours from different parts of the brain, but if there is one large tumour causing unpleasant symptoms (e.g., nausea, vomiting and vertigo), palliative surgery may help the patient to spend the last months of his life in comparative comfort. Prostatic metastases may respond to treatment with stilboestrol.

Secondary deposits of malignant **melanoma** may be found in the brain; they are small pinhead-sized black specks, so numerous that the condition is untreatable.

Other tumours which involve the brain and require surgical excision are **tuberculoma** (see p. 102) which is now very rare in Britain, but occurs in countries where tuberculosis is common,

gumma, a complication of syphilis (see p. 310) and **parasitic cysts** (see p. 110).

Tumours in the ventricles

The ventricles are lined with ciliated ependymal cells; an **ependymoma**, a rare intraventricular tumour, usually occurs in the fourth ventricle. Within each ventricle is a system of capillaries (the choroid plexus see Fig. 4.3) which produces CSF. A **choroid plexus papilloma** (Fig. 7.4) which causes excessive production of CSF and may be associated with infantile hydrocephalus (see p. 79), is attached by a stem to the wall of the ventricle (lateral or third) and because of its mobility as it floats in the CSF may momentarily block the ventricular system. This will cause a rapid rise in the intraventricular pressure (hydrocephalic attack) with sudden severe headache, clouding of consciousness or even death, or a 'drop attack' when the patient falls limply to the ground without loss of consciousness. A **colloid cyst** which arises usually within the third ventricle, behaves in a similar manner. Meningiomas occasionally grow within the ventricles.

Intraventricular tumours, though they are benign and usually very small, are difficult to remove, being in the central core of the brain, near the hypothalamus and the centres of consciousness, respiration and heart action. Radiotherapy is necessary following surgery.

The **medulloblastoma** is a highly malignant tumour growing in the vermis of the cerebellum

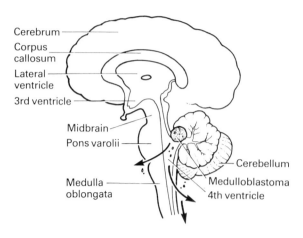

Cerebrum

Corpus callosum

Lateral ventricle

3rd ventricle

Midbrain

Pons varolii

Cerebellum

Medulla oblongata

Medulloblastoma

4th ventricle

Fig. 7.5   Medulloblastoma seeding into CSF pathways.

(Fig. 7.5) and invading the roof of the fourth ventricle; it seeds into the CSF and is therefore spread throughout the cerebrospinal fluid pathways. This tumour mainly affects young children and adolescents, in particular young boys. It is possible for the primary lesion in the fourth ventricle to be totally removed, but metastatic spread may have already taken place and surgery needs to be followed by irradiation of the entire CSF system in the brain and spinal cord. Though these tumours are very sensitive to radiotherapy, they sometimes recur.

Tumours of blood vessels

An **angioma**, a benign congenital tumour of blood vessels, may act as a space-occupying lesion or cause subarachnoid haemorrhage (see pp. 81, 134 and 264).

An **haemangioblastoma** is a rare tumour arising from the wall of a blood vessel. It is often cystic with a tumour nodule in the wall of the cyst and arises mainly on the surface of a cerebellar hemisphere; occasionally the tumour is solid and composed mainly of blood vessels. The cyst usually subsides when the tumour nodule is removed but surgery is difficult when the tumour is solid and very vascular. Polycythaemia may accompany the condition and subsides when the tumour is removed. The prognosis is good when there is a solitary lesion, but when the condition is familial there may be associated tumours in the retina, pancreas or kidney.

Tumours of cranial nerves

Tumours of the cranial nerves are rare.

An **optic nerve glioma** is a tumour of childhood which grows within the optic nerve enlarging the optic foramen (Fig. 7.6); vision in both eyes is affected if it spreads to the optic chiasma and the child will become blind if the tumour reaches the other optic nerve. Excision of the tumour will sacrifice sight in the affected eye though the eyeball itself is spared for cosmetic reasons. **Retinoblastoma**, a very rare, highly malignant tumour which occurs only in young children, affects both optic nerves and metastasises through the lymph glands to distant organs.

An **acoustic neuroma** (schwannoma) is a slow-growing tumour, seen mainly in older women; it arises in the region of the internal auditory meatus, eroding and enlarging the meatus and spreading into the cerebello-pontine angle (Fig. 7.6). The tumour causes deafness and is close to the facial nerve enveloping it as it grows, causing facial weakness and inability to close the eye and blink. Other neighbouring cranial nerves are gradually affected leading to sensory loss of the face and cornea (trigeminal nerve palsy), diplopia due to inability to turn the eye outwards (VIth nerve palsy), and dysphagia and dysphonia (IXth and Xth nerve palsies); the function of the cerebellum is also disturbed causing ataxia and loss of balance. When the tumour enlarges, compression of the pons varolii displaces the aqueduct of Sylvius and the fourth ventricle, and blocks the ventricular system resulting in hydrocephalus and raised intracranial pressure. Most of these symptoms will resolve when the tumour has been excised except unilateral deafness and facial weakness which may be permanent; the facial nerve is sometimes sacrificed to ensure total removal of the tumour. A permanent facial weakness may be partly cured by anastomosis of the damaged nerve to a branch of the hypoglossal or spinal accessory nerves. Acoustic neuroma may be bilateral and associated with neurofibromatosis (von Recklinghausen's disease – see Chapter 14).

Tumours of the endocrine glands

There are two endocrine glands in the skull, the pituitary gland and the pineal gland (Fig. 7.7). **Pinealoma** is extremely rare; the function of the pineal gland is unknown and the tumour obstructs the ventricular system.

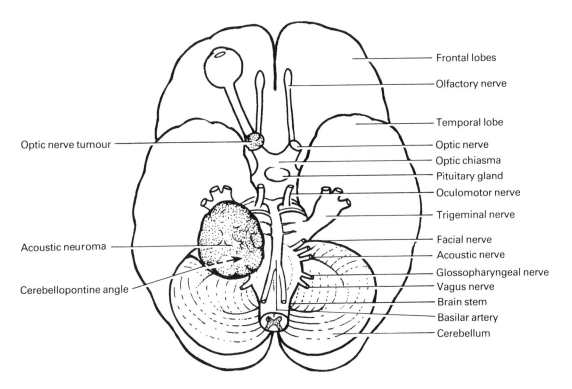

Fig. 7.6 Inferior view of the brain showing tumours of the acoustic (VIII) and optic (II) nerves.

The pituitary gland is the control centre of all the endocrine glands and is itself controlled by the hypothalamus. It lies at the base of the skull enclosed in the sella turcica (part of the sphenoid bone) and is surrounded by the arteries of the circle of Willis from which it receives its blood supply; above it lies the optic nerve chiasma (see Fig. 8.5). The pituitary gland is closely related to the ventricular system and the cavernous sinuses (see Figs 8.6 and 8.7) through which pass the cranial nerves which innervate the eyes and face; venous blood from the pituitary gland drains into the cavernous sinus. The gland consists of two lobes, the anterior lobe secretes hormones which stimulate secretions from all the other endocrine glands and the posterior lobe secretes pitressin, (the antidiuretic hormone which enables the kidney tubules to re-absorb water), and pitocin which causes uterine contractions.

The anterior lobe of the pituitary gland is the larger and is composed of three types of cell, acidophil, basophil and chromophobe. The exact

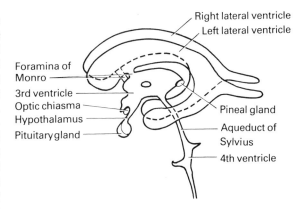

Fig. 7.7 Pituitary and pineal glands in relation to the ventricular system.

function of each cell is unknown, but is probably as follows.

1   Acidophilic (eosinophilic) cells secrete the growth hormone, and multiplication of these cells (tumour formation) causes an oversecretion producing gigantism in young people (before the epiphyses have hardened) or acromegaly in adults. These tumours are usually confined within the sella turcica and do not cause compression of the optic chiasma. Bitemporal headache is a symptom, probably caused by pressure within the sella turcica, which may resolve when the tumour ruptures the roof of the sella or following a course of radiotherapy.

2   Basophilic cells probably secrete the hormones which stimulate all the other endocrine glands. An increase in the number of these cells (a tumour) and in their function, leads to hyperpituitarism and will produce over-stimulation of the endocrine system, especially the adrenal glands, with symptoms of obesity, excessive growth of hair, purple striae of the abdomen, amenorrhoea in women and hypertension (Cushing's syndrome). These symptoms used to be treated by adrenalectomy though they are caused by a small pituitary tumour which only extends beyond the confines of the sella turcica to affect vision after 20 years or more. Adrenalectomy left the patient dependent on synthetic cortisone preparations for the rest of their life, without natural reserves to combat illness or shock and still with the possibility of further symptoms caused by the continued growth of the pituitary tumour. For these reasons the chosen treatment for a basophilic pituitary tumour is excision or radiotherapy.

3   Chromophobe cells are probably connective tissue, as they have no other known function. Tumours of these cells, **chromophobe adenoma** are of the utmost importance as they suppress the activity of the hormone-producing cells leading to hypopituitarism. This gives rise to hypogonadism (impotence in men, amenorrhoea in women, loss of libido, deficiency of body hair including the beard in men, and a reduction in 17-ketosteroid excretion), hypothyroidism which is unlike that of classical myxoedema (the patient does not have falling hair, coarse skin or an abnormal blood cholesterol) and adreno-cortical insufficiency with anaemia and hypoglycaemia. When the activity of

the hormone-producing cells of the pituitary gland is suppressed, the adrenal glands no longer receive sufficient stimulation; insufficient cortisone is produced and the patient has a low blood pressure. Any additional stress, infection, radiological investigation or surgery, cannot be met by an increased cortisone output and the patient will collapse extremely shocked. In addition to suppressing the hormone-producing cells, chromophobe adenoma enlarges beyond the confines of the sella turcica, causes pressure on the optic chiasma and needs to be removed or it will cause blindness. The pressure is often exerted on the centre of the chiasma producing a visual disturbance in both eyes (bitemporal hemianopia), but usually the vision in one eye is affected before that of the other. The lower fibres of the optic pathway are involved first and as these transmit visual impulses from the upper visual fields the disturbance, which may be very slight initially, is of the upper outer quadrant of vision (see Fig. 2.12). When a tumour is present early symptoms of visual and endocrine disturbance may pass unnoticed by the patient. Other symptoms depend on the size of the tumour and the direction in which it protrudes from the sella turcica; ocular nerve palsies occur as the result of pressure on the nerves as they pass through the cavernous sinus. Blood supply to the gland may be reduced if the tumour compresses the blood vessels from the circle of Willis; hydrocephalus and raised intracranial pressure develop if the ventricular system becomes obstructed.

Pituitary apoplexy occurs if there is sudden bleeding within the gland, an event which closely resembles subarachnoid haemorrhage both in its symptoms (sudden severe headache, rapid deterioration of vision, ocular palsies, mental confusion and even loss of consciousness) and in the possible presence of blood or xanthochromia in the CSF.

A chromophobe adenoma is usually surgically excised before a course of radiotherapy is given.

Congenital tumours
See Chapter 4

Signs and symptoms of intracranial tumour

The signs and symptoms of a brain tumour can be as various as the functions of the brain and may be spread over a very long period or compressed into a few weeks.

Tumours above the tentorium cerebelli

The following is an over-simplification of the function of the cerebral hemipheres; it is usual to attribute certain functions to particular areas of the brain, but it must be remembered that the brain functions as a whole and that each part is dependent on the others.

The most common supratentorial tumours are gliomas and secondary metastases, less common are meningiomas, pituitary and cranial nerve tumours.

A frontal lobe tumour may be silent for some time until mental changes are noticed (see p. 10), or the patient has a focal or generalised fit, or develops contralateral facial or limb weakness.

A parietal lobe tumour causes sensory disturbance in the contralateral limbs and face, and a distortion of the patient's own body image (a limb may feel enormous or the patient may not recognise a part of his body as his own, even though he sees it); there may be sensory epilepsy. There are silent areas of the parietal lobes whose functions are unknown; a tumour in one of these regions will be asymptomatic for some time.

A temporal lobe tumour gives rise to disturbance of behaviour (confusion, outbursts of irritability and sometimes even aggression), anosmia, deafness and pyschomotor epilepsy. The patient's ability to recognise an object by the sense of touch (stereognosis) is also impaired.

An occipital lobe tumour is rare, symptoms will be of visual disturbance (see p. 5).

Tumours in the dominant hemisphere cause dysphasia, a very valuable localising sign. The visual pathways pass through each cerebral hemisphere, any intracerebral space-occupying lesion is likely to affect these pathways producing an homonymous hemianopia (see Fig. 2.11).

When the pressure above the tentorium cerebelli rises to such an extent that there is nowhere left to accommodate the expanding brain, it will squeeze through the tentorial opening into the posterior fossa (uncal herniation – see Fig. 3.5).

Tumours below the tentorium cerebelli in the posterior fossa

The posterior fossa contains the cerebellum, brain stem and the origins of most of the cranial nerves; the cerebellum co-ordinates movement and maintains equilibrium, the brain stem contains all the pathways to and from the brain and the nuclei of the cranial nerves (in the medulla are the centres controlling heart action and respiration). The cranial nerves enable the patient to hear, taste, feel a speck of dust in the eye, cough and swallow (see Chapter 2).

Tumours within the posterior fossa will interfere with the functions of the cerebellum and the patient becomes inco-ordinated in his movements and loses his sense of balance. Cranial nerve involvement depends on the site of the tumour, whether the tumour is of the nerve (when it frequently affects several adjacent nerves), or whether it is in the cerebellum or brain stem. The signs of cerebellar and cranial nerve involvement are all on the same side as the tumour (ipsilateral).

When the pressure within the posterior fossa rises the contents are squeezed out, mainly through the foramen magnum, to compress the medulla and arrest respiration and heart action (medullary 'coning', see Fig. 3.5).

Tumour growth and raised intracranial pressure

A slow-growing tumour may reach a proportionately enormous size (the size of a tennis ball) before it causes obvious signs and symptoms because there is such gradual displacement of structures and the brain compensates remarkably. Mental change may be gradual and pass almost unnoticed until the patient acts in an unacceptable way, undressing or urinating in public or upsetting his family by disturbing behaviour. Limb weakness may be so slight that it only causes clumsiness and is attributed to rheumatism. An occasional 'blackout' may not have been investigated. Even a rapidly infiltrating tumour whose signs and symptoms appear to have been compressed into the space of a few weeks or months must have been present for very much longer to have spread throughout almost a whole hemisphere.

There comes a time when the patient's condition rapidly deteriorates and headache, unrelieved by simple analgesia, becomes a persistent feature, sometimes associated with vomiting. The enlarging tumour is stretching blood vessels and meninges, may be interfering with the venous drainage and CSF production and absorption, and is causing local ischaemia and oedema which will considerably increase the size of the lesion and its effects. Unless the patient receives treatment the intracranial pressure will unrelentingly increase and he will lose consciousness. Sudden rupture of fragile pathological blood vessels or rapid expansion of tumour cyst will cause a sudden and unexpected collapse.

For signs and symptoms of raised intracranial pressure see page 47.

Admission to hospital

A patient with neurological symptoms or who has had curious attacks, focal or generalised epilepsy (see Chapter 19) which suggest a possible brain tumour, will be referred to a neurologist for thorough examination and investigation. Early diagnosis is important to avoid the risk of irreversible brain damage due to raised intracranial pressure. The introduction of computerised axial tomography (CAT scan) which can be performed at an out-patient appointment has simplified the investigation of a cerebral tumour and saved the patient from the unpleasant procedure of air encephalography. When preliminary investigations have confirmed the presence of a brain tumour the patient will be admitted to hospital for further investigations and surgery. Most of the tumours of childhood are found in the posterior fossa and give rise to early signs of raised intracranial pressure and a child is always admitted to hospital urgently. Many patients with a short history of headache before the onset of rapidly advancing neurological signs are urgently admitted to hospital when a doctor's examination reveals papilloedema, an important early sign of raised intracranial pressure.

History and examination
(See Chapter 2)

A detailed general and neurological examination of a patient with suspected cerebral tumour will help to localise the lesion to a particular part of the brain; the doctor questions the patient and his relatives and probes deeply for information which will lead to a diagnosis. There is often a history of raised intracranial pressure with headache (made worse by coughing, straining or bending), the vision may become blurred, or there is sometimes

projectile or effortless vomiting especially in children. Urgent measures to relieve raised intracranial pressure (see p. 48) will take precedence over a detailed examination. It is vitally important to maintain a clear airway if the patient is unconscious or has respiratory complications as anoxia increases intracranial congestion and causes cerebral oedema.

The patient's general health, appearance, gait, posture and behaviour give valuable information. There are many helpful clues:

i   emaciation, skin pallor and discolouration suggest carcinoma;

ii   proptosis may be caused by tumours behind the eye;

iii skin lesions are associated with neurofibromatosis, melanoma and angiomata; and

iv   signs of endocrine disorder or neurosyphilis.

The doctor will feel the skull for abnormal lumps and will listen over the blood vessels for bruit. He will systematically examine the function of each cranial nerve and the motor and sensory functions of the whole body. Examination of the optic nerve with an ophthalmoscope gives vital information about raised intracranial pressure. Papilloedema, however slight, indicates oedema has been channelled along the optic nerve sheath from the brain (see Fig. 2.13); this important sign always leads to urgent investigation and treatment.

Investigations

It is important that the investigation of a patient with a suspected brain tumour is thorough; investigations proceed through a series of tests and radiological procedures described in detail in Chapter 2. The selection of investigations depends upon the condition of the patient and the suspected nature of the tumour, commencing with tests which are the least disturbing to the patient. Small deep-seated tumours are difficult to detect and careful follow-up and repeated investigations will be necessary.

There is always urgency to complete these tests as soon as possible, especially if the patient is unconscious. The nurse should always be aware that a patient with a brain tumour, though fully conscious on admission, may rapidly deteriorate even to the point of death.

Treatment

The aim of treatment is to completely remove or destroy the tumour without damaging healthy brain tissue; if the tumour is untreatable the aim is to try to improve the quality of the patient's life so that he passes his last few months comfortably and in his right mind. The physician needs to determine that the lesion is a tumour, locate its situation, discover the nature of the tumour (whether it is benign, encapsulated, infiltrating or malignant) and whether there are multiple lesions. This information is gained from the history, examination and radiological investigations. There is often consultation with other specialists; the advice of an endocrinologist may be necessary and an ophthalmologist will be asked to assess the patient's visual defect and advise regarding the need for urgent treatment to prevent irreversible blindness when there is a pituitary tumour. A patient with secondary intracranial carcinoma will be seen by a general or thoracic surgeon to assess the possibility of removing the primary growth. A patient with a suspected acoustic neuroma will be seen by an ear, nose and throat specialist who will perform caloric tests. When the surgeon has enough information about the tumour he will decide upon treatment. His choice lies between surgery for partial or complete removal of the tumour, palliative surgery to relieve hydrocephalus by the insertion of a ventriculo-peritoneal drain or Torkildsen's operation, radiotherapy or cytotoxic chemotherapy, a combination of surgery and radiotherapy or, a decision hard though it is to make, to do nothing at all. This latter decision can only be made when the tumour has been positively identified.

Slow-growing tumours give a good prognosis, but as the symptoms develop so slowly, possibly over a period of ten years or more, they may not be diagnosed until they have grown quite large. Infiltrating tumours give a bad prognosis, sometimes as little as a month or two, during which time the patient suffers distressing symptoms of raised intracranial pressure and paralysis before drifting into unconsciousness; dexamethasone will relieve the unpleasant symptoms of headache, nausea and vomiting by reducing cerebral oedema. When the drug is no longer benefitting the patient, its sudden withdrawal will cause a rapid peaceful decline and death within a day or two.

Nursing care

The patient with a brain tumour feels ill, has a headache, is nauseated, may have vomited, his tongue is furred, his mouth has an unpleasant taste and he is worried about the future, his work, his home and his family and is anxious about the results of tests. He may suspect that he has a tumour and be terrified of the implications having known or heard of someone who died of one, and he may be very fearful of going 'barmy' or becoming paralysed. Personality changes may already be apparent, the patient is bewildered, inattentive and unamenable to reason, aggressive, unco-operative (especially if he thinks there is nothing wrong with him) and annoyed at the need for seemingly unnecessary tests. There may be a fluctuating level of consciousness with periods of confusion and disorientation which are worse at night and in the unfamiliar surroundings of a hospital ward. Visual defects, deafness, dysphasia and curious sensory disabilities which interfere with the patient's recognition of his position in space and the reality of himself and his surroundings, can make communication with him extremely difficult, communication which is so essential for giving comforting reassurance and for gaining co-operation.

When the patient is admitted to hospital his condition must be assessed carefully by an experienced nurse to provide a basis for comparison. Patients should be encouraged to continue normal activities in the ward as far as they are able. The extremely ill patient who is very drowsy, dehydrated and weak will need skilful nursing care to improve his fluid intake and frequent observation of neurological condition, temperature, pulse, respiration and blood pressure. While the patient is undergoing special radiological investigations, observations must be continued vigilantly, especially after anaesthesia, when cerebral oedema and raised intracranial pressure may be increased by carbon dioxide retention and ischaemia. Recovery of consciousness following these investigations may be delayed by the patient's deteriorating neurological condition or an unobserved fit.

(For care of a patient with disturbance of consciousness, visual acuity, communication and movement see Chapter 3.)

When nursing patients who have disturbance of the pituitary gland due to a tumour it is essential that the functions of the gland should be well understood; it is then interesting to observe the effect of endocrine changes as well as those of a compressing intracranial space-occupying lesion. Changes in the patient's appearance and personality – with pale expressionless face, general apathy and slowness to respond, especially when there is no limb weakness or paralysis and the patient does not seem ill – do not arouse sympathy and may be irritating unless the cause is understood. There may be mental confusion when the tumour affects the frontal lobes or the blood chemistry is altered, and careful observation and supervision of all the patient's activities will be necessary. A patient with a low basal metabolic level feels the cold very keenly and should not be ridiculed if he wears many layers of clothing or asks for additional bed coverings; if hormone deficiency manifests itself as myxoedema, hypothermic coma is a risk in very cold weather. The hormone tests for pituitary insufficiency involve 24-hour urine collections which have to be recommenced should one specimen be accidentally thrown away. It should be remembered that the period of starvation prior to radiological tests or surgery may precipitate hypoglycaemia. Visual field defects should be taken into consideration when approaching the patient, taking care not to startle him, giving quiet explanation of medical and nursing procedures and placing things within his range of vision. Unless there is optic atrophy, visual disturbances usually recover quickly once the compressing tumour is removed.

Care following surgery

The patient should be nursed in an intensive care unit where resuscitation equipment is available. The nurse who is allocated to care for the patient must know his history and preoperative condition and it is helpful to know something of his family background.

Craniotomy
(See Fig. 7.8, and for postoperative care page 136.) A patient who has had a brain tumour removed will be allowed to sit up in a chair on the first postoperative day if his immediate recovery has been satisfactory, and thereafter will proceed to full mobility as soon as possible depending upon his disabilities.

When a pituitary tumour is to be removed a high dose preoperative injection of hydrocortisone is given with the premedication as the patient is unable to produce enough cortisone to combat the shock of surgery. Large doses of intramuscular hydrocortisone will also be necessary for a few days postoperatively. Very careful observation is necessary during the immediate postoperative period as the patient's blood pressure, electrolyte levels and conscious level may fluctuate dramatically, the patient being fully conscious and talking one minute and deeply unconscious the next. After a few days the hydrocortisone is given orally and at the end of a week a gradual reduction begins to a small maintenance dose or the drug is discontinued. Thyroid replacement therapy is also necessary. An accurate record of fluid intake and output must be kept, as the patient may suffer from diabetes insipidus postoperatively (see p. 95), it usually lasts only a few days but occasionally persists. Patients with disorders of the pituitary gland need much stimulation and throughout their

(a)
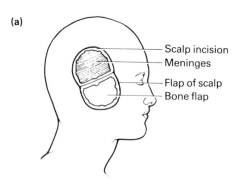

Scalp incision
Meninges
Flap of scalp
Bone flap

(b)
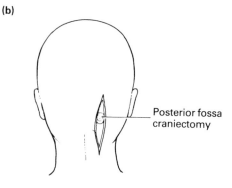

Posterior fossa craniectomy

Fig. 7.8 Cranial surgery. **(a)** Craniotomy. **(b)** Craniectomy.

stay in hospital efforts must be made to draw them into the community life in the ward, to encourage them to take meals with others at the table and join other patients in the day room. It should be realised that as restoration of hormone balance is a slow process, the patient will take several months to recover.

Posterior fossa craniectomy

On receiving the patient from the operating theatre, the nurse should find out details about the operation, any complications which have occurred and any special treatment which will be necessary. The nurse should appreciate that when the surgeon is operating, however carefully he manipulates the structures in the confined space of the posterior fossa, he may damage tissues causing oedema, ischaemia and possibly haematoma, which will compress the brain stem (medullary coning – see p. 38) and interfere with the function of the vital centres of swallowing, vomiting, respiration and cardiac function. It is because of this risk that the neurological assessment and record of vital functions (pulse, respirations and blood pressure) will be recorded quarter-hourly; the respiratory rate must always be counted for a full minute. The patient's respirations are an extremely important indicator of his well-being, they are often slow, but should be regular; should the respiratory rate fall to less than 10 per minute or develop an irregularity in rate or depth, the doctor must be informed immediately. The irregularity may be similar to Cheyne Stokes respirations, but there may be no definite pattern. Blood pressure levels may fluctuate markedly and the nurse should ascertain from the surgeon the acceptable upper and lower limits. It is likely that the patient will feel nauseated and may vomit; as the patient may also be dysphagic and risk inhalation pneumonia a prophylactic anti-emetic will be given. The patient may be conscious from the beginning. As soon as there is any sign of awareness, continual explanation and reassurance should be given distinctly and sympathetically; the nurse should face the patient while she is speaking as he may be deaf and already accustomed to lip-reading. The pupils are often small or pinpoint due to the unopposed action of the oculo-motor (III) nerve and the reaction to light will be very difficult to see. There may be cranial nerve palsies; when the ophthalmic branch of the trigeminal nerve is damaged, there will be loss of the corneal reflex and the eye must be protected by taping the eyelid closed (see p. 57) or using an eye bubble. Facial nerve weakness makes speech indistinct and distresses the patient if he cannot be understood; weakness of the glossopharyngeal and vagus nerves lead to dysphagia and difficulty in coughing or expelling vomitus, and suction is needed. It must be remembered, when testing the limbs, that the cerebellum controls the ipsilateral side of the body.

The first 24 hours of the postoperative period are the most crucial as the patient's condition is precarious. The quarter-hourly chart must be continued and the nurse must be alert and ready to summon the doctor if the patient's condition suddenly deteriorates; the patient may be alert and conscious one minute and within minutes, unconscious and near to death.

During the postoperative period the patient is usually nursed in the sitting position and should be well-supported with pillows (Fig. 7.9). Wound pain is often quite severe and an intramuscular analgesic (codeine phosphate) will be prescribed 4–6 hourly (morphine and pethidine are never given because they cloud the level of consciousness and affect the pupil reaction). Care should be taken that the wound is relieved of direct pressure and that the patient's head is carefully supported and his neck kept in alignment with his body. The wound dressing is inspected at frequent regular

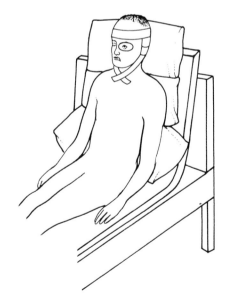

Fig. 7.9 Upright nursing position following posterior fossa craniectomy. Note eye bubble used to protect the eye.

intervals for seepage and may need additional packing. The patient must be turned slightly from side to side at 2-hourly intervals during the immediate postoperative period, being moved carefully by at least two nurses. Though the patient will find it painful, this is a useful opportunity to encourage deep breathing and coughing and suction should be used if necessary. Respiratory infection is likely because the operation is near the respiratory centre, the patient has had an anaesthetic, his cough may be feeble and respirations shallow; it is a very serious complication which might easily cause death, but with skilled nursing care can be avoided.

An intravenous infusion is set up preoperatively and continued for approximately 48 hours (dextrose and/or saline); for the first 12 hours nothing is given by mouth. The patient's mouth should be inspected and cleaned thoroughly every 2 hours; he is prone to develop a dirty mouth owing to weakness and sensory loss on one side of the face and secretions and vomit which cannot be expelled, collect in the throat and mouth unless effective suction is used.

The patient may be sluggish to respond to verbal requests and painful stimuli due to akinesis; if his condition is otherwise satisfactory, the nurse should not unnecessarily badger him nor inflict excessive painful stimuli.

After approximately 12 hours when the patient's condition has stabilised, the nurse will make observations about the patient's ability to swallow, to decide whether the patient is able to commence oral fluids. An experienced nurse should be present when the first sips of fluid are given in case the patient chokes and inhales the fluid. Only a very small amount of water should be given and though he manages on this occasion nurses should remain vigilant, as the patient may have occasional episodes of dysphagia. It is important that he is always in a comfortable upright position before taking a drink, as his swallowing ability will be severely handicapped if his chin is on his chest. The intravenous infusion will be continued until the patient is able to take adequate oral fluid – usually no longer than 48 hours. Should oral fluid intake continue to be insufficient, intragastric fluids may be given as a supplement, or if the patient is unconscious or completely dysphagic, as a full regime of 3-hourly feeding. When the patient's general condition improves, a further attempt must be made to give oral fluids and diet and every effort made to create the right conditions and give the patient confidence; it may be easier for the patient to swallow semi-solid substances than fluids, for example liquidised foods.

Within three or four days of operation, the patient will begin to sit out of bed and gradually increase his activities. He will need reassurance that the giddiness and unsteadiness he experiences when he first gets up is not unusual. He should not do too much too soon; each time the patient tries to walk it demands great concentration and effort which is exhausting. It is far better that he has several short spells in a chair with periodic short walks, than that he has one exhausting burst of activity and spends the rest of the day slumped wearily in a chair. Ataxia may be very severe at first and often two people are necessary to support the patient, (at this stage a walking frame is a useless aid). Patience and perseverance are needed for a long time, while nerve tissue recovers or retraining enables the patient to be fully independent.

Radiotherapy and cytotoxic chemotherapy

Those who are to undergo a course of radiotherapy or chemotherapy for treatment of cerebral tumour are admitted to a special unit. The patient will already have undergone preliminary investigations, identification of the tumour and in some instances surgical removal of part, or what appeared to be the whole, tumour.

Radiotherapy is a useful form of treatment which arrests the multiplication of malignant cells, destroys tumour cells and can be curative. Great care is taken to safeguard healthy brain tissue from exposure to the rays by preparing an individual plastic mask which directs the beam to the exact treatment area on every occasion.

The plan of treatment and its probable duration should be explained to the patient and his next-of-kin. They should be warned that the treatment will cause the patient's hair to fall out; some patients arrange to purchase a wig or obtain one through the National Health Service. The patient should be warned that he may feel tired and unwell during treatment; if he is not warned, he may be very disappointed that he feels worse than he did following his operation or before he began treatment.

The patient's activities are limited as little as possible during a course of radiotherapy, which lasts no more than one or two minutes daily on five days of each week for about six weeks. If the patient is well enough he will be more comfortable up and dressed and spending his time in the day-room or garden and will be able to spend weekends at home when home conditions permit. Occupational therapy and physiotherapy are continued unless the treatment is causing such intense fatigue or other unpleasant side effects that it is reasonable for the patient to rest in bed. However, a watchful eye must be kept that the patient does not take to his bed unnecessarily, as some patients are apathetic, lethargic and depressed and need encouragement. Throughout this form of treatment the morale of patients, staff and relatives must be maintained in every possible way, e.g. pleasant surroundings, good food and flexible visiting hours.

The nursing care will be adapted to the patient's needs; the problems most commonly met are those concerned with skin care and nutrition. The irradiated skin area must not be washed until two weeks after treatment has ceased nor must any other application be used, for the skin may break down; patient and relatives must be aware of this risk and a careful watch must be kept if the patient is confused. Should the skin become red and sore in spite of precautions, the doctor may prescribe an application of calamine and tannic acid; as this contains no metal component it does not interrupt treatment. Patients who are emaciated, whose blood chemistry is disordered or who spend much of the day in bed are at great risk of pressure sores and preventative measures must be taken. Nausea and vomiting sometimes occur but may be relieved by antiemetic drugs; metoclopramide (Maxolon) is particularly effective. A patient who has lost his appetite, has nausea and vomiting will need a light, nourishing and nicely flavoured, attractively served diet with extra fluids between meals.

The results of radiotherapy depend on several factors; as would be expected the earlier the tumour is diagnosed and the lower the grade of malignancy the better the results. In addition certain tumour cells are more radiosensitive than others. Sometimes, though the tumour recurs, treatment may relieve the patient of intolerable symptoms in the terminal stages of his illness.

Systemic cytotoxic chemotherapy is thought to select and destroy malignant cells and these drugs are given in combination with other forms of treatment, including radiotherapy. The patient will feel unwell during treatment.

Regular weekly blood counts are necessary during both forms of treatment and will be repeated more frequently if the results are abnormal; a blood transfusion may be necessary. Involvement of the bone marrow further disturbs the blood picture.

Interviews with relatives

The patient's relatives are seen by the medical officer when he is first admitted to hospital and at this time the doctor will prepare them for the procedures and investigations which are to follow and may be able to discuss the subject of brain tumour so that they are aware of the various possibilities of treatment and prognosis. The sooner the relatives are brought into the picture the better. Explanation needs to be clear and simple; almost any medical facts can be expressed so that a layman can understand them if patience, thought and a certain amount of time are taken. Time taken at this stage is well spent and a relative who is satisfied that everything possible is being done spreads a more tranquil, accepting attitude to the patient and other relatives and friends who visit him. When tests and investigations are completed the results should be discussed with the patient's next-of-kin as soon as possible, even if they are inconclusive. When a definite diagnosis has been made and treatment planned, there should be discussion with the patient and his relatives. They should be told about the operation or treatment and discussion should continue at intervals during rehabilitation and before the patient is discharged from hospital or transferred for care during the terminal stages of the illness.

When the patient's condition is deteriorating persistently in spite of treatment, relatives will be less alarmed if they know approximately what to expect at each stage and realise that the patient will have treatment or medication to relieve suffering throughout the course of the illness. The medical officer and a senior member of the nursing staff must always be available to answer questions and must not avoid such interviews because they are distressing, because they do not know what to say, or feel ashamed that their hospital cannot give curative treatment or for any other reason.

8

Intracranial Vascular Disorders

Brain cells need oxygen to survive and if they are completely deprived for more than three or four minutes, they will die. The cells also need glucose; these two essential elements are supplied by normal blood cells and blood chemistry, and a constant blood flow which is maintained by normal heart action, blood pressure and blood vessels. Circulatory impairment, whatever the cause, will lead to inefficiency of the brain which may affect consciousness, reasoning, judgement, memory or mood and impair the power of movement, co-ordination and sensation of any part of the body, depending on whether the disturbance is localised or widespread. Circulatory disturbance sometimes irritates brain cells causing an epileptic discharge.

Vascular disturbance may be sudden and catastrophic or insidious; haemorrhage disrupts and destroys cells and fibres whereas ischaemia leads to infarction and necrosis. A small lesion affecting a vital blood vessel can have disastrous widespread consequences whereas, by comparison, a large lesion in one cerebral hemisphere will cause paralysis in only one half of the body and in time the patient may recover. The patient's symptoms and disability will depend upon how much brain tissue is irreparably damaged, how much will in time recover given the right conditions, which functions of the damaged part can be undertaken by other healthy neurones and whether the cause of the circulatory disturbance is likely to persist or recur.

The incidence of cerebrovascular disease increases with age; after the age of fifty, in the presence of atherosclerosis, hypertension or hypotension, the cerebral circulation is often affected. The changes in the cerebral blood vessels may be present for many years before they cause symptoms, there may be continued gradual deterioration, or intermittent or sudden 'stroke'. The

risks of ill-health caused by obesity and the value of early recognition and treatment of hypertension, heart disease, diabetes mellitus and syphilis are known by laymen and medical practitioners alike; treatment of these conditions will reduce the risk of cerebral complications.

The outlook for someone who has suffered a 'stroke' has improved as, except in extreme old age accompanied by general ill-health, the patient may have many years of active useful life ahead, even after quite a severe 'stroke', if he receives the right

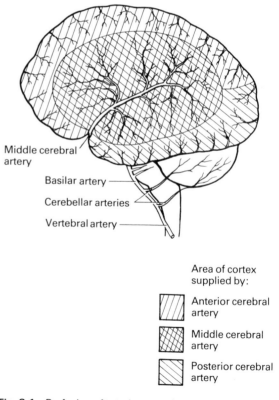

Middle cerebral artery

Basilar artery

Cerebellar arteries

Vertebral artery

Area of cortex supplied by:

Anterior cerebral artery

Middle cerebral artery

Posterior cerebral artery

Fig. 8.1 Profusion of arteries over the cortex of the brain.

treatment and early, well-planned rehabilitation. This is in contrast to the attitudes of a few decades ago when following a 'stroke' the patient was resigned to remaining in bed and being waited on 'hand and foot', leading a miserably restricted life for several years, outliving his spouse and causing his family much work, fatigue and curtailment of freedom.

Anatomy and physiology

The brain is unable to store nutrients and must therefore receive chemicals and glucose in a form ready for use by the neurones; oxygen, carried by the haemoglobin, is essential for the oxidisation of glucose. The health of the neurones is dependent upon a constant flow of nutrients to the cell bodies and as these are predominantly in the cortex of the brain (grey matter) it is here that a profusion of blood vessels pass over the entire surface, dipping into the cortex to supply the highly convoluted surface area (Fig. 8.1). Other blood vessels pass through the brain substance to supply the basal ganglia, cranial nerve nuclei and other nuclei at the base of the brain and in the brain stem.

Blood rich in nutrients is pumped from the heart via the aorta, innominate artery and subclavian arteries to the common carotid and vetebral arteries in the neck. The common carotid arteries divide at the angle of the jaw to become the internal and external carotid arteries (Fig. 8.2). The external carotid arteries supply the external parts of the head, the face, scalp, skull and dura mater. The internal carotid arteries enter the skull to supply blood to the brain; they pierce the petrous temporal bones of the skull, pass through the cavernous sinuses just behind each eye, give off the ophthalmic arteries (one to each eye) and then pass through the meninges to enter the subarachnoid space where each internal carotid artery divides into the anterior and middle cerebral arteries. The anterior cerebral arteries carry blood to the medial parts of the frontal and parietal lobes (Figs 8.1 and 8.3)

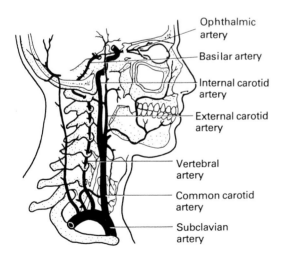

Ophthalmic artery

Basilar artery

Internal carotid artery

External carotid artery

Vertebral artery

Common carotid artery

Subclavian artery

Fig. 8.2 Blood supply to the brain.

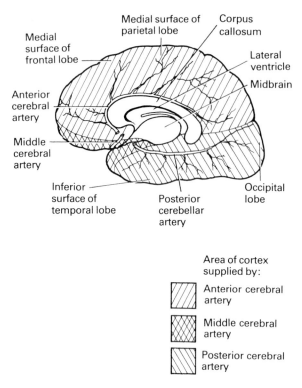

Medial surface of parietal lobe

Corpus callosum

Medial surface of frontal lobe

Lateral ventricle

Midbrain

Anterior cerebral artery

Middle cerebral artery

Inferior surface of temporal lobe

Posterior cerebellar artery

Occipital lobe

Area of cortex supplied by:

Anterior cerebral artery

Middle cerebral artery

Posterior cerebral artery

Fig. 8.3 Sagittal section showing arterial supply to medial and inferior surfaces of the cerebral cortex.

lobes and the under surfaces of the temporal lobes (Figs 8.1 and 8.3).

A small anterior communicating artery links the two anterior cerebral arteries, and the anterior and posterior cerebral circulations are united by the two posterior communicating arteries, creating the circle of Willis (Figs 8.5 and 8.12) which provides a cross-flow of blood (collateral circulation). Many small arteries (perforating arteries) leave the circle of Willis and pass into the brain to supply the hypothalamus, pituitary gland and other vital structures. The circle of Willis lies in the subarachnoid space beneath the cerebral hemispheres, above the tentorium cerebelli and immediately in front of the brain stem; it is closely related to the pituitary gland and optic chiasma.

The arteries divide into arterioles and capillaries, forming a network of vessels over the whole surface of the brain in the subarachnoid space. Venous capillaries carrying deoxygenated blood from the cortex, pass through the pia mater, enter the subarachnoid space and form a similar network. After passing through the arachnoid mater and inner layer of dura mater they enter the venous sinuses which are spaces formed between the two layers of dura mater (Fig. 8.6).

The system of venous sinuses returns the blood to the heart for reoxygenation. The superior sagittal sinus, which is also responsible for the reabsorp-

and the middle cerebral arteries to the lateral parts of the temporal, parietal and frontal lobes (Fig. 8.1). Small thread-like branches of the middle cerebral artery pass through the brain to the basal ganglia (Fig. 8.4).

The two vertebral arteries are given off by the subclavian arteries (Fig. 8.2) and pass upwards from the clavicular region through the foramina of the transverse processes of the cervical spine to supply blood to the posterior part of the brain. They are long arteries, with slightly tortuous loops at the base of the skull (to allow movement of the head and neck without undue stretching) and on passing through the foramen magnum they wind round the brain stem to unite at the front as the basilar artery. Small but vitally important arteries branch from the vertebral and basilar arteries to supply blood to the brain stem nuclei and cerebellum. At the upper end of the brain stem the basilar artery divides into the two posterior cerebral arteries which supply blood to the occipital

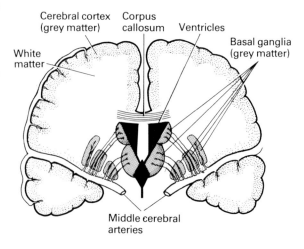

Cerebral cortex (grey matter)

Corpus callosum

Ventricles

Basal ganglia (grey matter)

White matter

Middle cerebral arteries

Fig. 8.4 Middle cerebral arteries in the Sylvian fissures supplying the basal ganglia.

tion of cerebrospinal fluid (see p. 70), arises at the base of the frontal bone (just behind the nose) and passes in the upper border of the falx cerebri to the occipital region. At the unification of the falx cerebri and tentorium cerebelli it becomes the right transverse sinus, which lies beneath the occipital bone in the tentorium cerebelli. The right transverse sinus leaves the skull through the jugular foramen where it becomes the right jugular vein, pouring venous blood back into the right atrium of the heart (Fig. 8.6). The inferior sagittal sinus in the lower border of the falx cerebri, after curving over the dividing partition of the lateral ventricles

(septum pellucidum) joins the straight sinus at the unification of the falx cerebri and tentorium cerebelli (Fig. 8.7). The straight sinus unites with the superior sagittal sinus, and becomes the left transverse sinus, pouring venous blood into the left jugular vein and thence into the right atrium of the heart. At the base of the skull is a network of small sinuses (cavernous, sphenoid, petrosal sinuses and basilar plexus) draining blood from the eyes, nose, ears, mastoid processes, pituitary gland, the inferior parts of the cerebrum, cerebellum and brain stem. These sinuses unite to drain into the transverse sinuses and the jugular veins.

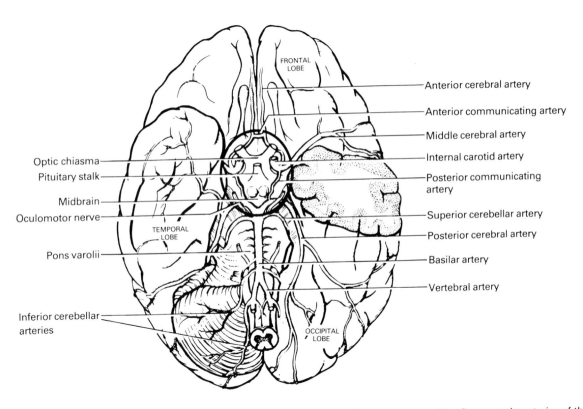

Fig. 8.5 The circle of Willis. Arteries enclosed within the bold ring just above the centre of the figure are the arteries of the circle of Willis.

Causes of cerebrovascular accident

Cerebral haemorrhage Haemorrhage may be arterial, capillary or venous, it may be in the subarachnoid space or in the brain, or burst from one to the other. Haemorrhage is caused by:

i hypertension associated with arteriosclerosis or a vascular anomaly;

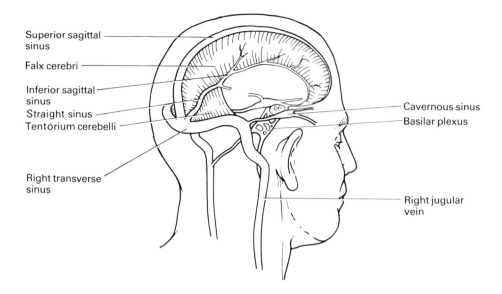

Superior sagittal sinus

Falx cerebri

Inferior sagittal sinus

Straight sinus

Tentòrium cerebelli

Right transverse sinus

Cavernous sinus

Basilar plexus

Right jugular vein

Fig. 8.6   The venous sinuses.

ii   aneurysm;

iii   arterio–venous malformation (angioma, see pp. 81, 134, and 264);

iv   certain cerebral tumours; fragile pathological blood vessels suddenly rupture;

v   drugs, e.g. anticoagulants and monoamine oxidase inhibitors;

vi   blood dyscrasias, e.g. haemophilia.

Cerebral ischaemia   Ischaemia is caused by any interruption in normal blood flow, or serious reduction or abnormality of the red blood cells. It may be due to:

i   hypotension, e.g. syncope and Stokes–Adams attack;

ii   anoxia associated with heart and lung diseases, respiratory obstruction and cardiac arrest;

iii   blood disorders, e.g. anaemia or polycythaemia;

iv   systemic disease which damages the arteries, e.g. diabetes mellitus and renal disease;

v   compression or stretching of cerebral blood vessels by space-occupying lesions;

vi   narrowed atheromatous cerebral arteries;

vii   partial or complete circulatory obstruction to part of the brain caused by:

(a)   cerebral thrombosis;

(b)   cerebral embolus from a diseased cerebral artery or carried in the circulation from another part of the body, e.g. a fat embolus from a fractured femur; or

(c)   cerebral arterial spasm which narrows a blood vessel, this may be caused by hypertension or accompany subarachnoid haemorrhage.

History and examination
(See also Chapter 2)

All patients who have had a cerebrovascular accident need a very detailed examination; 'stroke' takes many forms, may involve any part of the brain and there are a number of contributing conditions. An accurate history of the events leading to the present illness must be obtained from the patient if he is conscious, and from a reliable witness. Particular enquiry should be made into any past event which might have been a vascular incident, the family history, history of heart

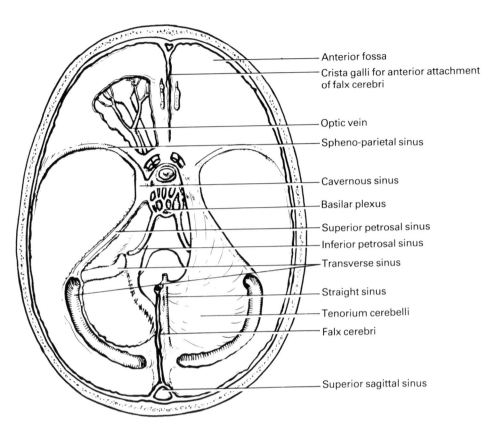

Anterior fossa

Crista galli for anterior attachment of falx cerebri

Optic vein

Spheno-parietal sinus

Cavernous sinus

Basilar plexus

Superior petrosal sinus

Inferior petrosal sinus

Transverse sinus

Straight sinus

Tenorium cerebelli

Falx cerebri

Superior sagittal sinus

Fig. 8.7   The venous sinuses of the base of the skull.

disease, hypertension and diabetes mellitus and whether they have been treated, if the patient has habitually suffered from headaches or migraine and whether there have been blackouts or fits, whether any drug treatment had been prescribed (including the contraceptive pill), whether there has been any change in mood or behaviour and if there were any factors which seemed to precipitate the illness. The witness may also know whether the patient's conscious level has improved or deteriorated from the onset of this illness until the present time.

General examination will include inspection for surface naevi of the head and face which may be communicating with or suggest an intracranial angioma, evidence of head injury which may have been sustained when the patient collapsed, or signs of a blood dyscrasia. Auscultation will be performed over the head and neck in a search for bruits, and the major blood vessels in the neck will be palpated; the cardiac and respiratory systems will be carefully examined.

Neurological examination will reveal many and various adverse signs which assist diagnosis, though they are sometimes misleading in localising the site of haemorrhage, haematoma or occluded vessel unless they are interpreted in conjunction with other tests and X-rays. The signs are also important for assessment and comparison; there is usually some alteration in the level of consciousness, but following ischaemic 'stroke' there is rarely complete loss of consciousness. Deterioration in the patient's conscious level and mental state indicate rising intracranial pressure. The ocular fundi commonly show hypertensive changes (exudates and retinal haemorrhages) and there may be papilloedema. There may also be aphasia or dysphasia, visual field defects (hemianopia), cranial nerve palsies and hemiparesis or hemiplegia with both motor and sensory disturbance. Other symptoms associated with brain stem and cerebellar disturbance are dysarthria, nystagmus and ataxia.

Investigations

1 Blood tests
(a) Full blood count, Wassermann reaction and Kahn test. Contributing conditions may be discovered, e.g. anaemia and syphilis
(b) Blood sedimentation rate – this will be higher than normal if there is arteritis
(c) Blood urea – this will be raised when there is kidney disease associated with hypertension
(d) Electrolyte levels
(e) Blood cholesterol

2 Lumbar puncture. This procedure is necessary to confirm subarachnoid haemorrhage; though the CSF pressure is extremely high immediately after haemorrhage, over 600 mms of water, lumbar puncture is permissible unless there is papilloedema; the raised pressure is due to the increased volume of subarachnoid fluid (blood and CSF) and not to a blockage in the CSF pathways. Lumbar puncture will reduce the intracranial pressure and to some extent relieve headache when some of the irritating blood-stained fluid is withdrawn. Three

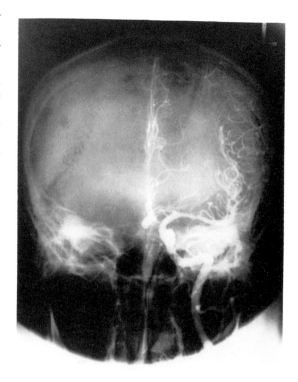

Fig. 8.9 Carotid angiogram showing anterior communicating aneurysm.

consecutive specimens of CSF should be obtained and if lumbar puncture is performed soon after haemorrhage, all three will be equally and obviously blood-stained. After a few days the CSF will be xanthochromic due to the breakdown of red cells; xanthochromia persists for 2–3 weeks. When a xanthochromic specimen is allowed to stand, red cells will settle and will be seen by the naked eye; for up to 9 days they will be found by laboratory testing. The protein content and white cell count will be slightly increased. When a primary intracerebral haemorrhage has ruptured into the subarachnoid space or ventricular system, red cells are present in the CSF. When there has been cerebral infarction following cerebral thrombosis or embolism the CSF may be normal or there may be xanthochromia and a raised protein level and white cell count.

3 Skull X-rays may show displacement of the pineal gland indicating a space-occupying lesion (haematoma, oedema or a large unruptured aneurysm); very rarely an aneurysm calcifies and can be seen on X-ray.

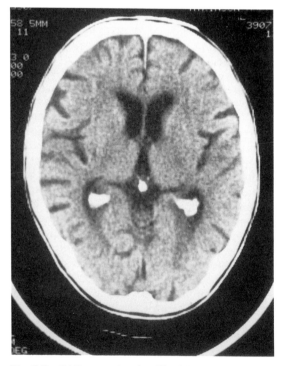

Fig. 8.8 CAT scan showing blood in the ventricles and subarachnoid space.

4 Chest X-rays may show pulmonary lesions or cardiac enlargement caused by hypertension which contraindicate the use of general anaesthesia for radiological investigations.

5 A CAT scan can differentiate between a haematoma and the generalised swelling caused by vascular spasm and its resulting oedema; it may localise a large aneurysm acting as a space-occupying lesion, reveal a tumour or angioma, demonstrate an area of infarction, or suggest the side on which a haemorrhage originated (Fig. 8.8).

6 Angiography is the most conclusive investigation as it demonstrates the condition of the blood vessels (Fig. 8.9). It is particularly helpful when there has been subarachnoid haemorrhage; bilateral angiography is always necessary as aneurysms are often multiple.

7 Electroencephalogram. When angiography has demonstrated multiple aneurysms, this test may help to determine which aneurysm has bled.

8 Electrocardiogram. This is used to determine the efficiency of the heart and exclude myocardial infarct.

9 Intravenous pyelogram may be necessary to examine the condition of the kidneys if the patient is hypertensive.

Cranial haemorrhage

Cerebral haemorrhage more often affects men than women, though subarachnoid haemorrhage is more common in women; there is a familial incidence. It is very much more common after the fifth decade when it is usually due to the effects of hypertension and atherosclerosis.

Intracerebral haemorrhage

The walls of the intracerebral arteries are often weakened by sclerotic changes thought to be partly caused by hypertension. Branches of the middle cerebral arteries are most commonly affected and bleeding is usually into the brain substance, but may leak into the subarachnoid space. The haemorrhage begins in the external capsule (Fig. 8.10), is large and forceful, causes severe cerebral oedema, compresses surrounding brain tissue especially the internal capsule, and disrupts the function of the whole cerebral hemisphere, even exerting pressure on the other cerebral hemisphere. The haematoma usually remains confined in the cerebrum, but may burst into one of the lateral ventricles where it may clot and cause sudden hydrocephalus and death, or rupture into the subarachnoid space where it may clot or be dispersed into the CSF. The intracerebral haematoma is gradually absorbed until only a neuroglial scar or

a cavity containing yellow serous fluid remains; sometimes another massive haemorrhage occurs which is rapidly fatal.

Haemorrhage into the cerebellum is very much less common, but because it occurs in the posterior fossa the condition is much more critical; unless the haematoma is removed the patient will die.

The patient may have had little warning of impending collapse; he may have had a headache and felt slightly 'off colour' during the day, prompting him to lie down, within a few hours a

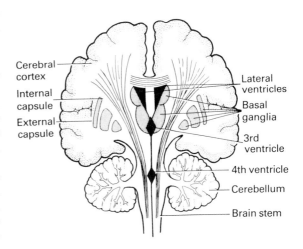

Fig. 8.10 The external and internal capsules.

dramatic deterioration will follow and the general practitioner will make a diagnosis of cerebrovascular accident and arrange for urgent admission to hospital. On arrival the patient, who may be florid, obese and hypertensive, is often in an extreme state of collapse with advanced signs of intracranial disturbance; he may be deeply unconscious or very drowsy, possibly aphasic and usually hemiplegic with dilated, unequal, sluggish or unreactive pupils, stertorous respirations, slow pulse and raised blood pressure.

Treatment

Measures to reduce raised intracranial pressure are essential and dramatic improvement may be seen after the administration of mannitol and dexamethasone. The blood pressure recordings will be watched carefully and the doctor will decide when a known hypertensive patient should resume anti-hypertensive therapy. Other patients whose blood pressure is persistently high will need investigations to check kidney and adrenal function to eliminate the possibility of treatable renal conditions and phaeochromocytoma before anti-hypertensive therapy is commenced.

Surgical removal of an intracerebral space-occupying haematoma is not the first choice of treatment because the patient is often elderly, obese, hypertensive, arteriosclerotic, a bad surgical and anaesthetic risk, and surgery will destroy more brain tissue and increase cerebral oedema. Most patients show some signs of recovery within ten days of the haemorrhage due to natural resolution of the haematoma and subsidence of cerebral oedema. Deterioration in the patient's condition in spite of measures to reduce intracranial pressure, or failure to make any improvement within ten days, suggests the need for surgical intervention.

The patient must receive physiotherapy and speech therapy as soon as possible if he is to regain his independence and powers of verbal communication and must have an intensive course of rehabilitation.

Subarachnoid haemorrhage

The networks of cerebral arteries and veins previously described, lie in the subarachnoid space and should one of these vessels rupture it will cause sub-

arachnoid haemorrhage. Haemorrhage is most commonly due to rupture of an aneurysm on the arterial circulation, less commonly rupture of an arterio–venous malformation or very rarely the result of haemorrhagic disease or anticoagulant therapy; occasionally the cause is not discovered. Bleeding from a vascular anomaly, partly buried in the brain substance, may cause an intracerebral haematoma as well as a subarachnoid haemorrhage. Subarachnoid haemorrhage, which usually affects women more than men between the ages of 30–45 years, occurs either when the individual is at rest or following strenuous activity. The symptoms and signs of subarachnoid haemorrhage are due to a sudden increase in intracranial pressure and severe irritation of the meninges by blood in the CSF. When the blood vessel ruptures there is usually sudden very severe headache of bursting intensity followed by collapse and possible loss of consciousness; the haemorrhage may be so severe that the victim dies soon after. Nausea and vomiting are common symptoms and the patient is photophobic, irritable and resentful of interference. Neck stiffness and a positive Kernig's sign develop 24–48 hours after the haemorrhage and the patient will complain of pain in the nape of the neck, lumbago or sciatica, caused by meningeal irritation. There is usually moderate pyrexia and tachycardia; the blood pressure is often high at first, but this is not always indicative of hypertensive disease and may settle within a few days. Mild glycosuria is common for a few days after subarachnoid haemorrhage. Localising signs will be seen if there is arterial spasm, cerebral ischaemia, oedema or an intracerebral haematoma. An epileptic fit may occur at any time during the illness and if it passes unobserved the ensuing unconsciousness may be wrongly attributed to another haemorrhage. When there has been severe subarachnoid haemorrhage the patient will be deeply unconscious with slow, laboured, irregular respirations, a slow pulse and raised blood pressure; hyperpyrexia occurs when the hypothalamus has been damaged.

Aneurysm

It is an interesting fact that during the natural development and formation of the arterial system there is an inherent weakness at the artery junctions, where the circular muscle fibres divide. The muscle layer of the artery walls (media) is thin or

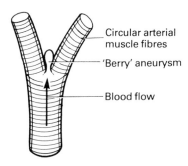

Circular arterial muscle fibres

'Berry' aneurysm

Blood flow

Fig. 8.11 Development of a 'berry' aneurysm.

absent; it is thought that the constant pressure of normal blood flow against this weak point stretches and further weakens the artery wall which then begins to bulge into a balloon-shaped projection, known as a 'berry' aneurysm (Fig. 8.11). This explains why the aneurysms are sometimes referred to as congenital and occur only at bifurcation points. Certain individuals have a tendency to premature degeneration of the arterial system with mild hypertension, which may contribute to the development of an aneurysm and to its rupture, but hypertension need play no part in the development or rupture of these anomalies. Other infective conditions (subacute bacterial endocarditis, polyarteritis nodosa and syphilis), lead to aneurysm formation, when a circulating infective embolus lodges in a peripheral cerebral artery. An aneurysm may be asymptomatic for many years, may suddenly rupture or occasionally act as a space-occupying lesion. Most aneurysms are found on the arteries of the anterior part of the circle of Willis, rarely on the posterior blood vessels; they vary in size from a pin head to a small plum; those that rupture are often the size of a pea.

When an aneurysm ruptures, bleeding may be severe and instantly fatal. The haemorrhage (1–30 ml) is insufficient to cause shock, but in such a confined space a small bleed dramatically increases intracranial pressure. Bleeding is momentary and will cease once the intracranial and intra-arterial pressures equalise. A clot then forms in the ruptured vessel which prevents further haemorrhage for a few days, but as it begins to break down and is reabsorbed there is a risk of further haemorrhage. The first haemorrhage may be small, causing headache but no loss of consciousness or

obvious neurological abnormality, the second is often catastrophic causing unconsciousness, adverse neurological signs or even death within the hour. Up to 40% of patients die within 24 hours of the first haemorrhage; of the remainder some will not recover consciousness and will ultimately die, some will recover to some extent, but will have permanent neurological disability, and others will recover completely. Unless the aneurysm is treated, the risk of a second haemorrhage will remain.

Aneurysm localisation

The location of an aneurysm which has ruptured can often be determined by clinical examination, but it is necessary to confirm its exact situation, size and shape by angiography (see p. 29), which will also demonstrate whether there are other similar lesions; occasionally no abnormality is seen as the aneurysm is too small to be detected, may have collapsed after bleeding or may be filled with blood clot preventing the entry of the radio-opaque dye.

Anterior communicating artery aneurysms are the most common and occur at the junction of the anterior communicating and anterior cerebral arteries (Fig. 8.12). The anterior cerebral arteries supply large parts of the frontal lobes and other small blood vessels leave this part of the circle of Willis to supply the hypothalamus and pituitary gland; haemorrhage causes spasm, and constriction of these arteries disturbs the blood flow and severely interferes with brain function. The patient may be confused, disorientated, apathetic, akinetic, unresponsive or even mute; there is often incontinence. When the hypothalamus and pituitary gland are affected there will be severe disturbance of the electrolyte levels which affects the patient's consciousness and behaviour (see p. 120).

Middle cerebral artery aneurysms are less common; they arise at the division of the middle cerebral and anterior cerebral arteries or where the middle cerebral artery divides into three branches (Fig. 8.12). Each middle cerebral artery passes between the frontal and temporal lobes in the fissure of Sylvius (in the dominant hemisphere it is close to the speech centre) and supplies blood to part of the sensory and motor cortex of one hemisphere (see Figs 8.1 and 8.4) and the basal ganglia. When haemorrhage occurs the middle cerebral artery constricts in spasm, the cerebral hemisphere becomes oedematous and if the aneurysm is buried in the brain substance, rupture will give rise to an intracerebral haematoma.

The symptoms of rupture of a middle cerebral artery aneurysm are contralateral hemiparesis and hemianaesthesia which is worse in the arm than in the leg (the cortex for the leg is supplied by the anterior cerebral artery; see Figs 2.6 and 8.3) and dysphasia if the lesion is in the dominant hemisphere. When there is an associated intracerebral haematoma all the symptoms are worse and there is greater involvement of the leg as, though its cortex has an independent blood supply, its fibres are compressed by pressure from the haematoma and oedema.

Posterior communicating and **terminal carotid artery aneurysms** are in closely related situations at the junction of the internal carotid and posterior communicating arteries (see Figs 8.5 and 8.12) close to the oculomotor (IIIrd) nerve. When the aneurysm ruptures the patient experiences the symptoms of subarachnoid haemorrhage and is found to have a partial third nerve palsy (ptosis and fixed dilated pupil, see page 16) on the same side as the aneurysm, and possibly contralateral hemiparesis. Arterial spasm can occasionally affect the ophthalmic artery causing temporary or permanent blindness. An aneurysm in these situations, even without rupture, may compress the oculomotor nerve.

Other aneurysms on the posterior cerebral circulation are rare (Fig. 8.12); they occur close to the brain stem, at the termination of the basilar artery, the origin of the cerebellar arteries and on the vertebral arteries. Subarachnoid haemorrhage accompanied by nystagmus and ataxia suggest a lesion in this area.

A micotic aneurysm is a very rare complication of a systemic infective disorder, is found on a peripheral cerebral blood vessel and may cause subarachnoid haemorrhage; the infective source must be treated.

Angioma

The cause of subarachnoid haemorrhage in a child or young person is often an angioma (arterio–venous malformation, see Chapter 4); these anomalies may occur on any part of the cerebral circulation and nearly always bleed at some time, usually early in life. They may be very small or so extensive that the blood vessels covering the whole of one cerebral hemisphere are involved; they may be superficial or enfolded deep within the brain and may include blood vessels which supply vital structures. An angioma (Fig. 8.13) is a space-occupying lesion which increases in size as the blood vessels become more dilated and tortuous; the pathological circulation deprives the cortex of blood as arterial blood is pumped directly into the venous circulation, by-passing the normal capillary structure. Epilepsy is a common feature. When the angioma ruptures it causes a subarachnoid

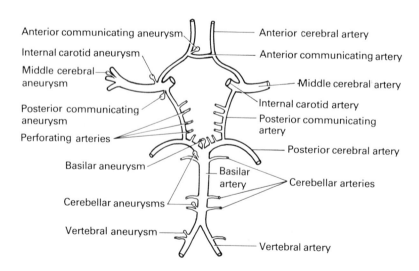

Fig. 8.12 The circle of Willis showing sites of aneurysm.

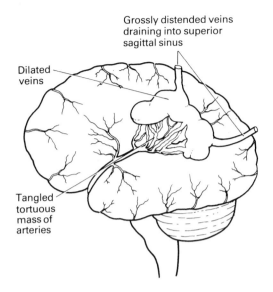

Grossly distended veins
draining into superior
sagittal sinus

Dilated
veins

Tangled
tortuous
mass of
arteries

Fig. 8.13 Angioma (arterio-venous malformation).

haemorrhage possibly associated with an intracerebral haematoma which sometimes completely envelops the abnormal blood vessels. A patient with a cerebral angioma may have other congenital abnormalities, in particular facial naevi (Sturge–Weber syndrome).

Treatment depends upon whether the angioma is superficial or deep, which and how many blood vessels are involved and whether the haemorrhage has obliterated the malformation. Surgical removal of the angioma is preferable to prevent further haemorrhage, but if this is not possible some benefit may be obtained by ligation of some of the feeding vessels. Surgery may be impossible if the angioma is exceptionally large or deeply situated, and if the vessels feeding the angioma also supply vital structures, e.g. the speech area or brain stem. Medical treatment is 6 weeks bed rest; radiotherapy is sometimes given to shrink the angioma.

Haemorrhage associated with drug therapy

Haemorrhage resulting from the use of drugs such as anticoagulants or monoamine oxidase inhibitors is investigated as described for aneurysm; the source of haemorrhage is rarely found, though an intracerebral haematoma may be demonstrated. Treatment includes discontinuation of drug therapy, examination of blood clotting times, bed rest and in some instances, if the patient has a haematoma and his condition does not improve, some benefit may be achieved by surgical removal of the haematoma.

Treatment following subarachnoid haemorrhage

A patient who has had subarachnoid haemorrhage must have complete rest in bed for a period of 6 weeks or until the source of the haemorrhage has been surgically treated. Headache will be relieved using analgesics (see p. 137). During the first few days following haemorrhage when there is a high risk of an aneurysm rebleeding, a drug tranexamic acid (Cyklokapron), may be given by intravenous infusion to prevent the breakdown and reabsorption of blood clot. A very ill patient will require an intravenous infusion to maintain fluid and electrolyte balance. Raised intracranial pressure will be relieved by administration of mannitol and dexamethasone; occasionally dextran (Rheomacrodex) is given to relieve arterial spasm. When the aneurysm has been located, its shape and size defined radiologically and it is known whether there are one or more aneurysms, a decision is taken between medical and surgical treatment depending upon the patient's age, general health and neurological condition

Surgical treatment

While an aneurysm is unprotected there is a constant risk of further haemorrhage which may be fatal. The sole purpose of surgery is to prevent another haemorrhage; the operation cannot reverse paralysis, speech disturbance or other neurological symptoms, the results of brain damage sustained at the time of the subarachnoid haemorrhage. The outlook following surgery has improved mainly as the result of careful selection of patients. A subarachnoid haemorrhage causes brain 'shock' and general metabolic disturbance in addition to its local effects, and the patient needs time to recover before being subjected to the further shock of major surgery. Very careful timing is necessary so that the operation is performed when the patient is physically at his best and before the aneurysm has a chance to rebleed. The use of Cyklokapron which prevents the breakdown of the blood clot which has temporarily sealed the aneurysm after rupture, gives greater safety during this waiting period. The success of surgery also depends upon the surgeon's skill enhanced by the use of a microscope and the close co-operation and assistance of the anaesthetist. Good oxygenation and elimination of carbon dioxide reduce the intracranial pressure and lessens brain swelling, and maintenance of a steady low blood pressure (sustained controlled hypotension) throughout the operation reduces the risk of sudden rupture of the aneurysm and aids haemostasis.

Preparation for craniotomy
Preoperatively it is necessary for blood to be grouped and cross-matched, the patient's relatives must be interviewed, an explanation of the proposed operation given to the patient and his relatives, and consent for operation obtained. The patient must fast for at least four hours and a premedication is given half an hour to 1 hour before the operation; at each stage of preparation the patient's identity must be checked with his nameband. A head shave is performed when the patient has been anaesthetised.

Surgical treatment of an aneurysm involves placing a small clip made of tantalum across the neck of the aneurysm and reinforcing its walls by wrapping with small pieces of muslin to promote fibrosis. Access to these aneurysms is difficult as they lie beneath the brain, close to the brain stem and other vital structures and brain tissue must be retracted. The aneurysm is often very small, it may rupture, one of the perforating vessels may be clipped with the aneurysm or thrombose, depriving vital central structures of their circulation. The use of a microscope during surgery enables the surgeon to magnify and work in very close proximity to these small but vital blood vessels greatly reducing the risk of accidental damage.

Some aneurysms, particularly basilar artery aneurysm, are more easily reached using the transphenoidal oral route.

Care following craniotomy
The nurse designated to 'special' a patient following craniotomy should know the patient's history and preoperative condition and it is helpful to know something of his family background. When the nurse receives the patient from the operating theatre she will be given details of the operation, any complications which have occurred and instructions relating to aftercare. During the immediate postoperative period the patient's neurological condition, vital functions and blood pressure level must be recorded every half hour. Deterioration following surgery may be due to cerebral oedema, arterial spasm, or haemorrhage, symptoms will be identical in each instance and must be reported immediately so that corrective measures can be taken. At each assessment attempts should be made to draw the patient into conversation, out of semiconsciousness into reality; he needs rest and when he regains consciousness and his condition stabilises, observations will be performed less frequently.

An intravenous infusion will be set up at the commencement of the operation in case blood transfusion or mannitol be urgently required; blood is only necessary if there has been profuse haemorrhage. The infusion (dextrose and/or saline) is continued until the patient is able to take sufficient oral fluids to prevent dehydration; sips of water are given at frequent intervals once the patient has regained consciousness and is able to swallow. During this transitional period a careful fluid balance record must be kept to prevent over-hydration. Nausea and vomiting may be present in the early postoperative period, but usually responds to the administration of an anti-emetic.

When the patient is roused for his assessment he should be encouraged to breathe deeply, to try to cough and expectorate; the nurse will need to use suction if the patient is obviously 'chesty' and unable to co-operate in this care. The patient will be encouraged to move himself and help when his position is being changed; a regime of 2-hourly turning from side to side is necessary for the very ill patient and those who cannot move themselves. All general nursing care must be given (see Chapter 3).

The craniotomy wound will have been sutured using fine black silk in each layer from meninges to scalp and a redivac drain is inserted into the wound to prevent the swelling caused by serous fluid draining into the eyelid; some surgeons use skin staples. Alternate scalp sutures or staples are removed on the first and second postoperative days and the drain is removed. The scalp receives such a good blood supply that healing is rapid and underlying layers of sutures prevent the wound from re-opening.

After approximately one week of bed rest, according to the surgeon's instructions and the patient's condition, he will be gradually mobilised.

Medical treatment

Patients who are considered unsuitable for surgery, those whose general and neurological conditions are poor or who have multiple aneurysms, will be prescribed total bed rest for a period of 6 weeks; medical treatment leaves a continuing risk of haemorrhage especially during the first 2 weeks. Rest is easy to prescribe but sometimes difficult to enforce, especially if the patient is confused. To help the patient to rest, headache must be relieved. The most useful analgesics are oral or intramuscular codeine phosphate alternating 4-hourly with paracetamol, but the first dose of codeine phosphate may be ineffective; pain relief may be obtained by giving paracetamol 2 hours later. Pethidine and morphine are avoided because of their sedative action and the risk of missing a relapse into unconsciousness. Other discomforting symptoms should be treated; a cough will worsen headache, urinary frequency and retention will cause restlessness, and constipation (a common problem due to immobility and the administration of constipating drugs such as codeine) should be avoided by the regular use of a gentle aperient. The period of complete rest should be followed by mobilisation with reassurance, and then early discharge from hospital with advice to return to full-time employment. This sequence of treatment and attitude of optimism will prevent unnecessary invalidism and neurosis. The more handicapped patients may benefit from a period of intensive rehabilitation.

Hydrocephalus as a complication of subarachnoid haemorrhage

The meninges are always irritated by blood in the CSF and occasionally adhesions form between the pia and arachnoid mater of the basal cisterns, blocking the CSF circulation and causing obstructive hydrocephalus. This is suspected when a patient remains mentally retarded and possibly incontinent in spite of good physical recovery. When a CAT scan shows dilatation of the ventricles the insertion of a ventriculo-peritoneal drain may be helpful.

Cerebral ischaemia

(This section should be read in conjunction with Chapter 9 as there is a close overlap between ischaemic and degenerative disease of the brain.)

Disease of the cerebral arteries is only part of widespread circulatory disorder which often also involves the coronary arteries and the peripheral circulation.

The brain is normally well supplied with blood, the blood vessels so arranged in the circle of Willis that they supply a good collateral circulation, and reflex postural control of blood pressure is usually most effective; even so, fainting, the simplest example of cerebral ischaemia, is common. (For causes of cerebral ischaemia see p. 128.)

After the age of 50–60 years, ageing processes begin to limit physical activity and gradually the whole circulation slows up. Cerebral atherosclerosis is very common, it develops gradually and the collateral circulation of the brain compensates for deficiencies for a number of years. Even when symptoms of early dementia and personality change develop they can easily be overlooked (see p. 153). Symptoms of transient cerebral ischaemia are quite common in later life because the heart is a less efficient pump, the blood vessels are narrowed by atheroma, damaged by hypertension and diabetes, and the individual may be receiving medications which further lower the blood pressure (tranquilliser, antidepressant, hypotensive and levodopa drugs); a systolic pressure of 130 mm/Hg may be too low for someone aged 70.

The two vertebral arteries which unite to form the basilar artery, are long, narrow and tortuous, they travel through the vertebral foramina, close to the articulating joints of the cervical vertebrae (see Fig. 8.2). The arteries suffer from the effects of ageing; they become furred with atheroma and lose their elasticity, and are affected externally when they are compressed by osteophytic outgrowths from arthritic joints (see Chapter 16). Neck movement may kink the vertebral arteries and temporarily reduce or cut off the blood supply to the brain stem, cerebellum and occipital lobes (vertebro-basilar insufficiency); this causes vertigo, visual disturbance (hemianopia, cortical blindness or diplopia), ataxia and nystagmus, or a 'drop' attack when the elderly victim falls momentarily unconscious to the ground, recovering instantly on reaching the horizontal position. Symptoms of vertebro–basilar insufficiency may also arise when there is subclavian or innominate artery stenosis or occlusion; blood is then drawn in a reverse direction from the vertebral artery during excessive arm exercise (subclavian 'steal' syndrome).

The common carotid arteries are liable to become completely blocked by atheromatous deposits; occlusion of one carotid artery may be present for some time without any obvious symptoms, providing the collateral circulation is satisfactory. Any additional burden on the circulation such as narrowing of the other carotid artery or a vertebral artery, or a fall in blood pressure due to overfatigue or illness may bring on an ischaemic attack which is most likely to affect the territory of the middle cerebral artery.

When there is atherosclerosis the lumen of the blood vessels are narrowed by the development of fatty plaques in the lining of the arteries which cause a general roughening and furring up; the blood swirls and pools around these irregularities (Fig. 8.14) and a thrombus may form. A piece of thrombotic material or atheromatous plaque may break away to form an embolus which is carried to a smaller distal artery; blocking of this artery deprives an area of brain of its blood supply and an infarct develops, an adjacent oedematous area increases the size of the lesion and the severity of its effect.

Cerebral emboli

An embolus may lodge in the ophthalmic artery causing blindness (the embolus can sometimes be seen in the retina through an ophthalmoscope) or in the internal carotid, middle cerebral or anterior cerebral arteries causing sudden hemiparesis, haemianaesthesia or dysphasia; the patient may have a fit. The first embolic episode may seem trivial if it is slight and short-lived, but the implications of arterial disease are serious. The second episode may be instantly fatal or leave the patient completely hemiplegic or aphasic. Sometimes there are many small incidents at unpredictable intervals, each tending to be more severe than the one before,

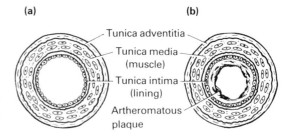

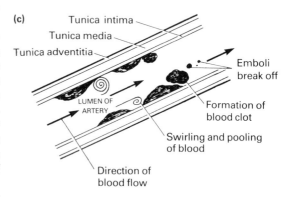

Fig. 8.14 (a) Cross section of a normal artery. (b) Cross section of an artheromatous artery. (c) Artheromatous artery showing pooling and swirling of blood.

leaving the patient progressively more disabled ('stuttering' hemiparesis).

Cerebral thrombosis

The onset of a thrombotic 'stroke' is usually during the night or early hours of the morning when the blood pressure is low, or at any time of day on getting up from a lying or sitting position. The brain may have managed for years on a restricted blood supply when some other factor tips the balance and the blood pressure becomes too low to maintain an adequate cerebral circulation. A thrombus forms in a cerebral artery and an infarct develops; the symptoms, sometimes preceded by over-fatigue, dehydration caused by a bout of diarrhoea and vomiting, an enema, influenza or poor neck posture during sleep, develop gradually over an hour or two, for example a tired business man, after an exhausting and stressful week may have a thrombotic 'stroke' when tension is relieved at the weekend (the 'Saturday morning stroke').

In almost every instance of ischaemic 'stroke' there is some lowering of the level of consciousness, but complete loss of consciousness is unusual; the patient often complains of a persistent dull headache, is usually confused, has a poor grasp of the situation, is monosyllabic and slow to respond verbally. Dysphasia, hemiparesis, facial weakness and hemianopia are variable depending upon the part of the brain most affected. Ischaemia of the brain stem, cerebellum and areas supplied by the posterior cerebral circulation may cause loss of consciousness and signs of cranial nerve and cerebellar disturbance, diplopia, nystagmus, dysarthria, dysphagia, vertigo and ataxia; vomiting often occurs.

Influencing factors and prevention of cerebrovascular disease

There are genetic factors and natural ageing processes which are unavoidable, but the incidence of cerebrovascular accident could be reduced if a healthy lifestyle were adopted. Regular exercise and a well-balanced diet, low in animal fats and containing calories not in excess of requirements, will help to avoid obesity, heart disease, hypertension, diabetes, anaemia and atherosclerosis. Smoking should be avoided as it damages the heart and lungs, has an adverse effect upon the circulation and is a contributory factor in coronary artery disease. Careful selection of patients for treatment with the contraceptive pill will lessen the risk of thrombosis, and thorough treatment of rheumatic fever and subacute bacterial endocarditis prevents the development of faulty heart valves with the risk of cerebral emboli. Before a person reaches retirement age he should be encouraged to give some thought to keeping himself healthy, active and occupied when he stops work; there are helpful pamphlets available which give such advice. In many areas there are good community services which arrange clubs and outings for the elderly and provide for regular medical check-ups. Many elderly people experience symptoms of transient cerebral ischaemia though they never have a 'stroke'; anyone who is having ischaemic episodes, however brief, should be seen by their general practitioner who will check blood pressure levels, examine the heart, test the urine for sugar, send blood samples for routine testing and possibly arrange for X-rays of the cervical spine.

Most victims of ischaemic 'stroke' are elderly; many elderly people live alone, watched over by kindly, but often equally elderly neighbours; loneliness leads to depression, unsatisfactory nutrition with long periods without food, in winter months increasing isolation, a lowered general health and possibly hypothermia. Many 'strokes' occur at night when the house is securely locked; the victim is often unable to get up from the floor after falling, cannot reach the telephone or get help and it may be many hours later that alarmed neighbours, finding curtains still drawn and getting no answer to their knock, call for help from the police who find the victim extremely cold and severely disabled lying on the floor. All elderly people living alone would feel more secure and their relatives less anxious if they were equipped with an emergency call system linked to their telephone.

Treatment

There is little that can be done to improve the condition of diseased cerebral arteries or remedy damage already sustained by the brain, but treatment aims to improve cerebral circulation and prevent situations which diminish cerebral blood flow. When an infarct has caused cerebral oedema a course of dexamethasone will be given to reduce raised intracranial pressure.

When the cause of cerebral ischaemia is due to stenosis or occlusion of one carotid artery, when collateral circulation and the patient's physical condition are good and there are minimal abnormal neurological signs, reconstructive or by-pass vascular surgery will be considered.

Anticoagulant therapy may be recommended for a small number of patients who have repeated transient ischaemic attacks and in whom there is no demonstrable carotid lesion, a stenotic lesion which is unsuitable for surgery or when there is a known cardiac or pulmonary embolic focus.

Taking into account the patient's past medical history and possible causes which led to the 'stroke', (poor general health, bereavement and prescribed drugs which may have had a hypotensive effect) and the result of blood tests, the aims of treatment are to improve general health, maintain blood pressure at a satisfactory level and begin a gradual rehabilitation programme, bearing in mind that the patient is elderly, needs time to adjust to changes of posture when he first gets up in the morning, has limited powers of concentration and tires easily.

Nursing care following cerebrovascular accident

The nursing care of someone who has had a 'stroke' is important and always demands skill, gentleness, patience, perseverance and understanding. It ranges from the care of a patient with subarachnoid haemorrhage (who has such severe headache, he would if he had the strength, hit the nurse who thoughtlessly slams down a metal tray on the locker) to the deeply unconscious patient who is extremely aged and will obviously never regain consciousness. There are some patients who will make a complete recovery from a slight stroke though the future remains uncertain, some who though critically ill will recover completely or partially to enjoy a few years of relatively normal happy life, others who can live only a dependent existence, unable to speak, understand or move, while others will die. In many instances there come vexed ethical problems of how long nursing and medical staff should seek officiously to keep alive a frail wreck of humanity who has lost all senses, is paralysed and totally dependent. Is it right to give antibiotics or start intragastric feeding to prolong life in these circumstances? Questions which are much discussed and have no definite answers.

It is impossible for every elderly patient who has had a 'stroke' to be admitted to hospital. Many patients who have sustained mild 'stroke' will recover spontaneously within a few days and will remain in their own home in the care of their general practitioner who will examine the patient fully, treat any chronic infection, review medication (in particular drugs used to treat cardiac conditions), mobilise community services (district nurse, meals-on-wheels and home help) and arrange for the patient to receive physiotherapy. He will advise the patient to take life more easily (call in the professional decorators and let the son-in-law mow the lawn) and will encourage him, if he lives alone, to give some thought to future sheltered accommodation. There will be discussion with the family so that all will know what the patient should and should not do.

Reasons for admission to hospital

1   To investigate the cause of cerebrovascular accident and to give intensive rehabilitation therapy.
2   For medical and surgical treatment which includes treatment of contributory conditions.
3   Nursing care of the extremely ill or disabled when there is no-one to care for them at home.
4   A further course of rehabilitation.
5   Social reasons – to allow relatives to take a holiday or when circumstances temporarily make it impossible for the patient to remain at home; alternatively residential care may be arranged in a private or local authority nursing home.

Immediate nursing care

After a severe 'stroke', whatever the cause, the first priority is to prevent the patient's condition deteriorating due to anoxia; careful observation of his general and neurological condition will detect the first signs of deterioration and rising intracranial pressure, which must be reported immediately to the medical staff so that counter-measures can be taken (see Chapter 3). Constant observation is essential as the patient's neurological condition is likely to change suddenly; he may lose consciousness or have a fit, the unconscious patient's airway may become obstructed or the confused or forgetful patient, attempting to get out of bed, may fall owing to weakness or unsteadiness. Records of the patient's temperature, pulse, respiration and blood pressure are kept throughout his stay in hospital, the frequency depending on his condition. The possibility of hyperpyrexia when haemorrhage affects the hypothalamus has already been mentioned. The very aged patient suffering from malnutrition and neglect may be hypothermic; mild pyrexia usually accompanies cerebral haemorrhage but may suggest deep vein thrombosis, respiratory or urinary infection. The patient's pulse may show irregularities when mitral valve disease has led to cerebral embolus and may also be significant when there is coronary artery disease. The character and rate of the patient's respirations are an important index to his condition and should never be ignored or recorded automatically at 20/minute; the ill patient who has had a 'stroke' so often develops respiratory complications. Blood pressure levels are particularly important and may fluctuate markedly; they are relevant in all conditions affecting the cerebrovascular system and must be promptly and accurately recorded in spite of technical difficulties when the patient is mentally disturbed. An attempt should always be made to allay the patient's natural anxiety about this procedure by commenting that it is a routine observation and avoiding a look of alarm should the recording be abnormal. On many occasions if the nurse's approach is calm and decisive and she is able to distract the patient into talking of other things, a blood pressure recording is possible. Those patients who are hypertensive, those taking hypotensive drugs and those in the postoperative period must have blood pressure recordings of greater frequency.

When the cause of the 'stroke' is known, a programme of total care is planned to suit each individual; this involves the surgeon, physician, nursing staff, physiotherapist, speech therapist, occupational therapist, medical social worker and the patient's relatives. All must know the aims and objectives of treatment, which are to return the patient to full and active useful life in the community (Fig. 8.15).

Complete bed rest, for the treatment of subarachnoid haemorrhage, is not always clearly understood nor the care thoughtfully arranged. There is a risk of further haemorrhage especially during the first fortnight, and in this time the patient must be kept quiet and as restful as possible; he should be shielded from bright light as he will have photophobia, but it is unwise to isolate the patient in a darkened room, because he must be constantly observed. The nurse should always speak quietly at

her approach, be careful not to jolt the patient's bed and always allow time for him to change his position slowly, as any sudden movement intensifies headache. He should be nursed in a comfortable recumbent position with one or two pillows and relieved in every possible way of any tendency to restlessness or the need to exert himself. The nurse may need to repeat instructions if the patient is inattentive or drowsy, and repeatedly explain the reasons for his admission and care; although the patient appears to understand he often fails to take in or retain information. The patient who is totally irrational presents a difficult problem as he is unable to co-operate and will be overactive and disturbed. Good anticipatory nursing care can sometimes prevent uncontrollable behaviour and allow the patient to rest quietly without the use of drugs; restlessness should always be noticed and the cause relieved immediately if possible. The patient may be either confused or too drowsy to complain of headache, a wet bed or a full distended bladder; oral analgesics may be effective for the relief of headache if they are given regularly before the headache has advanced to its severest intensity. When a patient remains restless despite these measures, a tranquillising drug may be the only solution.

The paralysed limbs of any patient who has had a 'stroke' must be carefully positioned (see p. 55 and Figs 3.6, 8.16 and 8.17) at all times and given passive exercises from the beginning until active physiotherapy is permitted. For some patients mobilisation will be delayed or given cautiously for several weeks because of the nature of their illness or combined illnesses, such as subarachnoid haemorrhage, heart disease or cerebral ischaemic attacks. For all other patients mobilisation starts early. The patient first sits up in bed, using plenty of pillows piled up straight as this will prevent misalignment of the trunk and strain on the paralysed shoulder – not in an armchair arrangement (Fig. 8.16).

A patient with a right hemiplegia usually has difficulty with speech and comprehension which makes it difficult for him to follow instructions about posture and movement. The patient with a left hemiplegia might seem to be less seriously afflicted, but be may be far worse off if he has lost spatial perception and joint awareness (see p. 7), as he does not notice when his body is in a grossly abnormal posture and cannot therefore correct it; the loss of body image may be so complete that

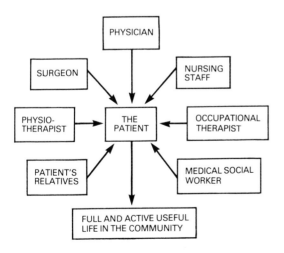

Fig. 8.15 Total care programme.

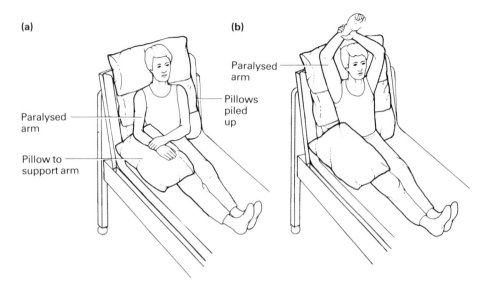

(a)

Paralysed arm

Pillow to support arm

(b)

Paralysed arm

Pillows piled up

Fig. 8.16   (a) Grasping wrist of paralysed arm. (b) Raising the paralysed arm above the head.

even when shown his own arm he will not accept it as his and confusion between right and left sides of the body is common. Homonymous hemianopia is associated with hemiplegia which increases the tendency to ignore the paralysed limbs and any activity beyond his range of vision. The patient's attention must be directed towards the paralysed side; this is achieved by bombarding the patient with stimuli from the side he would otherwise ignore and is helped by placing the bedside locker on the side of the paralysed limbs and siting the bed so that all interesting activities and approaches are automatically from that side. At first it would seem that these practices are unkind, making life even more difficult for the patient, but in the long run they will be doing him a great service to retrain the awareness of this side of his body as he cannot take any active part in his physiotherapy until he accepts these limbs as his; the reasons for this practice must be explained to the patient and his relatives.

Physiotherapy is the most important aspect of the patient's care; everything that is done with and for the patient is a form of physiotherapy and nurses must take advantage of every opportunity to reinforce the teaching of the physiotherapist, as it is they who spend most time with the patient; it is therefore most important that information given by the physiotherapist on the treatment of each patient is conveyed to both day and night nursing staff. To care for this patient well the nurse must

have the right equipment; the bed must be adjustable in height and have a firm base, bedsides if needed must be retracted or easily removed, a bedcradle is essential as are plenty of pillows. A ripple bed is unsuitable for a patient undergoing training in sitting balance as it is too unstable, and a 'monkey pole' hoist should never be used as it can only be grasped with the good hand which accentuates the misalignment of the trunk and is likely to induce spasm in the paralysed arm and leg. **No one should ever pull on the paralysed arm when moving the patient as this causes irreparable damage to the shoulder joint and sets up severe spasm.** The patient and nurse therapist must always be aware of the insensitive or paralysed arm and ensure that every time the patient is moved he does not roll or lie awkwardly on it. It should be appreciated that correct methods in rehabilitation are time-consuming, but when taught correctly the patient will need the help of only one nurse instead of two, will be less accident-prone and will achieve independence and go home sooner.

There are some advantages in having a ward designated solely to the care of patients who have suffered 'stroke' as a continuous programme can be especially geared to their needs.

Stages of physiotherapy

1   Passive movements and chest physiotherapy.

2 Combined passive and active movements. The patient must master each stage before being allowed to progress to the next.

i Rolling from side to side in bed to enable the patient to turn over.

ii 'Bridging' – lying flat on his back, the patient learns to lift his buttocks off the bed, a necessary manoeuvre for getting onto a bedpan.

iii Achieving balance when sitting unsupported.

iv Achieving balance when standing unsupported.

v Learning to walk and manage stairs.

The unconscious patient should be positioned as shown in Fig. 3.6 (p. 40) and his care is given in detail in Chapter 3. At first, treatment will be given in the ward as the patient is not yet ready to attend the physiotherapy department. The physiotherapist is only able to visit her patient once or twice a day for a period of up to 20 minutes each time and the patient must not be tired out when she arrives; the physiotherapist's time is valuable and there should be no interruption during treatment sessions or distraction from noise or ward cleaning. The patient must be encouraged to use any existing muscle power on both sides of his body and to protect the paralysed or weak limbs from bad postures which cause muscle spasm (spasm which starts in the trunk will spread to the shoulder, arm and then leg on that side); once it has occurred it is difficult to eliminate and can rapidly lead to permanent joint contractures. The patient should be encouraged from the earliest moment, to grasp his paralysed hand with his good one and with both arms straight, raise them above his head (Fig. 8.16) regularly and frequently throughout the day. When sitting in bed or in a chair he should always be upright with his trunk and shoulder in correct alignment and his paralysed arm supported on enough pillows to raise the shoulder to the correct height to stretch trunk muscles (Fig. 8.17); it is often necessary to place a small cushion in the 'small' of the back to keep the patient comfortable and prevent slouching; if this position is correct it will not trigger spasm.

Each physiotherapy manoeuvre is designed to show the patient how to achieve natural useful movement even though he is paralysed and has sensory loss. One of the important exercises to be mastered enables the patient to get on to a bedpan. The therapist works from the patient's paralysed

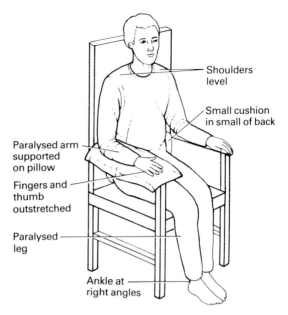

Fig. 8.17 Patient seated in armchair.

Shoulders level

Small cushion in small of back

Paralysed arm supported on pillow

Fingers and thumb outstretched

Paralysed leg

Ankle at right angles

side – with the patient in the supine position, his arms straight at his side, palms on the bed, fingers straight, knees bent well up with feet firmly planted on the bed at right angles, and with the therapist holding the paralysed foot in place, the patient raises his buttocks off the bed ('bridging'; Fig. 8.18); at first the patient will need some help.

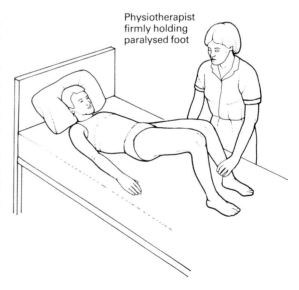

Physiotherapist firmly holding paralysed foot

Fig. 8.18 Patient raising buttocks off the bed – 'bridging'.

The patient will also be taught to roll from side to side and turn over in bed; he first grasps his paralysed hand with his good one, stretches both arms forward and on turning flexes the hip and brings the leg over (Fig. 8.19). This is difficult when turning on to the good side and help will be needed to initiate the rolling movement. From this position, the next step is to help the patient to the sitting position on the edge of the bed: the helper, facing the patient who is resting on his paralysed side, reaches under the patient's chest to his scapula with one hand and with her other hand under his knees, helps him to raise his trunk, take his weight on his paralysed elbow and swing his legs over the edge of

the bed to the sitting position (Fig. 8.20). The bed must be at the correct height so that the patient's feet are firmly planted on the floor.

The patient will be able to sit up in a chair long before he has achieved sitting or standing balance. The chair must be placed in the position usually

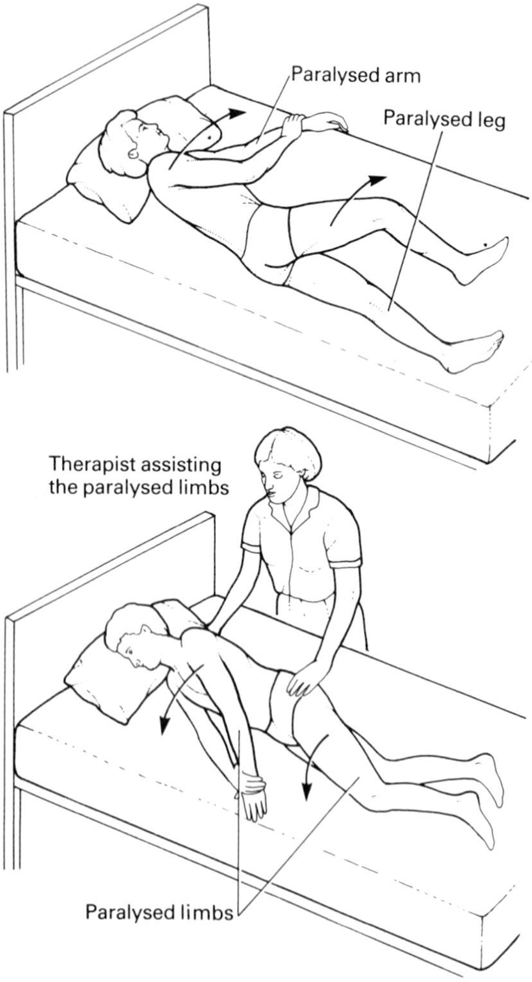

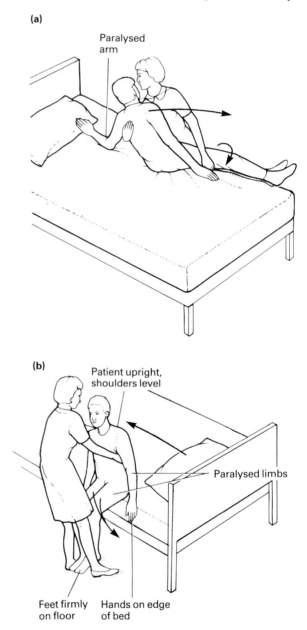

Fig. 8.20 Assisting the patient by **(a)** swinging him into a sitting position, to **(b)** enable him to sit on the edge of the bed.

Fig. 8.19 Patient rolling from side to side.

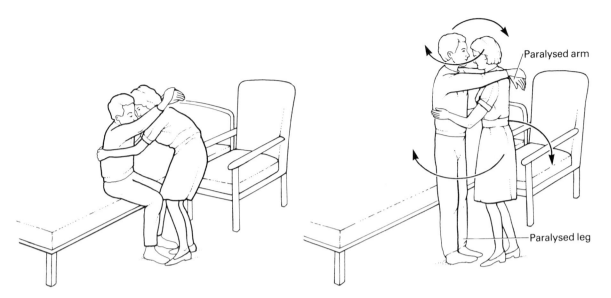

Fig. 8.21 Assisting paralysed patient to stand prior to seating in an armchair.

occupied by the patient's locker. To transfer the patient from bed to chair, the helper places the patient's arms on each side of her shoulders and with both arms round his chest beneath the scapulae, she places her feet against his feet, her knees braced against his and with her own body counter-balancing his she eases the patient into the standing position (Fig. 8.21), then turns him to lower him gently into the chair using the same counter-balancing manoeuvre in the reverse direction.

The patient must achieve controlled sitting balance before he is taught to stand, and controlled standing balance before being taught to walk. The patient may be rather disappointed that in spite of all his efforts and progress during the early weeks of physiotherapy, he has still not begun to walk; the importance of thorough groundwork to strengthen weak muscles prior to walking must be explained, for one faulty posture will destroy all that has been achieved and bad habits which are so easily acquired are difficult to correct. When the physiotherapist decides the patient is ready to walk, relatives will be asked to bring a pair of the patient's low-heeled, well-fitting walking shoes which must be worn every time the patient walks.

Routine general nursing care
(see Chapter 3)

Nutrition and elimination

During the first 24 hours following a 'stroke' it is wise to give only small amounts of fluid as the patient is likely to vomit, but from this time on, efforts should be redoubled to ensure a daily intake of at least 2½ litres to prevent dehydration, which is especially likely if the patient is apathetic and mentally and physically slow. Skill is needed to ensure that the patient who is feeling so ill takes and

retains enough fluid. Care must be taken when the nurse gives fluid to the patient, that it is something he likes and at the right temperature. **Piping hot drinks must never be placed within the reach of a confused, paralysed or very ill patient** as it is all too easy for him to burn himself because he reaches for it from an awkward angle and does not appreciate he has a weak or inco-ordinated hand and arm. Ill patients who are nauseated and drowsy should have small amounts of fluid often, throughout the day and night; the nurse should always take the opportunity to give the patient a drink following any nursing procedure. Clothing and bedding must be protected from spills, and flexible straws or specially adapted beakers are useful drinking aids for patients lying flat or those with a hemiplegia or facial weakness. As soon as possible a normal china cup should be introduced. Diet should be light, attractive, palatable and cut into manageable-sized pieces so that the patient can feed himself one-handed. A patient who is allowed to sit up in bed should be comfortably supported in an upright position before any food or fluid is given. Meals should be placed on a bed table in front of the patient and within his field of vision, if this is restricted. The plate must have a rim and may need a water-heated compartment if the patient is a slow eater; a non-slip mat is helpful. All these aids will help the patient to feed himself. Eating and drinking are difficult when there is facial weakness and loss of sensation of the face and mouth, even if there is no dysphagia; some patients are helped to feed themselves with less mess if a mirror is positioned on the table in front of them. Variety of diet is important for the elderly as they have so often, especially those who live alone on a restricted income, formed the tea and biscuit habit and will not easily be persuaded to take other food.

A patient who has suffered an ischaemic 'stroke' is likely to have signs of early dementia associated with cortical atrophy. The person may appear superficially normal, but it is noticed that the natural courtesies of everyday life ('please', 'thank you', 'excuse me', etc.) are forgotten and at meal-times there is lack of table manners and a tendency to bolt food or cram in too much; this, combined with periodic difficulties with swallowing and a depressed cough reflex, leads to episodes of choking and extreme cyanosis, necessitating the use of suction. The nurse, knowing her patient, should be careful of giving certain foods which provoke these attacks (coarse mince, rough cereal, salad, etc.), should avoid fish with small bones and supervise the patient during meals. Liquidised meals are more easily swallowed by someone with severe dysphagia.

A very few patients need supplementary or full intragastric feeding because they are unconscious, very drowsy or have severe dysphagia.

Many elderly victims of 'stroke' never regain their previous mobility, lose initiative, sit around all day inert, may overeat because there is no other interest, become obese, constipated, 'chesty' and prone to pressure sores. The diet should contain foods rich in vitamin B and roughage (including unprocessed bran) with limited carbohydrate and plenty of fluid.

There are some patients who are heavy, paralysed and confused and unable to get on to a bed-pan without help; no nurse should try to lift a heavy patient on her own, but it will be easier to roll the patient on to the bedpan taking care not to pinch or scrape the skin and making sure that the bedpan is well under both buttocks to prevent spillage; the patient is rolled off the bedpan in the same way. Unless the patient is having complete rest she will be able to help with this manoeuvre and can be taught the physiotheraphy method of 'bridging' (see p. 143); she may develop a preference for a particular shape of bedpan (conventional, 'slipper' or 'duck'). When the patient finds it impossible to use a bedpan she may be allowed up to a bedside commode; sometimes catheterisation is necessary because the patient is too ill to be allowed out of bed, has retention of urine, pressure sores or is incontinent. In many instances the patient need not be incontinent if given frequent opportunity to pass urine, receives prompt attention on request and has good bowel management (is neither constipated nor has diarrhoea). Incontinence may be the sole reason why someone cannot be cared for at home and it is reasonable to resort to an indwelling catheter to retain the patient's self respect and help to prevent odour. Some patients who have stress incontinence will feel more confident if they wear protective pants. It is important that the patient is taught how to get out of bed on to the commode so that when he goes home he can be safely independent at night; beds and commodes must always have good brakes.

Nurse–patient communication

The patient whose brain has suffered as the result of cerebrovascular disease will be mentally as well as physically handicapped. Extra patience is necessary especially with the elderly to encourage independence and bear with rather childish behaviour. There may be some degree of deafness as well as slowness of understanding, and memory impairment is especially trying when it is variable and the patient seems to hear and remember what he wants to; there may be dysphasia, aphasia or dysarthria. The nurse must beware of attending solely to the basic current needs of the patient and must bear in mind the possible need of new spectacles, dentures and hearing aid; she must make time to talk to him even when he does not respond, as she may be the patient's only contact with the outside world. The elderly patient may be bereft of close family or friends, unable to hear or understand the television, to see well enough to read the newspaper, or comprehend the plot of a book. The patient is so cut off by his inability to communicate that he will be comforted by a friendly arm round his shoulders, the grasp of a hand or the reassuring smile of a nurse.

It is better to underestimate the patient's abilities than to cause him to become agitated through excessive demands, though a little stretching of those expectations is necessary for any progress to be made. The patient with an ageing brain may be frankly neurotic, unreasonably fearful of being alone, panicky about going out and of new situations, suspicious of everyone's intentions and – through misinterpretation – paranoid and irritable, this behaviour being either uncharacteristic or an exaggeration of his previous personality. Emotional lability with a tendency to cry or laugh disproportionately to the circumstances, is an embarrassment due to damage to the inhibitory functions of the brain; nurses must realise that inappropriate behaviour may not be deliberate.

Mobilisation and rehabilitation

There is more nursing skill necessary to get the patient up and about than is often realised; many patients suffer from arthritis and even a day or two in bed makes all their joints stiffen and become very painful; diabetes mellitus and peripheral vascular disease are disorders often associated with age when the circulation to legs and feet is seriously impaired. Old people sitting about can get chilled extremities, they should be warmly clad in long woollen underpants and ladies might be persuaded to wear trousers. Great care must be taken of legs and feet as the skin is fragile and even small injuries may lead to infection, necrosis and gangrene. A trained chiropodist should attend to the patient's feet, never a nurse as she has not the right instruments, though she is responsible for regularly inspecting the feet, noticing cracks between the toes or tinea infection (athlete's foot), and making sure the feet are thoroughly dried without using clogging talcum powder. A surprising number of elderly people have had amputation of one or both legs which has followed years of deteriorating peripheral circulation; these patients are likely to have a 'stroke' as their cerebral arteries are also narrowed by atherosclerosis, this could paralyse their remaining limbs.

When the helpless patient is allowed to sit up in a chair for the first time, the way the nurses approach, help him out of bed into a chair, the length of time they leave him there and whether he is so placed that he can see activity in the ward and receives encouraging smiles or other attention once he is up, influence the speed and quality of his rehabilitation. The patient who is frightened when he is suddenly hauled out of bed, left sitting uncomfortably in a chair for an excessive length of time, becoming saddle-sore, cramped, tired and miserable will lack confidence and enthusiasm during physiotherapy, may develop pressure sores, ankle oedema and even have a further cerebrovascular accident due to hypotension.

Care must be taken not to overtire the patient as this might cause a fall in blood pressure with dizziness, which will undermine the patient's confidence when he is being mobilised, may cause a fall and risk an extension of any ischaemic area in the brain. Should the patient have a 'fainting' episode he should lie down for at least an hour to improve the cerebral circulation and when feeling better should get up slowly. These episodes are more likely to occur at night because the blood pressure is already lower and the elderly patient, getting out of bed to go to the lavatory, may fall or collapse with a 'stroke'. Nurses should show a sympathetic but matter-of-fact approach to any small incident, fall, or a day when the patient is less able than usual and more help is necessary, but in the event of a fall the doctor must be notified as he will want to examine the patient. In hospital there must always be unobtrusive observation of the patient day and night; there are some patients who very obviously must be protected by bedsides throughout the 24 hours, but others are only at risk at night when lights are dim and they are under sedation. Any patient who has had night sedation should never get out of bed without a nurse in attendance and this should be made clear to each patient.

Many patients with cerebrovascular disease are subject to acute anxiety, agitation and depression, and this is often treated with antidepressant or tranquillising medication. The nurse must observe the effect these medications have on the patient as they may cause excessive drowsiness, or more importantly, the gradual development of subtle changes in the patient's demeanour and behaviour; deterioration in the patient's ability to walk unaided, feed or dress himself can easily be overlooked or attributed to general organic factors. A dramatic improvement is sometimes seen when the offending drug is discontinued.

Mobilisation must start gradually, chairs must be suited to the patient and support given to paralysed or weak arms. The patient should be encouraged to move his feet and legs as much as he is able at frequent intervals while he is sitting down and if his memory is impaired he should be reminded or helped to do this. His newspaper, spectacles and a drink should be placed on a table within reach. It should be possible to observe him from the nurses' station and if he needs help to stand and walk, he must be encouraged to ask, rather than risk a fall. Confused patients with limb weakness should be so positioned that they cannot get out of their chair without a nurse being quickly available. Close co-operation between the nursing staff, physiotherapist and occupational therapist at all stages of the patient's recovery is very important and undoubtedly makes for smoother progress. The patient who has been up for too long before going to the physiotherapy department will be too tired to concentrate on instructions for regaining his balance and ability to walk. The patient's time-table for the day must be planned and he should be encouraged to take an interest in the programme, perhaps making suggestions to suit his own needs. The programme should be flexible as the patient and his vascular system are living variable forces; he may need more rest some days than others.

Some patients will have an opportunity to experience independent living in a self-catering flatlet near the ward before being discharged from hospital.

Relatives will need much support and advice (see Chapter 3); whether the patient is old and has had an ischaemic 'stroke', or is young and has had a subarachnoid haemorrhage, the relatives have responsibilities which may prove an unbearable burden and strain family relationships. The next-of-kin should be seen regularly by the doctor and must be aware of the risk of relapse or threat to the patient's life. They should be kept informed of planned treatment and expected date of discharge. The relatives need to be warned against overprotectiveness; they and the nursing staff may even need to kindly badger the patient a little as there is often apathy, lethargy and depression. Unnatural fear may make a patient afraid to be left alone; in the early days following a cerebrovascular accident it is reassuring if the patient can see other people and activity around him, but gradually 'time alone' must be introduced or he will be demanding and his fears may make unbearable demands upon his family.

When hospital treatment has brought the patient to the point where he is able to return home, he and his relatives will be given advice by the doctor and other members of the therapeutic team. Patients who have made a full recovery will need a period of convalescence before returning to work. Those whose job involves much responsibility and stress may be wise to find something which subjects them to less pressure, but this may be impractical advice. It is often a trait of the patient's personality which drives him on and whether at work or retired, these tensions are almost impossible to alter without the aid of tranquillisers. These factors play an important part in the treatment of hypertension; sometimes a mild cerebrovascular accident almost safeguards the patient, as it forcibly slows down his activities.

Patients in the younger age group who leave hospital with some residual disability may be fortunate enough to have the opportunity to go to a rehabilitation centre, but these centres are few and far between. Ideally, physiotherapy, occupational therapy and community care should combine to enable the patient to return to as normal a life as possible, to return to work whether this is the same occupation or a new one suited to his capabilities; for the housewife, the opportunity to learn how to adapt and run her own home. Relatives need advice, they should certainly be encouraged to treat the patient as naturally as possible, to avoid any emphasis on the new situation and it is helpful if there is someone, medically or socially skilled, who has time to discuss objectively any problems which may crop up. The general practitioner or district nurse, by their counselling, may be able to avert a major family crisis.

There are some small points of practical advice which should not be overlooked. Patients who have shown evidence of basilar insufficiency should be advised to take care when looking upwards as this may further diminish the circulation and lead to an episode of unconsciousness which can be dangerous if they fall from a height. The vertebral arteries are easily occluded and another familiar situation is that of the middle-aged or elderly motorist who is reversing his car out of the garage with neck craning round to see where he is going and then has a 'blackout'. Cervical arthritis aggravates this situation. Patients should be warned to avoid sharp turning movements of the neck. It is quite common for elderly people who have cerebrovascular disease to feel giddy and ill when they first get out of bed in the morning. If they sit up gradually and enjoy a cup of tea in bed they will avoid this unpleasant sensation. Sudden standing from the sitting position is also inclined to cause fainting and should be avoided.

'Strokes' most commonly affect the elderly and for this reason many additional problems are met. These are the normal accompaniments of old age: mental frailty, deafness, failing vision and stiff joints, loss of old friends and relatives which sometimes means solitude and loneliness; the married partner may be in equally frail health and there are often limited financial resources. Relatives need time to make arrangements for the patient's homecoming, preparing a room downstairs and borrowing equipment; hospital nursing staff can smooth the way by making all necessary arrangements well in advance and by sending a detailed report to the district nurse.

Care of the elderly is the responsibility of the community and an increasing problem with the normal life span being lengthened as it is by modern medicine and other factors. It is a subject in itself and all that can be said here is that wherever possible the patient should be allowed to remain in his own home, as he is likely to be happier there and his mind is less likely to deteriorate or his mental state become confused when in familiar surroundings with responsibilities and ordinary household tasks to occupy the day. Sometimes the conditions appear far from ideal especially if he lives alone, but it is 'home' to the patient and if he has friendly neighbours and there is planned visiting and help, this situation may continue happily for some time. Relatives must be given advice and persuaded to accept any offered assistance which will lighten their burden, each family and situation must be considered individually.

Home care following a mild cerebrovascular accident

Many elderly patients suffer a mild thrombotic 'stroke'. They wake in the morning with a hemiplegia, are usually mentally alert and will remain in their homes attended by their general practitioner. The district nurse will call daily to help care for the patient and will assess the need for special nursing equipment (bed cradle, incontinence sheets, urinal, bedpan, commode and Zimmer walking frame), and will assist and advise relatives about mobilisation and rehabilitation. It must be made quite clear that, though the patient looks awful and seems so helpless, from the very beginning he must be encouraged, in a kindly way, to be independent even though this takes a long time and seems a harsh attitude. He must wash his face, brush his hair, shave, put on his spectacles, and put in his dentures, feed himself and try to relearn old skills single-handed; he must try to move himself in bed, turn over and sit himself up, and exercise his paralysed or weak limbs (see Figs 8.16–8.20). A domiciliary physiotherapy service will be very helpful in the early days and then arrangements will be made for the patient to attend a physiotherapy department or day centre for rehabilitation. From the beginning the relatives should be warned not to discuss the patient within his hearing though he seems to be sleeping or uncomprehending (this includes in the next room or on the telephone). The district nurse should advise the relatives to contact the community social worker who will visit and advise on financial assistance available for the disabled.

1   Rates relief, which includes a reduction of the rooms used exclusively by the disabled person and a percentage of the rateable value for central heating, and garage if the car is used for transport
2   Attendance allowance, which becomes payable after 6 months but should be claimed in advance
3   Mobility allowance
4   Supplementary benefit

5   Grants to extend or modify premises to accommodate a disabled person, e.g. installation of a ground floor shower and lavatory

The social worker will also contact the occupational therapist who will visit and assess the need for aids to daily living including, for example, long-handled gadgets for picking up objects from the floor and putting on socks and shoes, feeding and bath aids, handrails, etc. There may be major problems if the disabled person cannot be left unattended and the social worker may be able to arrange voluntary sitters-in, or put the family in touch with local organisations and Church community.

In a family of several generations there is often conflict of interests and lack of understanding on both sides; elderly people need a set routine, meals at a certain time and retire to bed either early or very late, which makes it difficult for the housewife if she also has the interests of her children to consider and when her routine needs to be flexible. Youngsters make a lot of noise which is intolerable to the elderly, but conversely the television may need to be painfully loud because the old person is deaf. Old people can be extremely wearing to live with, repetitive, querulous, obstinate, fussy and demanding. Relatives are emotionally closely involved, busy, tired and cannot go 'off duty'; theirs is a 24-hour day.

9

Degenerative Disorders of the Brain

Degenerative disorders of the brain are usually progressive and diffuse, leading to dementia, a permanent irreversible loss of intellectual capacity. Specific changes in memory, mood, behaviour, speech and comprehension depend upon the part of the brain affected and are influenced by the patient's previous personality and intellectual endowment. There are many factors essential to maintain healthy brain cells (see Chapters 8 and 26) and if the cells are deprived of essentials they will either function inefficiently or die. Permanent brain damage with some degree of dementia is caused by factors which impair oxygen supply to the brain, disturb brain cell metabolism or overwhelm the brain with poisons and toxins (see Chapter 27).

It is known that many thousands of brain cells die daily once a person passes the age of twenty-five years. These cells are not replaced, but mental capacity is not noticeably affected as there are millions of cells in reserve, though it is an acknowledged fact that as one gets older it is less easy to learn and to adapt to new situations. Throughout life there are factors which may cause premature death of brain tissue. A few children succumb to rare genetically-determined conditions which result in brain degeneration; other genetic disorders develop in middle age. Some families seem to have a susceptibility either to conditions which contribute to brain degeneration or to premature ageing of the brain, becoming slow and incompetent at a comparatively young age compared with others who remain healthy and retain their mental faculties well into their nineties. Throughout life, accident or illness may rob a previously healthy person of their intellect, and the brain can be irreparably damaged by the cumulative effects of head injuries, chronic anoxia, cerebral ischaemia, liver failure, deficiency disorders or poisoning. Inexplicably a very few people become demented in middle age, (pre-senile dementia), whereas a greater number gradually develop the natural mental frailty of old age, in extreme intances known as senile dementia.

Anatomy and physiology

The normal loss of brain cells causes no appreciable change in the macroscopic appearance of the brain. When for any reason the brain degenerates, the meninges thicken, the brain shrinks and therefore the ventricles become large and spaces appear between the gyri over the surface of the brain (Fig. 9.1); there is a non-obstructive hydrocephalus and the ventricular CSF pressure is normal. The brain shrinkage may be localised or widespread and the frontal lobes, the seat of intellect and reasoning, are usually most extensively affected. Microscopic changes within the brain depend upon the cause of degeneration; senile plaques and dying cells are evidence of senile dementia and sclerosed blood vessels, old haemorrhages and softened areas of brain are indicative of atherosclerosis.

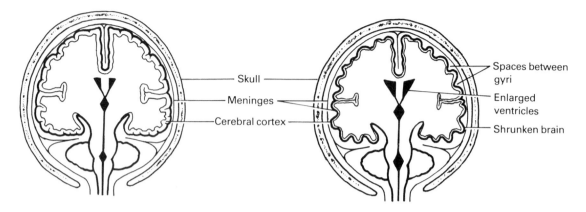

Fig. 9.1 (a) Normal brain. (b) Cerebral atrophy.

Dementia

Causes of dementia

1 Kernicterus
2 An idiosyncratic response to certain vaccines
3 Genetically-determined conditions, e.g. lipidosis occurring in childhood and accompanied by epileptic fits, and porphyria (see p. 326) which develops in middle age
4 Incidents causing acute brain anoxia – near-drowning, respiratory and cardiac arrest, failed suicide attempt and anaesthetic catastrophies
5 Severe head injuries or constant repeated battering of the brain as sustained by professional boxers and those with severe epilepsy; the latter also have repeated episodes of anoxia
6 Encephalitis and meningitis
7 Cerebral haemorrhage

⎱ Adhesions in the basal subarachnoid space may be the cause of dementia (see pp. 102 and 137)

8 Poisons – especially carbon monoxide, lead copper and alcohol
9 Chronic liver failure – excessive intake of alcohol is a factor
10 Deficiency disorders – deficiency of vitamin B complex including vitamin B_{12}. Excessive intake of alcohol is an important contributory factor
11 Thyroid deficiency disorders – cretinism and myxoedema
12 Cardio-respiratory disorders – severe congenital heart and lung abnormalities may affect the brain in infancy; acquired cardio-respiratory disorders in later life cause cerebral anoxia
13 Neurosyphilis – general paralysis of the insane (see Chapter 24)
14 Persistent high blood pressure damages cerebral arteries which reduces blood flow and oxygen supply to the brain (hypertensive encephelopathy)
15 Cerebral arteriosclerosis (see Chapter 8)
16 Unknown factors which cause pre-senile dementia:
 (a) Alzheimer's disease
 (b) Pick's disease
 (c) Other described syndromes
17 An ageing brain due to a combination of many factors, which include genetic predisposition, diminished blood flow, poor cerebral oxygenation, poor nutrition and loss of brain tissue (senile dementia)

Signs and symptoms

The onset is similar whatever the cause of dementia, though the rate of decline varies from a few months to several or more years and there may be associated physical symptoms and signs. Degeneration of the basal ganglia is not usually accompanied by dementia except when there is widespread cerebral arteriosclerosis and in Huntington's chorea (see Chapter 20).

Degeneration of the brain (cerebral atrophy) affects the entirety of the patient's mind and physical abilities leading to:

1 Intellectual deterioration with failure of
   (a) memory
   (b) concentration
   (c) comprehension
   (d) reasoning
   (e) insight
   (f) orientation
2 Emotional changes – the emotions become too easily stimulated and the patient has reduced control over laughter or tears
3 Deterioration of personality – there is an increasing tendency to selfishness and egocentricity with lack of consideration for other people's feelings. Personal habits, table manners, toilet habits and hygiene deteriorate and sexual offences may be committed
4 Weakness and inco-ordination of limbs
5 Disturbance of speech
6 Epileptic fits

Intercurrent illness often accelerates overall deterioration and relatives may notice for the first time that, 'he has not really been himself for a long time', or the general practitioner realises that (even taking into account the present illness, possible anxiety about his condition or his advanced age) the patient's comprehension and responses are slow, his memory for recent events extremely poor, his agitation excessive and his plans unrealistic. The history of deterioration will come mainly from relatives, though the patient himself may complain of fatigue, lack of interest, depression, a poor memory for names and recent events, a vague feeling of confusion about 'what is going on' and anxiety as to whether he will be 'able to cope'. Someone still in business or employment,

especially if the work is not of a routine nature, may become irritable and inefficient because he is being stretched beyond his limit, and there may come a point when, though the person lacks insight, it is obvious to the employer that a less demanding job or early retirement are necessary. Difficulties at home may develop gradually and if the individual is living alone it may be some time before anyone is aware of his inability to manage his own affairs, nutrition, personal hygiene, home care and finance; there may on the contrary be a sudden crisis when the person creates a disturbance at night, being unamenable to reason or, confused and disorientated, is found wandering out-of-doors incompletely clad and possibly causing a commotion.

Arteriosclerotic dementia

The commonest form of dementia is caused by cerebral arteriosclerosis (see Chapter 8). There is usually a history suggesting recurrent episodes of brain ischaemia (syncopal attacks, temporary weakness of a limb or visual disturbance). On examination there may be signs of residual pyramidal tract damage, weakness of face or limbs, or abnormally brisk reflexes. The severity of dementia may be difficult to assess if dysphasia is present, when it is important not to underestimate the patient's comprehension. Intellectual and physical deterioration may run a fluctuating course with features of anxiety and depression, the patient usually retaining some insight into his limitations. Some patients appear mentally normal, but more detailed questioning will reveal surprisingly limited mental abilities and when under pressure, the patient may show extreme agitation and distress or ill-temper.

Senile dementia

Senile dementia is characterised by the insidious onset of symptoms which have often been present for some years before their severity necessitates medical care. Most of these patients will be cared for in their own home.

Symptoms

i Reduction in initiative

ii Easily induced fatigue

iii Depression

iv Failure of concentration and attention

v Gradual failure of memory, especially for recent events

vi Failure of grasp and judgment

vii Confabulation, which may be described as the patient's inaccurate reminiscences coloured by a litte of his wishful thinking

viii Disorientation

ix Insomnia with night-time restlessness, confusion and a tendency to wander

x Acute delirious states occur with extreme restlessness, excitement and disorientation, persecutory ideas, resistiveness and complete insomnia

xi Paranoid or grandiose delusions are sometimes expressed

xii The elderly senile person may appear bland and stupid, unaware that he is behaving abnormally

Pre-senile dementias

Differences in the onset and progression of early dementia have led physicians to attempt classification, but although a variety of names are used for description, signs and symptoms vary and overlap and it is the constant feature of rapidly progressive and profound dementia in middle age which identifies pre-senile dementia.

Alzheimer's disease is characterised by extremely rapid deterioration with failure of memory, disorientation and disintegration of intellect. There are periods of intense restlessness, anxiety and useless overactivity, the pattern of the activity often being based on the patient's previous occupation. Speech becomes jargon, and apraxia and agnosia are apparent, showing the total degenerative involvement of the parietal lobes.

Pick's disease follows a similar rapid course of deterioration of memory, intellect and judgement, the patient showing a fatuous complacency. There is restlessness and disordered speech and writing; the patient, like a record that has stuck, constantly repeats the same word or meaningless phrase (perseveration) or echoes that which he has heard (echolalia). Dementia beginning in the prime of life

progresses relentlessly uninfluenced by any known form of treatment. A truly pathetic vegetative state is reached within about five years. The patient will need hospital care and physical decline ends in death.

Korsakow's syndrome is a condition which may be recognised during the course of several types of degenerative disease of the brain, and mainly affects young middle-aged women. There is gross impairment of memory and a unique degree of confabulation and, although the patient shows no impairment of comprehension, there is loss of insight, confusion and disorientation. Polyneuritis (see Chapter 25) may suggest the nature of the disorder which is commonly associated with chronic alcoholism.

Creutzfeld–Jakob disease is a condition in which there is a rapid progressive dementia and paralysis to death within six months, possibly attributable to a 'slow' virus.

History and examination of a patient with dementia

A thorough history and examination of the patient (see Chapter 2) is nowhere of more value than when the doctor is confronted by the problem of a patient showing signs of dementia, as the causes are diverse. A correct diagnosis is important, not only for the few patients whose dementia is due to an operable meningioma or remediable dietary deficiency, but also because, being assured that no treatable condition is being missed, relatives will be able to accept the situation more realistically and plan more effectively. Plans involve schooling, employment, finance, home and family arrangements and – only when absolutely necessary – institutional care.

Parents of affected children will be asked about their forebears and any known incidence of mental disorder, about pregnancy and parturition, the mother's health and drugs taken during pregnancy. Questions will be asked regarding the child's progress from birth onwards, facts concerning feeding, sleeping, activities, vaccinations, any normal landmarks, when it was first noted that the child was not making progress or was regressing, showing lethargy, lack of interest and comprehension at home or at school. Were there any physical accompaniments to the mental condition, did he have an illness or injury, has he had fits?

Relatives may show reluctance to disclose a history of venereal disease, the forerunner of neurosyphilitic dementia, and close questioning may also be necessary to elicit a history of head injury or the fact that the patient took part in boxing bouts some years before; the incidents may have been forgotten or thought to be irrelevant. Difficulty may be experienced in obtaining an accurate history if the next-of-kin is also aged or has some degree of dementia, or if the patient has lived alone for a long time; then the duration of the illness can only be guessed. Details about the patient's employment are important, firstly to exclude any possibility of its contribution to his present condition and secondly to understand the nature of the job and its demands.

Examination begins with observation of the patient's height, build, posture, gait, size and shape of head, evidence of endocrine disorder (cretinism and myxoedema), general appearance, state of dress and hygiene; personal neglect is common and dirty feet are almost symptomatic of chronic alcoholism, even in the face of vigorous denials from the patient and his relatives that he ever 'touches a drop'. Other specific relevant signs are the yellow pallor of vitamin B_{12} deficiency, the skin lesions associated with tuberous sclerosis, the stigmata of neurosyphilis, or signs of misshapen nose or cauliflower ears which suggest boxing injuries.

Investigations

All patients with dementia are carefully investigated to ensure that no treatable condition is overlooked; simple investigations may be performed at an out-patient appointment. Preliminary investigations include straight X-rays of the skull and chest, full blood count, haemoglobin, blood urea, Wassermann and Kahn reaction, serum B_{12}, tests for diabetes mellitus and thyroid deficiency and an early morning specimen of urine is analysed for urinary prophyrins (see p. 328). A CAT scan and EEG are helpful in excluding space-occupying lesions and give some indication of the size of the ventricles and sufficiency of blood flow to the brain. Psychological tests assess the patient's mental ability and emotional reactions and the first test provides a baseline for future assessments. Brain and rectal biopsies are sometimes used to classify dementia in young children and enable the doctor to discuss prognosis.

Assessment, management and treatment of a patient with dementia

Many patients first come to the notice of the medical team when they are admitted to hospital because they are unable to look after themselves, are dehydrated and malnourished, have had a fall, are suffering from hypothermia, have had an episode of cerebrovascular insufficiency or an acute illness which has revealed dementia (e.g., bronchitis, congestive cardiac failure, urinary infection). The immediate condition will be treated, general health improved by re-hydration, regular diet, vitamin supplements, a warm environment, company and encouragement. The cause of dementia will be investigated and specific treatment given, for example replacement therapy for endocrine disorder, vitamin B_{12} injections, cardiac regulators and diuretic medication, treatment for hypertension and supportive therapy for the alcohol-dependent patient. Medication will be necessary to prevent insomnia and relieve excessive anxiety or depression. Drugs sometimes have a cumulative effect causing daytime drowsiness, an increased risk of falls, incontinence and a greater dependence on others for help with every activity; the drug dosage will need adjustment to suit the individual. Treatment of respiratory disorders and physiotherapy will ensure optium oxygenation through the lungs and assist the heart in its task of pumping blood to the brain to relieve cerebral anoxia. Surgical intervention may benefit a few patients. A ventriculo–peritoneal drain may improve the patient's condition and prevent further deterioration when dementia is the result of hydrocephalus caused by adhesions of the meninges with blockage of the CSF pathways at the base of the brain; this can be a complication of head injury, subarachnoid haemorrhage and meningitis. Surgery is also necessary for excision of frontal lobe tumour or chronic subdural haematoma in the elderly, conditions which also cause dementia. The patient will be referred to a neurologist, psychiatrist and geriatrician for assessment and on the basis of these reports there will be discussion about the patient's future care between the ward sister, doctor, social worker and relatives. There is no specific treatment for many patients suffering from dementia and thought must be given to the future. Whenever possible the patient should be brought into the discussion so that his feelings and preferences are known. A patient who is slow in comprehension, hard of hearing or partially sighted understandably mis-interprets or only half understands conversation; he will be suspicious of the motives behind other people's plans, indecisive and even unrealistic because he lacks insight.

Is the patient fit to go home and live alone? Should he go to live with relatives? Can relatives perhaps rotate care? Can anyone come to live with him? Is warden-supervised residential accom-modation necessary? Deterioration can to some extent be delayed by enabling the person to remain in their own environment. Who will be at home, will the patient be alone for long periods? Is there suitable ground floor accommodation with a lavatory nearby? The occupational therapist will visit the home to assess home safety, adaptations and the need for aids to independence especially if the patient has physical disabilities. The nursing staff can show relatives by their example the best approach to the patient, and the ward sister will give helpful advice about the patient's manage-ment; she will explain how necessary it is to encourage independence by planning and estab-lishing routines for the patient which include getting up and dressed each morning and attending to his own toilet, regular meals, having responsi-bility for simple tasks in the home as he is able, taking regular exercise, a rest after lunch and going to bed at a reasonable hour. She will point out that the patient will often need to be gently reminded what to do next and will advise relatives that they must make their expectations clear to the patient and then insist upon certain standards of hygiene and behaviour at all times. They should be advised to contact their general practitioner if there is any deterioration in the patient's condition. They should also be asked to contact the community social worker who will liase with the community occupational therapist, put the patient's name on the disabled persons' register, arrange for day care or attendance at a day centre and voluntary sitters-in if the patient cannot be left alone at home, and accommodation in a residential home for the elderly while the family take a holiday. She will also give advice about financial allowances, maintain contact with the family to reassess their needs and give advice whenever the patient has a spell at home.

Before the patient leaves hospital the nursing staff will contact the district nurse if any nursing procedure is necessary, and arrange for meals-on-wheels and home help services if there is a need. When all arrangements have been made the patient will be discharged from hospital. A report will have been sent to the general practitioner who will visit the patient on his return home from time to time, to assess his condition and detect any underlying ill-health which would cause deterioration in mental health. The relatives will then be reassured that they are not shouldering the whole burden, that everything possible is being done and they will have an opportunity to discuss problems with their doctor who, being in close touch with the family, will realise when the patient can no longer be managed at home. Occasionally it becomes neces-sary to admit a very disturbed patient to hospital on a compulsory detention order, under the Mental Welfare Act; there are strict laws protecting the patient and his property. **However mentally deranged the patient, no-one should discuss his condition within his hearing**.

Those patients who cannot be cared for at home have few options; if finances permit they may be cared for in a private nursing home, otherwise they will be looked after in a local authority home for the elderly or a geriatric hospital, depending upon the severity of their disability. It is important that the relatives continue to visit the patient regularly and if possible arrange regular outings and visits home.

Nursing care in hospital

Nursing care for these deteriorating patients should never cease to be a stimulating challenge to every skill the nursing staff can summon. A dementing patient, confused and disorientated, bewildered, agitated, restless and incontinent may be admitted to a general ward where it is not possible to give the patient the ideal of 'freedom with supervision'. In this unfamiliar environment his behaviour is likely to be even more disturbed, he may endanger himself and other patients in the ward, pull down an intravenous infusion or remove carefully applied bandages, will fail to co-operate with his treatment, keep other patients awake all night or make constant efforts to escape. Restraint may be essential, but care must be taken to handle the patient gently as there is risk of fractures in these elderly demented patients who resist with almost superhuman strength and may have brittle bones; nurses restraining a patient to give him a sedative injection must be sure to grasp the patient over major joints. The patient must be transferred as soon as possible to a neurological or geriatric unit where disturbed behaviour is accepted and understood and facilities are adapted to meet these needs, otherwise such heavy sedation will be given that it will soon lead, for example, to a sequence of extreme drowsiness, immobility, incontinence, pressure sores, catheterisation, urinary infection and further mental deterioration.

Each nurse must know her patient well, his past, present, and an outline plan for future treatment; only then will she be able to contribute usefully and gain satisfaction in her difficult task which needs to be done well. Some think that looking after a demented patient is simply a matter of keeping him fed, clean, dry and out of trouble; there is more to it than that, though no doubt these are important factors.

Communication is a vital factor in this patient's care, but it can be very difficult because the patient is out of touch with reality, often hard of hearing, partially sighted and deluded. He should always be addressed by an acceptable formal or informal name which he would like under normal circumstances and this should be conveyed to everyone who meets the patient. Speech should be not too fast, distinct but not necessarily loud and abstract ideas should be avoided. Communication is also in the nurse's pleasant expression (not necessarily a smile which may be interpreted as derisory), and in the way she includes (or does not exclude) him in conversation though he cannot take an active part. The patient should never be addressed in the third person, a point that the nurse will need to convey to relatives, ancillary staff, voluntary workers and visitors, for example the chaplain. Her understanding care is also clearly expressed in her manner as she changes the patient's dirty clothes or soiled bed; she must never express abhorrence even if she discovers body or head lice.

Communication with relatives is all-important and may even make the difference between continued regular visiting and outings and the patient being abandoned in a strange hospital environment to the complete care of strangers. Relatives may have had a very difficult time, either visiting daily and never being quite sure what they will find, or living with the patient and fitting his care into their own busy lives. They are likely to be agitated, distressed and on the defensive, perhaps not wanting to know that someone in their close family is becoming demented and feeling that this reflects adversely on them. No manner of expression can soften this unpleasant fact; they may unreasonably expect the doctor to effect a complete cure and be quite aggressive about further deterioration. Alternatively, relatives can be extremely embarrassed and apologetic for the patient's behaviour. Sometimes doctors unjustifiably label a patient with a diagnosis of dementia and the relatives then pick upon any little quirk or habit to prove there is deterioration; this unkind attitude robs the patient of his self-respect and spoils relationships. The whole situation demands patience, courtesy, thoughtfulness and tolerance in the face of possible abuse and lack of co-operation; the patient may be querulous, outspoken, use foul language, bite and spit and have other unpleasant habits and irritating ways. Those whose minds have deteriorated may either look obviously abnormal or to outward appearance normal in spite of quite severe dementia.

The patient's care is often shared over a period of years, between home and the community services, and hospital. As time goes on it becomes apparent that the gradually deteriorating condition of the patient and the home situation is making it more difficult for this patient to be cared for at home, and hospital admissions become more frequent until ultimately admission to a long stay unit becomes necessary. Home and hospital environment are different and each has its advantages and disadvantages, one offering familiarity and family love (though this may be so tried as to be almost extinguished), and the other skilled care, less spoken criticism and more encouragement, company, young nurses and a generally stimulating atmosphere, but unfortunately some wards for the elderly have an atmosphere more conducive to depression, deterioration and decay – the attitude and morale of the staff are all-important (see p. 364).

Sometimes when the patient is admitted to hospital he is withdrawn and depressed through sheer lack of interest and stimulation at home and has given up trying; he may be feeling there is nothing in store for him but life in an institution, 'so what's the use of bothering at my age?'. Dementia is sometimes very patchy and even if the thoughts are not put into so many words, they may still influence the patient's behaviour. Some patients become resentful and unamenable to reason and especially to their relatives' suggestions; at the worst they are extemely negativistic about everything. Perhaps partly to show their independence, they want to lie in bed all day, or on the contrary (due also to disorientation), to stay up at night doing their washing, which can be as difficult for relatives at home as it is inconvenient in hospital. The patient is often resistant to the idea of any change of routine and has a phobia about leaving the house and meeting strangers, refusing even to go to the day centre. It must be insisted that he takes the offered opportunities and he will agree more readily to an idea put forward by his general practitioner or social worker than by his custodial relative. Some patients are reluctant to have help with their personal toilet though they cannot manage alone; being proud, resenting the inference that they need a bath or change of clothing, seeing no necessity for either, being modest or feeling too weary to be bothered. It is always helpful to try to understand the patient's way of reasoning and see his point of view.

Regarding hygiene, in hospital it is comparatively easy to organise a routine which includes a regular bath or shower, but at home relatives may find the matter a problem, though someone of the same sex to assist may overcome the patient's resistance. Nurses too must not assume that a patient is managing all right because he has been in the bathroom or appears to have dressed himself (of course there is always the possibility that he did not completely undress to go to bed and may not have done so for a long time). When admitted to hospital a patient may be found to be dirty, smelly and to have skin lesions and this may happen even after a period in hospital if he has not been adequately supervised. It is the patient who is up and about and apparently independent who may neglect personal hygiene as, if there is physical disability, it is easier for the nurse to offer assistance than it is when the patient's limitation is only of reasoning. Tact is certainly necessary in this instance and also if the patient is incontinent and ignores his damp or dirty clothes. Unobtrusive

supervision will be necessary throughout the day to ensure that the patient takes a nourishing diet and good fluid intake. In some instances it will be necessary to suggest regular visits to the lavatory, give assistance with clothing (it is particularly common for demented patients to forget to fasten trousers) and remind the patient to wash his hands, so important to prevent gastroenteritis. As the patient becomes more child-like, supervision becomes essential to safeguard him from danger and ensure that prescribed medicines are swallowed; demented, paranoid patients characteristically become crafty and deceitful and in their attempt to outwit the staff or relatives, will hide pills, matches, money and other commodities. Another important factor is to notice when the patient is 'off colour', he may not complain and may continue to eat normally, yet for example may be vomiting frequently. In spite of his apparently stoical behaviour, whatever the illness, whether a common cold, influenza, or something much more serious, pneumonia or carcinoma, the demented patient must receive as good medical care as someone in their right mind. When the patient is ill he should be allowed a day or two in bed, but this period should be as brief as possible.

Any patient whose intellect is deteriorating must be regarded as accident-prone, and foresight will safeguard both him and others. Falls are common and the patient's environment must be checked for potential dangers: polished floors, slip mats, trailing flexes, stairs and other hazards. Prevention of serious falls is assisted by good supervision throughout the twenty-four hours, provision of suitable walking aids in some cases (though these can prove more confusing than helpful to some patients), good lighting, bed, chair and commode at the same level so that the patient can get from one to the other easily. Some patients are so confused that they forget they need help to walk and do not call for assistance. Physical restraint always seems unethical, but so long as someone is within earshot it may be essential for the patient's safety for him to be confined by the table fixture of his chair with the chair tipped back slightly to prevent him slithering out. Fire precautions must be religiously observed, open fires guarded and smoking discouraged, but if the patient insists, he must be supervised on every occasion. Gas taps and fires are dangerous and even radiators should be fitted with guards.

A short spell in hospital (at least twice a year) will

enable relatives to have a holiday, and benefit the patient by giving an opportunity for a medical check-up, a stimulating change of environment and greater appreciation of home comforts when he returns. A new look at problems may suggest a solution; does the patient need his vision or hearing tested, are his ears blocked by wax? When senses are failing it is important to ensure that every available aid is given to sharpen what remains, many of the elderly need the assistance of spectacles, magnifying glass, large print books and a hearing aid. Does the patient wear his dentures – if not why not? Perhaps they no longer fit after thirty years or so and he needs new ones, which will improve his appearance, help him to speak more clearly and enable him to eat a normal diet instead of mush. Poor appetite may be helped by change of diet; an attempt may be made to remedy obesity, a fairly common problem due to inactivity, boredom and lack of normal inhibition which may even lead to gluttony. Total restriction of the patient's favourite foods is unreasonable, but relatives should be advised not to over-indulge the patient with fattening titbits. Diet also plays a part in the treatment of constipation, and fibre in the form of bran should be introduced daily; when diet, exercise and habit training (never rushing the patient out of the toilet) achieve regular bowel evacuation, it will prevent the disastrous effects of excessive use of aperients. Incontinence (see pp. 178 to 180) may be the sole factor which makes it impossible for someone to live at home, the patient often becomes totally preoccupied, anxious and agitated and will not go anywhere where a toilet is not easily accessible. Intractable incontinence of urine can be investigated; if it still persists when a urinary infection has been treated and constipation remedied, an indwelling catheter may make home management possible. Retention of urine may be a neurological disorder associated with brain stem ischaemia or due to an enlarged prostate gland; in either, there may be an overflow dribbling incontinence. When organic conditions have been treated, after a suitable interval (3 months) the patient should be given an opportunity to dispense with the catheter. How well can the patient get about, can he walk to the toilet? Has he a history of falls? A lack of suitable walking shoes may be the hazard; no-one should slop about in slippers. This may be a good opportunity to introduce a walking frame.

Time in hospital can be useful for observation and treatment which will lengthen the period of time the patient is able to live at home, possibly improve the quality of his life there and relieve already overcrowded, under-staffed hospitals of another patient. It should be appreciated that though the relatives may resume care of the patient feeling refreshed after their holiday, less inclined to be irritable and intolerant and better able to face their responsibilities, they may on the contrary have found how good life is without the burden. This is a time when they particularly need encouragement and appreciation – appreciation which the patient can neither express nor perhaps feel, these patients often being at their worst with those who are closest to them.

Environment is a most important factor in the care of all patients, even more so for 'long stay patients' with deteriorating mental faculties, to whom the ward will become 'home'. A happy atmosphere, bright, pleasant normal surroundings and the niceties of life will encourage more normal behaviour. One instance of this was an observation that some patients who were previously incontinent did not soil the floor when a fitted carpet was introduced instead of linoleum. (Did the staff also make more effort perhaps, reminding and taking patients to the toilet regularly?) Rather as children often produce the behaviour expected of them, so will deteriorated patients react if an environment is created which is obviously adapted to the worst expectations rather than the best.

The objects of treatment and care are similar to those recommended for any rehabilitation programme (see p. 62) coupled with the realisation that deterioration and increasing dependence are eventually inevitable. Every effort must be made to maintain general physical and mental health, taking into account the patient's age and other unavoidable limitations, helping him to remain independent, well occupied, comfortable and happy and trying to avoid institutional attitudes. The patient should wear his own clothes which can be kept in a bedside dressing table/wardrobe. He should be encouraged to display treasured knick-knacks and family photographs; a group photograph of the patient with his family is a constant reminder to the staff of what the patient was like before his illness, and their responsibility towards him and his family. Some patients hoard what might be considered rubbish, but nurses must resist the urge to tidy up or nag the patient – some can be tidied away while the patient is in the bath.

The patient's day must be as near normal as possible without a feeling of regimentation and with encouragement and assistance when necessary. The patient should get up and dressed, take his meals in a dining area, go for walks or take part in some chosen outdoor activity, engage in other forms of occupation (making scrapbooks, Christmas or birthday cards, colouring pictures, etc.). He should have a rest period after lunch, spend time with his visitors in quiet private surroundings, have an opportunity to watch television or listen to the radio if he wishes and finally go to bed at a normal hour, not be put to bed at 5 o'clock to be out of the way when fewer staff are on duty. There should be a routine for the day, as routine gives the patient a feeling of security, helps his failing memory and keeps things running smoothly. The day must have landmarks which will help orientation: newspapers should be available, clocks should have a clear dial, be placed in a prominent position and set at the right time. Clearly printed calendars also help orientation and the day can perhaps be emphasised by a hand-painted notice 'TODAY IS TUESDAY'. In the same way as one talks to small children when going about the house, speaking of the plan of activities for the day will help some patients to keep in touch 'it will soon be lunch time, just an hour's time, Janet will be here this afternoon', not necessarily expecting a reply though giving time always for the patient's slow thought processes to bring forth comment; there is nothing to be lost by chatting and a kindly voice is always reassuring and comforting rather than the isolation and atmosphere created by grim silence. This distraction may keep the slightly paranoid patient in pleasant mood preventing his mind wandering to persecutory thoughts, but always a nurse must be sensitive to her patient's reaction and ready either to speak of something else or keep quiet if that appears to please the patient.

Weekly landmarks must be deliberately arranged to give each day a different character, 'hair-do', mobile shop and library days, birthday celebrations, singsong evenings possibly arranged by voluntary workers, an occasional film show, fetes and sales of work, Sunday services; the aim should always be to encourage the patient to activities away from the ward if possible. Interests in the ward and dayroom are pictures on the walls, picture books and current magazines, possibly a fish tank, budgerigar or ward cat.

Always remember the patient is out of touch and forgetful and warn relatives of accidents and fire hazards (patients with dementia should not be allowed to carry cigarettes and matches). There are many extremely demented patients who will respond best if they are allowed a feeling of freedom and to wander their own sweet way, unharrassed by the interference of overhelpful staff, and they should be left to their own devices as much as possible, being firmly prevented only when their activities are antisocial or dangerous, or for the every day essential routine which includes forms of rehabilitation or training truly likely to benefit the patient.

All these comments may seem too elementary for a textbook, but it is just such simple observations and approaches which bring rich rewards. It is on the basis of experience that nursing staff are able to advise relatives how to manage situations at home.

Part II
Disorders of the Spine

10

Disturbances of Sensation and Power

Anatomy and physiology

The vertebral column is composed of thirty-three bones (7 cervical, 12 thoracic, 5 lumbar, 5 sacral and 4 coccygeal) which articulate with each other for mobility. In the cervical region there is lateral rotation, flexion and extension. The thoracic spine has little mobility in any direction, the lumbar spine mainly movements of flexion and extension. The adult spinal column when seen from the side has four curves (Fig. 10.1); the cervical curve develops as the infant is able to lift his head and learns to sit up and the lumbar curve as he learns to walk. When the body is upright the weight should be evenly distributed on the hips and an imaginary perpendicular line drawn from the ear through the shoulder and hips to the ankle denotes the centre of gravity.

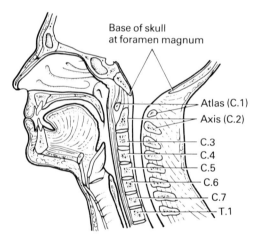

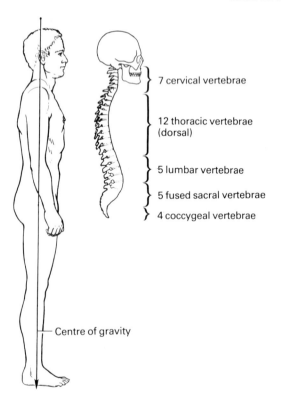

Fig. 10.1   Spinal curves and centre of gravity.

7 cervical vertebrae

12 thoracic vertebrae (dorsal)

5 lumbar vertebrae

5 fused sacral vertebrae

4 coccygeal vertebrae

Centre of gravity

Base of skull at foramen magnum

Atlas (C.1)
Axis (C.2)
C.3
C.4
C.5
C.6
C.7
T.1

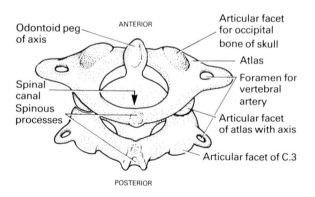

Odontoid peg of axis

ANTERIOR

Articular facet for occipital bone of skull

Atlas

Foramen for vertebral artery

Spinal canal
Spinous processes

Articular facet of atlas with axis

Articular facet of C.3

POSTERIOR

Fig. 10.2   Base of skull showing atlas and axis.

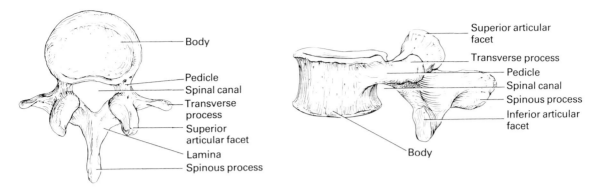

Fig. 10.3 Lumbar vertebra.

There are seven cervical vertebrae; the first, the atlas, is a ring of bone supporting the head, the second, the axis, has a peg (the odontoid process) which extends upwards into the atlas permitting lateral rotation of the head (Fig. 10.2). The remaining vertebrae each have a body which is small in the cervical region, increasing in size to the first sacral vertebra, then decreasing to the coccyx. A pedicle projects from each side of the body and from each pedicle, a transverse process. Two laminae connect the transverse processes to the spinous process, completing the circle of bone which protects the spinal cord (Fig. 10.3); the vertebrae each have two pairs of articulating facets, superior and inferior. There are slight variations in the structure of certain vertebrae, the cervical bones have a foramen in each transverse process for the passage of the two vertebral arteries (see Figs 10.2 and 8.2), the thoracic vertebrae have articulating facets for the twelve pairs of ribs (Fig. 10.4) and the sacral vertebrae are fused together into a large triangular-shaped bone which articulates with the iliac bone (sacro-iliac joints, Fig. 10.5). The vertebrae are cushioned from each other by the intervertebral discs and are held

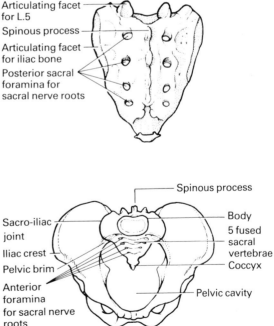

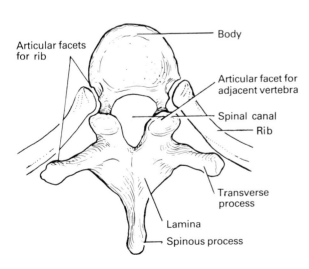

Fig. 10.4 Thoracic vertebra.

Fig. 10.5 The sacrum and pelvic girdle.

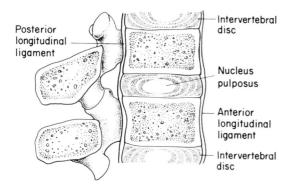

Fig. 10.6 Section through vertebral column showing intervertebral discs and ligaments.

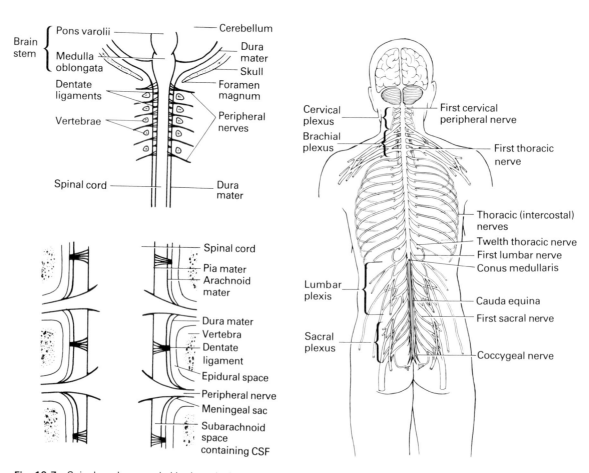

Fig. 10.7 Spinal cord suspended in the spinal canal.

Fig. 10.8 Spinal cord and peripheral nerves.

together by numerous ligaments (Fig. 10.6); the posterior and anterior longitudinal ligaments run the entire length of the vertebral column supporting the vertebral bodies, the ligamenta flava are short ligaments joining adjacent laminae, the supraspinous ligament joins the spinous processes and there are many smaller ligaments between the vertebrae.

The spinal cord, approximately 15 mm in diameter, is suspended in the spinal canal of the vertebral column (see Fig. 10.7). It is closely encased in meninges, a continuation of those surrounding the brain, and is tethered to the dura mater on either side by the dentate ligaments. The

cord is a continuation of the brain stem and ends as the conus medullaris at the level of the first or second lumbar vertebrae. A thin strand, the filum terminale, tethers the cord to the base of the spinal column. The shock-absorbing cerebrospinal fluid which circulates in the subarachnoid space is produced by the ventricular system and after circulation around the spinal cord, returns to the surface of the brain to be reabsorbed. The peripheral nerves which contain motor and sensory pathways, leave the cord in pairs (31 pairs in all), one pair from each segment of the spinal cord (see Chapter 25), throughout its length (Fig. 10.8); each nerve emerges from the meningeal sac which forms

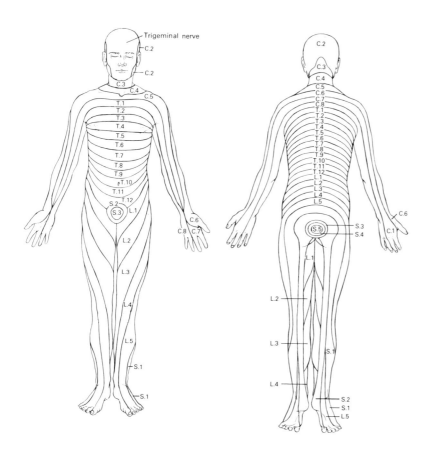

Fig. 10.9 Dermal representation of nerve root distribution.

a short sleeve one third of an inch long (see Fig. 10.7), before passing from the spinal canal through a foramen formed by two adjacent vertebrae. Nerve roots from the cervical cord supply the neck, upper thorax and most of the arms, the thoracic nerves supply a band down the centre of each arm and the remaining part of the chest wall and abdomen, and the nerve roots of the cauda equina (horse's tail) which fills the spinal canal below the conus medullaris, supply the lower back, legs and external genitalia (Fig. 10.9).

The spinal cord receives its blood supply from the anterior spinal and two posterior spinal arteries which lie within the subarachnoid space and run the length of the spinal cord (Fig. 10.10) and are branches of the vertebral arteries at the base of the

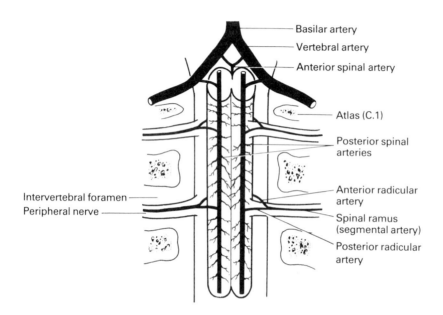

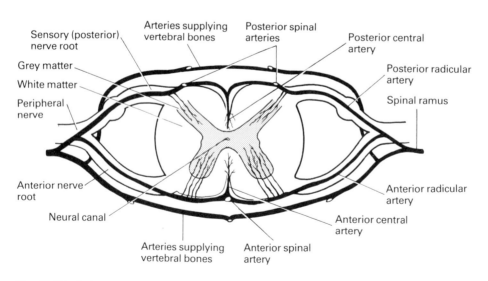

Fig. 10.10   Spinal arteries and section through spinal cord showing grey and white matter.

skull. Other segmental arteries enter alongside each nerve root, unite with the spinal arteries and increase the blood supply; fine branches of these arteries dip into the grey matter of the spinal cord to supply nourishment to the cell bodies of the neurones. The cord has no means of storing nutrients for future use and must receive a constant blood supply; cessation or diminution of this supply for even a short time will cause permanent spinal cord damage. A network of venous plexuses, throughout the length of the vertebral column, some within the subarachnoid space and some between the dura mater and the vertebrae, drain de-oxygenated blood from the spinal cord and return it to the venous system.

The cell bodies of the neurones are arranged in a characteristic H-shaped area in the centre of the spinal cord (Fig. 10.10) and are surrounded by the white fibres which also enter, leave and cross the grey central area throughout the entire length of the cord.

Sensory impulses of touch, temperature, pain, posture and joint position arise in the skin, muscles, tendons and joints of the whole body and pass along the sensory nerve pathways in the peripheral nerves to the sensory root ganglion and are relayed to the posterior part of the spinal cord. The nerve pathways of each sensation travel a separate course to the brain, some immediately crossing to the other side, some ascending a few segments before crossing while others ascend and then cross in the medulla. All but the nerve pathways to the cerebellum carry their impulses to the sensory cortex in the opposite cerebral hemisphere; here they are interpreted and messages are transmitted to the motor cortex which sends impulses down the motor pathways in the brain and spinal cord to the lower motor neurones of the peripheral nerves which transmit impulses to the muscles. At every level in the spinal cord there are links between the sensory neurones and the lower motor neurones forming the reflex arcs (see Fig. 2.4), thus enabling reflex muscular activity to take place without conscious control, e.g. when a person touches a burning hot object he will withdraw from the stimulus almost before he has had time to notice the intense heat and pain, the brain simultaneously interpreting the reflex action and the pain.

Impulses of sensation and motor power are carried in known pathways in the spinal cord, though the grouping is not as clear-cut as is shown for convenience in diagrams. The fibres carrying

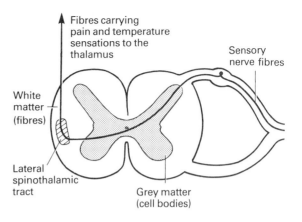

Fig. 10.11 Pain and temperature tracts.

sensations of pain and temperature (see Figs 10.11 and 17.1) travel upwards for a few segments then cross to the opposite side of the spinal cord and continue upwards in the lateral spinothalamic tract to the brain, terminating in the thalamus; other neurones carry the impulses from the thalamus to the sensory cortex of the brain. Sensations of touch and pressure are transmitted along fibres which immediately cross to the opposite side of the cord, but are carried in the ventral spinothalamic tract to the thalamus and thence to the sensory cortex (Fig. 10.12). The sense of position and movement of bones, muscles, joints and tendons (joint position sense) is transmitted to the sensory cortex through the posterior (dorsal) columns

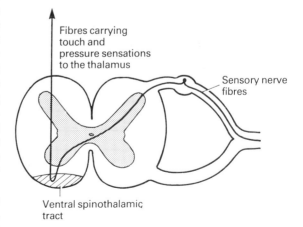

Fig. 10.12 Touch and pressure tracts.

(Fig. 10.13). The fibres ascend to the medulla, cross to the opposite side, then messages are relayed via the thalamus to the cerebral cortex. The spinocerebellar tracts carry impulses from all parts of the body to the cerebellum (Fig. 10.14); most of these fibres ascend to the ipsilateral cerebellar hemisphere, a few cross to the opposite side.

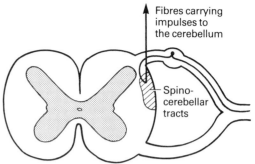

Fig. 10.14 Spino-cerebellar tracts.

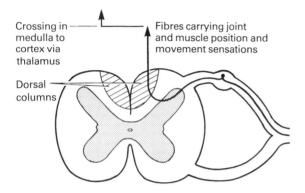

Fig. 10.13 Joint and muscle position tracts.

The descending motor pathways commence in the motor cortex of the frontal lobes, pass through the internal capsules of the brain to the brain stem, where they cross to the opposite side in the medulla. They continue to descend in the lateral motor pathways (pyramidal tracts; Fig. 10.15) of the spinal cord, and terminate in the anterior horns of grey matter where they synapse with the anterior horn cells (lower motor neurones). Impulses from the cerebral cortex are passed out to all parts of the body along the motor pathways of the peripheral nerves, to initiate voluntary movement. There are other influences which affect the function of the motor neurones; impulses are relayed from the vestibular part of the eighth cranial nerve, the cerebellum and the red nucleus in the midbrain, exerting a co-ordinating influence on the muscles of the trunk and limbs and allowing reflex adjustments in posture. The nerve fibres descend in the vestibulo-spinal and rubro-spinal pathways of the spinal cord (Figs 10.16 and 10.17) to the anterior horn cells (lower motor neurones). The extra-pyramidal system (see Chapter 20) controls muscle tone, posture and initiation of movement.

The autonomic nervous system comprises two chains of ganglia outside, on either side and running the whole length of the vertebral column,

one pair of ganglia communicating with each segment of the spinal cord (Fig. 10.18). This system supplies the involuntary control of the thoracic and abdominal viscera (heart, lungs, bladder and abdominal organs), the eyes, endocrine glands, salivary glands, sweat glands, blood vessels, erector muscles of each hair and the external genitalia. These organs are controlled by a careful balance between sympathetic (which excites) and parasympathetic (which subdues) systems. The autonomic nervous system, an integral part of the central nervous system, is under the control of the hypothalamus yet almost functions as a separate entity and is influenced by strong emotions when the sympathetic system responds by preparing the body for 'fight or flight'. Some of the

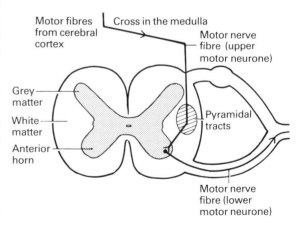

Fig. 10.15 Pyramidal (motor) tracts.

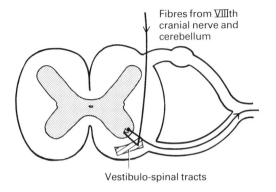

Fibres from VIIIth cranial nerve and cerebellum

Vestibulo-spinal tracts

Fig. 10.16 Vestibulo-spinal tracts.

cranial nerves form the parasympathetic part of the autonomic nervous system, namely the oculomotor nerve which constricts the pupil, part of the facial nerve to the submaxillary gland, part of the glossopharyngeal nerve to the parotid gland, and the vagus nerve which innervates thoracic and abdomal viscera and slows the heart and subdues the activity of abdominal organs. The sacral nerve roots, which control the bladder and external genitalia, are also part of the parasympathetic nervous system.

Symptoms and signs of spinal disorder

The severity and duration of paralysis and sensory loss depends upon the extent of damage to the spinal cord or cauda equina and whether any part can recover; **once the spinal cord is destroyed it cannot regenerate, but providing the destruction is not total there can be considerable recovery; the peripheral nerves can very slowly regrow providing the nerve cells and myelin sheaths remain intact** (see Chapter 25). The distribution of loss of function depends upon the level or levels of disorder in the cord or cauda equina, whether the lesion compresses the cord from within or without, affects only one side, is a disease of the insulating myelin coverings of the nerve fibres or affects the nerve cells or the peripheral nerve roots. The lesion is 2–3 segments higher than the sensory level would suggest because of the overlap between adjacent peripheral nerves. When the cord is severed or irreparably destroyed by disease, the lower section is isolated from the rest of the cord and brain, but will continue to receive information from the

peripheral nerves and autonomic nervous system, and reflex activity continues unmodified. A transecting lesion of the cervical cord causes paralysis and sensory loss of all four limbs (quadriplegia, tetraplegia; Fig. 10.19), a lesion at the level of the tenth thoracic vertebra causes paralysis and sensory loss below the level of the umbilicus (paraplegia), a lesion in the cauda equina causes disturbance in the buttocks and legs. A lesion in one side of the cord causes paralysis on the same side of the body below the lesion and sensory loss on the other (Brown-Séquard's syndrome; Fig. 10.20). Sensory or motor disturbance will depend upon the disease, e.g. in poliomyelitis which affects the anterior horn cells, though there may be complete paralysis, all forms of sensation are spared. In syringomyelia which involves the fibres of pain and temperature as they cross the centre of the cord, there are at first only sensory symptoms, later, as the syrinx enlarges, motor symptoms develop; rapidly compressing lesions of

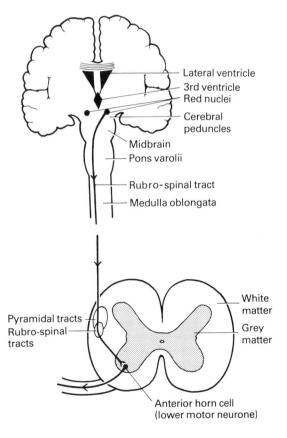

Lateral ventricle
3rd ventricle
Red nuclei
Cerebral peduncles
Midbrain
Pons varolii
Rubro-spinal tract
Medulla oblongata
White matter
Pyramidal tracts
Rubro-spinal tracts
Grey matter
Anterior horn cell (lower motor neurone)

Fig. 10.17 Rubro-spinal pathways.

the spinal cord such as abscess, will produce severe and rapid paralysis and sensory loss. Lesions affecting the cauda equina (entirely peripheral nerve roots) will disturb all forms of sensation and power as these are the final pathways to and from the lower trunk and legs and are a major part of the reflex arc. Bilateral lesions at any level will generally disturb bladder function as the bladder receives its nerve supply from both sides of the spinal cord. Some chronic diseases, for example multiple sclerosis, affect one side of the cord more severely than the other and the patient will retain some voluntary control over bladder function until the cord is completely destroyed. Lesions affecting the lower segments of the spinal cord and cauda equina cause impotence, but higher lesions causing paraplegia leave these segments intact, and though there are problems of mobility, sexual intercourse is still possible; a woman with paraplegia can conceive and bear a child.

Causes of weakness and sensory loss

1   Congenital
    (a)   Meningocele, myelomeningocele and syringomyelocele
    (b)   Angiomata
    (c)   Dermoid cyst
    (d)   Syringomyelia and syringobulbia
    (e)   Diastematomyelia
2   Traumatic
    (a)   Prolapsed intervertebral disc
    (b)   Fracture dislocation
    (c)   Knife and gunshot injuries

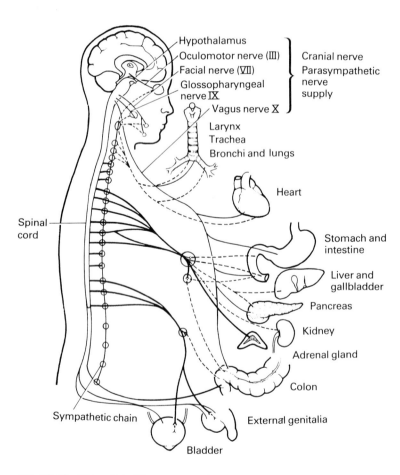

Fig. 10.18   The autonomic nervous system.

3 Infective
   (a) Osteomyelitis
   (b) Arachnoiditis
   (c) Myelitis including poliomyelitis
   (d) Spinal abscess
   (e) Spinal tuberculosis
   (f) Tabes dorsalis (neurosyphilis)
4 Neoplasia of the vertebrae, meninges, spinal cord, nerve roots, blood vessels or the neural canal
5 Vascular
   (a) Haemorrhage
   (b) Haematoma
   (c) Thrombosis
6 Degenerative
   (a) Spondylosis
   (b) Spondylitis
   (c) Paget's disease
7 Demyelinating diseases
8 Motor neurone disease
9 Peripheral nerve disorders – polyneuropathy

10 Disorder affecting the neuromuscular junction – myasthenia gravis
11 Muscle diseases
   (a) Polymyositis
   (b) Muscular dystrophy
   (c) Myopathy
12 Vitamin deficiency diseases – subacute combined degeneration of the cord
13 Cerebral lesions
   (a) Tumours in the parasagittal region
   (b) Lesions affecting the brain stem
14 Poisons and toxins

Admission of a patient with spinal disorder

It is not always possible for the nurse to know the exact extent of the patient's weakness or paralysis when she is awaiting his admission. When seen as an out-patient or in the casualty department the

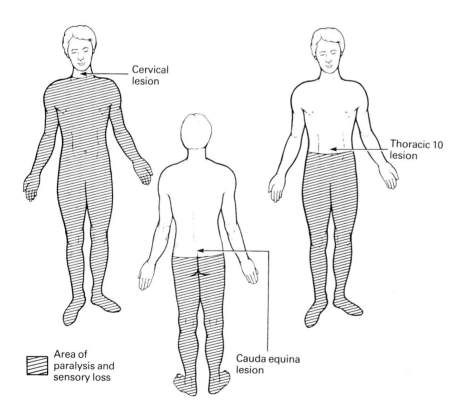

Fig. 10.19 Paralysis and sensory loss with cervical, thoracic and cauda equina lesions.

term paraplegia or quadriplegia may have been loosely used to describe disorders ranging from slight weakness to complete paralysis, or the patient's condition may have deteriorated considerably since he was last seen; whereas then he had very slight weakness, on admission he may be unable to walk. The nurse must be prepared for every circumstance; the following equipment should be available when a patient with spinal disease is to be admitted.

i   A bed with an integral wooden base or a full-length fracture board.

ii   Sandbags to support the head and neck if there is instability of the cervical spine.

iii   A small firm pad for use under the neck to maintain the natural curve of the cervical spine when there is a cervical fracture.

iv   A full length sheepskin and sheepskin bootees.

v   A bed cradle, always essential if there is weakness or paralysis of the legs.

vi   Plenty of pillows and a sorbo-rubber wedge for good positioning of the patient.

vii   A neurological examination tray.

viii   Suction apparatus and resuscitation equipment if the disorder affects or might affect the cervical cord or brain stem as the nerve supply to the intercostal muscles and the diaphragm could be impaired. An artificial ventilator should always be available and maintained in good working order at all times.

ix   Intravenous infusion, lumbar puncture and catheterisation trolleys.

Even the calmest patient may be alarmed if he sees elaborate equipment at his bedside; it is better that resuscitation and suction apparatus is near at hand yet out of sight. A patient who needs resuscitation and maintenance of respiration by an artificial ventilator may be mentally very alert yet unable to speak, able to understand and misunderstand a great deal of what is said at the bedside and suffer extreme distress; clear explanations must always be given to him.

The immediate nursing care, when the patient is admitted to the ward, will depend upon the cause and severity of the disorder, e.g. a patient admitted with a fracture dislocation of the upper cervical spine whose respirations are severely laboured and whose life is threatened, will need urgent resuscitation, whereas one with suspected cervical spondylosis whose only symptom is of mild progressive quadriparesis may remain fully ambulant, independent and require little immediate nursing care. Before the patient arrives the nurse should try to discover something of his history and symptoms and on admission she must make a thorough assessment. Should there be any doubt about the cause of paralysis it is always best to position the patient on his back without a pillow, but with a small firm pad under the nape of the neck until he has been seen by a doctor. The doctor should be notified immediately a patient is admitted with acute paraplegia, quadriplegia or rapidly progressing weakness, so that he may examine the patient (see Chapter 2), determine the level of the lesion and avoid delay in diagnosis and treatment. Delay may mean unnecessary permanent paralysis from spinal cord compression, or ascending lesions which can threaten the patient's respirations, may progress unseen and catch the staff unprepared.

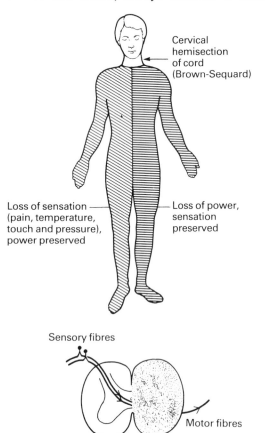

Fig. 10.20   Brown-Séquard's syndrome.

Observations

What observations can the nurse make? If the patient is ambulant, how does he walk, does he drag one or both legs, is there footdrop? Is the limb movement spastic or flaccid? When seeing the patient on his bed, which limbs are weak or paralysed and is there flexor or extensor spasm in response to stimulation? Is there muscle wasting? The nurse should test the patient's limb movements very carefully, this will be a guideline to future changes, improvement or deterioration. It sometimes helps the patient to move an apparently totally paralysed limb if the weight is supported, overcoming the pull of gravity. Are the arms affected as well as the legs, indicating disease in the cervical region? Lesions high in the cervical cord in the region of cervical 3, 4 or 5 will damage the phrenic nerves and affect the upper motor neurone supply to the intercostal muscles. Lesions in the lower cervical and the thoracic regions affect the intercostal nerves (see Fig. 10.8).

The nurse must bare the patient's chest and have a good look. Is there difficulty in breathing? Are both sides of the chest wall moving equally? Is breathing mainly diaphragmatic with little or no chest movement? Are there any indications of respiratory infection?

Does movement of any part of the body cause pain? Where is the pain; is it in the distribution of one or more nerve roots or is it localised to a particular part of the spinal column? What form does the sensory disturbance take; is there inability to determine temperature, touch, pressure, vibration and posture? All forms of sensation may be individually or severally affected. What is the degree of sensory disturbance; it may be only slight paraesthesia or complete numbness? The patient whose body feels no discomfort is very susceptible to pressure sores; is there discoloration of the skin over the pressure areas, are there sores, burns, ulcers or swollen painless joints?

Has the patient noticed any disturbance of micturition? How long has there been disturbance and what is its nature – hesitancy, dribbling, incontinence or complete retention? Is there distension of the abdomen due to retention of urine; when a urine specimen is obtained or if there is incontinence, is there evidence of infection?

Questions relating to bowel function should always be asked. The nurse should find out whether the patient has constipation, how often he has his bowels open and whether defaecation is difficult. Is there diarrhoea? This is often a complication resulting from impacted faeces due to sluggish bowel action; a rectal examination may be necessary to discover the cause. Diarrhoea, on the other hand, may be due to excessive use of aperients or a variety of intestinal conditions.

The patient's temperature, pulse, respiration and blood pressure will be recorded on admission. A raised temperature may be the result of urinary, respiratory or wound infection, deep vein thrombosis, or infection of the spinal cord, meninges or spinal column. The respiratory rate should be carefully checked for a full minute as patients suffering from high cervical disorders are in danger of respiratory paralysis; this applies particularly to fracture dislocations and to such diseases as poliomyelitis and syringobulbia where the upper cord and brain stem may be acutely affected.

A careful record of fluid balance is necessary to assess kidney function and when there are urinary difficulties. Should retention of urine be suspected, the doctor should be notified at once and preparations made for catheterisation. When urinary infection is suspected a urine specimen should be sent for laboratory testing; chronic urinary infection is common among women.

Without delay the bedridden patient should begin a 2-hourly regime of turning and skin inspection. Those who are mobile must not be forgotten, as if there is any sensory disturbance they are just as susceptible to sores and skin and joint injuries as an immobile patient, and careful lifting and turning are essential. No patient should sit for long periods in one position and patients should be taught how to raise themselves from the chair seat frequently and be encouraged to stand or walk with help at regular frequent intervals. Continuous nursing care is essential while tests and investigations are being done, and there should be nursing supervision and care when the patient spends a long period in the X-ray department.

When there is acute traumatic or infective spinal paralysis the patient is confined to bed. All patients should be visited by the occupational therapist and the physiotherapist who will assess, plan and begin a programme of treatment to suit each individual. The medical social worker should be contacted and a brief resumé of the case will enable her to anticipate the problems that may arise though it is possible she can do little at this early stage (see p. 194).

Patients admitted with chronic disorders, though they are very disabled, should be encouraged to continue their usual activities while tests and radiological investigations are performed. There is a risk in a busy ward that a patient who needs less urgent and constant attention will feel neglected and think the staff are less interested in him than in their more acutely ill 'interesting cases' and the patient may harbour unnoticed anxiety and loneliness. Extra care should be taken to ensure that he is given ample opportunity to see and speak to both medical and nursing staff, that he should see their interest and concern for him and be kept well informed about investigations and plans for his treatment. When the staff are exceptionally busy it is most helpful if there is a good morale and camaraderie among the patients, then no-one will feel left out.

Investigation

A full and detailed history of the illness is often the most valuable part of any examination and may enable the doctor to make a diagnosis; it is supported by a complete general and neurological examination (see Chapter 2). The functions of the brain are examined in addition to those of the spinal cord, as paraplegia, though most commonly caused by spinal lesions, may also be caused by a lesion in the brain (e.g. parasagittal tumour) or by a condition which involves both brain and spinal cord (multiple sclerosis). In his examination the doctor maps out the area of disturbance and then, bearing in mind the complexity of the sensory and motor pathways, he endeavours to localise the lesion to a particular level in the spinal cord.

Blood tests
Haemoglobin, white cell count, ESR and blood grouping are important as transfusions and treatment for anaemia may be necessary. Vitamin B_{12} estimation is necessary to exclude subacute combined degeneration of the cord (see Chapter 26). Wassermann and Khan tests for syphilis are always performed and blood urea levels and electrolyte estimation will be a guide to kidney function and general health.

Chest X-ray
Chest X-ray is always essential, it may reveal primary carcinoma and tuberculosis suggesting the nature of the spinal lesion, and show other respiratory disorders; there may be congenital heart disease associated with congenital disorder of the spine and spinal cord.

Spinal X-rays
These may show:
1   Congenital abnormalities, e.g. spina bifida
2   Fractures with or without dislocation
3   Narrowing of the disc space between two vertebrae when an intervertebral disc has prolapsed
4   Evidence of infection and collapse of vertebral bodies
5   Areas of calcification, erosion of bone or enlargement of foramina in the presence of neoplasia
6   The position of foreign objects, e.g. a bullet
7   Degenerative changes in the bone associated with spondylosis, spondylitis and Paget's disease
8   The evidence and extent of previous surgery

The spinal cord and peripheral nerves cannot be visualised by plain X-rays and in diseases such as multiple sclerosis or poliomyelitis the X-rays are normal.

Lumbar puncture
Lumbar puncture (see p. 32) is performed:
i   to obtain a specimen of CSF for laboratory analysis;
ii   to measure the CSF pressure;
iii to introduce radio-opaque substances.
For normal CSF see p. 33.

In the presence of a partial or complete block in the flow of CSF in the spinal subarachnoid space, changes take place in the stagnating fluid below the level of the blockage.

   (a)   The protein increases particularly when the compression is from outside the spinal cord (extramedullary).

   (b)   The fluid may be xanthochromic and clot rapidly.

   (c)   The pressure may be below normal and the normal pulsations corresponding to pulse rate and respirations are reduced or absent.

   (d)   Queckenstedt's test may show a slow rise and fall of CSF or no response when there is a partial or complete block in the spinal subarachnoid space because pressure is applied at a level above the lesion, whereas pressure on the abdomen below the level of the lesion may cause an exaggerated increase in the CSF pressure.

(e) The CSF cell count will only be increased if the cause of obstruction is inflammation.

When blockage to the flow of CSF in the spinal theca is due to a tumour, lumbar puncture, through lowering the pressure, it may exacerbate the symptoms and urgent surgery becomes essential.

Myelography

Myelography (see Chapter 2) outlines the shape of the spinal cord, cauda equina and the intraspinal section of the peripheral nerves. The radio–opaque dye may slowly drip past a partial obstruction. If the obstruction is complete, it will stop at the lower level; cisternal myelography will then be necessary to show the extent of the lesion. Abnormalities in the region of the foramen magnum are demonstrated best by air myelography.

Nursing care of a paralysed patient

The common usage of the term 'paraplegic' to describe someone whose legs have been paralysed for years, who is well used to his condition and able to instruct those who help him in every detail of his care, can easily lead to the wrong approach. There should be a sense of urgency; this condition is always an emergency until a definite diagnosis has been made. In many instances the paralysis is due to a lesion compressing the spinal cord; if the cord is relieved of pressure almost immediately it will recover and the patient will regain the use of his limbs. The likelihood of complete recovery decreases with every hour that the compression is allowed to persist. The nurse is responsible for the crucial hour-by-hour observations and must report to the medical staff as soon as she notices increasing weakness of a patient's legs, if he mentions that his appreciation of sensation has altered or if he complains of difficulty in micturition or has not passed urine. It is tragic when after much delay, the patient has an operation for a benign compressing lesion, e.g. a spinal meningioma, yet, because the cord has been compressed for too long, paralysis persists and the patient is forced to lead a wheel-chair existence for the rest of his life. This is equally important for the elderly and those whose general prognosis is bad, for surely no-one should unnecessarily lose the use of his legs. There are many conditions which, even though they are treated promptly and correctly, will leave permanent paralysis; then the nurse must be intensely aware of the many complications which persistently threaten to spoil or shorten the patient's life.

Paraplegia may be acute in onset, for example fracture dislocation, or develop slowly, for example a slow-growing neoplasm or cervical spondylosis. With the onset of acute paraplegia there is a period of up to six weeks when the cord is in a state of shock and paralysis is flaccid. As this stage passes, spasticity develops with accompanying muscle spasms and the existing risk of pressure sores can be complicated by friction sores and joint contractures. In the chronic form of paraplegia there is spasticity from the onset: this increased muscle tone can sometimes be useful, enabling the patient, whose legs are otherwise useless, to bear his own weight while transferring from chair to toilet or bed, giving greater independence. As early as possible the patient must be encouraged to be independent; it is fruitless for him to lie back and wait for recovery which may never come. From the beginning, even when the patient is lying inactive, shocked and depressed, the foundations of good rehabilitation can be laid by good optimistic attitudes towards independence and skilled nursing to prevent complications which will threaten independence.

Prevention of complications

The nurse must be aware of the complications which threaten a patient who is paralysed, in order to prevent them.

Pressure sores and skin abrasions

There are a number of reasons why paralysed patients are extraordinarily prone to develop pressure and friction sores and these factors may also delay healing:

(a) total immobility;
(b) loss of skin sensitivity;
(c) interference with the autonomic nerve supply to the blood vessels which impairs circulation;
(d) reflex sweating which makes the skin soggy;
(e) muscular spasms which cause friction and bring skin surfaces into close and forcible contact.

A normal healthy person, whether standing, sitting or lying, makes frequent slight adjustments to his position and weight distribution all the time; the paralysed patient cannot make these adjustments. There must be adequate staff to ensure that the patient is moved absolutely regularly at frequent intervals day and night, a trained nurse should always be available to provide supervision and advice, and full use should be made of any available mechanical aids to facilitate lifting. The ward temperature should be comfortably cool, a bedcradle is needed to ensure circulation of air to the patient's body, his bedding kept to a minimum, he should wear cotton garments in preference to nylon and have a daily bath or shower. Observation of the skin is of great importance and there must be good lighting; during the night a powerful torch should be used to inspect the skin carefully each time the patient is moved. The nurse should plan exactly how the patient is to be lifted and positioned before going to his bedside, as too much discussion over his head is likely to cause anxiety. Moving and positioning the patient must always be performed with great care as the consequences of negligence or faulty technique are serious; should a sore develop, it is so easy for each individual to lay the blame on someone else.

The patient must be turned two-hourly throughout the 24 hours using supine, prone and both lateral positions if his condition permits (see Figs 10.21, 10.22 and 3.6). When a reddened area persists even after a two hour rest, the patient must not lie on that area until the skin returns to normal; the same applies to any area which is blistered, bruised, grazed or in any way abnormally marked. Four people may be required to lift the patient, particularly following fracture dislocation and cervical spinal surgery when it is vital to maintain the patient's head and spine in correct alignment; the patient must always be lifted clear of the bed, chair, commode or hoist seat whenever he is moved to prevent his skin being stretched, dragged or bruised. Creased sheets must be smoothed, crumbs and other particles brushed out of the bed and indwelling catheters carefully positioned, as these may rapidly cause blistering and skin abrasions, which may become infected and produce a necrotic festering sore; once the skin has broken, scar tissue forms, which is always more susceptible to future breakdown. Care must be taken when lateral positions are used to prevent one limb resting on another; in the supine and prone positions when the powerful hip adductors are working unopposed, a small pad will be necessary to keep the knees apart

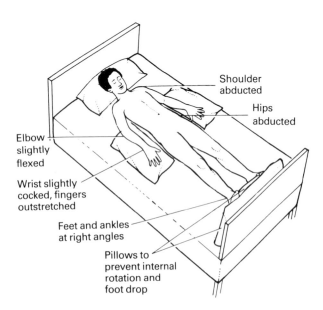

Fig. 10.21 Supine position for patient with quadriplegia.

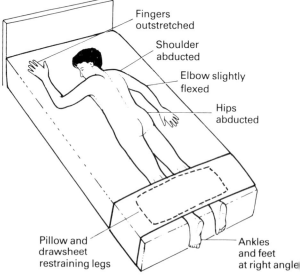

Fig. 10.22 Prone position for patient with quadriplegia. The legs are restrained to prevent flexion contractures.

and when the patient is lying prone, pressure upon the toes can be relieved by allowing his feet to hang clear of the end of the bed.

Special beds and turning frames relieve the nursing staff of some heavy lifting; in other than specialist units, it may be impossible to find four able-bodied nurses to lift and turn patients every two hours. There are several ways of relieving pressure: sheepskin rugs and bootees are useful as are alternating pressure mattresses and water beds; pack beds made of thick sections of foam rubber or several pillows bound together in a draw sheet can be arranged to relieved pressure to suit each individual patient's needs.

The skin is a delicate organ and must be treated gently. A heavy-handed nurse can unknowingly cause damage; long fingernails, rings and wrist watches so easily scratch insensitive skin; hot water bottles should *NEVER* be used. Vigorous rubbing, as sometimes practised by some people, can cause untold damage to the deep tissues; the skin may remain intact for some while, but suddenly a large dark area appears beneath the skin and the underlying tissue breakdown comes to the surface as a necrotic sore. Gentle applications of oil to a dry skin will prevent cracking. The skin should be kept cool and dry and unless the patient suffers from incontinence, talcum powder is helpful. The patient is no longer able to walk and the skin which is normally shed from the feet builds up to become a thick, hard, cracked pad over the undersurface of the foot increasing the risk of pressure sores on the heels, sides of the feet and toes; this problem also affects the hands of a patient with quadriplegia. Should the cracking be deep enough to cause an open wound there is risk of infection. The care of the feet and hands is important, including regular washing and soaking in soapy water, thorough drying, especially between the fingers and toes, and frequent application of arachis or similar bland oil to soften and remove dead skin. Callouses already formed will respond to similar treatment, or if the patient is allowed out of bed, a good soaking of his feet in a bowl of warm water, followed by the application of arachis oil should hasten the removal of dead skin. The fingernails of a patient who has quadriplegia should be kept short to prevent them digging into the palms of his hands.

Occupational therapy and physiotherapy play an important part in preventing pressure sores by developing useful muscles which enable the patient to lift himself clear of the bed when turning, assist

him to transfer easily from his wheelchair without injuring himself and to lift frequently and regularly, clear of the seat when sitting in a chair, to allow better circulation to sacral areas. There is an assortment of anti-pressure cushions (foam or water) for use in wheelchair or armchair; these are particularly useful for elderly and quadriplegic patients who cannot lift themselves in their chair.

Unfortunately pressure sores sometimes develop; a sore, however small must be treated as a surgical wound and sterile dressings should be applied using an aseptic technique. The sore should be thoroughly cleansed, necrotic tissue must be removed before healing can take place and desloughing solutions such as aserbine should be used to break down necrotic tissue and keep healthy tissue clean as it heals. A light packing dressing may be necessary when a cavity is present, but care must be taken not to pack the cavity too firmly as this will impede circulation, delay healing and through pressure on healthy tissue, may even cause further necrosis. Healing should be a gradual process of granulation from the base and sides of the cavity, the surface skin should never heal while there is a cavity and necrotic tissue within, otherwise it will only break down or develop into a discharging septic sinus. During treatment, all pressure must be eliminated from the area. Since most sores involve the sacral and hip areas, and it is impossible to relieve them of pressure if the patient sits in a chair, mobilisation must be postponed – a totally demoralising situation for any patient when he may be bedbound for many months. Skin grafting may be the only solution.

Anaemia is a fairly common problem especially if there are pressure sores; blood transfusions, a high protein diet and vitamins are given to improve the patient's general health and assist the body's natural healing powers.

The patient with quadriplegia cannot help himself at all and is dependent upon nursing staff and relatives, who must be trained in lifting and turning techniques.

Contractures

The muscles used to flex limbs are stronger than those for extension; when spinal cord disease leads to paralysis of a limb, reflex movement develops; this is more often flexor than extensor and usually called spasm. Flexor spasms are the most troublesome, as untreated the patient will rapidly develop the characteristic posture seen at its worst and most pathetic in a patient with quadriplegia who, with contractures of all four limbs, lies in a curled up position with arms and legs rigidly bent against his trunk. Good positioning is vital; in the supine position (Fig. 10.21) the knees can be extended, without being hyperextended which damages the joints and puts increased strain on muscles and tendons. The hips should be slightly abducted and the feet at right angles to the legs, a position maintained by the use of a pillow and board across the end of the bed; care must be taken to prevent internal rotation of the foot. When there is quadriplegia the arms should be slightly abducted at the shoulder and the elbows slightly flexed by placing a pillow under the forearm, the wrist should be cocked and the fingers and thumb outstretched. Contractures of the knee joints caused by flexor spasms can be prevented by restraining the knees with a pillow and tightly stretched draw sheet (Fig. 10.23). In the prone position (Fig. 10.22) the same posture of joints applies and the legs may need to be restrained; the feet can only be kept at right angles if a pack bed is used or the feet hang over the end of the bed. In the lateral position (see Fig. 3.6) knees should be slightly flexed, the uppermost leg supported on a pillow and the ankles at right angles. Should the patient be quadriplegic his uppermost arm should also be supported on a

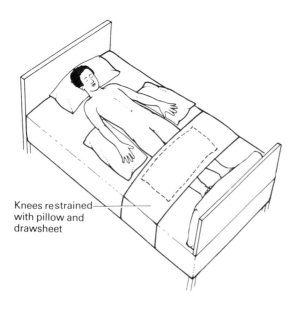

Knees restrained with pillow and drawsheet

Fig. 10.23 Restraining knees when flexor spasms threaten to cause contractures.

pillow, the elbow slightly flexed, wrist cocked and fingers outstretched. **These positions must be correctly maintained throughout the 24 hours** and all instructions from the physiotherapist must be conveyed to the day and night staff.

Physiotherapy
The paralysed joints must be put through a complete normal range of movements at least twice a day; nurses should watch the physiotherapist so that they can supplement the treatment themselves while giving nursing care, or be fully responsible for it at weekends and during holiday times. Should the nurse be unsure of the range of movement required, and normally possible in any particular joint, she should examine the movement of her own joints and then simulate this degree of movement on the patient. A nurse should always feel free to ask the physiotherapist for advice about a patient's treatment. When contractures are already present, physiotherapy and good positioning will prevent them getting worse; gradually the muscles and tendons will be stretched until a full range of movement can be achieved. Systemic infection, particularly urinary tract infection, increases muscle spasms and should be promptly and adequately treated.

Muscle relaxant drugs and hydrotherapy will help control flexor spasms and reduce spasticity, but in some progressive diseases flexor spasms may become uncontrollable. When the diagnosis of incurable disease is certain, and only then, it may be beneficial for the patient to undergo the operation of tenotomy (when the tendons of muscles causing spasm are deliberately cut), or the nerves of the cauda equina may be destroyed by injections of phenol into the lumbar theca.

Urinary tract infection and renal failure

Urine is excreted continuously by the kidneys and passes down the ureters to be stored by the bladder until there is sufficient urine to stimulate the sensory stretch receptors in the bladder wall. These receptors relay impulses along the sensory sacral nerve roots to the lower spinal cord and impulses are then transmitted to the brain where they are interpreted as a pressure discomfort within the bladder and the desire to pass urine. Motor impulses are then relayed to the bladder which contracts, and to the external sphincter which opens voluntarily and urine is passed. The neck of the bladder remains open only while urine is being passed, then closes automatically. The brain has the power to suppress sensory impulses many times before pressure in the bladder becomes so great that the messages can no longer be ignored and urine has to be passed.

Micturition is fundamentally reflex involving the nerve roots of the cauda equina, the lower segments of the spinal cord and the autonomic nervous system. In infancy it is totally reflex, the bladder emptying when in contains a certain volume of urine; as the infant grows he learns to understand the sensations and usually achieves control of micturition, day and night, by the age of three years. Several factors interfere with control of micturition at any age:

i   infection – cystitis;
ii   laxity of the pelvic floor muscles;
iii muscle relaxant drugs;
iv   loss of inhibitory cerebral control;
v   disturbance within the sensory and motor nerve pathways of the cauda equina and spinal cord.

Bilateral lesions of the cervical and upper thoracic cord which cause quadriplegia or paraplegia spare the reflex arcs of micturition, and the bladder becomes spastic, irritable and frequently empties small amounts of urine automatically. A patient who has partial bladder control will experience urgency and precipitancy of micturition with incontinence. In either circumstance the patient is likely to have retention of urine. Bladder function is surprisingly well retained when the cord lesion is unilateral. Lesions of the lower segments of the cord and of the cauda equina affect the reflex arcs of micturition, and the bladder which is no longer able to transmit or receive nerve impulses becomes flaccid (atonic), fills beyond normal capacity without causing any discomfort and then overflows causing incontinence. It empties incompletely and large quantities of urine stagnate in the bladder. Whenever there is retention of urine, there is a serious risk of urinary tract infection. Recurrent urinary infections, dilatation of the ureters, renal calculi and hydronephrosis cause renal failure and the premature death of patients with paraplegia and quadriplegia. Most of these urinary complications can be avoided if certain precautions are always taken.

1   The bladder must be emptied at regular intervals to prevent stagnation of urine and back-pressure on the ureters and kidneys.

2   A high fluid intake of at least 3 litres per day; the more fluid is flushing through the urinary system, the less likely are infection and renal and vesicular calculi. Every nurse must be aware of this essential need and should encourage her patients and their relatives to see the wisdom of the regime and ensure that it is always maintained, as it must be for the rest of the patient's life.

3   Catheterisation must be a strictly aseptic procedure and all urinary and drainage apparatus should be sterile.

4   Urine specimens should be sent to the laboratory once weekly for analysis and if at any time there should be the slightest suspicion of infection – (clouding of urine, offensive odour or unexplained pyrexia) – for pathology and sensitivity to antibiotics; antibiotics are not used prophylactically.

Catheterisation
Catheterisation is necessary when there is retention of urine. During the first 48 hours after the onset of acute paraplegia or quadriplegia, catheterisation is necessary to assess returning kidney function as there is usually a period of oliguria caused by hypotension (the result of haemorrhage from multiple injuries), or the effect upon the sympathetic nervous system of a high cervical lesion (see Fig. 10.18). A small-sized self-retaining catheter should always be used. Leakage around the catheter sometimes occurs due to partial or complete blockage by debris, or occlusion of the eye of the catheter when it is pulled into the urethra; the catheter must be replaced with one of the same size. The nurse should not be tempted to insert a larger catheter as urethral dilatation causes further leakage, and incontinence when the catheter is no longer required. When a catheter is used adequate drainage must be maintained and this can be achieved by:

1   Intermittent catheterisation.
     Each catheterisation must be performed under strictly aseptic conditions. The patient is first given the opportunity to void naturally, then whether he passes urine or not he is catheterised, the bladder emptied and the catheter removed. This procedure should be performed every 6 hours and in this way returning bladder function or development of an 'automatic bladder' can be detected at the earliest possible moment. When the residual urine is less than 100 ml, the frequency of catheterisation is gra-

dually reduced until it is discontinued entirely. Two more weekly assessments of the residual urine should be made.

2   Closed-circuit open drainage.
The catheter is attached to a sterile one-way drainage bag, the risk of infection is reduced as the bladder is constantly empty and there is no stagnant urine.

Intermittent catheterisation, if correctly performed, can keep the urine sterile for a period of up to twenty days, but after this, infection invariably occurs. This method is therefore only useful if the bladder is expected either to regain normal function or become automatic within three weeks. When there is no recovery of bladder function after a lengthy period, open drainage is the method of choice as infection is less likely; a high fluid intake, continuous drainage and a weekly bladder washout using a gravel solvent should prevent collection of debris. A silicone-covered cathether is used and the urethral orifice must be cleansed carefully each day; the catheter need not be changed for 3 months unless it becomes blocked. Once the patient begins to be mobile (in a wheelchair or on his feet) and is dressed he will be fitted with a holster or sporran day drainage bag; these bags hold approximately 400 mls and will be changed for a larger bag holding 2000 mls at night. The bags are washed thoroughly using running cold water and used again, each bag lasting about a week.

Disorders of bowel function

Patients with paraplegia and quadriplegia almost always have some disorder of bowel function. Inactivity and loss of muscle tone cause constipation, weakness of the anal sphincter muscle leads to loss of control and incontinence and poor muscular control to difficulty in evacuating the bowel. Many problems can be averted if sensible measures to prevent constipation are taken from the very beginning of the illness. The patient's co-operation and intelligent understanding of the problems will help him to train his bowel to evacuate at regular times even when there is considerable degree of dysfunction.

Management
i   The diet should include plenty of fibre, e.g. bran and vegetables.

ii   A high fluid intake is essential.
iii   The patient should be encouraged to try to evacuate his bowel at a regular time daily or on alternate days. Nursing staff must be prepared to give the patient prompt assistance when he wishes to go to the toilet, as repeated delays lead to failure in habit training.
iv   The gastro-colic reflex is normally stimulated immediately following a meal or hot drink; this is the best time for the patient to attempt bowel evacuation.
v   Aperients (faecal softeners and purgatives) should be given to regulate bowel function and adjusted to suit the patient's needs; they should be introduced gradually and great care exercised to ensure that an excess of aperients does not lead to diarrhoea; seasonal fruits can be a cause of diarrhoea. It is extremely difficult for the patient to prevent incontinence as the anal sphincter is weak and there will also be difficulty in retaining enemata; for this reason suppositories are often more suitable. Diarrhoea and incontinence, often the result of careless attempts to 'get results' are most distressing and will bring a catastrophic lowering of morale and cause skin soreness. There is a danger in a spinal injured person of paralytic ileus, then the administration of enemata is contraindicated (see p. 212).
vi   The patient can assist defaecation by
(a)   deep breathing which increases the recto-anal pressure
(b)   massaging the left side of the abdomen over the descending colon
(c)   inserting a gloved finger into the anus
vii   Digital evacuation should be performed if defaecation does not occur spontaneously.

On admission to hospital, the patient may already have severe faecal impaction; the faeces should be softened by the use of suppositories or a small enema followed by a digital evacuation taking care not to overstretch the anus. When impaction is severe a high colonic enema may be necessary. Once the bowel is empty, training can begin according to the above list. When a regular bowel evacuation is established the patient with paraplegia will learn self-care; this will be simplified once he has achieved balance and is able to transfer from wheelchair to toilet. The patient with quadriplegia may never achieve this independence; should regular digital evacuation be necessary when the patient returns home, this becomes the responsibility of a relative or the district nurse.

Overweight

Any paralysed patient should be encouraged to 'watch his weight': obesity will decrease mobility, make lifting more difficult, sweating more likely and increase the risk of pressure sores; it may also contribute to heart disease and aggravate breathlessness. Caloric intake should be controlled to a level in keeping with the patient's physical activity, otherwise he will steadily put on weight, especially if boredom and depression lead to compulsive eating.

Rehabilitation

(See also pp. 62 and 362)

No-one would choose to lose the ability to walk, to lose their independence or in some instances to become even more helpless than a child, yet this does happen to people of all ages, some of whom have experienced the joys of youth, the pleasures and responsibilities of running and maintaining a home and garden, parenthood and the satisfaction of a successful career; others have regrets over missed opportunities. At whatever age a person is robbed of their freedom by spinal disaster (because most patients retain their intellect and awareness) there are always tremendous psychological reactions and adjustments especially when the patient has others dependent upon him. Some people will accept their lot and find new interests and challenges, whereas others constantly dwell on the past and call to mind things they can no longer do. Nurses and therapists are in no position to criticise; they need to be sympathetic, sensitive to the patient's variable mood and approachable so that the patient feels quite free to express his frustations, emotions and anxieties; the staff need to give encouragement and try to draw the patient out of his despair. The patient may relate particularly well to one number of the staff; this can be a good thing, but the patient needs more than one therapist and the rehabilitation team must all pull together with everyone informed of the patient's programme and progress.

The patient may be able to come to terms with his disability when it develops gradually, but a constant or sudden additional deterioration, especially if his hopes have been raised by improvement, will cause deep depression. When someone has suddenly become completely paralysed he may bravely face the circumstance, but at any time, provoked by a seemingly trivial incident, the realities of the situation may come home to him and he will give way to uncontrollable grief. The outburst will give emotional relief and the patient must be given privacy to have a good cry; these crises may come at night because the patient, unable to sleep, has time to think. A young person suddenly robbed of all power and caged within his motionless body with the volatile emotions of youth, prospects of love and marriage blighted, is unable even to let off steam by slamming the door and storming off. What internal turmoil there must be. Nurses must be tolerant of irritability, childishness and petty jealousies and constantly try to create a peaceful, caring, good-humoured therapeutic atmosphere among a group of patients (and also their therapists) whose ages, interests, personalities and social backgrounds are different. Patients should be encouraged to take an interest in each other as this helps mutual understanding and prevents a patient becoming engrossed in his own condition and treatment to the exclusion of all else. Noise is a nuisance, but if there is mutual understanding it should be possible to have periods of quiet interspersed with times of banter and light-hearted jocularity, music, radio or television.

Rehabilitation aims to return the patient to independence as soon as possible, firstly, personal independence and later, independence which enables the patient to resume a useful role in society. For the housewife and mother this means caring for her home and family, for others, returning to work or finding a new job, and for the paralysed child, it is the beginning of a whole new way of life. Plans for rehabilitation should be made from the beginning whatever the cause of paralysis, even if there is a possibility that the patient's condition may suddenly or continuously deteriorate, as for him it is extremely important that he is independent for as long as possible. Though the patient sees no future for himself, a positive realistic approach to rehabilitation will challenge him, and the very fact that plans are being made will give him hope; relatives should be drawn into the planning. The patient will have good and bad days and more harm than good is often done by being too rigid; there are occasions when a nurse should give help though she knows the patient could perform the task himself, this may not be a retrograde step but rather increase goodwill and encourage further endeavour. Certainly a patient must learn to manoeuvre his wheelchair and open doors, for example, but normal courtesies should not be forgotten and meeting occasional helpfulness, he will go on his way more speedily and in better heart; there are of course patients who are naturally inclined to be lazy and helpless, who will need firm, good-humoured chivying and praise.

Some patients can begin an active programme of rehabilitation immediately, for others mobilisation may be delayed for weeks or months; this valuable time should not be wasted. The occupational therapist plays a very important part; she can do much to keep the patient mentally, and as far as possible, physically occupied, building up his strength for the time when he begins more active rehabilitation. When he can sit out of bed he will be taught by the occupational therapist to use the various aids that will help him with his personal toilet, dressing and feeding; these aids are particulary useful for the patient with quadriparesis to enable him to use any residual movement (see Disabled Living Foundation, p. 366). When the patient tires less easily he will begin to attend the occupational therapy department daily where he will continue to practise the skills of personal independence he has begun to learn in the ward and then progress to using tools and machinery designed to exercise and strengthen existing useful muscles. A housewife, mother or someone who lives alone, should have ample opportunity to learn how to use the many gadgets devised to help in the kitchen and learn the art of cooking 'paraplegic style'. The occupational therapist will have many opportunities to observe progress and will be able to advise medical staff when it is desirable for the patient to be retrained for future employment.

The physiotherapist will visit the patient twice daily while he is immobilised in bed, to teach breathing exercises, exercise weak muscles, prevent deep vein thrombosis and the development of con-tracture deformities in paralysed and semi-paralysed limbs and teach exercises which will strengthen muscles, even those with only slight residual movement. The patient will be shown how to do his exercises (sometimes using tension springs) and told how often to do them; nurses should encourage these activities, notice improvement and praise the patient for his perseverance. When the patient is able to sit up, the physiotherapist will participate more actively in teaching him how to achieve balance; elastic stockings or crepe bandages firmly applied from toe to groin, are often necessary to prevent venous pooling in the legs and hypotension when the patient first gets out of bed. Once he has mastered balance, the patient will learn how to transfer from his wheelchair to the bed, toilet, car, etc., how to get back into his chair if he inadvertently falls out and how to manoeuvre his wheelchair up and down kerbs. A few fortunate patients can be taught to walk short distances with the aid of a spinal support and leg calipers. Local fund-raising efforts have enabled some young patients with paraplegia to purchase and learn to use computer-controlled brace and calipers.

Hydrotherapy has a useful role as warm water relaxes muscles and gives buoyancy to the limbs which can then be moved more freely. The patient with paraplegia can be taught to swim, giving him additional freedom of movement; as well as being of therapeutic value it is a great morale booster. Swimming is one of the best ways of strengthening shoulder and arm muscles and improving breathing control. Suitable sporting activities, archery, weight-lifting, swimming and table tennis, will be encouraged and the competition can be enjoyable and give a sense of achievement.

The medical social worker should be consulted soon after the patient's arrival in hospital (see p. 194). She will be asked for advice and practical help in dealing with a variety of problems. At first financial matters take priority, but plans for home adaptations or rehousing take a considerable time and must be put in train as soon as possible. It is an expensive time for families as the patient may be in one of the few specialist rehabilitation centres far from home, transport for visiting is costly, the patient's income may have stopped when he became incapable of continuing his job, he may have a wife and children to support and hire purchase and mortgage commitments. A mother may have the anxiety of young teenagers arriving home to an empty house and scarcely old enough to fend for themselves, or young children separated and cared for by various relatives and friends or taken into the care of a local authority home. The medical social worker can be a useful link for a single-parent family, she will ensure that children are happy and well cared for and will arrange for children to visit their parent. She is also the link between the patient, his employer and the disabled persons' resettlement officer (DRO) and at an early stage can assess the possiblity of the patient being reaccepted by his employer when he is fit to resume work, whether the employer's attitude would allow him to find a suitable position for his employee even if he remains disabled, or whether it will be necessary for the patient to seek or train for a totally different type of work. She will also advise and assist the patient in claiming the financial assistance to which he is entitled.

The home may need adaptations for the convenience of someone in a wheelchair, wider doorways, ramps, handrails and raised toilet seats; a commode may be necessary when a lavatory is inaccessible. The kitchen may need considerable alteration, for example, lower working surfaces and a sink with space beneath to fit knees and wheelchair. These are but a few examples, there are many more mechanical aids (see Disabled Living Foundation, p. 366) available.

The patient may need a car to go to work and his own car can be adapted to hand controls; though previous driving experience is helpful, the disabled person will need to learn to drive a hand-controlled vehicle. The patient will be able to claim a mobility allowance.

Children of school age will need educational facilities while they are in hospital. The law states that all children over the age of five years must be educated according to their mental and physical abilities. A programme of study may be provided by the child's own school teacher as soon as the period of acute illness is over, and the occupational therapist and nursing staff can arrange for a suitable time to be set aside for quiet and study. The mobile library will help by providing a regular supply of books. A child will be at considerable disadvantage when he returns to school unless provision is made; this necessity is now appreciated by all paediatric units. Plans for future education will be necessary if the child is likely to remain handicapped (see pp. 201 and 350). The responsibility for educating disabled children now lies with the education authorities though all too often it falls to the parents to see that their child is educated in the right establishment, preferably near his home though this is not always possible if there is mental subnormality as well as physical disability.

It may be necessary for a District Nurse to attend the patient on his return home; it is helpful if she is able to visit him in hospital to learn first hand exactly what his care entails and for patient and nurse to get to know each other. Some patients will need little help, while others are much more dependent and need assistance every day with washing, dressing, getting up and going to bed.

During rehabilitation, there will be discussion concerning the patient visiting his own home. He may already have been out for a drive when staff, who are used to helping him, are available on his departure and return to help him in and out of the car. The first visit home is a very emotional experience; the patient has longed for the day yet it can so often fall below expectations, even be calamitous, as he feels his disability even more keenly in familiar surroundings where he was previously able to move about freely and normally. There are many personal adjustments to be made in family relationships and these will take time; it would be unwise to do other than reintroduce the patient to his family and home gradually, for a few hours, a day, a weekend, a week. During this time unforeseen problems will occur and there will be an opportunity to discuss and resolve them while the patient and his family are still in close touch with the rehabilitation team. While he is in hospital the patient will have learnt the complications which may arise as a result of spinal paralysis and how best to avoid them. He should be instructed when to contact his general practitoner; there is a danger that through ignorance or a desire for total independence, the patient will feel the necessity to soldier on when complications threaten, rather than seek medical help.

Sexual relationships should be discussed; there may be fear of sexual intercourse, fear of an unwanted pregnancy, or ignorance which deprives a couple unnecessarily of a normal part of life. A man with paraplegia may think that he is no longer fertile, a woman with paraplegia may unwisely presume, because of her paralysis or a very irregular menstrual cycle, that she cannot become pregnant. The decision to have a child when one or both partners have paraplegia should not be taken lightly, though paraplegia alone is not a justifiable reason for denying parenthood.

Finally the patient will be ready for discharge from hospital where he has had a protected environment suited to his needs and where he has had the constant company and support of those he has come to regard as friends. As he leaves hospital, instead of the expected feeling of happy anticipation, he may well be filled with anxiety and have a sudden acute lack of self-confidence despite everyone's efforts to prepare him for the occasion. A great deal depends on the way the rehabilitation team have gradually withdrawn their support, the patient's personality and the home circumstances to which he is returning. Those who are able to go out to work are less likely to feel a sense of isolation, but even they may be glad to be put in touch with a club for disabled persons. The community is becoming more aware of the needs of the disabled and much publicity has been given to the problems they experience in finding suitable accommodation, parking their vehicles, using wheelchairs along the pavement and gaining access to shops, libraries, public conveniences, cinemas, theatres and other public buildings. Local authorities are understandably unable to remedy all the mistakes of the past, they are limited by lack of funds when they consider making drastic alterations for a minority, but attempts are being made to ensure that all new public buildings have lifts and easy access for wheelchairs, and leaflets are being printed to keep the public informed of the location of these facilities. There are many organisations to help the disabled who, through force of circumstance spend much of the day alone, or live alone. Some are able to attend a day centre where they meet others and take part in various activities. Those who remain at home need regular visitors who are prepared to help with shopping and meals. A home help and 'meals-on-wheels' may be supplied, but these services are heavily overburdened and informal help from neighbours is often willingly given, some will even arrange a rota of helpers once their interest has been aroused. Some schools encourage sixth formers to adopt a disabled person, and 'task force' will undertake spring cleaning, painting, decorating and other help. The most important feature of all these forms of assistance is the company they give the housebound person. There are occupations which the patient can pursue in his own home, some bring small remuneration, others are for pleasure and interest; they range from addressing envelopes, assembling small parts for factories, rug making, carpentry and making jewellery. Even the individual with quadriplegia, with the right equipment can lead a busy life. 'Possum', the name given to Patient Operated Selective Machinery, enables the severely paralysed patient to lead an 'active' life. It is possible to operate such sensitive machinery by an almost imperceptible twitch of a small bundle of muscle fibres or a puff of expired air. This machinery is very costly, but it enables severely disabled people to manoeuvre wheelchairs, turn the pages of a book, write by means of typewriters, to 'converse' when speech is destroyed, to select television and radio programmes and most important of all, gives them a reason for living by keeping them mentally alert when they would otherwise vegetate. Machines of this nature are in an area of scientific development and are likely to become smaller and cheaper to produce.

After leaving hospital the patient will continue to receive regular medical supervision by his general practitioner, and by periodic attendance at outpatient clinics and specialist units. Readmission to hospital may be necessary for the following reasons:

1   To re-investigate the disease causing paralysis
2   To give a further course of rehabilitation
3   To treat pressure sores, urinary or respiratory infections
4   For operative treatment to the urinary tract
    (a)   removal of calculi
    (b)   transplantation of ureters
5   For other medical or surgical reasons
6   To allow relatives to take a holiday

The burden on the family is almost always a heavy one; a disabled person is probably even more subject to moodiness than the average individual and holidays are essential both for the patient and his family. There are special holiday homes for the disabled or if a family wish to go on holiday together, accommodation suitable for someone who uses a wheelchair can sometimes be found in the country or at the seaside. Sometimes the patient is readmitted to hospital for two weeks to enable relatives to get away; the period should not be longer or all the home arrangements are likely to break down and the patient may become reluctant to leave hospital.

With improved medical services, operative techniques, nursing care and understanding of the long term problems of paraplegia and quadriplegia, the patient's life expectancy is now much better than it once was.

11

Congenital Spinal Disorders

(This chapter should be read in conjunction with Chapter 4 as the two subjects closely overlap.)

In early embryological development the vertebral column forms as an enclosed tube containing a primitive spinal cord; the column closes posteriorly by fusion of the two halves of the spinous processes (Fig. 11.1). Many congenital disorders of the spine and spinal cord are the result of incomplete union of the vertebrae and incomplete closure of the neural tube and most of the lesions are obvious when the baby is born; they are usually found in the lumbo-sacral region, but occasionally affect the cervical or thoracic spine. Congenital disorders of the spine and spinal cord are the commonest form of congenital malformation and may occur in as many as 1 in 300 births; unfortunately the more severe lesions are the most common. Abnormalities produced by incomplete closure are:

Spina bifida occulta The two halves of the spinous process fail to unite (Fig. 11.2); the condi-

tion may be suggested by the presence of a tuft of black hair, pigmentation of the skin or a dimple on the back overlying the bony defect. The spinal cord and nerve roots are not usually involved, but sometimes the development of symptoms suggests either tethering of the nerve roots, which prevents the normal ascent of the cord within the spinal canal as the child grows, or other congenital lesions (dermoid cyst or lipoma) which cause pressure on the cord or cauda equina. Persistent enuresis is a significant symptom especially when it occurs during the day as well as at night.

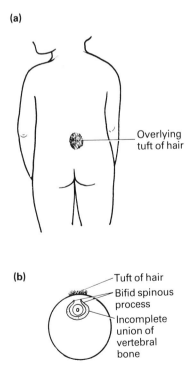

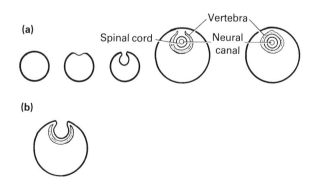

Fig. 11.1 Embryological development of vertebral column. **(a)** Enfolding of ectoderm and normal development of primitive vertebral column. **(b)** Faulty closure and union of spinous process.

Fig. 11.2 Spina bifida occulta. **(a)** External appearance suggesting presence of the disorder. **(b)** Section of vertebral body showing bifid spinous process.

(a)

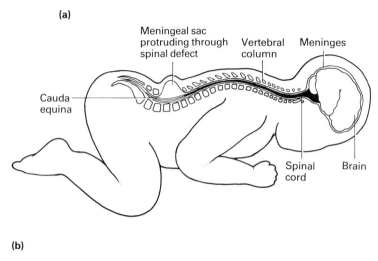

(b)

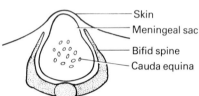

Fig. 11.3   Meningocele. **(a)** Longitudinal section. **(b)** Transverse section.

Meningocele   The meninges, containing cerebro-spinal fluid, bulge through the bifid spine; the sac is only partially protected by skin, and the central, exposed, unprotected portion may rupture and leak CSF (Fig. 11.3).

Myelo-meningocele   The most common of the deformities; the protruding meningeal sac also contains spinal cord and nerve roots (Figs 11.4 and 11.5).

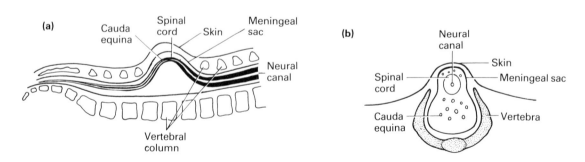

Fig. 11.4   Myelo-meningocele. **(a)** Longitudinal section. **(b)** Transverse section.

(a)

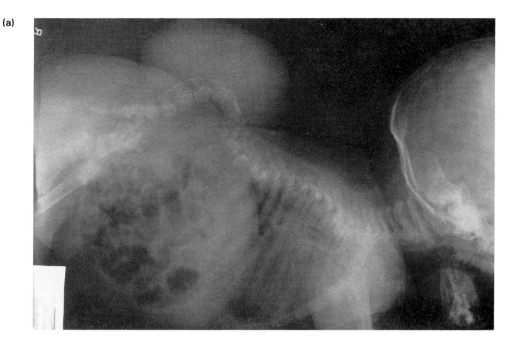

(b)

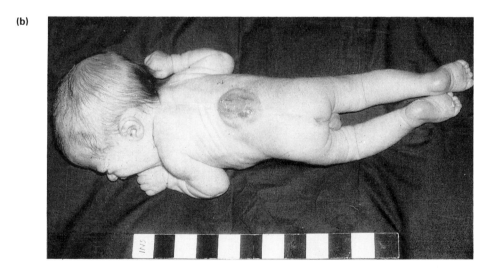

Fig. 11.5 (a) X-ray showing spinal deformity and myelo-meningocele. (b) Infant with myelo-meningocele.

Syringo-myelocele The posterior part of the spinal cord protrudes into the meningeal sac enlarging the central neural canal (Fig. 11.6).

Myelocele The skin, bone and meninges are completely absent and the spinal cord which has failed to unite posteriorly, is flat, opened out and lying on the surface of the baby's back (Fig. 11.7).

These deformities are sometimes accompanied by abnormalities of other organs (e.g., heart and kidneys); deformities of other parts of the vertebral column (kyphoscoliosis) are common and may also affect the rib cage. Deformities of the legs develop *in utero*, particularly talipes (Fig. 11.8 and p. 196)

due to the abnormal pull of opposing muscle groups, dislocation of the hip from constant flexion and adduction, and fixation of the knee joints from persistent extension of the legs.

Hydrocephalus often accompanies the severest forms of spinal abnormality (3 to 5 above) when:

i   there is incomplete development of the CSF pathways;

ii infection ascends through a ruptured meningocele causing basal meningitis and forming adhesions at the outlets of the 4th ventricle;

iii repair of a leaking meningocele dams up excess CSF within the ventricles;

iv there is Arnold Chiari malformation.

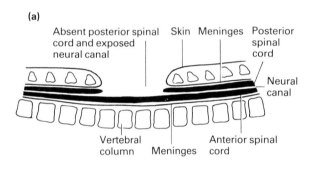

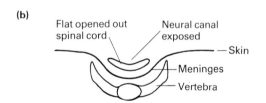

Fig. 11.6 Syringo-myelocele. (a) Longitudinal section. (b) Transverse section.

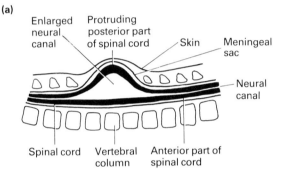

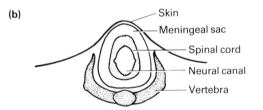

Fig. 11.7 Myelocele. (a) Longitudinal section. (b) Transverse section.

Spina bifida and myelo-meningocele

The cause of these forms of congenital abnormality is not yet known; viruses have been blamed, but there is no positive proof of their involvement. It is known that a woman who has given birth to an infant with myelo-meningocele is much more likely than other women to have another child similarly affected; this may be the result of a genetic factor or dietary deficiency in early pregnancy, possibly a folic acid deficiency. The mother of a child with spina bifida can have a test on the amniotic fluid during the early stages of subsequent pregnancies to discover whether the foetus is abnormal; should there be evidence of defect, abortion will be considered.

There is a decrease in the number of infants born with spina bifida; this may be as a result of abortion carried out when the foetus is known to be abnormal, but it is likely there are other unknown factors. This current trend may not be permanent.

The sad problem of babies who are born grossly deformed has aroused heated discussion for some years as advances in medicine and surgery have made it possible to keep them alive. Some have felt that were euthanasia legal these babies should be 'put down' as soon as they are born, but even they wonder who should be responsible for the decision and what degree of abnormality should call for such drastic measures. There are those who think more moderately, that the babies should not be kept 'officiously alive' by vigorous resuscitation and extensive surgery. Others think no effort should be spared to keep the baby alive at all costs using every conceivable operation to repair and reconstruct his malformed body.

At one time most of these babies died naturally soon after birth. Then came advances in medicine and surgery and every baby with spina bifida was operated on and many survived. Their survival brought many unforeseen problems, some of which could never be rectified. The initial repair of the defect in the infant's back involves replacement of displaced nerve tissue, repair of the meninges and plastic repair of the skin and subcutaneous tissue. CSF often leaks from the sac and infection enters causing meningitis. Hydrocephalus frequently develops within a few days even if it was not obvious at birth, necessitating a ventriculo-peritoneal or atrial shunt; the shunt may block, become infected and need to be removed (see p. 76). As the child grows the shunt must be changed to be proportional in length – yet another operation. Talipes equino varus and dislocation of the hips will call for surgical correction if the child is ever to walk or stand, but these children often remain paraplegic and there is an extreme susceptibility to pressure and friction sores; they also have paralysis of the bladder with the constant risk of infection, the common complication of hydronephrosis and the possibility of more reconstructive surgery. Then, in spite of all this corrective surgery, nothing can be done to change an inherent mental subnormality.

Medical and surgical management

It is unfortunately impossible to assess an infant's potential at the time when decisions are made regarding suitability for surgical repair. Even knowing the family background, no-one can be certain whether the baby will attain normal milestones, nor whether he has a resilient personality. Will he overcome all obstacles and go on to university or will he have 'a chip on the shoulder' and make no effort to be independent? One operation succeeds another, each causing parental anxiety, and the child who spends frequent periods in hospital suffers much pain and discomfort and missed schooling. This child who has undergone so much treatment may remain alive, but what quality of life will he enjoy? As a mentally subnormal child with paraplegia there is little or no future. Disabled children often appear quite happy and stoical, but when they reach adolescence they become increasingly self-conscious, have difficulty finding employment, their social life is restricted and their desire for marriage may be unfulfilled. There is always the hope that treatment will improve; research into the cause and prevention of abnormal foetal development continues to be of utmost importance. No-one can be sure of the right decision, yet decisions about treatment must be made soon after the baby is born, without unnecessary delay, and there can be no half measures. The paediatrician or neurosurgeon has a heavy responsibility and whatever their decision it is only reached after careful consideration. It is now generally considered that surgery is indicated only if the baby has a good expectation of a useful life and has no other major congenital abnormality. Should he have gross hydrocephalus, obvious deformity of the spine and rib cage, severe myelo-meningocele and paraplegia, surely the decision on whether to operate is less difficult? There are however, many shades between this extreme and those mildly affected babies who will obviously respond well to treatment. There are other factors, such as the parents' wishes and the family unit – the baby may be the sixth child and only girl, or the much-wanted baby born to parents who have been striving for a child for many years. The survival of the infant does not entirely rest on a decision for immediate surgical repair; should the baby unexpectedly survive without this early surgery, an operation can be performed at a later date.

The care of these babies is distressing for all concerned and not least for the nursing staff, physiotherapists and occupational therapists who are closely involved with the baby and his family. It is important from the beginning that there is frank discussion between the medical staff, parents and other members of the therapeutic team. The baby's condition must be fully understood and, with forethought for the future, stage by stage, short- and long-term plans for treatment and rehabilitation will be made.

When a baby is born with obvious spina bifida abnormality the mother should be told by the doctor or midwife in attendance. Some mothers do not know before the baby is born that there is anything wrong, but most mothers have thought of the possibility of their baby being in some way abnormal and often their first anxious question after the baby's birth is 'Is he all right?'. This preparedness of many mothers is a protection for the initial shock and though the mother may be exhausted after labour, if she asks, her question should be frankly and sympathetically answered; should she not ask, she must inevitably be told as soon as possible, choosing a time when her husband is with her for each to comfort and support the other. Careful handling and presentation of the facts may prevent the mother rejecting her baby. The mother should see her baby soon after birth and if possible, hold him in her arms to establish a bond; this must never be forgotten in the distress felt by doctor or midwife when they deliver an imperfect baby. The baby will need the loving care and acceptance of his parents and will continue to do so as he grows. The defect should not be understated, 'just a little cyst', nor should it be suggested that 'he will be quite all right when he has had a little operation'.

As soon as he is born the baby will be placed in an incubator to combat shock, keep him warm and reduce the risk of infection. Great care will be taken when handling this newborn infant to prevent rupture of the meningeal sac and he will be placed on his side; an active baby may need a small pad under his buttocks to prevent him rolling over on to his back. The whole meningeal sac will be lightly covered with a sterile, non-adherent dressing, overlaid by a layer of gauze soaked in saline and secured by a bandage. When the meningeal sac has been ruptured *in utero* or during the process of birth the risk of infection is very high and damage to the exposed spinal cord greatly increased. The baby will be seen as soon as possible by a paediatrician and within the first 24 hours of life will probably be transferred to a children's hospital or neurosurgical unit. A specimen of the mother's blood and blood taken from the baby's umbilical cord will be obtained before the baby is transferred as blood will be difficult to obtain if the infant arrives cold and shocked at the receiving hospital. It has often been the custom to ask the mother to sign a consent form for operation before the baby is transferred, but as she has hardly had time to recover from the birth nor had time to consider the implications of surgery this would seem unwise. Unfortunately because the specialist hospital is often a considerable distance from the place of birth, it allows no opportunity for the parents to discuss together the matter of surgical treatment. The baby will be transferred in a portable incubator and will be accompanied by his father and a midwife. The mother may also be transferred if there is a mother and baby unit.

Admission to the specialist hospital

When the baby arrives he will be settled into the ward incubator, preferably in a single room. He will be received by a trained nurse who has a good knowledge of the appearance and behaviour of normal infants. She will notice his response to her voice and to being picked up, whether he opens his eyes, cries or moves his limbs, the size and shape of his head and trunk, the appearance of the meningeal sac and the position of his legs and feet; has he any obvious hydrocephalus, spinal deformity, paraplegia or talipes? She will notice whether his colour is good and breathing satisfactory. The nurse will inspect the baby's skin very carefully for early signs of pressure sores and should she see any mark or reddening she should adjust the baby's position to relieve pressure and plan a more frequent turning regime. The umbilical cord will be inspected to ensure that it is clean and dry; if 24 hours have passed since the baby's birth, the plastic umbilical clamp will be removed and replaced by a ligature.

The baby's father must be approached sympathetically, as he has so recently sustained a severe shock and is likely to be bewildered and anxious. He should be shown to a comfortable waiting room, given refreshment and asked to wait at the hospital until the doctor has seen and examined the baby and is able to discuss his condition and treatment. To avoid asking the father too many questions the midwife should be asked to give as much information as possible before she leaves, regarding the delivery, the condition of the baby at birth, his weight, length and head circumference measurement.

The baby will be examined by the doctor soon after admission; X-rays of chest and spine may be requested. This completed, consultation will take place immediately and if operation is thought to be possible and likely to benefit the baby, the surgeon will interview the parents and explain the nature of the repair operation, the complications which may follow and any other possibilities which may affect the baby's future. The explanation should be neither too glibly optimistic nor too harshly pessimistic, for either extreme leads to misunderstandings which may erode a good relationship between the parents, medical and nursing staff. The baby's father will not be asked to sign the consent form for operation until he has been given an opportunity to ask questions, talk to his wife and consider the proposed treatment.

Some parents may have already decided that any child born to them with such an abnormality should not be operated upon; these parents may need more time to reconsider their earlier decision in the light of information they have been given.

When a baby is considered unsuitable for operation, his parents will be seen by a senior doctor. It is particularly important in this instance that a very clear explanation is given, stating the reasons why an operation is impracticable; it should be understood that were surgery undertaken, considerable suffering would be inflicted upon the child throughout his life, which in the end, would still leave him a helpless, mentally subnormal, paraplegic individual needing institutional care. The parents will need assurance that the baby will not be allowed to suffer, that he will be given every care, being fed when he is hungry and kept clean and comfortable and that, should circumstances change, an operation will be considered at a later date. A senior member of the nursing staff should be present at this interview; the parents may be so anxious and agitated that they fail to fully understand the doctor's discussion. Only if she was present at the time can the nurse know exactly what the parents were told and clarify points misunderstood. It may be difficult for some parents to accept the surgeon's decision; they should not be prevented from seeking a second medical opinion if they so wish, for otherwise when they have had time to think, they may blame the hospital for not operating on their baby. Very occasionally in spite of two medical opinions parents insist on treatment and, against his better judgement, the surgeon feels obliged to operate.

Preoperative care

Surgery is best performed in a unit where the anaesthetist can give full neonatal anaesthetic techniques with intubation. When operation is recommended surgery takes place within 24 hours of birth. The baby will not be fed during this interval and atropine and vitamine K will be given preoperatively. The baby will be transferred to the operating theatre in the incubator, which must be promptly plugged in to the electricity supply. To prevent undue heat loss, a heated mattress should be used during the operation.

Postoperative care

Following repair of the spinal defect the baby will return to the ward in the incubator in which he will be nursed for approximately ten days.

The baby's condition should be watched constantly to ensure that his airway is clear and his respirations and colour satisfactory. The incubator controls should be checked at regular frequent intervals and adjusted if necessary. Each baby should have his own set of equipment and every effort should be made to prevent cross-infection. He should be kept clean and dry and his position changed frequently to prevent pressure sores. All his nursing care should be given in a smooth sequence to avoid harassing the baby unnecessarily and when he is receiving attention the nurse should talk to him and, by her gentle care, convey a loving atmosphere. This is always necessary for a normal infant from birth onwards; how much more so for a baby deprived of close contact with his mother, to help him develop awareness and thrive. A more active baby whose restlessness, crying and general agitation threaten wound healing may need a mild sedative, but it is better to avoid sedation by contenting him in some other way.

Records   Rectal temperature, pulse, respiration, fluid intake and output and bowel evacuation must be recorded; pyrexia will alert the staff to the possibility of wound or urinary infection, or meningitis. Hyperpyrexia may give rise to febrile convulsions. The anterior fontanelle should be palpated when the baby is resting quietly and the head circumference measured daily, preferably by the same nurse to ensure accuracy; should there be any increase in the measurement, this must be reported to the medical officer as it is likely to be a sign of developing or worsening hydrocephalus.

Feeding   Immediately following operation, the intravenous infusion will be regulated according to the doctor's instructions; a paediatric intravenous giving set will be used, which accurately measures and administers small quantities of fluid. Each baby will be fed according to his requirements and should be weighed regularly; a small, poorly baby may need small, dilute 1-hourly tube feeds, whereas a stronger one may take bottle feeds 4-hourly. Weakly babies tolerate bottle feeding poorly and vomit after feeds, and the regime should always be introduced gradually. The baby who is a very slow feeder may need supplementary tube feeds; there may be vomiting when a feed has been given too quickly or when the feeding regime has been advanced too rapidly; there may be failure to gain weight or even weight loss.

Care of the urinary tract   A baby with spina bifida may have congenital renal abnormality and if he is born with paraplegia, is likely to have urinary retention due to bilateral spinal cord damage and may have developed hydronephrosis even before birth; careful observation of urinary output is necessary to prevent further complications. The baby's bladder should be emptied before each feed and digital compression may be necessary; this must be performed carefully by placing one hand beneath the baby's buttocks and with the other, exerting very gentle 3-finger pressure above the symphysis pubis. There are several observations which must be made during this procedure and recorded:

(a)   Had the baby passed urine before compression of the bladder?

(b)   If he had done so, was more urine obtained when the bladder was compressed?

(c)   Has the urine an offensive odour suggesting urinary infection? When the bladder is incompletely emptied urinary infection is likely; a specimen of urine will be collected for laboratory examination.

Catheterisation is occasionally necessary if, in spite of digital compression, there is retention of urine; it may also be necessary for a 24-hour urinary collection. An alternative for this collection is an adhesive urinary bag, but these bags are inclined to leak and may damage insensitive skin.

Care of the baby's bottom and groins   While the baby is being nursed unclothed in the carefully controlled atmosphere of an incubator it is easy to notice when he has passed urine or faeces and needs changing. The baby will lie on an incontinence pad which is more absorbent than a cotton sheet and when nappies are used, they should preferably be of the disposable one-way type so that the urine does not remain in contact with the skin. It is more than usually difficult to prevent nappy rash in these babies who constantly dribble urine and faeces. The same principles always apply; at each change of nappy the baby's bottom should be thoroughly washed with a mild soap and water; as soon as the wound is well healed the baby should be put in the bath regularly as washing cannot replace immersion. After a thorough wash, the skin should be dried carefully with a soft towel, special attention being paid to the skin folds; a liberal application of zinc and castor oil cream or petroleum jelly should be used on every occasion as a barrier to prevent urine and faeces coming into contact with the baby's skin.

Care of the umbilical cord The umbilical cord must be inspected, kept clean and dry with spirit or a suitable antiseptic powder, and religatured if necessary. When the baby is nursed in the prone position, which is desirable in many ways, the cord may get warm and soggy, which makes its care doubly important. While the plastic clamp is in use the prone position is unwise as pressure from the clamp may cause an abdominal sore.

Care of the wound There are several factors which affect satisfactory wound healing; the humid atmosphere in the incubator, a shortage of skin leading to tension on the sutures, and poor blood and nerve supplies to the tissues. Inspection of wounds and removal of sutures depends on the type of repair and suturing employed. The wound is sometimes left exposed, on other occasions a pressure dressing is applied which should be left untouched for 10 days unless it is moist, shows signs of CSF leak or the baby is unwell or pyrexial. The sutures are removed on the 10th day at the direction and under the supervision of the surgeon; the baby can then be nursed out of the incubator and 'up and dressed' for the first time if his condition is satisfactory.

Positioning The baby's position should be changed regularly, rotating through left and right lateral, semiprone and prone positions. Limbs and feet should be placed in as natural a position as possible each time the baby is moved and he should never lie on an area already reddened or blistered. Deformities of the legs may make positioning difficult, but foam pads can be used, for example a baby whose hips are fully flexed can be nursed prone with a pad under his thighs to help extend his legs.

Family involvement

The baby's mother should be encouraged to visit him as soon as possible and if she is able, stay with with him while he is in hospital. The longer the visit is delayed the greater the chance of weakening the normal maternal bonds which will harm the baby's relationship with his mother and his feeling of security, and it may lead to total rejection by the mother. She should be shown how to hold, feed, change and bath her baby and introduced to the physiotherapist who will show her how to position him correctly and exercise his paralysed limbs. Opportunities should be given for brothers and sisters to visit the new member of their family, then he will not be a total stranger when he goes home, and the whole family will accept him. They should be allowed to watch the baby being fed or bathed and, rather than just having a peep at him, should hold him to establish a closer contact.

The medical social worker

The medical social worker should be given an early opportunity to interview the baby's parents. They may need her immediate help and advice and it will take time for her to establish a good relationship with them, to understand fully how the birth of a handicapped child is going to affect this particular family and know the type of assistance they are likely to need now and in the future. The medical social worker will be a ready listener to the first expressions of their disappointment, guilt, despair and anxiety. She will be able to assure them that their present feelings are natural and are those experienced by all parents in this situation. At their first meeting she will understand that both parents are bewildered and distressed, the mother having not fully recovered from the physical effort of the baby's birth, the shock of his abnormality, and possibly also physiologically depressed; the mother will also be concerned about the welfare of her other children and how they will react to the news that their sister or brother is handicapped. While at the maternity hospital the mother will probably have felt envious of other mothers with healthy babies and will shy away from talking about her own. The father has been rushing hither and thither, to see his distressed wife, the new baby, possibly either looking after his other children or visiting them, and also trying to fit in a normal working day; all this in addition to anxiety about the future. The parents may wonder if they are in some way responsible for the baby's abnormality; if this thought occurs to them they may not speak of it, but instead blame each other. An opportunity to express all their anxiety and conflicting feelings to an outsider may prevent marriage break-up later. The medical social worker can, from experience, anticipate hurdles for those who are inexperienced in caring for a handicapped child; there will be no escape from the constant demands imposed on each member of the family. The mother should be warned that though this child may occupy much of her time and attention, she must try to arrange her day to leave some time available exclusively for her husband and other children, to keep them close to her and avoid a family break-up. A mother can be too self-sacrificing; she must have opportunities for complete relaxation with freedom from responsibility and it is here that the father, other members of the family and the community can do their part. Some parents try to deny their baby's handicap and make light of it, they hope for a cure though they have been told this is impossible and present a misleadingly casual, light-hearted exterior. They may be able to keep this up while the baby is very young and his care the same as that for any baby, but when he fails to keep pace with the progress of his contemporaries, they will no longer be able to disguise their disappointment and heartbreak; there is then sometimes complete collapse of parents who were thought to be coping well. A few parents reject their baby and push the experience aside, neither visiting the baby nor wishing to take any part in his care and treatment; this rejection may become permanent. It is impossible to force parents to love their baby, but their interest, sense of responsibility and caring can be gently encouraged and nurtured from the beginning if the situation is handled carefully and sensitively. The important factors are the way in which the mother is first told about her baby's abnormality and the opportunity she is given to see and hold him before he is transferred from the maternity hospital. Later, her fears will be allayed by the friendliness and encouragement she meets when she is shown how to care for her baby and the reassurance given her, that at each stage of the child's development there will be someone available to advise and offer practical help.

The medical social worker is mainly responsible for co-ordinating all available help (see p. 350) from

1   Hospital rehabilitation team
    (a) paediatrician
    (b) nursing staff
    (c) physiotherapist
    (d) occupational therapist
    (e) speech therapist

2   General practitioner
3   Health visitor
4   District nurse
5   Spina bifida society
6   Local authorities

The medical social worker will give advice and attend to matters concerning:

i   Financial assistance
     (a) cost of transport to and from the hospital
     (b) family income supplement
     (c) attendance allowance
     (d) grants available for purchase of essential equipment, e.g. a washing machine and tumble dryer
ii   Housing – if it is at all possible the family should have ground floor accommodation and they may need to move house; the local housing authority may need to provide suitable accommodation
iii Schooling – attendance at a normal school is preferable, but the child may need to attend a special school where there are facilities for children using wheelchairs, calipers and other appliances and opportunities for physiotherapy
iv   Aids and appliances from the national health service
v   Local authority assistance – the medical social worker will act as a link to obtain help in arranging for
     (a) installation of a telephone
     (b) home help
     (c) home alterations
vi   Holidays and convalescence – she will be able to provide lists of hotels and other accommodation where disabled children are welcomed and similar lists of convalescent homes

Physiotherapy

The physiotherapist should see and assess each baby with spina bifida as soon as possible, whether or not the spinal defect has been surgically repaired. It would be wrong for a baby who unexpectedly survives to be left with deformities of the feet which could have been corrected by early treatment. Her task will involve assessment, treatment, instruction of the nursing staff and the baby's mother and later, seeing the child regularly as an out-patient and when he is readmitted to hospital for a course of physiotherapy or for some other treatment.

When she first sees the baby, the physiotherapist will make a rapid assessment of muscle and movement and compile a muscle chart. She will also note and record any deformities present and will probably be able to see the infant's physical potential almost at a glance, planning his treatment accordingly. She will discuss the baby's treatment with the nursing staff and show them how they can help correct the baby's deformities when they position him and also discuss her aims in treatment and method of applying splints when these are used. Her daily treatment will start with passive stretching of the baby's hips, knees and feet; at first, the treatment, which will last for about ten minutes daily, will be performed as the baby lies in his incubator, later the physiotherapist will take him on her lap.

It is most important that the physiotherapist establishes a good relationship with the baby's mother, for it is she who will be giving him his daily treatment at home. The mother should be present when treatment is performed and allowed to give physiotherapy under supervision on a number of occasions before the baby is discharged from hospital.

Mental and physical development

Everyone responsible for the baby's care must realise from the beginning that once the wound is healed, they will need to stimulate and encourage him to make as much normal movement as possible. A very young baby needs visual and auditory stimulation, and toys need to be dangled within his reach; the baby will sense the approbation and smiles which greet his movements, at first groping and experimental and then purposeful. It will be very easy for this baby to be backward in his development unless he is shown the possibilities of enjoyment and exploration which open up to him when he makes an effort. It is important that the question of development is discussed with the baby's mother, that she knows when to expect him to roll over, pull himself into a sitting position, crawl or pull himself along, and does not think he is a good baby when he lies just where she puts him; if this is allowed he will not develop his perception of shape, size, texture, and other skills at the same rate

as mobile babies. A handicapped child will need even more love, encouragement and praise than a normal one, but his mother should be urged to treat him as normally as possible, neither overprotecting him nor treating him like a clinical curiosity; she must show displeasure at naughtiness and correct him in the same way as any other naughty child, but also give praise when it is due.

Most children with myelo-meningocele have urinary retention, and the child's mother is taught from the beginning the necessity for digital compression of the bladder, regularly throughout the day, to ensure that the bladder is empty. As the child develops there will be a need to dispense with nappies. Boys up to the age of 5 years can use a penile spout urinal, then they may successfully manage using a penile sheath attached to a drainage bag; an indwelling catheter is unsuitable as it sometimes causes stricture and the formation of false passages. Girls, on the other hand, have more success with an indwelling catheter. There has been recent interest in intermittent catheterisation for boys and girls; it is only suitable for intelligent youngsters who can catheterise themselves and who are able to remain dry for long enough to make it worthwhile. When successful it allows freedom from urinary devices and the youngster feels more normal; the catheter is rinsed under the tap and kept in a clean plastic bag, gross urinary infection is avoided because the bladder is emptied completely and there is no residual urine.

Complications

Hydrocephalus

Hydrocephalus (see Chapter 4) may be recognised by the baby's larger than normal head circumference at birth or when daily measurement shows a persistent excessive increase; this is especially likely when the spinal defect has been repaired and is very frequently associated with myelo-meningocele, less often with meningocele. Hydrocephalus should be relieved as quickly as possible as the longer it persists the more likely it' is to cause mental retardation.

Hydronephrosis

This is a common complication due to retention of urine and back-pressure in the ureters, pelvis and calyces of the kidneys. The condition often develops *in utero* and an early intravenous pyelogram may show the baby's kidneys to be grossly dilated. Observations will be made to find out if the bladder is emptying completely, catheterisation will be necessary if there is retention of urine and urinary infection will be treated with antibiotics. Any urinary infection must always be treated promptly to prevent further kidney damage.

Talipes equinovarus and congenital dislocation of the hip

These deformities develop *in utero* and are due to muscle imbalance caused by paralysis of some muscle groups. Talipes (Fig. 11.8) is difficult to treat; physiotherapy is necessary to manipulate the feet into their correct position which is maintained by the use of splints held in place with adhesive strapping. This simple treatment may not be fully effective and tendon transplants are then necessary to balance the muscles of the foot; several operations may be necessary and sometimes, on reaching the teens, triple arthrodesis is required to fix the

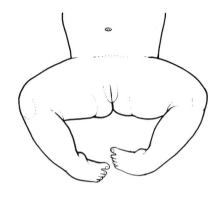

Fig. 11.8 Infants feet showing talipes equinovarus.

foot in a good position. Treatment for talipes is always important even if the child is paraplegic, as deformity creates difficulties when calipers are worn. Congenital dislocation of the hip is very commonly associated with spina bifida; as soon as the spinal wound has healed the dislocation is reduced and then splinted until the joint becomes stable.

Further care and rehabilitation

The baby with spina bifida and hydrocephalus is likely to spend the first 6 to 8 weeks of life in hospital. During this time he will be fully assessed, his spinal defect repaired and if necessary a ventriculo-peritoneal shunt will be performed. He will be given physiotherapy as a start to gradual correction of leg and foot deformities with use of splints if necessary. His feeding regime will be established though there may still be some problems, as babies with spina bifida are more inclined to vomit and generally less likely to thrive and make a steady weight gain. The infant may be quite alert, but is more often apathetic and less inclined to cry when hungry or uncomfortable than a normal infant. The nursing staff will take a pride in his survival and progress though they constantly wonder whether his mental state will be normal – it is so

hard to tell in a small baby; all babies develop at a different rate so comparison is always unreliable.

Some of the mother's anxiety and disappointment will have been dispelled through talks with the medical and nursing staff and medical social worker, and by coming to love her baby because of the contact she has had through visiting, feeding, playing with him and giving him his exercises, but she may still find it difficult to think of him as her baby and really one of the family, having had no experience of looking after him at home. Should this be her first baby the mother needs to be shown how to make up feeds, sterilise feeding equipment and bath her baby, in addition to special advice about the care of the ventriculo-peritoneal shunt. She will need to know the symptoms which indicate that the shunt has blocked (see p. 76); how to compress the bladder and when to suspect urinary infection. The physiotherapist will give the mother any necessary final instructions and reminders. All mothers should be given an appointment for the baby to be seen at the special clinic for babies with hydrocephalus and spina bifida, where he will be seen by all members of the rehabilitation team; the appointments will be at three-monthly intervals. Attempts should be made to co-ordinate the follow-up appointments so that the child is seen by each specialist during the one hospital visit and not repeatedly trailed back and forth to hospital. During the final weeks before the infant is discharged the parents should be seen by the doctor, and their child's future will be discussed in some detail; they will also be given an opportunity to ask questions and given an outline of future treatment which will include the following.

i   Regular attendance at the out-patient clinic.
ii Information about the shunt and when the child is likely to be readmitted for revision and lengthening of the tubing.
iii Discussion in general terms about the treatment he will be receiving for talipes and other deformities of bone and muscle, and when the child is likely to be readmitted to hospital for orthopaedic treatment. It is probable that at this stage the parents will want to know whether their child will learn to walk.
iv Discussion regarding problems of incontinence.
v   The necessity for intravenous pyelography at regular yearly intervals.

The parents will be advised to give their disabled child as normal an upbringing as they possibly can; it is far better to let him get 'mucky and dirty along with the rest' than to overprotect him and stunt his development.

This interview will be handled according to the parents' understanding and personality: some would obviously rather not know what is in store and will be content to rely on advice given when the time comes; others will be full of questions, doubts and fears, which can to some extent be dispelled by discussion. A full report of the baby's condition and treatment will be sent to the general practitioner and area health visitor who will make contact with the family.

The family

There are always adjustments to be made when a baby arrives home from hospital for the first time. The mother is inevitably more anxious about the handicapped baby, who takes much of her time and attention; the father and other children may feel neglected and jealous, they will feel less shut out if they are allowed to help look after the baby. An only child will be at some disadvantage, as his mother may become too completely absorbed in his care and very over-protective. She may smother him with affection to compensate for earlier feelings of rejection; there are then likely to be emotional difficulties when the child reaches an age of self-expression. A normal toddler tires his mother by the end of the day; there are added stresses to the care of a handicapped child who cannot rush off and hide when he feels cross after a battle with his mother, so shows signs of extreme frustration; he is heavy to lift and carry and instead of becoming more independent is quite clearly going to need as much attention as a baby for a long time. The prospect becomes daunting for the best of mothers: extra lifting, dressing when a normal child would be able to dress himself, the unpleasantness of incontinence and the feelings of shame that her child has no control over bladder and bowels, not to mention the offensive odour which hangs around the house, the tedious waiting often entailed by out-patient appointments and endless hospital visiting which may involve considerable time spent in travelling. The special care her child needs will prevent the mother going out to work and there may therefore be financial stress. All the problems will seem so much worse when she is tired, the strain on a marriage is often too much and there is a high rate of marriage breakdown. The child's development will have many setbacks due to recurrent separations from his family, unpleasant, frightening and sometimes painful procedures in hospital and eventually the realisation of his limitations and how different he is from other children; this becomes even more noticeable when he reaches adolescence.

The medical social worker at the hospital and the health visitor will continue to be adviser and friend to the family and will discuss problems as they arise, making suggestions which in various ways lighten the family's burden. There are those families who will not accept advice or help however tactfully the matter is approached, but in most cases the mother is willing to unburden her problems to the health visitor who, noticing perhaps signs of excessive strain may suggest the child attends a playgroup specially adapted to the needs of handicapped children or will begin to discuss suitable holiday arrangements. When the child is very severely handicapped or the family is completely unable to cope, in spite of all the help offered by the social welfare services, residential care will be considered and may be in the best interests of the child. It is essential that every effort should be made however to maintain the parents' interest in their child, that they visit him, have him at home for some weekends or part of the holidays and that he continues to keep in touch with other members of the family. It is sad that so many of these children after all they have gone through should be in residential care, neither seeing nor hearing anything of their parents, who are only too glad to forget they had an abnormal child and be rid of the burden of care; they are perhaps afraid that if they show any interest they will be expected to resume their responsibility.

Spina Bifida Association

From the time that her baby is a few months old, the mother of a handicapped child will probably be greatly helped by joining the Association for Spina Bifida and Hydrocephalus. She will then have an opportunity to meet other parents with similar problems, may get ideas of how to help her baby's development and mobility, how to keep him happy and amused, the location of the nearest toy library and the latest information about equipment and toys which are specially designed to contribute to the progress of a disabled child.

Reasons for readmission to hospital

1   Feeding problems
2   For periodic revision of ventriculo-peritoneal shunt because the system has blocked or the tubing requires lengthening because the child is growing
3   Treatment of sores and fractures
4   Physiotherapy
5   Small orthopaedic operations
6   Orthopaedic operations on the spine and hips
7   Serious urinary infections
8   Intravenous pyelogram
9   Urinary tract operations
10 Occupational therapy
11 Social reasons
12 Treatment of status epilepticus (see Chapter 19)

Whenever the baby with spina bifida is readmitted to hospital it gives a useful opportunity for a complete review of his progress and home situation. He should be kept in hospital no longer than absolutely necessary and all those who normally care for him should be encouraged to visit regularly and continue to help with his care, should be kept fully informed about the reasons for admission, likely length of stay, his progress if he is in hospital for longer than planned, and date of expected discharge. The nursing staff, with their close daily contact, can assess the child's activity and mobility, whether he shows interest in his surroundings, can sit up, feed himself, has bladder or bowel control and, when he is older, his ability to dress himself. He will be formally tested by a psychologist to assess his IQ at 6-monthly and then yearly intervals; this will be very helpful when decisions are necessary regarding his schooling and will prevent him being over-stressed if he is mentally retarded. The physiotherapist and occupational therapist will make their assessment and the parents will be seen by the medical social worker to discuss any problems the family have experienced.

Feeding problems

In spite of the fact that the mother has been shown how to feed her baby and supervised giving feeds while he is still in hospital, has attended Health Clinics and been visited at home where the health visitor has watched her give a feed, there may still be feeding problems. Problems may be intermittent and the feeding regime is ever-changing as the baby grows; an inexperienced mother may be tempted to give too much too soon, introduce solids before her baby is ready and this may lead to vomiting and failure to thrive. The health visitor cannot be present all the time and it is often more satisfactory to observe the baby in hospital for 2–3 weeks; during this time the baby's mother should continue to feed him with some supervision.

Revision of the ventriculo-peritoneal shunt

(See p. 76)

Pressure sores and fractures

From infancy onwards the child with spina bifida is susceptible to pressure and friction sores associated with his lack of skin sensitivity, poor nerve supply and deficient circulation mainly affecting his legs and feet. This is aggravated by immobility, splints and calipers, incontinence, tendency to excessive weight gain even in childhood, and later, in some instances, difficulty in maintaining a high standard of personal hygiene when he has to rely on other people for help and is probably unable to shower or bath as often as is necessary. Lack of muscular activity causes sluggish venous return from the lower limbs which feel cold to the touch, show purple discoloration and are subject to chilblains and sores. It is important that splints should be well padded with orthopaedic felt and that calipers are light weight and well-fitted to prevent friction.

The child and his parents must be taught to inspect his skin regularly, especially those areas where pressure or friction are most likely, and wall mirrors fitted at a low level are useful to enable the child to see all insensitive areas clearly; the parents should also know what to do if an area appears red, blistered or sore and how to treat the many abrasions and injuries sustained in play and when to seek medical advice. Injuries to the legs and feet should be avoided as even minor abrasions may be very difficult to heal. Small injuries may lead to fractures as there is poor ossification of bones in the paralysed limbs; because the child's injury is painless the mother must be alert for signs of joint dislocation or fracture. Advice will also be necessary about suitable clothing. The child will need to be more warmly clad than a normal active child; cotton and wool are better for all purposes than man-made fibres in spite of the apparent advantages of fabrics which are easily washed, dried and need no ironing, which for the mother of an incontinent child is such an important consideration. Cotton socks are preferable to stretch nylon as they are less cramping to the toes and allow better ventilation. To lessen the risk of chilblains, woollen socks and bedsocks should be worn in cold weather. Trousers are warm and protective, and give a young girl confidence by hiding unsightly legs.

It should rarely be necessary for a child to be readmitted to hospital for the sole purpose of treating a pressure sore, though sores which are extremely slow to respond to treatment at home may need intensive hospital care to:

1 Discover the precipitating factor, failure to follow previous advice, neglected hygiene, unsuitable clothing, obesity and ill-fitting appliances, and improve general health and hygiene.

2 Ensure continuity of treatment and observation throughout the day and night; it is often an impossible task at home or at school to change the position of a heavy paralysed youngster as frequently and regularly as necessary and relieve pressure from a sore area at all times.

3 Provide special treatments by the physiotherapist
(a) alternating infra-red and ultraviolet light;
(b) other treatment to stimulate the circulation.

4 Heal the sore quickly and take measures to prevent other sores so that the patient gets back to his normal routine as soon as possible.

Physiotherapy

The physiotherapist will see the child each time he is admitted to hospital; she will assess his progress, compare it with the development of a normal child, consider whether home treatment is correcting his deformities satisfactorily and whether it is developing weak muscles to their full extent. She will have discussion with the doctor about possible surgical intervention when there are obstinate deformities, or if she foresees that a deformity of the spine is likely to cause difficulty when fitting a brace. When the child reaches two-and-a-half to three years of age his degree of mobility will probably have developed to its full extent, and this is the time for the physiotherapist in consultation with the doctor, to decide the most suitable type of caliper; these will be made to measure, supplied and maintained by the National Health Service. Each child is very carefully assessed as an individual as no two children have the same deformities, personality, intelligence, height, build, muscle power, coordination or attitude to their disabilities. The child will be measured for his calipers at an out-patient clinic and when they are ready, it may be an advantage for him to have a short period in hospital for intensive physiotherapy where he will learn to walk using his calipers (Fig. 11.9) and his mother will be shown how to fit them. This training may be possible as an out-patient if the child lives near the hospital, but it should be remembered that getting a disabled child ready to go to the hospital takes a long time and daily attendance will put an impossible burden on an already harassed mother. However handicapped the child, every effort is made to enable him to stand and walk a few steps even when the process looks impossibly laborious to an observer. While standing at a workbench he will be supported in a harness (as shown in Fig. 11.9), or supported within the workbench (Fig. 11.10); not only does this posture help to prevent pressure sores and improve the general circulation but in so doing it assists kidney function. Hydrotherapy is a useful form of treatment and source of enjoyment.

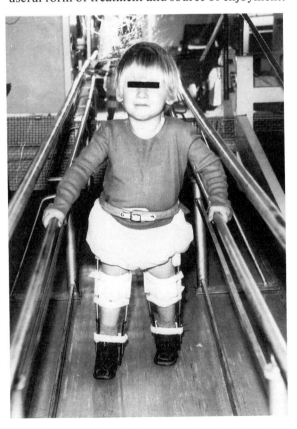

Fig. 11.9 Child with spina bifida learning to walk with calipers.

Intravenous pyelography and micturating cystogram

Admission to hospital may not be necessary for these comparatively simple radiological procedures which demonstrate the condition of the kidneys and functioning of the bladder.

Urinary tract management

Incontinence of urine is a greater problem for girls because they cannot wear external urinary collection devices; their alternatives lie between an indwelling catheter, intermittent catheterisation and operations to augment bladder function and improve sphincter control. The ileal loop operation, transplanting the ureters into an isolated loop of ileum which opens on to the surface of the abdomen, is less favoured than it once was; this operation allowed urine to drain into an ileostomy bag which was emptied at convenient intervals and the bladder became an extinct organ. This was a serious operation which even put the child's life at risk; some patients who had this operation have more recently had an operation to reinstate the bladder. Electrical stimulation of the bladder, or of the cord itself, is in an experimental stage and not yet in general use.

Occupational therapy

The occupational therapist, a member of the rehabilitation team, will see the child when he attends the clinic at three-monthly intervals. When he reaches the stage of being propped up and begins to take an interest in his surroundings and toys, the occupational therapist should make her first contact with baby and mother. She will be able to discuss stages of development, perhaps giving suggestions about constructive toys and the use of mobility aids (Fig. 11.10) when he is old enough. At a later stage, when he is 4–5 years old, she will concentrate on teaching him independence in dressing; he may be extremely slow to learn and perform this skill and the occupational therapist may discover that at home he is dressed by his mother who finds it much quicker. A child who has never had sensation in his legs may be totally unaware of their existence and will have problems about his own body image. His attention will be drawn to the appearance of his legs and their position in relation to the rest of his body; full-length wall mirrors are

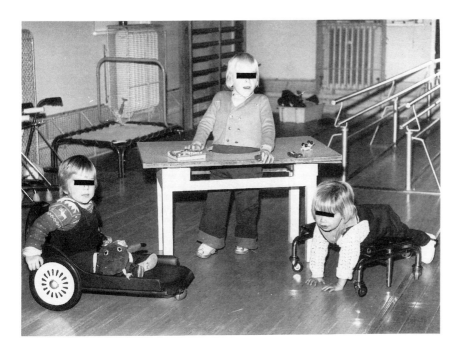

Fig. 11.10 Children using mobility aids and child wearing calipers supported in a workbench.

useful so that he can watch himself dress and walk with calipers. When the child is in hospital the occupational therapist will see him at intervals during the day, fitting in with the treatment programme, perhaps being present when he is having a bath or getting dressed to teach him methods which will lead towards independence. During free activity time before he begins regular school activities, she can help with constructive play.

Social reasons for admission to hospital

The reasons for admission primarily centre round the mother, for it is she who is essential to the child's welfare at home; if she is ill, in hospital, pregnant, during the period of childbirth and immediately afterwards or if for any other reason she is unable to look after her handicapped child, he will probably need to be admitted to hospital; he may also be admitted to enable the family to take a holiday. Finally, if despite all available community assistance the family are unable to cope, the child may be admitted to hospital to assess his condition and arrange admission to a residential home.

Education

The education of all handicapped children presents similar problems (see Chapters 10 and 28); answers to a series of questions about the child will show how normal facilities can be adapted or what special provision he needs.

1 Can he be ready for school punctually each day and tolerate a normal length day?
2 Transport – how can he travel, does he need help getting in and out of a vehicle and does he use a wheelchair? How independent is he when using his wheelchair?
3 Is he able to take his meals normally? Does he need a special diet?
4 Does he require assistance when going to the lavatory? Is he incontinent? Does he need help with an appliance?
5 Is the child, though partially independent, liable to have falls?
6 Is he physically backward or mentally retarded?

7   Are there any behaviour problems?
8   Is he subject to fits?

It will be a foregone conclusion that these children cannot go up and down stairs.

Can any of these children be accommodated in an ordinary school? A few with slight disability fit in quite easily with a little help and tolerance from teachers and other children. The best provision is when a special area in an ordinary school is designated for the use of handicapped children who can join in some classes and activities with normal pupils of their own age group, but also have separate activities. They will need a higher staff/pupil ratio or trained persons to give assis-tance as these children find it difficult to keep up with other children, for poor hand manipulation makes it hard for them to learn skills. Special courses in social development and independence are being set up throughout the country in an attempt to develop the independence of these children before they leave school. Day attendance or residence at a special school may be necessary for some children, but the disadvantage is that the child is isolated in an atmosphere of ill-health. A few severely handicapped children may need education at home. On reaching school-leaving age there remains the problem of further training and employment (see p. 267).

Syringomyelia

Syringomyelia is a rare disorder in which a cavity develops in the grey matter of the spinal cord, usually in the cervical and upper thoracic regions. The name is derived from syrinx (a tube) and myelos (the spinal cord). The cavity, which is irregular in shape and size, develops very slowly over a period of 10 to 20 years, it is filled with fluid and extends up and down the spinal cord. The cavity may be:

i   a projection from the central canal into the substance of the cord (syringomyelia; Fig. 11.11a);

ii   a simple dilatation of the central canal at any level of the upper thoracic or cervical cord (hydromyelia; Fig. 11.11b); or

iii   a dilatation of the central canal continuous with the 4th ventricle (syringobulbia).

The condition is probably congenital in origin although the symptoms usually appear between the ages of 25 and 40 years; it may occasionally be the result of haemorrhage or thrombosis within the cord, or arise in the immediate vicinity of an intra-medullary tumour. Other congenital abnormalities often accompany the disorder and may in fact be the cause of the condition by interfering with the circulation of blood and CSF at the base of the skull and in the upper cervical cord, and actually force the CSF to enter the neural canal, an other-wise vestigial channel. The commonest of these is Arnold Chiari malformation (see Fig. 4.10), but other congenital abnormalities, fusion of the cervical vertebrae (Klippel–Feil abnormality), atlanto-occipital fusion and basilar impression (basilar invagination), are occasionally found.

Symptoms

Syringomyelia affects young men more commonly than women; the symptoms are dependent upon the situation and direction of expansion of the syrinx; as it is in the centre of the cervical or thoracic spinal cord, sensory symptoms are noticed in the hands and it is the pain and temperature fibres which are damaged first, as they cross the centre of the cord (Fig. 11.11); one hand may be more seriously affected than the other. Other forms of sensation are usually spared at first, but there may be flaccid weakness and wasting of the hands due to internal pressure from the cyst upon the anterior horn cells in the spinal cord; the hand develops a characteristic claw-like posture. As the cavity enlarges other nerve pathways gradually become involved, the weakness and sensory dis-turbance in the hands spreading slowly up the arms to the shoulders. Later the lateral upper motor neurone pathways to the legs become compressed causing a spastic paraparesis; the weakness may be greater in one limb than the other or uniformly

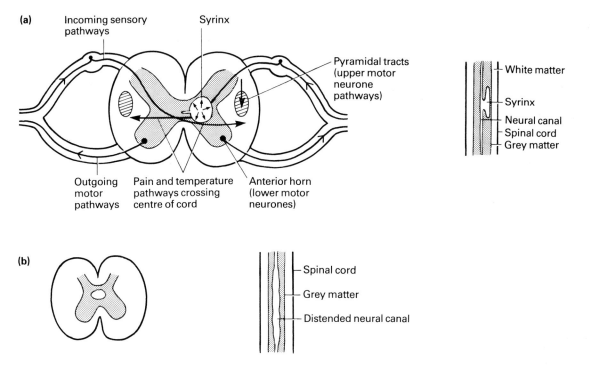

Fig. 11.11 Section through spinal cord showing nerve pathways affected in **(a)** syringomyelia and **(b)** hydromyelia.

affected. Sensation from the legs may be similarly affected. The symptoms, which are usually very slowly progressive, may be much more rapid if cavitation is caused by a tumour or when sudden haemorrhage into the syrinx (haematomyelia) increases the internal pressure upon the cord.

Symptoms have usually been present for some time before the patient seeks medical advice. He may have accepted as normal or not noticed gradual wasting and weakness of the hands, particularly if both hands are equally affected. Only when he finds that some of the finer movements of his fingers have become clumsy and it is becoming difficult or impossible to do up buttons, tie his shoelaces or perform similar simple skills, or when painless burns become infected, is he prompted to see his doctor.

Admission to hospital

Admission to hospital will be necessary for investigations to exclude other lesions such as tumour, to give treatment to halt the disease, for physiotherapy and to teach the patient to protect his affected limbs.

The doctor will take a detailed history, record the duration and progress of the symptoms and when he examines the patient will notice signs of congenital abnormality, an abnormally short neck with restricted movement. The functions of the cranial nerves will be tested carefully; when the rare condition of syringo-bulbia occurs, it will interfere with the functions of the cranial nerve nuclei near the 4th ventricle causing dysphagia, vertigo, sensory loss in the face and respiratory disturbance. Almost invariably the patient has a kyphoscoliosis and there may be evidence of spina bifida occulta suggesting the disorder is congenital. It may be noticed that the patient has scars or recent burns on the hands; one patient stated that he won bets with his work-mates that he would feel no pain if they stubbed out their cigarettes on his hand. Similarly joints which have been painlessly damaged may be swollen. The doctor will test the power of all the limbs noting the distribution of muscular weakness, and will map out areas of sensory disturbance. He will observe the character-istic texture of the hand which feels smooth, flabby and almost boneless. He will examine the tendon reflexes which are usually diminished in the hands and arms (lower motor neurone disturbance) and increased in the legs (upper motor neurone disturbance); the plantar responses are likely to be extensor.

Investigations

Chest X-rays will be performed and skull X-rays will include views of the base of the skull and cervical spine. A lumbar puncture may be performed to obtain CSF; the analysis will be normal unless there is severe block to the flow in the subarachnoid space, when the protein content will be raised. A myelogram is necessary to exclude obstructive lesions (tumours) and demonstrate abnormalities in the region of the foramen magnum.

Treatment

Sometimes the disease arrests spontaneously after about 10 to 20 years, otherwise it is slowly progressive, with lengthy, apparently dormant periods. It is usual for the patient to become totally paraplegic but the condition is rarely the cause of death. Treatment is aimed at arresting the gradual disease process before too much permanent damage has occurred; the various surgical measures that have been attempted have benefitted only a few patients. Treatment includes:

i   a decompressive operation at the base of the skull and the upper cervical spine when Arnold Chiari and other malformations are present, sometimes with incision of the syrinx;

ii radiotherapy has been used in an attempt to destroy the glial cells lining the cavity and thus shrink the cyst;

iii ventriculo-peritoneal shunt may benefit a few patients in whom no congenital abnormality has been found and whose disorder possibly results from the forcing of CSF into the neural canal by adhesions, the result of inflammation of the meninges around the 4th ventricle.

When the syrinx is caused by a cystic tumour symptoms can be relieved by removing the tumour followed by a course of radiotherapy.

Treatment is mainly palliative. The patient must be taught how to recognise and prevent situations which would cause injury to his pain-insensitive limbs, for example always using an oven glove when cooking, testing the bath water with a thermometer, and using a cigarette holder, changing to pipe smoking or giving up smoking to prevent burns. The patient should be instructed in the first aid treatment of burns and warned that falls and other minor accidents may seriously damage his insensitive joints; he should be asked to consult his doctor if he should notice a swollen joint or anything more than a simple burn.

Care will be taken when the patient with syringobulbia eats and drinks. Intragastric feeding will become necessary if dysphagia is present (see Chapter 3); the patient will be fully conscious and able to co-operate when the tube is passed and he will be very self-conscious about his appearance. The tube should be secured inconspicuously and the nasal passages cleaned regularly to remove encrusted discharge; petroleum jelly should be lightly applied around the nostrils. There is always a risk of respiratory failure when there is a high cervical lesion and an artificial ventilator must be available.

Physiotherapy and occupational therapy

Physiotherapy and occupational therapy play an important part in the treatment of syringomyelia. Exercise helps to strengthen weak muscles and the therapists can teach the patient how to use the many aids made for the disabled. The patient may find dressing becomes difficult, so clothing should be easy to put on and zips or velcro fastening used instead of fiddly buttons. Walking frames, sticks and elbow crutches may be unsuitable for the patient with syringomyelia, as the weight taken by his weak arms may damage or even dislocate his joints. Obesity puts an added burden upon weak limbs. A power-assisted wheelchair may become necessary if and when the patient is no longer able to walk.

Diastematomyelia

This is a rare condition in which a spur of bone prevents the normal ascent of the spinal cord within the spinal canal as the child grows; it is occasionally associated with spina bifida. Surgical removal of the spur of bone allows the cord to adopt its natural position.

Spinal angioma

A spinal angioma is a congenital malformation of blood vessels consisting of a tangled mass of distended veins surrounding the spinal cord partially within the subarachnoid space and the remainder within the cord itself. It is a very rare condition arising mainly below the mid-thoracic level but has been known to occur higher. The malformed blood vessels gradually become more distended extending over quite a large area of the spinal cord, possibly as much as two to three segments. Although congenital, symptoms of disturbance rarely appear before the teens and when they do it is because;

i part of the cord is deprived of an adequate blood supply due to either small haemorrhages or thrombosis of small vessels;

ii nerve roots are irritated by the presence of the angioma;

iii spinal subarachnoid haemorrhage produces severe spinal pain and nerve root irritation. Blood is found in the CSF;

iv The angioma acts as a space-occupying lesion causing cord compression;

v massive haemorrhage destroys the cord.

Symptoms are often of a remitting and relapsing nature similar to multiple sclerosis and may be aggravated by an additional strain placed upon the circulation, for example during pregnancy. The patient may have a subarachnoid haemorrhage which presents as sudden severe pain in the centre of the spine; later the patient will complain of headache as blood circulates in the CSF to the cerebral subarachnoid space. When the haemorrhage is into the substance of the spinal cord the patient will suddenly develop paraplegia or quadriplegia depending on the level in the spinal cord. Severe nerve root pain sometimes accompanies subarachnoid haemorrhage or occurs because the angioma is irritating a nerve root.

Investigations

(a) Blood tests
(b) X-rays of the spine
(c) Lumbar puncture to examine the CSF
(d) Myelography to outline the lesion

Treatment

The patient will have a period of bed rest. When the angioma has been located surgery may be possible to clip the feeding vessels. The outcome depends upon the level of the lesion and whether the spinal cord has been destroyed by haemorrhage or ischaemia; if not, the prognosis is good and the patient may make a complete recovery.

Nursing care

When the angioma has caused a subarachnoid haemorrhage the patient will have a period of six weeks' bed rest. When the angioma or haemorrhage into the cord causes paraplegia or quadriplegia the patient will be cared for as described in Chapter 10. Haemorrhage high in the cervical cord can be devastating, necessitating urgent resuscitative measures and the patient's respirations must be maintained with a positive pressure ventilator. Spinal and nerve root pain and headache must be relieved by adequate analgesia.

12

Spinal Injury

Acute injuries

The spinal cord is protected by a sturdy bony column held together by tough ligaments, it is suspended throughout its length by numerous small ligaments and cushioned by CSF (see Fig. 10.7). The spinal cord is a small soft structure, no thicker than a man's little finger, which is closely confined within the vertebral column without space to accommodate oedema, haematoma or foreign body. Any severe spinal injury which tears ligaments and fractures vertebrae will affect the alignment and stability of the protective column and will crush or sever the cord, disrupt its blood supply and cause oedema or haemorrhage. The cervical region is more likely to sustain injury because it has a greater range of movement, less protection from muscle and bone and it supports a weighty structure. The result of spinal cord injury is paralysis, sensory disturbance, loss of bladder and bowel control and sometimes serious suppression of respiration.

Severe spinal injuries which permanently disable previously healthy men and women in the prime of life are often the result of road traffic accidents, while others are the result of accidents in the home, at work, or during recreational pursuits and are common during wartime.

Accident prevention

Many serious accidents can be avoided; from school-days onwards members of the community should understand the purpose of regulations imposed in various spheres of life and be encouraged to adhere to them. There should be proper supervision of gymnastics, swimming, horse riding and other potentially dangerous activities; all safety equipment should be well maintained, safety harnesses used by those working at a height and apparatus in fun fairs and adventure playgrounds should attain certain recognised safety standards and receive regular inspection. Accident prevention should be taught and publicised. Publicity cannot be too graphic as even among intelligent people there is lack of awareness of the hazards of travel; many do not maintain their vehicles, think their driving is always perfect, are in a hurry, lack courtesy and disregard safety. The road user should keep to all the regulations designed for his protection including the use of safety belts, car head rests and safety seats and belts designed for children. Those obtained should meet official safety standards; drivers should be warned against excessive hours of driving without a set period of rest, and the effects of alcohol on judgment of driving conditions.

The risk of spinal injury is increased by:

1 Potentially dangerous occupations, e.g. window cleaners and scaffolders whose work involves heights, travelling salesmen who spend long hours driving, policemen and jockeys or others exposed to similar risks

2 Leisure pursuits, e.g. horse riding, swimming and karate

3 Age and general health – any condition which causes diminished concentration, 'giddiness', 'blackouts' or deterioration in visual acuity, balance and co-ordination increases the risk of accidents; heart disease, arteriosclerosis, diabetes mellitus and epilepsy are all contributory factors. Psychological factors include anxiety about domestic or financial matters and depression which may lead to attempted suicide.

4 Alcohol and drugs

Few accidents, if they were examined in detail, could be said to be uncomplicated and there is a fascinating interweaving of cause and effect which increases with the age of the victim, for example a travelling salesmen because he spends many hours daily on the road, is more likely than others to be involved in a road traffic accident, and becomes more accident-prone if his concentration is impaired by fatigue, depression, alcohol, marriage breakdown or when he develops heart disease because of the sedentary nature of his work. Another example is an ageing farm worker who since boyhood has been used to climbing about on trailers and hay ricks and becomes accident-prone as he gets older. His injuries are likely to be more severe: he may have episodes of momentary 'giddiness' or loss of consciousness due to arteriosclerosis, is likely to be arthritic and less able to correct his balance and when he falls his brittle bones are more likely to fracture; fragile blood vessels may thrombose or rupture. A depressed person may make a failed suicide leap and sustain severe spinal injury.

Anatomy of the spine
(See Chapter 10)

Direct injury

Direct injury is the result of a hefty blow on the back by a moving object, for example falling masonry, a blow from a passing vehicle or a mugging attack; the forceful blow fractures the spinous or transverse processes or laminae (see Fig. 12.3), but the vertebral bodies, articular facets and spinal cord usually escape injury.

A baby's spinal cord may be damaged by excessive neck extension during delivery.

Indirect injury

Indirect injury is sustained when a victim is hurled through the air and comes to a sudden halt on landing; he may be thrown from a vehicle, fall or jump from a height or dive into shallow water. In these incidents the body stops instantly at the point of impact, the oncoming directional force of the rest

of the body concertinas the vertebral column, exerting a great pressure which crushes vertebral bodies. If there is also rotation, sudden flexion or extension, ligaments are torn and articulating facets are fractured and dislocated. Like a spring which immediately recoils when released, so the spine may resume its normal position and alignment, but within these brief moments the spinal cord may have been crushed or severed and its blood supply drastically reduced or cut off causing irreparable damage. Whiplash injury is another serious type of indirect injury, often the result of quite trivial car accidents which suddenly send the head into motion; the victim's head is flung backwards and forwards tearing the anterior and posterior spinal ligaments (Fig. 12.1). Though the bones may not be fractured, dislocation of two adjacent vertebrae may crush or sever the spinal cord. The passenger in a vehicle is more often injured in this way as, unlike the driver, he is unaware of traffic conditions, is unprepared for sudden braking or impact and does not brace himself against them. Car seat-belts because of their restraint upon the body prevent many serious head

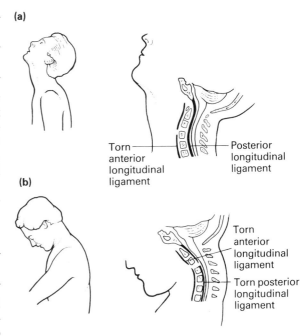

(a)

Torn anterior longitudinal ligament

Posterior longitudinal ligament

(b)

Torn anterior longitudinal ligament

Torn posterior longitudinal ligament

Fig. 12.1 Whiplash injury. **(a)** Sudden hyperextension of the neck. **(b)** Hyperextension followed by sudden hyperflexion – unstable spine.

and spinal injuries, but they may provoke whiplash injuries; these injuries can be dramatically reduced by using a head-rest of the type tested and approved by the motoring organisations.

There may be a combination of direct and indirect injury.

Penetrating injuries

Penetrating injuries from stabbing and shooting accidents may damage the spinal cord and foreign bodies sometimes lodge in or near the spine.

Management of spinal injury

There is always the risk of spinal injury with any accident on the road or fall from a height. Spinal injuries are most common in the cervical region and may be overlooked especially if the victim has sustained a head injury and is unconscious; injuries at the base of the skull involve the centres of heart and respiratory function in the medulla and often cause instant death. An injury above the 5th cervical vertebra is dangerous as it can seriously affect the phrenic nerves to the diaphragm which emerge from the 4th and 5th cervical segments, and the upper motor neurone supply to the intercostal muscles. The thoraco-lumbar junction is another common site for injury. Before the victim is moved his condition must be carefully assessed; he may be conscious or unconscious, lying on the ground or awkwardly slumped over the steering wheel and he may have multiple injuries with haemorrhage. It would be better and is sometimes essential to wait for skilled help before the victim is moved, but this is not always possible. If the circumstances of the accident dictate that the injured person must be moved, it must be remembered that his head, neck and spine must be kept in alignment and several competent people are required to lift the victim, one person assuming responsibility for the head and neck and directing the manoeuvre. When everyone is in position they should lift smoothly and simultaneously, all the while reassuring the patient and maintaining the body in normal alignment to prevent irreparable damage to the spinal cord; **a patient with a broken neck will lose any hope of recovery if his head suddenly flops.** The injured person should be laid flat on his back on the ground, but NO cushion or folded bundle should be placed under his head; should the neck be stiff and the head twisted, no attempt should be made to straighten it as a dangerous cause of this posture is a fracture of the odontoid peg with partial dislocation of the atlanto-axial joints (Fig. 12.3).

Clothing may conceal severe injuries and haemorrhage and should be cut away as this patient must not be moved.

It is vital that ambulance crews, police and other personnel called to the scene of an accident are aware of the risks involved in moving a person whose neck or back may be broken. The conscious patient should be asked if he has any pain in his back or neck, can he move his arms and legs and has he 'pins and needles' or tingling in his limbs? Weakness or complete absence of movement in all limbs with sensory disturbance suggests cervical injury, and weakness or lack of movement in the legs with sensory loss suggests the injury to be in the thoracic or lumbar spine. The first assessment should be recorded and used as a baseline for any subsequent improvement or deterioration. The patient may have sustained a head injury; if he is unconscious, irrational or restless the spinal cord can be damaged if he is lifted unskilfully or, in his confusion, struggles to move. Great care will be needed to lift the patient on to the stretcher, a manoeuvre facilitated by using a spinal board and collar which will prevent sudden flexion of the neck when the patient is moved; this equipment can even be used to safeguard someone who is being lifted from a damaged vehicle as it can be strapped on with the person in a sitting position (Fig. 12.2). To lessen the risk of complicating the patient's injuries, some ambulances – particularly those in

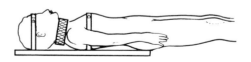

Fig. 12.2 Using a cervical collar and spinal board to immobilise a fractured cervical spine.

regular use on the motorways – are equipped with special stretcher canvases which, when used in conjunction with multi-purpose trolleys, convert into X-ray and theatre tables; this reduces the number of times the patient has to be lifted.

Admission to hospital

In the casualty department the patient should remain on the specially adapted stretcher-trolley-table until his history has been taken by the doctor, examination and X-rays completed, anti-tetanus immunoglobulin or tetanus toxoid administered and immediate surgery performed. The patient who has sustained multiple injuries will need extensive X-rays of the entire body; spinal X-rays will be taken from several angles as only careful study may reveal the important effects of hyperflexion and hyperextension. X-rays will demonstrate fractures and crushing of the vertebrae, dislocation, bone splintering and the presence of foreign bodies (Fig. 12.3); other important X-rays include those of the skull (especially the base of the skull), chest and injured limbs. The patient's clothes must be removed, if necessary by cutting, to facilitate thorough examination and observation; on no account should the patient sit up or struggle to undress. Close observation is necessary to ensure that the patient has a clear airway and that his respirations are satisfactory; the patient may have fractured ribs, 'stove-in' chest or his respiratory muscles may be paralysed by a cervical fracture. An endotracheal tube cannot be passed when the patient has a cervical fracture and should there be acute respiratory failure or obstruction (see p. 50) an emergency tracheostomy will be necessary and the patient's respirations will be maintained by a positive pressure ventilator. The nurse should inspect the patient's mouth carefully as teeth may have been broken or loosened in the accident. The casualty nurses will be available to calm and reassure the agitated patient, watch for and report any deterioration in conscious level and limb movement, care for intravenous infusion, observe for signs of internal bleeding, assist with wound toilet, bandages and plaster for immobilisation of limb fractures, give analgesics as prescribed and care for anxious relatives. The patient should at no time be lifted without the doctor's permission, nor should any attempt be made to lift him unless enough

people are available; one qualified person should always be available to assist and direct the lifting manoeuvre. All initial treatment should be completed in as short a time as possible, preferably within two hours, so that the patient's position can be changed, as his motionless, insensitive body is at serious risk of tissue damage at pressure points.

The ward nurses will receive information and will prepare all necessary equipment before the patient arrives (see Chapter 10). A trained nurse may be necessary to 'special' the patient, she will receive him and supervise his transfer from trolley to bed; the patient will be placed on a sheepskin and sheepskin bootees or foam leg channels used to protect his heels. Skull traction tongs may have been applied and a doctor or other experienced person will help to set up the traction apparatus using the correct weight and degree of counter-traction.

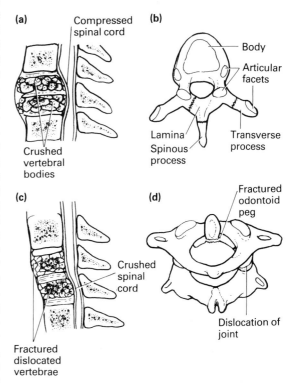

Fig. 12.3 Spinal fractures. **(a)** Crushed vertebrae. **(b)** Fractures of transverse and spinous processes and lamina. **(c)** and **(d)** Fracture dislocation.

Observations

The nurse will notice the patient's general condition, demeanour and whether he is in obvious pain; she will ask him a few relevant questions about the accident, mainly to assess conscious level and mental state and to establish rapport. A detailed history can be obtained from the doctor's notes to avoid cross-examining the shocked, exhausted patient. The nurse must always bear in mind the possibility of associated head injury with increasing intracranial pressure, and a deteriorating spinal cord condition and regularly perform a full neurological examination and record of vital functions; the respiratory rate must be carefully counted with the chest exposed to assess the depth of respirations, as a patient with a high cervical lesion can develop respiratory failure.

Relatives or a witness to the accident can give helpful information and should be seen by the doctor and a member of the nursing staff; a searching enquiry should be made into the patient's general and medical history. When a general medical disorder is thought to have caused an accident, certain investigations are necessary:

i   Haemoglobin – severe anaemia may have caused fainting.
ii Blood sugar levels – the patient may have had a hypoglycaemic or hyperglycaemic episode.
iii Electrocardiograph – cardiac dysrhythmias or myocardial infarction may have caused momentary unconsciousness.
iv Electroencephalogram – an epileptic fit may have caused the accident.

Treatment

The aims of treatment are to correct dislocation and maintain the patient's spine in a position which will prevent further cord damage, allow time for the tissues to heal, bones to unite and peripheral nerves to regenerate, during this time preventing complications and pursuing a course of planned rehabilitation (see Chapter 10). When a patient has sustained a spinal fracture he will be treated by immobilisation, the duration depending upon the severity of the injury and the rate of healing as shown on X-rays.

Simple cervical fractures

The patient is treated with bed rest; he should be nursed on his back without pillows, with his head and neck immobilised between sandbags. The patient's co-operation is essential; he should be told why this treatment is necessary and given an approximate idea of how long he will need to remain in this uncomfortable restricted position. After about one week, further X-rays will be taken and if these show satisfactory alignment of the fracture and signs of healing, the patient will be fitted with a collar and gradually mobilised using a soft collar in bed and rigid collar when he is up and about; he may be fitted with a plaster jacket with head and neck extension. The patient's activities will be guided by the physiotherapist.

Fracture dislocation in the cervical region

Treatment of fracture dislocation in this normally very mobile and critical region is more difficult and prolonged; not only must there be immobilisation, but also traction to separate and align the vertebrae and to relieve the spinal cord of pressure. Under local anaesthesia skull calipers are screwed into the outer table of the skull and are attached to a weight by a cord strung over a set of pulleys; usually 2.25 Kg (5 lbs) is sufficient to maintain normal alignment. Slight hyperextension is usually necessary and for this purpose a small pad is placed under the neck. After 24 hours X-rays will be taken to check that the correct degree of traction has been achieved; if there is too little or too much, the weight will be adjusted accordingly. The patient can be turned into almost any position providing one nurse is responsible for keeping the head in line with the body and attends to the change of pulley for each position adopted. An interval of several weeks will elapse before further X-rays are taken to check healing progress. In some centres where cervical fusion is performed early and when oedema has subsided, the traction is removed at approximately 6 weeks from the injury. Otherwise after a period of about 3 months when satisfactory bone union has been achieved, traction will be discontinued, the patient is fitted with a collar and then, always wearing his collar, he will be very cautiously mobilised; he may need to wear a collar for several weeks or months, in particular when travelling. When at last the patient is ready to dispense with the collar, he should get used to the feeling by leaving it off for short periods at first as he is likely to feel insecure without it.

Simple fractures of thoracic and lumbar vertebrae

These will be treated by a prolonged period of complete bed rest on a firm bed; the patient's head should rest on one pillow and a firm pillow should be placed in the small of the back to hyperextend the spine.

Fracture of the coccyx

The coccyx can be fractured easily when someone lands heavily on their 'tail'; this is a very painful condition and the sufferer cannot sit down. Recovery is spontaneous, taking several months.

Extensive spinal injuries

The long-term care of a patient who has sustained severe multiple spinal injuries presents many problems, not the least of these being the provision of the necessary staff to enable a trained nurse and three others to change the position of the patient every two hours, night and day for months. The Stryker turning frame is favoured by some doctors, but several nurses are still needed to turn the patient safely and the plaster bed is inclined to cause pressure sores. The most satisfactory solution is the provision of a very costly motorised bed with push-button control which effortlessly alters the patient's position.

Nursing care
(Read also Chapter 10)

The patient will be kept under particularly close observation for the first 48 hours after injury, as it is imperative that there is no deterioration in his already serious condition; weak respirations which suggest impending respiratory failure dictate the immediate need for artificial ventilation, and signs of increasing muscular weakness and sensory loss may be due to spinal cord compression by oedema, haematoma, foreign body or fragment of bone and indicate the urgent need for medical or surgical decompression. A course of dexamethasone is given to reduce oedema of the spinal cord. The nursing staff will have ample opportunity to talk to the patient while they attend to his comfort, they should try to allay some of his fears but must be wary of painting a falsely optimistic picture to the patient or his relatives. The outlook is hopeful if the patient retains some movement and sensation in his limbs or shows slight improvement when the transient conditions of spinal shock and oedema begin to resolve, but in many instances there will be no improvement and the patient's limbs will remain totally paralysed without sensation; the spinal cord does not regenerate, if any part has been destroyed the patient will have some permanent disability.

The frequency of neurological assessment and recording of vital functions will depend on the seriousness of the injury and at first will be half-hourly, the assessment being made while other care is given to allow the patient some restful intervals. Particular attention is paid to the amount of movement and sensation in the limbs and the very first observation must be accurate as weak muscles tire very quickly and comparison is often between mere flickers of movement. The depth and rate of respirations should be observed carefully by baring the chest to detect early signs of respiratory failure (see p. 51) which is likely if the lesion is above the level of the 5th cervical vertebra. The blood pressure recordings will be of value if the patient is very shocked. The patient's temperature will be recorded 4-hourly. An initial mild pyrexia is to be expected as a reaction to injury and to blood in the cerebrospinal fluid, which should settle within 48 hours. Any sudden rise in temperature may be due to respiratory or urinary infections, septic lacerations, wounds and compound fracture sites or deep vein thrombosis. Should the patient complain of sudden severe chest pain and his respirations become rapid and shallow the likely cause is a pulmonary embolus.

An intravenous infusion will have been set up in the casualty department and several pints of blood and plasma will be transfused to counteract the shock of severe blood loss from multiple injuries; other intravenous fluid will be given according to the patient's electrolyte balance and the infusion may be continued for about 48 hours. Care is taken not to overload the circulation during this time and the patient will not be pressed to take oral fluid as the autonomic nervous system which controls the kidneys may be in a state of shock and the patient may have oliguria. The patient will be catheterised to assess returning kidney function; once the kidneys have regained function fluids should be increased to 3 litres per day, then if the patient continues to have retention of urine and there is absence of bladder sensation a catheter will continue to be necessary (see p. 179). Similarly the nerve supply to the bowel may be in a state of shock (paralytic ileus); enemata must not be administered until this condition has resolved.

General hygiene, skin care, pressure area care, bladder and bowel care are of the utmost importance and are described in detail in Chapter 10.

When skull traction is used the scalp wounds should be inspected daily, if there are signs of infection a wound swab will be taken for culture and the appropriate antibiotic prescribed; infection of the scalp should be promptly treated as it could extend to cause chronic osteomyelitis of the skull.

A patient with a cervical fracture may have also sustained head injury with a fracture at the base of the skull, and facial injuries with fractures of the mandible, maxillae and nasal air sinuses. This combination of injuries presents many problems with the patient immobilised as he is with skull traction (see p. 210). A high protein fluid diet, sucked through a straw, will be necessary for the six week period that the patient's jaw is wired and the nurse will need patience and perseverance to ensure that nutritional needs are met, as lying in such an awkward position, maybe paralysed from the neck down, he will not at first manage nor have the appetite for large quantities of fluid at any one time. Nutrition is very important to promote healing which can be delayed by the metabolic disturbance caused by severe injury and the always present risk of tissue breakdown, pressure sores and anaemia. A variety of flavoured fluids should be offered to tempt the patient's palate, but nutritious drinks should be alternated with clear fluids to cleanse the mouth as oral hygiene is difficult.

Physiotherapy

The physiotherapist is the person most acutely aware of the patient's muscle power and ability, and will work in close consultation with the occupational therapist to devise methods which will enable the patient to be as independent as possible. An overhead mirror, prismatic spectacles and bookstands may help the patient with his occupational activities whilst he is having bed rest, and tension springs will strengthen hand, arm and shoulder muscles in preparation for the time when he will be able to use monkey pole hoists above the bed and lavatory, wall rails and ramps.

Medical social worker
(See Chapter 10)

Psychiatric advice

The patient who has attempted suicide should be seen by a psychiatrist who may recommend treatment for depression and give supportive psychotherapy. Psychological assessment may be required when head injury has caused brain damage or personality disorder, to guide those planning the patient's rehabilitation programme; assessment may also be necessary in connection with claims for compensation.

Rehabilitation
(See Chapter 10)

Relatives will need support and advice from medical and nursing staff and should be encouraged to participate in the patient's care throughout his time in hospital; they should continue to be given the opportunity to obtain the advice of at least one member of the rehabilitation team until the patient has completely recovered or is leading a satisfactory wheelchair life. Claims for compensation are protracted and unsettling for the patient and his family and may take several years to conclude.

Chronic spinal trauma

There have been literary allusions to lumbago and sciatica since as early as the fifteenth century, with some indication of its duration and the attempts which were made to treat the condition – rest, warmth and manipulation. In the 1930s it was realised that the cause of sciatica could be protrusion of an intervertebral disc pressing on the sciatic nerve and by 1945 came the realisation that it could also be the cause for lumbago; 'slipped disc' became a fashionable illness as soon as the description was coined, and to this day back pain is often wrongly attributed to disorder of the disc. The older generation who had put up with the discomfort of 'the rheumatics', a touch of 'fibrositis' or 'neuritis', a crick in the neck or just plain backache for so long, were sceptical about the new-fangled term rather glibly used by some medical practitioners. Their doubts increased when it became obvious that though there were occasional instant cures when the 'disc' was 'put back', often suffering continued for weeks or months in the old way until the trouble cured itself. Once the condition was given a name everyone expected treatment to be available and instantly curative; unfortunately the treatment of an episode of acute back pain is little changed and still involves discomfort and inconvenience for many weeks, prolonged sick leave, loss of earnings, disruption of family life and misery for someone who is forced to suddenly withdraw from his normal activities, responsibilities and social life.

Degenerative changes of the joints, ligaments and intervertebral discs are the result of normal wear and tear, minor stresses and strains and chronic inflammation. Many people suffer from periodic episodes of pain in the back and various factors have been suggested for the cause. Some dubious propositions, with consequently bizarre treatments, blame a single factor such as diet, but surely the condition must encompass other factors: heredity, climate, overweight, occupation, poor posture, pregnancy, age and excessive recreational and sporting activities, for example judo and gymnastics, especially when the body is immature.

Precipitating factors and preventative measures

In Great Britain chronic backache is a national disorder accounting for enormous loss of 'man' hours and incurring high expenditure in sickness benefit. 'Back trouble' seems to be more common and occurring at a younger age, which may seem strange when so many heavy tasks in the home and in industry have been taken over by machinery; the increased incidence is probably due to the current lifestyle, as so many people spend long periods sitting, they have sedentary occupations, travel to work by car and train, spend their leisure time watching television, have insufficient regular exercise, are overweight and engage in sudden bursts of over-enthusiastic activity at weekends and holidays when their body is out of training and their muscles are flabby. The nation would be well-advised to conduct a campaign to inform the general public how to avoid back strain and injury; this campaign starts with the very young. A baby's spine is examined at birth and parents should be advised not to be over-eager to sit their infant up nor make him walk before he is naturally ready. Periodic medical examination is necessary as the child grows to detect abnormal postures and give early treatment. Attention should be paid to the way children sit at school and to their general deportment, and they should be actively discouraged from lifting heavy weights which can damage immature joints and lead to premature degenerative changes. Satchels or rucksacks are better for carrying school books to and from or around school as the weight is distributed evenly on the shoulders and prevents distortion of an immature spine. It is thought that some people are born with a narrow spinal canal which makes them more likely to suffer from back conditions. It may be possible in the future to screen young persons to prevent unsuitable candidates from embarking on a career which involves heavy lifting; sometimes it may be sufficient to teach back strengthening exercises and give advice about lifting. The expectant mother should be given dietary advice, a benefit to herself and her unborn baby; she should also be advised on correct posture and suitable footwear as she will be carrying extra weight (more so if she carries other young children) and straining back ligaments slackened by hormonal changes. When attending her baby she should either sit with him on her lap or have the changing mattress at a suitable high level to prevent unnecessary back strain; she should be well supported in a comfortable armchair or lying on the bed when breast feeding. The effects of repeated spinal damage are seen at a surprisingly young age, even as young as the teens, but usually it is the middle-aged who develop back disorders, especially those whose occupation persistently strains joints and ligaments – farmers, storekeepers, builders, mothers of young children, nurses and those who sit for lengthy periods in badly designed seats. The absence of suitable equipment and desks or working surfaces at the wrong height, puts unnecessary strains upon the back and neck. There should be incentives to designers and manufacturers to produce beds, chairs and seats, including car seats, which give good support to the spine. Employers should be persuaded to purchase well-designed office equipment, give training in lifting techniques to employees, and provide and encourage the use of lifting apparatus and hoists.

Anatomy
(See also Chapter 10)

The stability of the spine depends upon a very complex structure of supporting ligaments (see p. 163) and strong muscles, and its mobility upon controlled freedom of movement at all the joints. Each vertebra articulates with neighbouring vertebrae above and below (two joints between each pair of vertebrae) and between the vertebral bodies is a shock-absorbing intervertebral disc (see Fig. 10.6); the thoracic vertebrae also have facets for the articulation of the ribs. The articulating joints are surrounded by an articular capsule and each joint is well supported by ligaments. The whole vertebral column securely contains and protects the spinal cord and its emerging nerve roots. The mobility of the spine is affected when the joints or discs or both are damaged, in each circumstance the symptoms

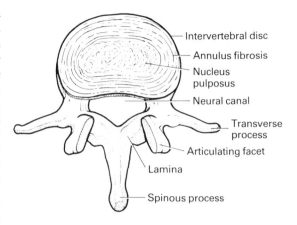

Fig. 12.4　Intervertebral disc.

are very similar. There is such mobility and so many joints which are subjected to daily strain for years that it is not surprising they are sometimes wrenched, which can set up such severe pain and muscle spasm that the patient may understandably think he has 'slipped a disc' or broken his back; he hardly dares to move for fear of pain and this tension increases muscle spasm which is likely to spread to involve other muscles.

A less common, more serious event is the rupture and herniation of an intervertebral disc. Each disc (Fig. 12.4) consists of a cartilaginous ring (annulus fibrosus) and gelatinous core (nucleus pulposus) and is adherent to the bone above and below and contained and strengthened by the anterior and posterior longitudinal ligaments. These structures are anterior to the spinal cord. The spinal column has a series of natural curves (see Fig. 10.1) and while these curves are maintained the discs are subjected to an even pressure throughout. When the spine is flexed the anterior part of the disc is squeezed and the backward pressure within the disc is towards the spinal cord or nerve roots (Fig. 12.5); as the disc ages, the annulus fibrosus becomes less elastic, brittle and, as there is no blood supply, cracks occur which never heal. Sudden flexion stress may:

(a) rupture the annulus fibrosus and detach a fragment which encroaches upon the contents of the spinal canal;

(b) rupture the annulus fibrosus and allow the unrestrained soft nucleus pulposus to ooze out and compress the contents of the spinal canal;

(c) both (a) and (b) may occur simultaneously.

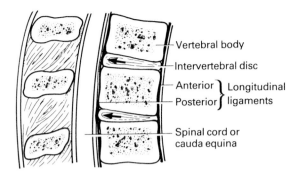

Fig. 12.5 Pressure within disc when spine is flexed.

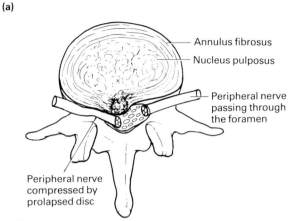

These changes may affect one or more discs. Lateral disc herniation is far more common than central protrusion; it compresses a nerve root, just before the nerve root passes through the intervertebral foramen (Fig. 12.6). A central disc herniation in the cervical and thoracic regions causes pressure on the spinal cord, and in the lumbar region the central nerve roots of the cauda equina. Cervical disc prolapse occurs mainly at C5/6; thoracic disc prolapse is extremely rare as spinal flexion is limited by the rib cage and sternum; prolapsed lumbar disc is the most common because there is greater strain in that region when bending and lifting, the disc is larger and the comparatively narrow posterior longitudinal ligament offers less restraint, the discs between L4/5 and L5/S1 vertebrae are the most vulnerable.

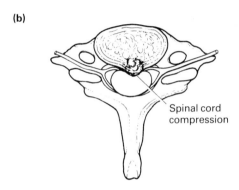

Lumbar spinal disorder

Most adults have at some time in their lives experienced one or more bouts of lumbago or sciatica. The onset of pain may be unexpected and cause inconvenience for only a day or two, or be more severe necessitating a few days in bed; pain may be the immediate result of a slight twisting movement or follow some strenuous sustained activity to which the person is unaccustomed, for example moving furniture, gardening or spring-cleaning. Sometimes there is a delay of several hours before the gradual onset of symptoms which are obviously related to a particular activity. Even when the discomfort is short-lived it may be an

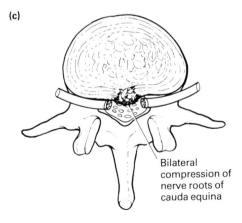

Fig. 12.6 Disc herniations. **(a)** Lateral lumbar disc prolapse. **(b)** Central cervical disc prolapse. **(c)** Central lumbar disc prolapse.

early warning sign of more serious trouble in the future. The patient must be assured that he will recover, as anxiety is a great hindrance to recovery and tension increases muscle spasm, but he should be warned that discomfort may last, not for 'just a few days' but may run into weeks or months. He will need to be patient and should follow certain important principles which will speed recovery and, if they become a life-long habit, will prevent recurrence.

1   Good posture is always essential. The patient should be shown the correct shape of the spine and must understand why he should always maintain these curves when standing or walking and why the small of his back should always be supported by a firm cushion whenever he is seated, including when driving his car. Unfortunately the manufacturers of most chairs and car seats pay insufficient attention to good supportive design.

2   Strain upon the back will be reduced if, when picking up objects from the floor the knees are bent or one leg is extended backwards (Fig. 12.7).

3   The bed and mattress should be firm; if the bed is unsuitable it would be better to sleep on a mattress on the floor.

4   All unnecessary bending or lifting should be avoided; if lifting is necessary, correct methods must be used.

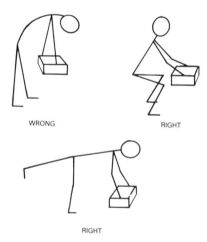

Fig. 12.7   Postures to be used for picking up objects from low down.

Warm clothing and the use of a soothing hot water bottle in the small of the back are helpful (the water must never be too hot or the bottle placed next to the skin); a hot water bottle is firm and just the right size to use in a chair instead of a cushion and the warmth may help the patient's muscles to relax and allow his lumbo-sacral spine to adopt its correct curve. Regular analgesic medication is necessary as relief of pain also helps the patient to relax and lessens painful muscle spasm; an analgesic is particularly necessary at night to ensure a good rest. Constipation, partly caused by the regular use of analgesics, should be avoided by taking sufficient fluid, a high fibre diet and if necessary a mild aperient; pelvic congestion from an over-full bowel or occurring during menstruation will aggravate back pain. A few patients do not recover or relapse as soon as they get up; resting in bed at home may prove ineffective as the temptation to get up to the lavatory and potter about is too great, and there may be no relative or friend available to help with domestic affairs.

A severe episode of back pain is often preceded by years of intermittent backache or episodes of lumbago or sciatica; the pain may be so sudden and severe that the patient is fixed in a stooping posture or collapses to the ground unable to move, the doctor is called to see him immediately and will administer an intramuscular analgesic and help the patient to straighten out into a comfortable position. He will recommend rest in bed and when the pain is under control will make a full examination to determine the level of the lesion and detect motor and sensory abnormalities. Straight leg raising will be tested cautiously as it causes very severe pain; limitation of straight leg raising and diminished or absent tendon reflexes in the legs are significant signs of nerve root involvement. A few patients will be admitted to hospital because they have adverse neurological signs or no-one to look after them at home. Most patients have a period of bed rest at home and, should this fail, an out-patient appointment will be arranged with a general physician, neurologist or orthopaedic specialist who will compare his examination findings with those of the general practitioner and assess any improvement or deterioration, perform a rectal or vaginal examination when there is an indication of a possible pelvic lesion and arrange for the patient to have spinal X-rays. A course of out-patient physiotherapy may be arranged or the patient will be admitted to hospital for further investigations and treatment.

Admission to hospital

A few patients with acute back pain are admitted to hospital on the first day they have ever experienced pain, but many have experienced repeated episodes of lumbago or sciatica with constant niggling pain or nagging ache for years and tiresome difficulties in everyday activities, for example it is impossible to reach their feet to put on socks and shoes or cut toenails, to get out of the bath even if it has been possible to get in, drive the car or meet the demands of young children whose constant clamouring has become a nightmare. Many patients have had various forms of treatment, bed rest at home, physiotherapy (heat, massage, traction and exercise) and analgesic and anti-inflammatory medications; X-ray examination being normal, the patient is left with the feeling that no one believes him, yet he still has pain. Some patients being stoical, have continued activities which aggravated their condition, others exaggerate their disability in a plea for help and understanding. Some patients are so accustomed to chronic invalidism that they almost relish it, exaggerating their suffering and using their 'back trouble' to gain sympathy and attention or as an escape from responsibility. Unfortunately backache and a stiff neck are regarded as comic and a person who excuses himself from every activity because of his 'back' is likely to be labelled neurotic and a bore; in very few instances does the complaint receive the compassion it deserves, especially as it is never fatal.

History and examination
(See Chapter 2)

It is very important to instil confidence in this patient who is at the end of his tether and may be feeling that there is little point in admission to hospital though he realises there is no alternative. The doctor and nurse must appear confident and optimistic and be undeterred by a gloomy disgruntled patient, full of complaints about previous unsuccessful treatment. A complete general and neurological examination is essential for every patient, as lumbar pain and sciatica are symptoms of many disorders. A detailed history is necessary to discover how long the patient has experienced symptoms, the duration, frequency and severity of episodes, whether there has been any previous treatment, when and how the present attack developed and whether anything relieves the pain. During the history and examination the doctor will assess the patient's reaction to his symptoms and the severity of the pain. Is the patient able to walk, does he drag his foot or admit to tripping, can he sit down or is the pain so severe that he has to lie down? Has he an abnormal posture (stooped or twisted sideways, positions which give some relief from pain)? Pain may be limited to the lumbar region or radiate into the buttock, down the leg or even into the foot, suggesting that the sciatic nerve is involved. Although the pain is limited to one area at the present time, questions will be asked about previous episodes and whether movement, coughing or sneezing increase the pain. The patient will be asked to describe any abnormal sensations he has experienced in his legs, tingling, 'pins and needles' or numbness and its distribution, as they are useful localising signs. Questions must be asked about bladder function and whether micturition is normal, as a central lumbar disc protrusion will affect both legs and may compress the bilateral nerve roots to the bladder; retention of urine is such a serious sign because normal bladder function, once lost, may never return. The doctor will examine the patient's spine, will notice flattening of the lumbar curve or the existence of abnormal spinal curvature. He will apply manual pressure to either side of the spinous processes to try to discover at which level there is pain. The doctor will test the mobility of the patient's spine in all directions and will persuade the patient to try to touch his toes to determine restricted and pain inducing movements. He will examine the patient's limbs in detail to demonstrate weak and wasted muscles, and map out areas of abnormal sensation (see Fig. 10.9) to help localise the lesion. The reflexes and plantar responses will be examined and may be diminished or absent in the affected leg. Straight leg raising is usually restricted to less than 90° in both legs but more noticeably in the leg affected by the lesion, because stretching the sciatic nerve induces pain.

Investigations

1   ESR – this will be raised if the patient is suffering from active arthritis.
2   Chest X-rays.
3   Spinal X-rays – spinal X-rays often appear

normal despite the patient's symptoms, they may show unrelated bony changes, there may be insignificant narrowing of one or more disc spaces or obvious narrowing indicating the level of a disc prolapse. An abnormality may be seen which suggests a space-occupying lesion (see p. 174), e.g. spinal tumour.

4 Lumbar puncture – the CSF protein is slightly raised when a prolapsed intervertebral disc is present (up to 80 mg/100 ml); this test is usually combined with myelography (see p. 32).

5 Myelography – this radiological investigation outlines a protruding disc; it is an essential investigation if there is any suspicion of neoplasia.

6 Radiculography (see p. 35) – a radiological investigation confined to a specific area of the spinal cord, but can proceed to a full myelogram if the need arises.

Treatment

The patient's successful treatment in hospital is greatly influenced by the attitude of the therapeutic team and each patient should be considered carefully as an individual – what have been the causative factors, have his occupation or normal activities aggravated the condition? Has anyone tried to explain to the patient why he has developed back trouble, what it is or how to prevent recurrence? Has the patient had any treatment, why did it fail? Is he excessively anxious about his condition because it threatens his occupation, causes domestic worry or because he thinks he has a tumour? It is very easy for a patient to conclude there is something sinister or unusual about his condition as the serious-faced medical staff ponder the right treatment. Do not let this patient be labelled 'difficult' (see p. 256).

Constant niggling pain or nagging ache causes irritability and the victim feels guilty for his continuing complaints, often unsupported by medical evidence. The first period of disablement and treatment for a sudden acute attack of sciatica or lumbago may be borne as easily as any other illness and the patient's life reorganised accordingly. Should the condition be resistant to treatment or recur after a few weeks with the prospect of many more weeks' bedrest and traipsing to and fro from hospital or physiotherapy clinic, the patient's morale will become low and his irritability reflected

in his attitude to treatment. Finally he may become so dissatisfied with the apparent ineffectiveness of treatment that after discussion with friends or acquaintances who have had similar experiences, he tries to find a quick cure by going to an osteopath or chiropractor; his decision may coincide with natural spontaneous recovery.

When it has been established that the patient is suffering from lumbar joint strain or a prolapsed intervertebral disc, alternatives of treatment will be discussed with the patient. Complete bed rest for a period of three to four weeks is usually prescribed, even for those who have previously had bed rest at home, and may be combined with pelvic or leg traction and epidural injections.

Complete bed rest
The aims of treatment are:

1 To relieve the spine of weight and movement.
2 To avoid the posture which is known to strain joints and increase pressure within the intervertebral disc, i.e. sitting, and adopt a posture which encourages the spine to regain its normal curves.
3 To allow time for irritated nerve roots to recover and muscle spasm to subside and prevent further herniation if there is a prolapsed disc.

Bed rest is a successful form of treatment given the right conditions and indications; it is essential for patients who are immobilised by very severe pain and it is the treatment of choice when discomfort and pain have persisted for many weeks. Medical treatment is prolonged and it would sometimes seem to disregard the value of the patient's time. It is easy to say 'health must come first', but prolonged ill-health except when it is welcomed as an escape, always leads to anxiety about employment, finance, family unity and frustration at loss of freedom. The patient's co-operation is essential and he must be encouraged to make all necessary arrangements at home and at work so that, free from anxiety, he can relax and settle down to 3–6 weeks' recuperative treatment. The medical social worker may be able to solve problems which might otherwise delay the patient's admission to hospital and will continue to see him at least once a week after his admission. Before he begins treatment the patient should be told exactly what is entailed and for approximately how long he will be confined to bed. He should be warned that it is quite usual for the pain to be a little worse during the first few days and that there is rarely significant improvement until the end of the second week. The patient should be given a regular daily opportunity to discuss his condition with the doctor or a senior nurse as, airing his anxieties, he will be more content. During this period the patient needs mental and physical rest without boredom. Analgesic medication should be administered regularly and, combined with a tranquilliser and muscle relaxant such as diazepam, will help the patient to rest more comfortably; inevitably much of the day will be spent dozing and most patients will find that after the first few days they will have adjusted to inactivity and time no longer drags. A non-steroid anti-inflammatory preparation will be administered to alleviate the inflammation of musculo-skeletal conditions. Some patients will require night sedation.

The patient should be nursed on a bed with a firm base and lie flat with one pillow under his head. A bedcradle is necessary to allow freedom of leg and foot movement and keep the patient comfortably cool. The bedside locker or bed table should be conveniently positioned and nurses should thoughtfully arrange things so that the patient can reach them easily. Before the nurse commences any procedure, clear explanation of the manoeuvre must be given to the patient to prevent him making any movement which will cause pain as he will instinctively try to move to be helpful. When he moves he must do so in one piece, the nurse at the ready and helping to maintain body alignment. Depending upon the patient's condition, some will be allowed to go to the lavatory once daily on a sanichair, others who ought to remain in bed all the time but who find using a bedpan causes pain will be allowed to use a bedside commode. Raising the buttocks on to a bedpan distorts the curvature of the spine; the patient can be made comfortable if his trunk is first raised by rolling on to two parallel pillows (Fig. 12.8).

When the patient has pelvic traction the usual daytime weight of traction is 11 kgs (25 lbs) which is reduced to 7 kgs (15 lbs) at night. Traction is usually started with the lesser weight but even this may not be tolerated at first; another trial will be made with the lesser weight or traction will be given intermittently. By the end of a week if there is no obvious improvement an epidural injection of methylprednisolone acetate (Depo-medrone) may be given; this can be repeated after a few days.

General care

The patient should be given a daily blanket bath, normal opportunity to wash face and hands, clean teeth and brush and wash hair; he must on no account reach up to a wash bowl nor do anything which causes him to move from a relaxed supine position. A dusting of talcum powder will give greater comfort at pressure points which should be inspected regularly, a sheepskin will prevent pressure sores. A pelvic traction corset may be removed when the patient is bathed, but must be correctly reapplied over the iliac crests. Temperature, pulse and respiratory rates will be taken if the patient is unwell. Daily physiotherapy, breathing and leg exercises will be given to keep the patient physically fit and prevent deep vein thrombosis; carefully fitted, full-length anti-thrombotic stockings are advisable.

A high fibre, low calorie diet is most suitable as it prevents constipation and weight gain. Some overweight patients need to be restricted to as little as 3200 kj (800 calories) daily; a diet will be a particular hardship as meals are one of the highlights of the day and should therefore be presented as attractively as possible catering for the patient's taste. Patients should be persuaded to take plenty of fluids and meals should be eaten slowly to avoid indigestion; an antacid may be necessary.

By the end of 3 weeks if the patient is symptom-free he will be very cautiously mobilised wearing

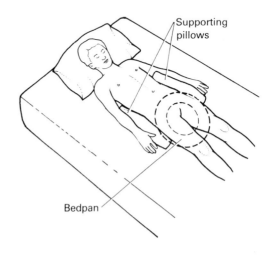

Fig. 12.8 Raising patient on pillows to enable use of a bedpan.

a surgical corset if this has been recommended. For the first week the patient will not be allowed to sit, but must either stand, walk or lie down. He will be given advice about after-care (see p. 216). Any patient who has experienced severe 'back' problems will need to seriously consider a change of occupation which avoids the need for strenuous activities.

A small percentage of patients with acute back pain are suffering from a prolapsed intervertebral disc; some will respond to complete bed rest and other forms of medical treatment, but a few will require surgery. A myelogram is always necessary prior to surgery.

Indications for surgery

i   Extreme intractable pain.
ii A central disc protrusion affecting bladder function.
iii Failure of conservative treatment.
iv Recurrent disc prolapse.

Surgical treatment

(a) Laminectomy – partial removal of two adjacent laminae on the side of the disc protrusion, or a microdiscectomy (a small hole bored through the lamina) allows access to the disc (visible behind the nerve root; Fig. 12.9) which can then be removed. More than one disc space may be explored; laminectomy in this instance will weaken the spinal column whereas with the microdiscectomy this is not so.

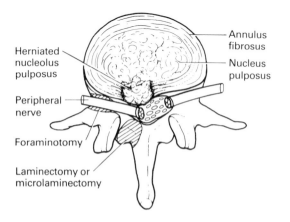

Fig. 12.9 Surgical procedures for removal of prolapsed disc.

Herniated
nucleolus
pulposus

Peripheral
nerve

Foraminotomy

Laminectomy or
microlaminectomy

Annulus
fibrosus

Nucleus
pulposus

(b) Foraminotomy – this operation is favoured by some surgeons as it does not weaken the supporting structure of the spine and the patient can be more quickly mobilised. The foramen is enlarged around the emerging nerve root and the prolapsed portion of the disc is removed.

(c) Spinal fusion – several lumbar vertebrae are fused together to limit flexion movement of the lumbar spine.

Postoperative care

Once the patient has regained consciousness he will return to the ward in his own bed; it is usual for the patient to be lying on his back as this will help haemostasis and keeps the spine in alignment. A record will be kept of temperature, pulse, respirations and blood pressure. An intramuscular analgesic will be given within the first hour, before the patient experiences severe pain, and this will relax the patient and prepare him for the first change of position; an analgesic will also be necessary to settle the patient for the night. At least two nurses will be needed to turn the patient (one of whom must be an experienced nurse), the patient must receive a clear explanation of the procedure and try to relax to co-operate with instructions, he will need plenty of reassurance.

The nurses must lift simultaneously and ensure that the patient is comfortably positioned. Thereafter the patient's position will be changed from side to side 2-hourly. At the next turn, if this is according to the surgeon's instructions, the patient will be allowed to turn himself with supervision. The easiest and least painful method is to turn over on to hands and knees while bedding is smoothed before lowering onto the other side; female patients will then find it more comfortable to adopt a kneeling position to use a bedpan (Fig. 12.10). All patients should be encouraged to pass urine after 4–6 hours. Retention of urine is a possible complication following spinal surgery. If the patient has not passed urine within the first 12 hours or is experiencing bladder discomfort he may be allowed to get up to a commode or stand by the bedside to use a urinal; should these measures fail the patient will be catheterised. A high fluid intake should be encouraged and a careful record of intake and output kept. The patient will be mobilised gradually according to the selected surgical procedure and the surgeon's instructions; some will be allowed up on the first postoperative day, others

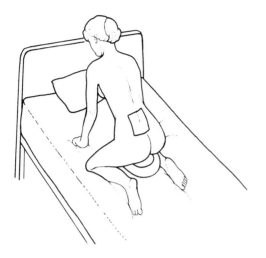

Fig. 12.10 Kneeling position for patient to use bedpan.

after 5–7 days and following spinal fusion the period of bed rest will be longer to allow time for the vertebrae to fuse. Sutures will be removed at the end of a week if the wound is well healed. Pyrexia or any complaints of increasing pain or tenderness in and around the wound area indicate the wound should be inspected as there may be haematoma or early signs of wound infection.

Cervical disc lesion

The cervical disc lesion is rare, affecting patients of any age; it is the result of degeneration of the disc, repeated minor trauma or a sudden wrenching injury; the most commonly affected disc is between C5/6 vertebrae, but degeneration can affect other discs, sometimes several simultaneously (see Chapter 16). Central disc protrusion will compress the spinal cord (see Fig. 12.6), the onset of symptoms is often acute, occurring spontaneously or after injury. Sometimes after injury there is a delay of several weeks before the acute or gradual onset of symptoms; the latter may be falsely attributed to a spinal tumour. Frequently the patient gives a history of recurrent bouts of neck and shoulder pain. This pain, which he wakes with in the morning, is usually very severe, fixing the neck in one position; after a day or two it disappears. After several relatively short-lived episodes of neck pain the patient suddenly experiences intense persistent pain, radiating into the shoulder or arm and associated with abnormal sensations in the arms, weakness of all limbs and stiffness in the legs, signs of spinal cord compression. The patient may complain of 'giddiness' (vertigo) if the vestibulo-spinal pathways are compressed.

Examination

Neck mobility is severely limited, the head may be fixed to one side and attempts to straighten it produce intense pain. The patient has difficulty walking and his legs are spastic, tendon reflexes are usually increased and plantar responses extensor (upper motor neurone). There will be weakness, muscle wasting and diminished reflexes in the hands and arms (lower motor neurone).

Treatment

Almost all patients suffering from prolapsed cervical intervertebral disc will respond favourably to medical treatment, which involves one or more of the following:

i   A correctly fitting collar to immobilise the neck and hold it in a slight degree of extension; a rigid collar will be worn during the day and a softer one at night. It may take several weeks for symptoms to subside and the collar should be worn constantly. This treatment may be combined with traction

ii   Traction is usually given in the out-patient physiotherapy department 2–3 times weekly

iii   Manipulation – in skilled hands manipulation can be dramatically effective, but is extremely dangerous if performed incorrectly, even producing irreversible quadriplegia.

Investigations

The patient will be admitted to hospital for investigations if:

(a) he has extreme pain with severe physical disability and bladder disturbance;

(b) the symptoms are progressive, suggestive of a tumour;

(c) conservative treatment fails.

Investigations will be performed as described on p. 217. A cisternal myelogram is usually necessary as a prolapsed cervical disc may cause a complete blockage to the flow of contrast medium in the sub-arachnoid space; the nature of the lesion may be uncertain until it has been outlined by cisternal and lumbar myelography.

Cervical laminectomy and postoperative care

Laminectomy will sometimes be necessary to remove the fragmented disc and relieve spinal cord compression; some surgeons prefer to use the anterior approach (see Fig. 16.3). Postoperatively this patient will be nursed flat and turned from side to side two-hourly. One nurse should be responsible for supporting the patient's head and neck whenever he is moved. Then, after 24 hours, taking care not to allow sudden flexion movements, the patient gradually sits up in bed, wearing a soft collar to give support to the neck. The patient will get out of bed for the first time after the sutures have been removed, on the 7th postoperative day. A rigid plastic collar with a chin support is then used during the day and the soft collar reserved for night-time use.

All general nursing care and rehabilitation will be given as for a patient with paraplegia (see Chapter 10).

13

Spinal Infection

Improved sanitation, pasteurization of milk, purification of water supplies, the widespread vaccination programmes of recent years and early treatment of infection with antibiotics have all played a major part in reducing the incidence of spinal infection, but in the developing countries where there is overcrowding, little or no sanitation, malnutrition and generally poor health in the community, there is still a high incidence of such diseases as tuberculosis and poliomyelitis. In these poorer countries children who contract infection either become immune or die. In more advanced countries the population often escapes the childhood infection which gives immunity and such normally infantile diseases as poliomyelitis then occasionally affect adults. When diseases appear to have been eradicated, parents become less concerned about vaccination and innoculation and do not have their children immunised; these unprotected children then risk serious disease. Fast air travel and the ease of travel from one continent to another must inevitably increase the likelihood of contagious diseases being brought into a country during their incubation period; immigrants may bring infection into a country otherwise free of the disease. Some causes of spinal infection are now reduced; self-induced septic abortion which used to lead to septicaemia and sometimes spinal abscess has become less common since the introduction of the Abortion Act. Tabes dorsalis, the spinal form of neurosyphilis, still occurs as, although treatment of syphilis is readily available, unfortunately there is ignorance and reluctance to seek help.

Spinal infection may be acute and reach the spinal cord within a few days of the onset of an illness, as in poliomyelitis, but it may be chronic, developing during many months as in tubercular disease of the spine. Infections of the spine and spinal cord are rare; they usually affect the thoracic and thoraco-lumbar regions and remain confined within that area, but sometimes track upwards in the cord to the brain stem as in ascending myelitis. The infection may involve only the vertebrae, also include the meninges or be confined within the spinal cord or nerve roots.

The patient who develops an acute infective disorder will be admitted to hospital very seriously ill, with high pyrexia, severe pain and rapidly developing paralysis; on the contrary someone with a chronic illness may seem generally well, but has a slowly progressive paralysis.

Infective organisms

i   Bacteria including the tubercle bacillus
ii Viruses
iii Spirochaetes

Mode of entry into the body is through:
(a) The respiratory system – droplet infection
(b) The alimentary tract – ingested in contaminated food and from feeding utensils and dirty hands
(c) Direct contact with the organism, e.g. the spirochaete of syphilis during sexual intercourse

Bacterial infection

Bacterial infection of the spine and spinal cord is rare, the causative organism is usually the staphylococcus.

Viral infection

Virus infections cause inflammation without pus formation:
i   They attack both grey and white matter of the brain and spinal cord (encephalomyelitis; see

Chapter 6) or their effect is localised to a section of the spinal cord (myelitis).

ii   They select and attack certain types of nerve cells:

  (a) the poliomyelitis virus has an affinity to the anterior horn cells;

  (b) the virus of herpes zoster selects the posterior sensory nerve root ganglia.

Anti-viral chemotherapy is in the early stages of development and production and many virus infections still run their full course; good nursing care is therefore vital and can save life and prevent permanent disability.

Syphilitic infection
(See Chapter 24)

The spirochaete treponema pallidum is transmitted during sexual intercourse. The evidence of primary infection in the genital area is often so slight that it passes unnoticed; should it remain untreated the patient may develop tertiary syphilis. The spinal form, tabes dorsalis, develops 8–12 years later.

Myelitis

Myelitis is an inflammatory condition of the spinal cord; the cause is often unknown, but may be due to

i   bacterial invasion of the cord

ii   meningo-vascular syphilis

iii   a demyelinating disorder

  (a) acute disseminated encephalomyelitis

  (b) neuromyelitis optica

  (c) an acute form of multiple sclerosis

iv   a variety of viruses, for example measles or the poliomyelitis virus.

Transverse and ascending myelitis

The inflammation affects several segments of the lower thoracic spinal cord and involves all the nerve pathways in a cross section, and the surrounding meninges; the cord swells, is congested with blood, there may be thrombosis and sometimes the infection is so severe that all nerve conduction in the spinal cord is interrupted. The severity of symptoms depends on the level of the inflammation and the degree of oedema. The term ascending myelitis is used when the inflammation spreads upwards in the cord to the brain stem.

Signs and symptoms

Transverse myelitis mainly affects the young to middle-aged. The onset is of a 'flu-like illness with pyrexia and central back pain, followed a few days to a week later by rapidly increasing weakness and sensory loss in the legs and lower trunk with re-tention of urine; within a few hours the patient's legs can be completely paralysed. The patient must be examined without delay so that the level of the lesion can be determined as there is always a possibility of the ascending form of myelitis involving the muscles of swallowing and respiration. Pain in the back is at the level of the lesion, paralysis is flaccid, all reflexes are diminished or absent and all forms of sensation are affected. As both upper and lower motor neurones are involved, spacticity and extensor plantar responses develop after a while.

Investigations and treatment

Blood tests will include a full blood count, ESR, Wassermann and Kahn, blood culture and viral studies. A lumbar puncture will be performed to exclude spinal block and to obtain CSF for analysis, spinal dynamics are usually normal unless myelitis is secondary to a spinal abscess. The protein and cell counts in the CSF are increased, the cells being both polymorphonuclear granulocytes and lymphocytes.

A broad spectrum antibiotic will be prescribed as the cause of the illness may be an unknown organism; a course of anti-inflammatory corticosteroid drugs are given to reduce inflammation and oedema of the spinal cord. Complete rest appears to be beneficial during the acute phase of the illness; it has been noticed that those patients who have been too active and have become overtired have developed more severe and extensive paralysis and when there have been signs of improvement, a relapse often coincides with overactivity.

Nursing care
(Read Chapter 10)

This is a grave illness which can lead to respiratory failure and a ventilator must always be available. If the patient survives the acute infection then a considerable degree of recovery should be expected though it will take many months and there may be some residual disability.

Poliomyelitis

Poliomyelitis is a notifiable disease, a serious illness which was once feared as there was considerable publicity about the after-effects and victims who spent the rest of their lives in an 'iron lung'. Since vaccination became routine and effective the disease seldom occurs and some parents being wary of the side-effects of any vaccination no longer see the need to give their children this protection.

The poliomyelitis virus attacks cells in the anterior horns of the spinal cord (see Fig. 10.15) and the motor nuclei of the brain stem (lower motor neurones), causing muscle paralysis without sensory loss and subsequent wasting of the affected muscles about 3 weeks after the onset of the illness. The usual route for entry of infection is through the alimentary tract. Outbreaks of poliomyelitis may be sporadic or of epidemic proportions, the disease mainly affecting children of 2 to 5 years of age, though it can affect other age groups if they have escaped immunity and have not been vaccinated. The incubation period is usually 7 to 14 days, but may be as long as 5 weeks. The throat is a common haven for the virus and when poliomyelitis is prevalent in a community it may be precipitated by an operation on the nose, throat or mouth, for example tonsillectomy or tooth extraction, which provide a portal of entry. The virus is found in the faeces in the early days of the illness.

Reaction to infection
i Immunity may develop
ii There may be a mild general infection followed by immunity
iii Severe general symptoms may develop without paralysis
iv A few patients run the full course of the illness with paralysis

Stages of the disease

1 Pre-paralytic
(a) Initial symptoms are those of fever, malaise, headache, drowsiness or insomnia, sweating, flushing, faucial congestion and gastrointestinal disturbance. These symptoms last 1 to 2 days after which there may be temporary relief for 48 hours, or the period may merge into the paralytic stage.

(b) Headache increases, pain in the back and limbs develops with hyperaesthesia of the superficial and deep tissues; there may be delirium. The neck will be stiff and the patient resistant to passive flexion of the spine as this causes pain. There is no paralysis or wasting of muscle at this stage, but muscle fasciculation may be seen. Complete rest is essential and may prevent development of paralysis; even so, some patients will pass into the paralytic stage.

2 Paralytic stage
This rapidly follows the pre-paralytic stage, maximum damage occurring within 24 hours though sometimes there is a later deterioration when the virus spreads upwards in the spinal cord, paralysing the intercostal respiratory muscles and destroying the nuclei of the higher centres of swallowing and respiration in the medulla oblongata (bulbar poliomyelitis). The facial, pharyngeal and laryngeal muscles become paralysed, making even the swallowing of saliva impossible and the patient will make gurgling sounds in his throat and will be on the brink of respiratory failure; anticipating such an emergency, suction apparatus and a respirator must always be available.

The pre-paralytic stage of this illness may be missed when there is just an isolated outbreak of the disease and it is normally not until the patient shows signs of weakness or paralysis that he is admitted to hospital. The patient will be admitted to an isolation ward where all staff are protected by vaccination and full barrier nursing precautions can be taken. On examination the patient looks very ill, has severe headache, neck stiffness, pain on movement, the muscles are tender and there is hyperpyrexia. Examination of the limbs will assess the extent of weakness or paralysis, which is sometimes asymmetrical. It will be noticed that the muscles are flaccid, tendon reflexes diminished or absent and there is no sensory loss. History and examination normally reveal the diagnosis which will be confirmed by lumbar puncture; the CSF pressure and cell content are increased, both poly-morphonuclear cells and lymphocytes are present (50–250/100 ml) at first, later only lymphocytes will be found. The protein rises moderately during the second week of the illness.

Nursing care

When the patient is acutely ill complete rest is essential; the bed needs to be firm to support the patient in a comfortable, relaxed recumbent position. Weak and paralysed limbs must be handled gently holding them at the joints without over-stretching or grasping the tender muscles, the limbs positioned and supported by sandbags and splints to prevent contractures. Lightweight bedding and a bed cradle are necessary. Splints should be removed regularly to inspect the skin and give gentle passive movements. Nursing procedures, spread throughout the day, will allow periods of rest and must never be pursued to the point of exhaustion. Analgesics are necessary and a mild sedative may be prescribed to avoid restlessness and unnecessary muscular activity; these measures will help to prevent muscle spasm. Those patients who develop bulbar palsy will be nursed in the semiprone position with their head lower then their trunk to facilitate drainage of secretions; suction will be necessary and an artificial ventilator should be available. Intragastric feeds will be given 3-hourly.

Observations

Temperature, pulse and respiratory rates should be recorded according to the patient's condition, half-to- hourly; he must be constantly observed for ascending paralysis and difficulty in swallowing and breathing. Children may not complain of diffi-culty in swallowing but simply refuse to eat or drink. Whenever the respirations are recorded the patient's chest should be bared for inspection; danger signs are shallow, rapid respirations. The nurse should notice whether the respirations are purely diaphragmatic or purely intercostal. Late signs of respiratory failure are the use of accessory respiratory muscles in the neck, splaying of the nostrils with each inspiration and cyanosis. This late stage should NEVER be reached.

A mechanical ventilator must always be avail-able when poliomyelitis is suspected and at the first hint of respiratory embarrassment the patient

should be prepared for the idea of mechanical assis-tance and shown the apparatus. One of two types of respirator will be used.

1 Negative pressure ventilator (iron lung) This type of ventilator is used when respiratory failure is due to paralysis of the muscles of respiration (inter-costal muscles and diaphragm). The patient's body is enclosed within a 'tank'; a vacuum is created around the thorax which draws out the chest wall and air is automatically sucked into the lungs. The patient will be able to speak with each respiratory expiration. This type of ventilator is unsuitable for patients with bulbar poliomyelitis as salivary secretions which the patient is unable to swallow will be sucked into the lungs.

2 Positive pressure ventilator (see Chapter 3) This is used when the patient has bulbar poliomyelitis or

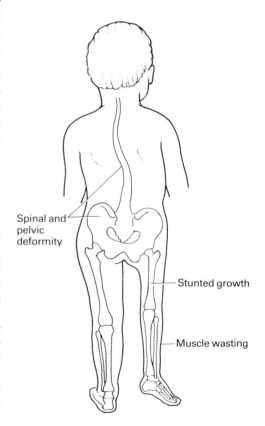

Fig. 13.1 Illustration to show wasting of muscles, stunted growth, pelvic and spinal deformity in a child following poliomyelitis.

a combination of bulbar and respiratory paralysis. The patient will need a tracheostomy and a cuffed tube will prevent inhalation of secretions.

Physiotherapy

The physiotherapist will give passive exercises extremely carefully and gently for only short periods; analgesics, necessary for the relief of pain, should be administered half an hour before the physiotherapist's visit. As soon as possible all the patient's joints should be put through a full range of movements; these exercises will be spread throughout the day and entirely adapted to the individual, depending upon how much pain the patient experiences and how tired he is. Improvement begins at the end of the first week when pain has receded and muscles show some signs of recovery. When opposing muscle groups are unequally affected, the pull of the stronger muscles leads to the development of contractures and deformities.

The patient will remain in the isolation unit until 3 consecutive stool specimens have been found to be free of the virus; sometimes the virus persists in the faeces and these patients will become carriers of the disease.

Rehabilitation is lengthy, calipers are necessary to support weak limbs and the growth of a child's affected leg is stunted leading to spinal and pelvic deformity (Fig. 13.1); these effects can be modified by the use of surgical appliances (shoes, braces and corsets) and corrective surgery at a later date. Arrangements will be made for a child to be educated while in hospital (see Chapter 11) to enable him to rejoin his peers at a normal school.

Arachnoiditis

Arachnoiditis is a chronic inflammation, the cause of which is not yet fully understood; it may develop spontaneously or follow spinal surgery. The symptoms are similar to those of prolapsed intervertebral disc.

Spinal abscess

Spinal abscess is a rare condition; the onset of infection is acute, usually arising at the thoracolumbar junction and likely to have followed a staphylococcal infection. The focus of primary infection may be a distant boil; a septic embolus, borne in the blood stream produces a small area of osteomyelitis in one of the vertebral bodies, pus gathers and an abscess forms between the vertebra and dura mater (extradural abscess). The abscess (Fig. 13.2) not only acts as a space-occupying lesion compressing the spinal cord, but it also causes tissue necrosis and thrombosis resulting in anoxia and oedema of the spinal cord; this may be the reason for sudden deterioration in the patient's condition.

The patient becomes feverish, complains of excruciating pain in the middle of his back radiating round his chest, his legs become progressively numb and weak and within a day or two will be completely paralysed; the spine is tender and the skin unusually sensitive at the level of the lesion.

Investigations, observations and treatment

i   Haemoglobin, full blood count and blood sedimentation rate – the blood sedimentation rate and white cell count are usually above normal.
ii Lumbar puncture – CSF is xanthochromic and the protein content increased; there may be a partial or complete CSF block.
iii Myelography is essential to outline the abscess.

Careful neurological assessment should be made and recorded as soon as the patient arrives in the ward and will continue half-hourly. Temperature, pulse, respiration and blood pressure recordings will be one-hourly or according to the patient's condition; hyperpyrexia will be controlled by fanning and tepid sponging. Constant observation of

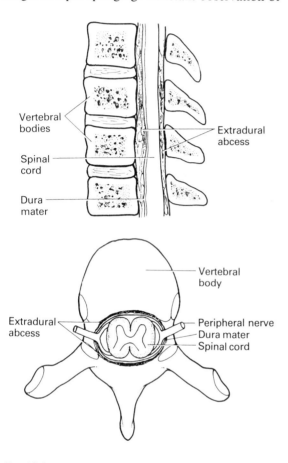

Fig. 13.2   Extradural abscess.

the patient is essential and any deterioration should be immediately reported to the doctor. A broad-spectrum systemic antibiotic will be prescribed. Lumbar puncture and myelography will be performed and when the abscess has been located the patient will undergo laminectomy for aspiration of the abscess. The success of treatment depends upon early drainage before the patient becomes completely paralysed, though tissue necrosis and thrombosis may continue to cause deterioration and will be the cause of incomplete recovery. An incision is made, usually in the thoracic region and extradural catheters will be positioned with their multi-perforated ends in the abscess cavity and open ends emerging from the upper and lower ends of the incision. These catheters are aspirated according to medical instructions (usually 6-hourly) when a dilute antibiotic is instilled into the extradural cavity. The pus taken from the abscess at operation will be cultured and this may indicate that a change of antibiotic is necessary; the catheters will be removed after 48 hours. A full course of systemic antibiotic will be given.

This is likely to be a long illness, the patient at first toxic, pyrexial, drowsy, depressed and anorexic with considerable pain. There may be delayed wound healing due to the debilitated condition of the patient and the presence of extradural catheters. A good fluid intake and a light high-protein diet should be given and the patient's general condition boosted as far as possible by pleasant surroundings, encouragement from the staff and as much help as possible in alleviating all anxiety. Expert nursing care is essential (see Chapter 10).

Spinal tuberculosis (Pott's disease)

This is a rare chronic infection of the vertebral column and is a notifiable disease; it usually starts in childhood with primary lung tuberculosis. The infection eventually reaches the spine, usually the thoracic region, and gradually spreads to involve several vertebral bodies and intervertebral discs (Fig. 13.3). The early symptoms of spinal involvement are slow and insidious with complaints of mild localised back pain and tenderness; when one or more nerve roots are irritated there may be pain and occasionally areas of increased sensitivity (hyperaesthesia) radiating round the chest. When

spinal tubercular disease is very advanced, vertebrae will be destroyed and the spinal column will collapse compressing the spinal cord and causing paralysis.

Causes of spinal cord compression:

i   an extradural tubercular abscess;
ii   vertebral collapse (hunchback) – this occurs at a late stage of the illness;
iii   infective thrombosis may damage the spinal cord and complicate *i* or *ii* above.

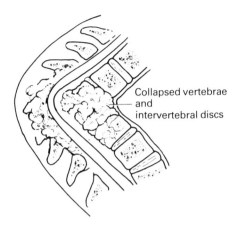

Collapsed vertebrae
and
intervertebral discs

Fig. 13.3 Spinal tuberculosis (Pott's disease).

Treatment

1 Bed rest
2 Anti-tubercular drugs
3 Surgery. Observations relating to limb movements, sensory disturbance and bladder function are very important as deterioration, however slight, indicates the need for surgical decompression of the spinal cord.

The patient will be isolated until it is certain that there is no active pulmonary tuberculosis. Chest and spinal X-rays will be performed and sputum specimens or gastric washings collected for analysis on three consecutive days. Rest is very important for the treatment of tuberculosis. The patient will be nursed in a plaster bed, with an anterior shell to allow turning and prevent pressure and plaster sores, but still maintain immobilisation of the spine. Rest combined with a long course of anti-tubercular drugs will cure some patients, but antero-lateral decompression of the spine will be necessary for any patient threatened by paraplegia; the operation removes any abscess or bony debris which is causing spinal cord compression without weakening further the supporting structure of the spine. Postoperatively the patient is nursed in his plaster bed for about three months or as determined by X-ray evidence of improvement. Physiotherapy, occupational therapy and schooling are important during this time to maintain physical fitness and keep the patient mentally stimulated. He will then gradually resume activity, but should have regular rest periods each day.

Since the introduction of anti-tubercular chemotherapy the prognosis has greatly improved, allowing surgery during the active stage of the illness and avoiding paraplegia by prompt decompression.

All contacts of the patient should be screened for tuberculosis.

Herpes zoster (shingles)

This common disease is an acute infection of sensory ganglia and sensory nerve roots caused by the virus of chicken pox. A child may contract chicken pox (varicella) from an adult with herpes zoster, whereas an adult who has had chicken pox is unlikely to contract herpes zoster from a child with chicken pox, but he will not be immune from herpes zoster as the organism is harboured in the posterior nerve root ganglia and at a time of stress or debilitation the disease will erupt. The virus attacks the sensory neurones of one or more posterior nerve root ganglia, the Gasserion ganglion of the trigeminal nerve (mainly the opthalmic branch) or the sensory geniculate ganglion of the facial nerve. The infection occasionally spreads from the ganglia to the spinal cord (myelitis), more rarely it affects the anterior motor nerve pathways to cause paralysis, or occasionally involves the brain and spinal cord (encephalomyelitis, see page 105).

The disease is common in both sexes, it never affects babies but most often affects those over the age of fifty. The incubation period is about 2 weeks. Herpes zoster usually appears without warning; the patient may have had a recent contact with chicken pox or have had a prolonged debilitating illness, or mention factors which have lead to a 'run down' state of health.

Symptoms and signs

The first complaint is often of hypersensitive skin on one side of the face or trunk, the patient can hardly bear the friction of their clothes, may loosen a belt or remove a brassière. Nothing abnormal can at first be seen, but the doctor's examination will show that the area corresponds with the distribution of one or more sensory nerves. The patient may complain of feeling generally unwell and have a mild pyrexia which is followed about four days later by a rash in the same area as pain (Fig. 13.4). The skin becomes red, groups of red papules develop, rapidly blister and the whole area is slightly oedematous and very painful. The blisters dry off, form crusty scabs and separate leaving scars; during this period there is sometimes intense skin irritation. The area is often numb for a long time after the rash has disappeared, but sometimes the skin continues to be hypersensitive to light touch. When herpes zoster affects the ophthalmic branch of the trigeminal nerve the cornea becomes insensitive; blisters which form on the cornea will cause blindness as, when they heal, they form opaque scars. When the virus affects the sensory part of the facial nerve it causes pain and rash in the ear, palate and throat, loss of taste on the anterior two-thirds of the tongue, facial weakness, giddiness and deafness; sometimes a cervical ganglion is also affected and the rash covers a more extensive area involving the lower jaw, upper part of the neck and occipital region.

Treatment

Few patients with this common disorder need to be admitted to hospital. Complete recovery is usual within 3 weeks though the pain may linger for considerably longer. The patient will be advised to keep the affected area cool and dry and to wear loose, smooth cotton clothing and warned not to apply home remedies. When the disease is mild, simple analgesics and sedatives will suffice, but if the infection is very severe or affects the face, the immediate use of oral cortisone (prednisolone) will terminate the acute stage of the disease which is a tissue reaction to the virus infection; this will also prevent the persistence of post-herpetic pain or hyperaesthesia. The use of steroids, however, may precipitate the appearance of the rash of chicken pox and slightly increase the risk of encephalo-myelitis.

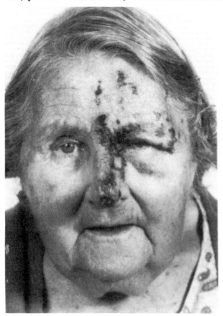

Fig. 13.4 Herpes zoster. From Coakes, R.L., and Holmes Sellers, P.J. *An Outline of Ophthalmology* (1985), John Wright & Sons, Bristol.

Nursing care

Admission to hospital may be necessary if the patient lives alone, is generally frail and ill, needs treatment for the complications which accompany herpes zoster when it affects the trigeminal or facial nerves, or in the rare instance when the virus infects the spinal cord or brain.

Initially a single room is advisable to provide quiet surroundings, to isolate the patient from others and protect him from the risk of secondary infection. Gentle sympathetic care is needed, the patient may be embarrassed by facial disfigurement caused by the rash or his inability to wash or shave; treatment must be explained clearly as this elderly patient may be deaf and so preoccupied by his pain that he lacks concentration. A patient with trigeminal herpes may be difficult to understand as he will speak quietly with as little facial movement as possible to avoid causing pain. The nurse should be attentive and try to anticipate the patient's needs to save him the necessity of speaking; he certainly should not have to repeat himself or raise his voice. Any patient who is confused, weak, has poor visual acuity, experiences giddiness or unsteadiness of gait should always be assisted when he gets up. Temperature, pulse and respirations should be recorded 4-hourly until pyrexia has settled, any signs of secondary infection must be reported. When herpes zoster affects the ophthalmic branch of the trigeminal nerve the patient should be warned not to touch or rub the insensitive eye. Four-hourly eye care should be given by an experienced nurse, the eyelids being kept clear of debris by irrigating with normal saline; antibiotic eye ointment may be prescribed to prevent secondary infection.

Mild analgesics should at first be given at regular 4-hourly intervals, a good night's rest will help the patient to bear his discomfort and night sedation may be necessary. It is not advisable to apply creams and powders to the rash unless there is secondary infection when an antibiotic cream will be prescribed.

Post-herpetic neuralgia

Post-herpetic neuralgia is an uncommon sequel to herpes zoster, especially since the use of steroids in the early stages of infection; the pain is severe, intractable and spasmodic, most often affecting the elderly and those who suffered from ophthalmic herpes. The pain which may persist for 1–2 years, sometimes indefinitely, is extremely demoralising, particularly for those who live alone and have no close relatives or friends – it may be so severe as to induce the depressed patient to think of suicide. Many forms of treatment have been tried, none completely effective; some relief has been obtained from treatment with phenytoin sodium and carbamazepine, local skin cooling, nerve stimulation, nerve destruction, radiation of the nerve root and operations on the spine and thalamus (see Chapter 17). Despite treatment there remain a few patients who continue to experience severe and persistent pain. Pain is occasionally exaggerated in an attempt to gain sympathy, but when depression is a factor the patient may benefit by psychotherapy and treatment with an antidepressant drug. Patients need encouragement to participate in activities which divert their attention from their pain and need to be put in contact with local community services. The patient must not feel he is abandoned because there is no further curative treatment; he still needs medical advice and psychological support.

14

Spinal Neoplasm

Anatomy and physiology
(See also Chapter 10)

Tumours affecting the spinal column, meninges and spinal cord are uncommon. They arise mainly in the thoracic region, least commonly in the lumbar region; they may be benign or malignant, primary or secondary and are classified according to their relationship with the spinal cord (medulla). Intramedullary tumours (Fig. 14.1a) grow within the spinal cord whereas extramedullary tumours (Fig. 14.1b), though they may compress the cord and interfere with its function, grow from the surrounding structures (meninges, blood vessels, nerve roots and bone). Benign tumours which do not infiltrate the spinal cord are fortunately the most common; the patient is likely to make a complete and lasting recovery if the tumour is diagnosed and removed before compression of the spinal cord has caused permanent damage.

The spinal cord is approximately 15 mm in diameter and fits snugly inside the spinal canal; it is anchored by the filum terminale and along its length by the meninges, the dentate ligaments and the emerging nerve roots as they pass through the foramina. Any neoplasm within the spinal canal, however small, must give rise to spinal cord compression and displacement; it interferes with the function of the nerve roots, reduces the circulation of blood to the cord by compressing and distorting blood vessels which may haemorrhage and thrombose, and the cord swells due to venous congestion. A slow growing tumour causes such gradual displacement that signs of cord compression are not evident for a considerable time.

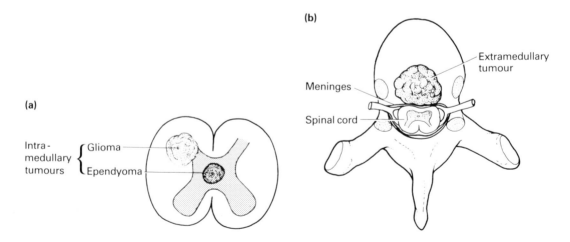

Fig. 14.1 (a) Intramedullary tumour compressing spinal cord from within. (b) Extramedullary tumour compressing spinal cord from without.

Tumours of the vertebral bones

Secondary carcinomatous metastases from the breast, bronchus, prostate gland, gastrointestinal tract, thyroid gland or kidney may spread to the vertebral column through the bloodstream or lymphatic system; there may be similar spread from myeloma, melanoma, lipoma, lymphosarcoma and Hodgkin's disease. The lesions are multiple (Fig. 14.2) causing direct pressure on nerve roots, and cord compression through pathological fractures or collapse of vertebral bodies. The onset of symptoms is usually acute with severe nerve root pain and rapid paralysis, sensory loss and sphincter disturbance. Decompressive surgical treatment and radiotherapy is palliative; it may prolong active life or only serve to relieve the patient of excruciating nerve root pain. Vertebral osteosarcoma is a rare tumour treated in a similar way.

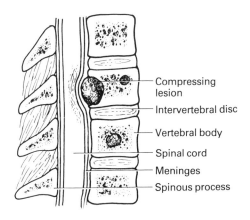

Fig. 14.2 Multiple spinal metastases (extramedullary).

Tumour of the meninges (meningioma)

This primary benign tumour arising from the dura mater (Fig. 14.3) usually occurs in the thoracic region; it grows slowly over a period of several years and mainly affects middle-aged women. The onset of symptoms is very gradual; there may be localised back pain, nerve root pain or slowly progressive weakness of the legs with sensory disturbance as the tumour presses into the spinal cord;

sphincter disturbance occurs when there is almost complete paraplegia. Treatment is by early surgical removal. Given time, though there has been severe paraparesis, complete recovery is possible.

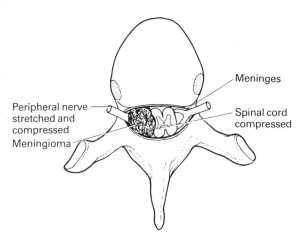

Fig. 14.3 Spinal meningioma (extramedullary).

Blood vessel tumours

Haemangioma

This is an uncommon tumour of blood vessels lying between the dura mater and the vertebrae (Fig. 14.4a). A 'port wine' naevus (Fig. 14.4b) is sometimes present on the back at the level of the haemangioma and may be connected to it. The spinal haemangioma will be surgically removed and the naevus treated with radiotherapy.

Angioma
See Chapter 11.

Tumour of the nerve root sheath

A neurofibroma develops from the neurilemmal cells surrounding the nerve fibres. It is usually a single tumour, but there may be multiple tumours in the spinal canal associated with other neurofibromata in the brain and subcutaneous tissues (neurofibromatosis; see Chapter 7). The spinal tumour often encircles a nerve root, may spread

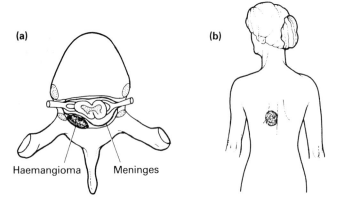

Fig. 14.4 **(a)** Spinal haemangioma (extramedullary); **(b)** 'port wine' naevus.

into the intervertebral foramen along the nerve root and even appear outside the spinal column (dumb-bell tumour; Fig. 14.5). Neurofibromata are the commonest of spinal tumours; they are slow growing, benign and produce symptoms of nerve root involvement; as the tumour enlarges it encroaches upon and compresses the spinal cord. The first symptom may be pain radiating into the chest or abdomen, caused by the part of the tumour lying outside the spinal column and it is not uncommon for patients with nerve root pain caused by neurofibroma, to be investigated for abdominal and thoracic conditions.

Laminectomy and surgical excision of the tumour is usually very successful, the weak insensitive limbs recovering completely, sometimes very dramatically; a thoracotomy or laparotomy may be necessary to remove the extraspinal extension of the tumour.

Tumours of the spinal cord

Glioma (Fig. 14.1a)

This is a malignant, rapidly growing, infiltrating tumour of connective tissue. The tumour first spreads through the substance of the spinal cord only causing symptoms when it becomes large enough to cause compression; the tumour may suddenly increase in size, due to internal haemorrhage, with dramatic onset of paraplegia. Treatment is palliative, a decompressive laminectomy and radiotherapy may give temporary relief.

Ependymoma (Fig. 14.1a)

This tumour arises from the ependymal cells which line the neural canal in the centre of the spinal cord; the neural canal is continuous with the filum terminale. An ependymoma is a benign, slow growing elongated tumour which presses upon the pain and temperature pathways as they cross the centre of the spinal cord producing symptoms similar to those of syringomyelia; a slowly progressive spastic paraparesis also develops. An ependymoma of the filum terminale presses upon the central nerve roots of the cauda equina; symptoms are similar to central disc protrusion, root pain and backache which may be present for some time before leg weakness and bladder disturbance develops.

Access to ependymomas within the cord is diffi-

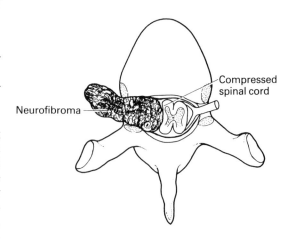

Fig. 14.5 Dumb-bell neurofibroma (extramedullary).

cult but they can be successfully removed using an ultrasonic aspirator; tumours of the filum terminale can be totally removed.

Other tumours

Epidermoid tumour, dermoid cyst, chordoma and cholesteatomas are congenital tumours (see Chapter 4) which may, very rarely, develop in the spinal region.

History and examination

A detailed medical history will be taken and particular enquiry made about any previous illness treated by surgery or radiotherapy. Examination will help to localise the lesion to a particular level in the spinal cord, differentiate between an extra-medullary and intramedullary tumour, help to determine the nature of the lesion (the patient's skin will be inspected for café au lait patches, neurofibromata or naevi) and assess the extent of neurological disturbance; further investigations are always necessary to confirm the diagnosis.

Investigations

When there are signs of rapidly increasing spinal cord compression, investigations and treatment must proceed urgently.

Routine blood tests include haemoglobin estimation, full blood count, blood sedimentation rate, blood urea and Wassermann and Kahn. Chest X-rays are helpful in revealing carcinoma of the lung, evidence of myelomatosis, and occasionally the shadow of a neurofibroma. Straight X-rays of the spine will be taken from several angles. Spinal tumours cause demonstrable bony changes:

i pathological fracture and collapse of one or more vertebral bodies;
ii erosion of a pedicle, widening of the space between two adjacent pedicles or of the intervertebral foramina;
iii calcification;
iv expansion of the bony spinal canal with narrowing of several pedicles;
v scalloping of the posterior surface of the vertebral bodies.

Lumbar puncture

When there is a tumour, manometry usually shows partial or complete obstruction to the flow of CSF in the subarachnoid space. The CSF is often xanthochromic, the protein content increased; it is particularly high (300 mg per cent or more) when a neurofibroma is present, the cell count is raised and the CSF coagulates on standing. Changes of pressure following withdrawal of CSF increase the patient's symptoms.

Myelography
(See p. 34)

This procedure, lumbar or cisternal or both, gives more detailed information about the position, size and nature of the tumour.

Treatment

Treatment depends on the situation of the tumour and whether it is benign or malignant. Laminectomy and surgical excision is often highly successful when the tumour is benign and accessible; when tumours are extensive it may be necessary to remove several laminae. Malignant tumours, some of which are cystics will be treated by radiotherapy, sometimes preceded by palliative surgical measures (laminectomy and cystic aspiration); radiotherapy is also given when excision of a tumour is incomplete.

Postoperative care
(See Chapter 12)

Mobilisation usually begins on the 7th post-operative day when the sutures have been removed and the wound has healed; bed rest may be prolonged for those patients who have vertebral collapse associated with secondary carcinoma. Following cervical laminectomy a collar is necessary and is fitted when the patient is to start sitting up in bed. Standing and attempts to walk will be for very short periods at first, help will be needed and suitable walking aids used. As exercise tolerance increases, a full programme of rehabilitation will be introduced (see p. 181). Patience and perseverance are necessary as, though progress may be very slow, it may continue for up to 2 years to full recovery.

15

Spinal Vascular Disorders

The spinal cord and nerve roots receive a good blood supply (see Chapter 10). Vascular disorder of the spinal cord is a rare condition.

1 Haemorrhage Haemorrhage in and around the spinal cord is either the result of injury or less commonly of spontaneous haemorrhage. The causes of spontaneous haemorrhage are:

i rupture of congenital vascular anomalies (angioma) and the pathological blood vessels of malignant tumours;

ii syringomyelia;

iii blood dyscrasia, e.g. haemophilia; the haemorrhage may also be the result of minor injury;

iv treatment with anti-coagulant drugs.

Haemorrhage may be extradural, subdural, subarachnoid or intramedullary.

2 Thrombosis of the anterior spinal artery.

History

The onset of symptoms of haemorrhage and thrombosis of the blood vessels supplying the spinal cord are sudden, destructive and compressing; it is often difficult for the doctor to be sure of the cause of spinal disorder though the level is obvious. A detailed medical history may suggest the likelihood of vascular disturbance; there may be a family history of blood dyscrasia, the patient may be known to have haemophilia or have had episodes of haemorrhage or thrombosis. There may be a history of minor injury or a fall or it may be known that the patient is taking anti-coagulant drugs.

Examination

Subarachnoid haemorrhage

When there is blood in the CSF the patient will be generally ill and pyrexial; blood irritates the meninges and nerve roots which causes severe backache and pain radiating into the arms, round the chest or into the legs; headache developing after backpain suggests that the haemorrhage has originated in the spinal theca. There will be neck stiffness and a positive Kernig's sign.

Intramedullary haemorrhage

Scattered petechial haemorrhages cause minimal symptoms which usually clear up completely. Massive haemorrhage into the spinal cord causes cord compression from within and is totally destructive, it extends longitudinally within the grey matter of several segments and causes complete paraplegia or quadriplegia with loss of sphincter control. Paralysis will at first be flaccid and later when the period of spinal shock has passed, spasticity develops. The blood will be reabsorbed, but it is replaced by serous fluid (hydromyelia). A haematoma confined to one side of the cord produces a Brown Séquard syndrome characterised by weakness or paralysis, loss of touch, vibration and joint position sense on one side of the body, and loss of pain and temperature sensation on the other (see Fig. 10.20).

Thrombosis

When the patient has sustained thrombosis of the anterior spinal artery there will be paralysis and loss of sensation, except for those sensations transmitted in the posterior columns, joint position and vibration sense. The symptoms depend on the level and extent of the thrombosis.

Investigations

1 Blood tests – full blood count, estimation of haemoglobin, blood sedimentation rate, blood urea, Wassermann and Kahn, prothrombin and blood clotting times.
2 Chest X-rays.
3 Spinal X-rays will reveal fractures, or abnormal channels in the bone caused by the dilated blood vessels of an angioma (see p. 205).
4 Lumbar puncture may show increased pressure and partial or complete block in the flow of CSF. The fluid may be heavily bloodstained or xanthochromic and the protein content raised. Following anterior spinal thrombosis, spinal dynamics and CSF analysis are normal.

5 Myelography is necessary when the cause of spinal cord compression is uncertain.
6 Spinal angiography will demonstrate the circulation of the spinal cord.

Nursing care

(See Chapter 10)

Bed rest is necessary until the diagnosis has been made, the patient's condition has stabilised or there are signs of improvement. The patient will be attended by the physiotherapist and occupational therapist during his period of rest and both will assist in his full mobilisation and rehabilitation programme; the chances of recovering full power are greater if some slight movement has always been retained, but is unlikely if dense paralysis persists for more than a week. When quadriplegia from a spinal vascular cause affects an elderly person, the prognosis is poor as the individual is likely to rapidly succumb to any of the complications which can occur.

16

Spinal Degenerative Disorders

Degenerative disorders of the spine are common, affecting, to some degree, almost everyone over the age of fifty, though most remain free of serious symptoms. It is a gradual process probably aggravated throughout life by repeated minor strains and injuries often related to occupational factors. The joints and discs of the cervical and lumbar vertebrae are most likely to sustain damage as they are more mobile than the thoracic vertebrae.

Cervical spondylosis

The joints and ligaments of the cervical spine are damaged by injury and arthritic inflammation over a period of many years, and the damage is repaired by osteophyte formation which results in the gradual development of bony protrusions at the margins of each vertebra and enlargement of the articular facets. The nerve roots sustain repeated injury and become adherent to their meningeal sheaths which tether the cord and restrict its mobility during normal movements of the head and neck; the intervertebral discs collapse and protrude, stripping the ligaments from the margins of the vertebral bodies (Fig. 16.1). When these degenerative changes are mainly lateral, pressure is upon the nerve roots and radicular arteries, where-as central degenerative protrusions compress the spinal cord and anterior spinal artery. The spinal canal is narrowed by these ridges and protrusions at each disc space affecting the function of the spinal cord which is further threatened by an inadequate blood supply; widespread ischaemia causes softening of the cord and impairment of function. Despite this gloomy picture the symptoms are not always as bad as might be expected.

Cervical spondylosis may:

i give rise to no symptoms or only slight discomfort attributed to 'old age' or 'rheumatism';

ii produce signs which only the doctor detects

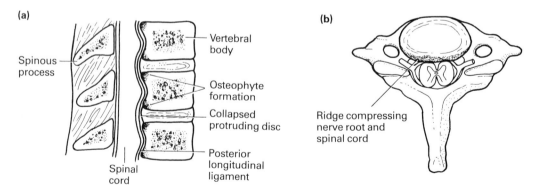

Fig. 16.1 Degenerative spinal changes. **(a)** Section through vertebral column showing osteophytes and collasped disc. **(b)** Cervical vertebral illustrating areas of compression.

(spasticity, increased reflexes and very mild sensory changes);

iii cause symptoms related to nerve root (brachial neuropathy) or spinal cord (cervical myelopathy) disturbance; these structures are often affected simultaneously.

Brachial neuropathy

Brachial neuropathy is a common acute disorder often caused by irritation of nerve roots by long standing cervical spondylosis. The symptoms of aching neck and shoulder and severe arm pain develop over a period of hours or days, gradually increasing in intensity; sudden severe pain shooting down the arm with paraesthesiae extending into one or more fingers or the thumb, is related to movement and posture. Episodes of acute pain persist for several weeks and there may be long periods (a year or more) before another similar episode is experienced, although the sufferer may describe burning and tingling sensations which are troublesome at night and due to the adoption of an awkward position in bed. The patient can sometimes attribute the onset of symptoms to a particular sustained activity.

On examination there may be restriction of active and passive neck movements, crepitus, and local tenderness over the spine and in the affected muscles. The doctor may find no abnormal neurological signs or only very slight lower motor neurone signs in the affected arm. Though the patient describes episodes of sensory loss, they may only be related to movement and not demonstrated on examination.

Investigations include blood sedimentation rate to exclude active arthritis, and spinal X-rays to demonstrate osteophyte formation and narrowing of the disc spaces. Oblique views are necessary to show narrowing of the intervertebral foramina; these changes may be apparent in the cervical and lumbar regions though the latter is usually asymptomatic.

Cervical myelopathy

The onset is usually insidious, the patient in the 60–70 age group complains of increasing difficulty in walking with a tendency to trip, and of painful neck stiffness and clumsiness of his hands for fine movements such as fastening buttons. Though myelopathy develops over a period of time, the symptoms sometimes suddenly appear or increase markedly when the patient's neck has been suddenly jerked or hyperextended, the result of a fall, minor car incident or induction of anaesthesia, which cause acute disc protrusion or sudden occlusion of a spinal artery.

On examination the patient's spastic gait may be obvious and his shoes excessively worn at the toes. Neck movements will be restricted and painful, with crepitus. There may be mixed upper and lower motor neurone signs in the arms because the lesions are compressing the nerve roots (lower motor neurones to the arms) and the spinal cord, but only upper motor neurone signs in the legs (see p. 24). Slight sensory loss affects the arms more than the legs.

Investigations include routine blood tests, serum B_{12} estimation to exclude subacute combined degeneration of the cord, and spinal X-rays. Lumbar puncture and myelography (Fig. 16.2) are sometimes necessary to exclude an operable disc lesion or spinal tumour.

Treatment of cervical spondylosis

Most patients suffering from cervical spondylosis are elderly and have widespread spinal degeneration, they may be hypertensive, their general circulation affected by arteriosclerosis, and cerebral circulation impaired by vertebral insufficiency (see p. 137); treatment can only be symptomatic. These patients suffer much discomfort and inconvenience, but will be reassured if their general practitioner gives them a thorough general and neurological examination, confirms the diagnosis with blood tests and X-rays, and discusses in simple terms the disorder, recommended form of treatment and its expected duration. The patient will be less aggrieved by his chronic condition, with its distressing persistence or recurrence of pain and weakness, if he is satisfied that he is not missing curative treatment. The patient should be advised to remain active, but avoid movement or postures which aggravate pain and paraethesiae. A regular non-addictive analgesic is necessary to control pain, help the patient to relax and so relieve muscle

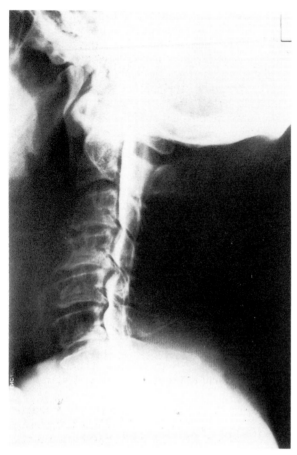

Fig. 16.2 Myelography showing osteophytic ridges in cervical spondylosis.

spasm; a muscle-relaxant tranquillising drug may be beneficial. The patient should be advised to sleep on a firm mattress in a posture which prevents kinking of his neck or cramping his shoulder and arm, and if necessary night sedation will be given to ensure a good night's rest. A collar must be worn day and night for 2–3 months to keep the head and neck in the correct position and prevent excessive movement. Most patients require physiotherapy twice or three times a week as an out-patient; radiant heat, shortwave diathermy and gentle massage aim to relieve pain and spasm by relaxing tense muscles and freeing 'seized up' neck joints. When a nerve root is being nipped or cervical disc lesions are causing severe pain, intermittent traction is sometimes recommended and some patients find dramatic relief from pain. Exercises are

necessary to maintain or regain neck mobility, prevent painful 'frozen shoulder', keep the patient mobile and strengthen weak limbs; the patient is asked to continue these exercises daily at home. Though the patient should be encouraged to give each form of treatment a fair trial, he will be referred back to his doctor if his symptoms get worse or he develops new ones. Most patients respond favourably to conservative treatment though recovery is slow, may be incomplete and symptoms sometimes recur necessitating further treatment. When the patient has made no progress in spite of treatment he will be referred to a specialist for a complete review of his condition.

Reasons for admission to hospital

1 Severe intractable pain.
2 Signs of acute or increasing cord compression.
3 An intensive course of rehabilitation; these elderly patients may be living alone or have an equally elderly spouse and it is essential that they retain their independence for as long as possible.
4 Surgery.

In hospital the patient will be thoroughly examined, blood tests and spinal X-rays will be repeated, changes compared and a myelogram may be recommended. Analgesic medication may be changed and the patient will be observed day and night to assess his disability, discomfort and reaction to his symptoms. A period of continuous traction may be given to a patient with severe pain, especially if he has shown some response to intermittent traction as an out-patient. When conservative measures fail or the patient is admitted with an acute exacerbation of symptoms, possibly due to the prolapse of an intervertebral disc, surgery will be considered.

Operations to relieve nerve root compression are not necessarily effective as much of the trouble is the result of long standing trauma and lies within the nerve itself; similarly various surgical measures that have been tried to decompress the spinal cord have met with disappointing and sometimes short-lasting results. These operations involve several vertebrae and include laminectomy to free the cord by cutting the dentate ligaments on one side, laminectomy for removal of bony ridges and degenerate discs, and an anterior spinal operation to fuse two or three vertebral bodies and remove bony

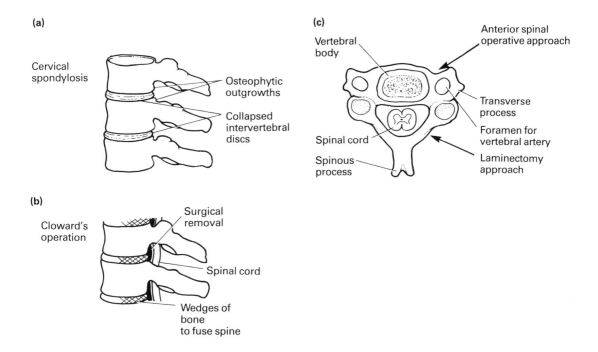

(a)

Cervical spondylosis

Osteophytic outgrowths

Collapsed intervertebral discs

(b)

Cloward's operation

Surgical removal

Spinal cord

Wedges of bone to fuse spine

(c)

Vertebral body

Anterior spinal operative approach

Transverse process

Foramen for vertebral artery

Laminectomy approach

Spinal cord

Spinous process

Fig. 16.3 Operative measures for cervical spondylosis. **(a)** Cervical spondylosis. **(b)** Cloward's operation. **(c)** Laminectomy approach.

protrusions and prolapsed discs (Cloward's operation; Fig. 16.3). The latter is preferred as it makes for easier access to the operative site and does not weaken the vertebral column. On the whole the results of the lengthy and difficult pro-cedures are no better than conservative medical treatments, except in specially selected instances, and it is considered undesirable to subject most of these elderly patients to major surgery with such uncertain results.

Ankylosing spondylitis

Ankylosing spondylitis is a generalised disorder which may result in severe spinal deformity. It tends to be familial and affects men more often than women, starting in early adult life, sometimes following a back injury. There are a variety of apparently unconnected early symptoms (iritis, urethritis or pain and tenderness of the joints) accompanied by mild fever, fatigue, lack of energy and loss of weight; low lumbar backache develops often waking the patient from sleep. The sacroiliac joints are affected in the early stages and they and the vertebral bones become fused and inflexible; these changes can be seen on X-ray. When the disease is severe there is marked kyphosis of the cervical, thoracic and lumbar vertebrae and chest expansion becomes limited due to fusion of the costovertebral joints.

Treatment

1 Analgesics to relieve pain.
2 Anti-inflammatory drugs, e.g. phenyl-butazone and steroids.
3 Physiotherapy, paying particular attention to posture; swimming is a useful exercise.
4 Radiation to halt the disease process.
5 Surgery to correct major bony deformity and help the patient to lead a more useful life.

Spondylolisthesis

In this condition the 5th lumbar vertebra is partially displaced forwards on the sacrum which kinks the cauda equina.

Paget's disease

Paget's disease is a common condition, whose cause is unknown, occurring equally in men and women over the age of fifty. The skull, vertebrae, long bones and pelvis may be affected; there are areas of increased thickness and density in the bones with adjacent thinned patches and increased vascularity where the bones are thick, and here the covering tissues feel exceptionally warm.

The patient usually has no symptoms, but headache may accompany skull deformity and there may be pain in other bones; the disease is often discovered accidentally when X-rays are taken for some other condition. Fractures may occur spontaneously or following only minor injury; they usually heal quite well. The vertebrae may collapse causing spinal cord compression.

There is no specific treatment for Paget's disease, but analgesics may be necessary. Steroids or radiotherapy may relieve severe or intractable pain.

Part III

Other Disorders of the Nervous System

17

Pain

Pain is a conscious experience which we have from birth, a protective mechanism without which survival would be improbable.

The problem of pain has been acknowledged since early days, much has been written on the subject of its relief and all manner of remedies tried from herbal cures and drugs to complicated surgical procedures; both have held their risks, addiction on the one hand and permanent damage to personality or nerve supply on the other. Witchcraft and hypnosis have played a part and suicide or euthanasia have in some cases been a last resort. Even in this century when such great advances have been made in medicine and surgery, other ancient forms of treatment, for example acupuncture, still have a place and the only relief from intractable and insufferable pain may be death. Many a discussion centres on whether it is right to allow a person continued suffering, excruciating persistent pain which they feel unable to bear, when animals are relieved of their misery by being 'put to sleep'.

In all walks of life, especially after middle age, pain is a common, almost daily experience and topic of conversation, when all the body's systems begin to show signs of wear and tear, joints and muscles creak and groan, spinal nerves are nipped and such conditions as haemorrhoids, bunions and gout are more likely to occur. Even the younger age group experience pain, headache, dysmenorrhoea, cramp, stiffness and pain following unaccustomed sporting activities or athletics and the pain of childbirth.

Some cultures and societies encourage a stoical attitude to pain and discourage any mention of ill-health, for others it becomes a preoccupation, particularly for those who are bored, lonely or find it difficult to capture the attention of their family, friends or acquaintances in any other way; then the question, 'How are you?' leads to a long rigmarole associated with pain, ill-health and medical or surgical treatment.

Pain is a symptom and only the patient can feel its intensity. Each person's reaction to their own pain is unique and many factors influence how keenly they feel it and how well they bear it (pain threshold), factors which every nurse should bear in mind whatever type of pain is described and whatever its cause. Judgements must never be made; one patient may appear to be complaining excessively about the slight discomfort caused by a curable illness, while the patient in the next bed makes little complaint in the face of severe pain from an incurable disease. The one may be experiencing pain for the first time, have been cosseted in childhood, may be a naturally timid person, have a low pain threshold, be frightened in the hospital environment where he may previously have had his complaints of pain ignored, have no close family or friends, lack the support of religious belief and live alone in poverty; the other with all the support he needs may uncomplainingly suffer and accept his lot.

The factors influencing reaction to pain are too many to enumerate, they vary according to race and creed, availability of medical treatment, sex, occupation and financial status, marital happiness, outlook and general contentment with life. Fatigue and depression are well known to lower an individual's tolerance of pain.

There is almost always anxiety and fear associated with pain; imaginative man suffers in advance and when he feels pain, begins at once to question its cause, wonders if he will die as the result, whether an operation will be necessary, and with those thoughts come all the others relating to care of the family, earning ability and fear of disablement. Anyone whose occupation holds an element of danger and risk is prepared for injury and usually better able to withstand pain. A soldier prepared physically and psychologically for battle may continue to fight heedless of severe wounds and often recovers more rapidly than the civilian, because his bravery will receive recognition and his future is secure; the civilian will receive no medal and is more anxious about his livelihood.

A child's parents, particularly his mother, play an important part in his reaction to pain. The toddler falls, how does his mother react? Does she give him a cuddle, rub and kiss the hurt, matter of factly clean the wound and apply a dressing, all the while encouraging the child and telling him that it is not serious, will soon be better and complimenting him on his bravery; or does she show acute anxiety, becoming obviously flustered and shocked; a child can hardly understand this unspoken fear, but the mother's anxiety may be reflected in his adverse reaction to pain or to admission to hospital. Another child may discover that his mother in her

efforts to pacify him, gives special treats or he becomes the centre of attention and this may set the pattern for every trivial incident. Pain may also be felt, elaborated and exaggerated as an escape from school or any unwanted activity; in later life this response persists as an automatic, unconscious escape from unpleasant or difficult situations or as a plea for attention. The underlying cause for repeated visits to a general practitioner may be a cry for help, though the patient complains of pain the real nature of the problem may be obscure, marital or other difficulties; the patient must not be labelled hysterical for there may be a serious underlying organic cause; even if this is not so, without treatment the patient will get worse.

Anatomy and physiology

Pain is a symptom of disease or injury, 'felt' by the thalamus, interpreted by the cerebral cortex and localised to a particular part of the body. The pain from some diseased internal organs may be experienced elsewhere (referred pain), for example from appendicitis it is felt in the epigastric region and from the heart it radiates down the left arm.

The sensory nerve fibres in the peripheral nerve roots transmit impulses from the sensory receptors to the posterior horns of grey matter in the spinal cord. The pathways of pain ascend a few segments in the cord and then cross through the centre of the grey matter to the opposite side to continue their

ascent to the brain. In the thalamus they synapse with other sensory neurones which carry the impulses to the sensory cortex of the cerebrum (Fig. 17.1) where they are interpreted on the basis of past experience learned since infancy. Pain is an unpleasant experience appreciated in a number of ways; from childhood we learn to differentiate between the discomforts of bruises, cuts and grazes and later the more painful experiences of toothache, colic, strained joints, wrenched muscles and cramp; upon these past experiences we judge the degree of pain.

Headache

Headache is a common painful symptom suffered by the entire population to a greater or lesser extent at some time during their lives. The brain itself is totally insensitive to pain, but there are certain structures in the central nervous system which are extremely sensitive.

i   Large intracranial blood vessels and venous sinuses
ii   Large extracranial arteries
iii   The meninges
iv   The cranial sensory nerves

Causes of headache

1 Psychological factors
There are a large number of patients who complain of headache for which no organic cause can be found; these patients may be unable to cope with life's stresses and strains and there may be obvious or unrevealed problems at work or in the home causing anxiety. The patient may not acknowledge that he has any problems or anxiety nor relate them

to his headache; it is likely that this type of head-ache is produced by physical tension centred in the scalp and neck muscles. Others who complain of various unpleasant sensations in the head, parti-cularly 'pressure on top of the head', 'tight bands' or 'nails being driven in' become preoccupied with their pain, allow it to dominate their lives and cons-tantly seek a cure going from one doctor to another. The patient may respond to the assurance that there is nothing organically wrong, and treat-ment with tranquillisers or anti-depressant drugs,

but in some instances the pain is intractable and the individual may be attention-seeking or have another motive for persistent headache. Headache may persist following head injury when the patient is expected to return to work before he has fully recovered or is seeking compensation for his injury (see Chapter 5).

2   Dental decay and diseases of the eye and nasal sinuses

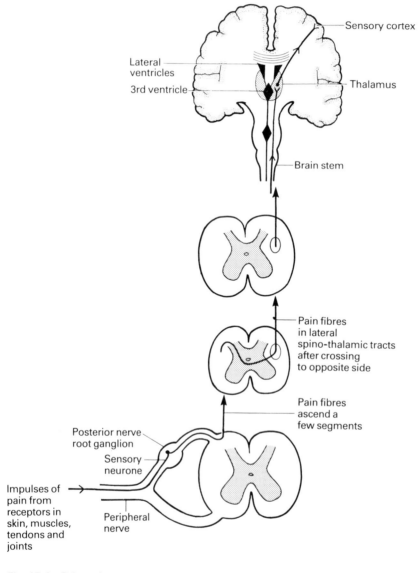

Fig. 17.1 Pain pathways.

Pain and tenderness are usually localised, but there may also be headache.

3 Disturbance in the sensory nerves

This causes neuralgia; the pain is usually paroxysmal, short and sharp, along the distribution of a nerve root. Particularly notable is trigeminal (Vth cranial nerve) neuralgia; occipital neuralgia may occur when the greater occipital nerve is nipped by outgrowths of bone in cervical spondylosis.

4 Changes in the tension within large intracranial blood vessels

It is well known that migraine, malignant hypertension, toxaemia and displacement of blood vessels by intracranial tumours cause headache as a result of changes in the intra-arterial pressure.

5 Inflammation of extracranial arteries – temporal arteritis (see p. 252)

6 Changes in tension upon the meninges

This may be the result of low or high intracranial pressure caused by:

    (a) dehydration
    (b) fluid retention
    (c) intracranial space-occupying lesions (see Chapter 7)
    (d) intracranial haemorrhage (see Chapter 8)
    (e) following lumbar puncture (see Chapter 2)

7 Inflammation of the meninges

Headache is very severe in meningitis and subarachnoid haemorrhage (see Chapters 6 and 8).

Migraine

Migraine is one of the most common neurological disorders suffered by approximately 5% of the population; it is more common in women than men. The first episode usually occurs soon after puberty but a child may have had cyclical vomiting; episodes become less frequent and less severe as age advances and disappear in middle life though there may be an exacerbation at the menopause and occasionally the disorder continues into old age. It is hereditary, affecting those with a fairly high level of intelligence who also have an intense, perfectionist, conscientious disposition. If these susceptible individuals eat certain foods, for example chocolate, citrus fruit, cheese or wines (food containing amines which cause dilatation of blood vessels), or if they go without food for long periods, migraine may develop. Some individuals have a pattern, attacks occurring rhythmically once a week, once a fortnight or once a month; others have no particular cycle.

The headache of migraine is often severe; it is caused by dilatation of the branches of the external carotid artery which supply blood to the meninges (see Figs 5.3 and 8.2). Preceding the headache many patients experience an aura due to a period of arterial constriction causing temporary ischaemia of parts of the brain. The aura lasts about half an hour and is usually visual as the occipital cortex is most often affected. The disturbance involves the homonymous fields of vision, partially or completely (see Fig. 2.11); in these areas vision becomes misty and there may be shimmering lights (teichopsia) and jagged lines (fortification spectra). Ischaemia due to constriction of the middle cerebral artery produces an aura of abnormal sensation and weakness of one arm and dysphasia; the third cranial nerve may be affected by ischaemia causing ptosis and a fixed dilated pupil. When the basilar artery is affected, brain stem and cerebellar ischaemia will produce symptoms of giddiness, dysarthria, ataxia and possibly loss of consciousness. These less common forms of aura may persist from several hours to a day or two. Ophthalmoplegic migraine, a rare condition, is characterised by repeated attacks of headache accompanied by transient paralysis of the oculomotor muscles; this may lead to irreversible paralysis.

There are many variations and combinations of aura and symptoms; some patients experience headache without aura, others aura without headache. Each individual experiences his own particular aura, which is usually the same in each attack, but may affect either side of the head depending upon the area of the brain which is ischaemic. As the aura subsides the headache begins, increasing in severity until it is so severe that the sufferer is compelled to lie down in a quiet darkened room; there is often accompanying nausea and sometimes vomiting. Headache is usually unilateral, but may spread to involve the whole head in a throbbing pulsating manner; anything which increases intracranial pressure (stooping, sneezing, coughing, vomiting) intensifies the headache.

There are many sufferers of migraine who 'ride out' their attack and receive no medical treatment. The headache may last for a day or two, and may be relieved by vomiting or sleep; analgesics such as paracetamol and aspirin if taken during the period of the aura may avert headache, but they are ineffective once the headache has begun.

Investigations

Investigations are usually unnecessary as the history and familial tendency are in most instances conclusive. When the diagnosis is in doubt further investigations will be necessary to exclude the following organic lesions:

i   Angiomatous malformation (see Chapter 8); the symptoms of migraine are then consistently on one side.
ii Intracranial neoplasm; the headache may have some of the characteristics of migraine, but episodes of monoparesis and sensory disturbance persist for longer periods.
iii Vascular disease causing temporary ischaemia (see Chapter 8).

Treatment

When a general practitioner first sees the patient during an attack of migraine, he may know little of the patient's background and simply prescribe suitable analgesic medication, but should the child or adult suffer from repeated attacks, the doctor will consider the patient's life situation in more detail; he will arrange a further appointment to see the patient and, in the case of a child, a separate interview with the parents.

A careful history will be taken including a detailed account of the first attack of migraine and any variation in subsequent attacks, their frequency and any common factors which precede them. The doctor will discuss and try to reveal possible causes of stress, migraine being only one of several disorders known to be stress-related and particularly brought about by seemingly insoluble situations in which the patient feels trapped; he will be encouraged to talk about himself, his family, work, leisure pursuits and his hopes and fears. Considerable time, persistence and a certain amount of probing may be necessary to reveal the one situation which is the crux of the matter. Patients are reluctant to admit that they cannot cope, are meticulous to a fault, and are creating

some of their own problems through setting excessively high standards; a child's migraine may be caused by her parents' unreasonable expectations of career success. Possible causes of anxiety include:

i   School studies, homework and examinations combined with parental pressure to 'do well' or 'get on'.
ii   Employment – unsuitable work, lack of job satisfaction or fear of redundancy.
iii Adverse relationships at school or work.
iv   Marital problems.
v   Fear of unwanted pregnancy.
vi   Financial matters.
vii Problems concerning teenage children.
viii Poor relationships with 'in-laws' and problems created when aged parents live in the same household.

The doctor will need to show great understanding and considerable tact if he is not to upset the patient; he may for example begin by emphasising the patient's capability, pointing out the characteristics which he knows him to possess – exactitude, conscientiousness and boundless energy, how admirably he has managed in a situation which would have caused many an individual to crack up and the doctor will go on to explain the effect the patient's stressful life is having on his physical system.

The migraine subject is often an obsessional personality who is immaculately groomed, whose employment demands accuracy and perfection (an accountant, personal secretary or executive), who carries similar standards of perfection into his personal life, home, garden and leisure time; he often tries to fit too much into one day, rushing frantically from one engagement to another, with hasty meal times or long periods without refreshment, and little or no relaxation until forced to rest by a severe attack of migraine. 'Saturday morning migraine' is a familiar sequel to a trying week possibly following drinks on a Friday evening and foods to which the individual is susceptible, a bar of chocolate on the way home or fruit, cheese and wine with the evening meal.

Recommendations and medication

1   Diet – care should be taken to avoid long periods of fasting and foods known to bring on an attack. Heavy wines, e.g. sherry and port, should be avoided. Some sufferers find benefit

from eating a few leaves of the feverfew plant daily.

2   Eyesight should be tested and spectacles provided to counteract any refractive errors.

3   The patient should think of ways to create a calmer daily routine and take practical measures to relieve life's pressures; his talk with the doctor may have uncovered difficulties which the patient was reluctant to admit or of which he was unaware; viewing them now in an objective way, he must, with the help of doctor, priest, employer or Citizens' Advice Bureau try to alter attitudes and situations.

4   Drugs
i   A mild sedative or tranquilliser may be prescribed – taken regularly at first to break the circle of tension and circumstance, and then occasionally when the patient knows he is under strain.
ii   An analgesic such as aspirin may relieve a mild attack of migraine.
iii   Antihistamine preparations taken at night may be helpful if the migraine is due to allergic reaction.
iv   Diuretics will be of value when migrainous headache is due to pre-menstrual fluid retention.
v   Vaso-constricting drugs, e.g. ergotamine tartrate, often combined with other medications to enhance its effect – Cafergot (a combination of caffeine, ergotamine and belladonna) and Migril (ergotamine, caffeine and cyclizine); these should be taken as soon as there is warning of an attack. When the headache is very severe or the patient is nauseated and vomiting, intramuscular ergotamine tartrate may be the only successful form of treatment (ergotamine preparations are contraindicated during pregnancy or if the patient has arterial disease).

Migrainous neuralgia

The symptoms of this painful condition have many of the features of migraine. The pain around and behind one eye is intense, lasting an hour or two and occurring several times a day; it may extend to the forehead, temple and face, but is not accompanied by nausea and vomiting. When the attack reaches its peak there is nasal congestion, conjunctival injection and tears will stream from the eyes, particularly on the side of the headache. There may be a regularity about its occurrence and it may repeatedly wake the sufferer at night. After a period of several days there is freedom from pain which may last for months or years.

The ingestion of amines such as cheese are known to precipitate an attack and should be avoided. The treatment consists of the administration of oral or intramuscular ergotamine tartrate; patients whose attacks are at night may find cafergot suppositories helpful.

Trigeminal neuralgia (Tic douloureux)

Trigeminal neuralgia is a chronic disease of unknown origin occurring in later life; women are more often affected than men. The pain is usually on one side of the face, is very severe and lasts only a few seconds; it may occur several times a day for several days and then disappear only to recur days, weeks or months later as suddenly as it ceased. The remissions get progressively shorter until the pain becomes scarcely bearable, it may be so severe that the patient commits suicide. When the disorder affects a younger person or if it has on separate occasions affected each side of the face, it may be associated with multiple sclerosis (see Chapter 18) and evidence of this disease will probably be found in other parts of the nervous system.

The trigeminal (Vth cranial; see Fig. 2.10) nerve is mainly sensory, transmitting sensation from one half of the face and the front of the head including the eye, mouth, palate, teeth, maxillary sinus and the anterior two-thirds of the tongue (Fig. 17.2). It is divided into three roots.
1   The ophthalmic branch – sensation from the cornea is conducted along this nerve pathway
2   The maxillary branch
3   The mandibular branch – this also carries a small motor root to the muscles of mastication
Beneath the temporal lobe close to the brain stem these three branches unite to form a large ganglion (Gasserian ganglion) which transmits impulses along the posterior sensory root to the pons varolii. The motor nucleus is in the floor of the 4th ventricle; the motor nerve root emerges from the

pons varolii, travels with the mandibular branch of the sensory nerve and innervates the muscles of mastication, the soft palate and middle ear.

Patients suffering from this disease adopt a very characteristic posture (Fig. 17.3) during a spasm of pain with their shoulders hunched, head bowed and hand shielding, but not daring to touch the face. The eye on the affected side may close and tears stream from it during an attack; there may be a visible tic. Elderly ladies usually wear a soft woollen head scarf pulled forward to protect the face from draughts, men are sometimes unshaven and the face may be dirty on one side; each patient is aware of circumstances which trigger their pain, for example washing, shaving, touching the face, a draught, eating or even just talking.

Treatment

Any condition which causes facial pain should be investigated and treated; pain from sinusitis and dental decay may aggravate episodes of trigeminal neuralgia or lead to a wrong diagnosis.

The pain of trigeminal neuralgia was once difficult to control as common mild analgesics had little effect and the powerful addictive drugs could not be used because of the chronic nature of the disorder. An anticonvulsant phenytoin sodium was sometimes found helpful, but for total relief from pain many patients ultimately required surgical destruction of the nerve (trigeminal nerve root section or alcohol injection) which renders the face permanently numb and the cornea insensitive. With the advent of carbamazepine in the early 1960s medical treatment has become more successful, most patients are either pain free or find their pain bearable, the addition of phenytoin sodium is

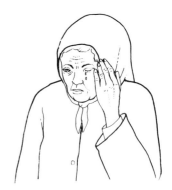

Fig. 17.3   Patient during a spasm of trigeminol neuralgia.

sometimes necessary to enhance this effect. Surgical treatment is reserved for a very few carefully selected patients who in spite of medical treatment continue to find their pain unbearable.

Surgical procedures

During discussion about possible operative treatment great emphasis is always laid on the unpleasant after-effects, and throughout the interview the doctor will try to assess the patient's personality. A few individuals are psychologically unsuitable for surgery as they will not be able to accept loss of facial sensation, becoming so obsessed with it that they are resentful of their treatment and, forgetting the severity of their previous pain, may even try to sue the doctor.

i Peripheral nerve blocking procedures (Cryoblock) – the peripheral portions of the nerve are inactivated, anaesthetising the painful area of the face.

(a) Access to the ophthalmic branch is through the supraorbital foramen.

(b) The maxillary branch is reached through the infraorbital foramen.

(c) The lingual approach is used to reach the mandibular branch.

The infraorbital nerve block for pain in the distribution of the maxillary branch achieves the best results.

ii Central nerve procedures

(a) Destruction of nerve pathways in the Gasserian ganglion by thermocoagulation, alcohol or glycerol injection. The patient is starved prior to surgery and given a premedication as the operation

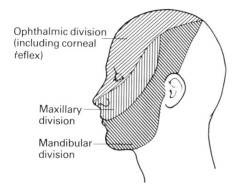

Ophthalmic division (including corneal reflex)

Maxillary division

Mandibular division

Fig. 17.2   Cutaneous distribution of the trigeminol nerve.

is performed under intermittent general anaesthesia. The coagulator or needle is inserted through the cheek into the foramen ovale at the base of the skull – its correct placement is aided by X-rays taken during the procedure. A successful operation brings immediate and lasting pain relief but the face will be permanently numb. Whenever possible the ophthalmic branch of the trigeminal nerve is spared to avoid loss of the corneal reflex.

(b) Posterior fossa exploration and microvascular decompression using foam padding to insulate the trigeminal nerve from the adjacent basilar or cerebellar artery, the pulsation or spasm of which triggers the trigeminal nerve.

The advantage of a Gasserian ganglion block is that surgery is relatively minor but it has the disadvantage of leaving permanent facial sensory loss and possible loss of the corneal reflex. On the other hand a posterior fossa exploration for microvascular decompression leaves no sensory loss but carries all the risks of major surgery with the additional risk of postoperative intracranial haematoma. It is unsuitable for many of the sufferers of trigeminal neuralgia because they are old and frail. The choice of surgery therefore depends on the age and fitness of the patient and the distribution of the pain.

Nursing care

Many patients suffering from trigeminal neuralgia are aged, some have been widowed, live alone and suffer not only paroxysms of intolerable pain, but also loneliness and sometimes poverty. They live in a state of apprehension, waiting for the next attack of pain and may become extremely depressed, neglecting personal hygiene, nutrition and their home; they may take to their bed or become suicidal.

The patient will be seen by the general practitioner who will usually recognise the disorder from the history and prescribe carbamazepine; the doctor will explain to patient and relatives that the drug may at first cause giddiness and unsteadiness and advise additional care. Tottery aged patients should be supervised by their relatives or by regular visits from the district nurse who will help the patient to bath; this will provide an opportunity to notice whether the patient is depressed, confused or malnourished, to enquire whether tablets are being

taken regularly and ensure that there are satisfactory arrangements for renewal of prescriptions. There may be an opportunity to report the patient's needs to her doctor, encourage neighbours to pop in or call in community services; relatives may need the nurse's advice. The patient and her relatives should be given an opportunity to express any particular anxieties or problems when they see the neurologist at an outpatient appointment.

The patient will discover some protective measures from bitter experience, and will stay indoors when there is a cold wind, keep out of draughts, drink tea lukewarm and avoid cold foods; she may fear to wash her face or clean her teeth even when free of pain, but should be shown how unwise it is to neglect oral hygiene and encouraged to take a nourishing diet to 'keep up her strength' though she is miserable and has no appetite. Nurses must always be careful not to ridicule any little eccentricities or apparent fussiness and should never attempt to press their attentions on a patient during a paroxysm of pain nor try to extract a reply until the attack is over.

Care following trigeminal thermocoagulation or injection

The patient may undergo a trigeminal nerve block as an out-patient or during a one day stay in hospital; it must be remembered that the patient is likely to be elderly and frail and may be a little tottery on her feet after the injection. As soon as possible the patient should resume all normal activities.

Especial care is necessary when the cornea is deliberately desensitised; precautions must be taken to see that corneal ulceration does not occur. Preoperatively a detailed explanation should be given to the patient about the care of her eye as unnoticed particles of dust or grit, or accidental touching of the cornea will cause damage; spectacles should be fitted with a transparent side shield. Repeated warnings not to touch the face will be necessary as the patient may feel a compelling need to rub her insensitive face. A mirror will be helpful whenever the patient washes her face to avoid touching the eye with the flannel and she should inspect the eye daily for any redness which should be reported promptly to her doctor. Keratitis may develop and unless this is treated promptly with antibiotic eye drops or ointment, corneal ulceration is likely. Tarsorrhaphy is usually unnecessary unless the facial nerve is damaged during the operation; inability to close the eye and the absence of protective tears increases the risk to the insensitive cornea and tarsorrhaphy then becomes essential.

The patient's mouth, tongue and gums will be insensitive on the side of the operation and she may unknowingly chew her cheek or tongue when eating, be unaware of ulcers caused by ill-fitting dentures or of food particles collecting beneath the denture plate. After each meal the patient should be advised to remove and rinse her dentures, swill her mouth with warm antiseptic mouthwash and inspect cheek, gums and tongue for signs of abrasion.

Glossopharyngeal neuralgia

The glossopharyngeal (IXth cranial) nerves (see Chapter 2) provide sensation and movement to the throat. Neuralgia in this region is triggered by swallowing and the pain which is sometimes not excessively severe will be felt in the throat, tongue or ear on one side; when the pain is severe the patient stops eating and drinking and rapidly becomes undernourished and dehydrated, a particularly dangerous condition in the elderly. The disease is very rare and has long remissions; usually only one glossopharyngeal nerve is affected, but occasionally the disorder may affect both nerves or be associated with trigeminal neuralgia. Transient syncope may accompany the pain as the glossopharyngeal nerve supplies the carotid sinus.

Treatment with carbamazepine may bring complete relief from pain; should nerve section be necessary a posterior fossa craniectomy will be performed. It is not possible to treat bilateral pain by operation as loss of both glossopharyngeal nerves would make swallowing impossible.

Atypical facial pain

This term is used to describe facial pain which has been present for a long time and whose cause and cure have evaded all the doctor's investigations. The behaviour and distribution of the pain does not fit into the pattern of a recognisable disorder, nor can it be traced to a particular organic cause (temporal arteritis, tabes dorsalis, syringobulbia, dental decay, abscess or sinusitis); only time will

tell whether the cause of pain has been an undetected tumour. Facial pain is not uncommonly associated with depressive illness and anxiety states, especially where there are obsessional traits in the patient's personality and when there is fear of cancer.

Treatment

Successful treatment of psychiatric illness may cure facial pain and patients with persistent pain often need supportive psychotherapy; their depression may be the result of pain rather than its cause when antidepressant drugs will be less effective. Injections of alcohol and neurosurgical operations are often ineffective though the patient may urge the doctor to try these measures. Local physical treatments, freezing the skin or using a vibrator may bring greater relief; drugs used in the treatment of trigeminal neuralgia (carbamazepine and phenytoin sodium) may be given a trial but usually prove ineffective. These patients who are dogged by pain constantly see different doctors to try to find the cause and cure and, failing to find relief, will need sympathetic understanding.

Temporal arteritis

Temporal arteritis occurs in old age. The symptoms are the result of inflammation of cranial arteries causing narrowing and ischaemia. This is a widespread, generalised disorder which may affect arteries in any part of the body. The patient complains of headache and pain in the temporal region especially at night, or of sudden blindness preceded by headache and possibly by other symptoms of vague malaise, loss of appetite and aching limbs. On examination the doctor will find that there is extreme tenderness in the temporal region on the affected side and palpation of the temporal artery on either side reveals thickening and absent pulsation. The patient may have complete loss of vision in one or both eyes.

Investigations

The diagnosis is usually obvious from the history and examination, but may be confirmed by:
  (a) raised blood sedimentation rate;
  (b) temporal artery biopsy showing characteristic cell changes.

Treatment

Steroid therapy, which must start urgently, will rapidly relieve headache and possibly save sight, though it will not restore sight once lost. The maximum dosage of oral prednisone will be administered for one month and dosage will then be tailed off gradually and discontinued at the end of 6 months unless there is a recurrence of symptoms.

Relief of severe and persistent pain

Severe and persistent pain is associated with skeletal, vascular and nerve disorders, for example arthritis, peripheral vascular disease with gangrene, scar pain and following herpes zoster, but malignant disease is the chief cause of severe and intractable pain resulting from the invasion of the lymphatic, skeletal and peripheral nerve systems by malignant cells. Some patients with malignancy will only live a short while, whereas others may have an almost normal life span. Pain must be controlled, but if the patient is likely to live for years rather than months, the powerful addictive drugs are not prescribed until all other avenues have been explored. Referral to a pain clinic is often helpful. The objects of treatment are to:

1 Cure the condition causing the pain, e.g. by using anti-inflammatory medications and joint replacement for arthritis.

2 Relieve the pain with a non-addictive analgesic which does not cause side effects; several analgesics may be tried before the most suitable is found. Simple analgesics include paracetamol, di-hydrocodeine and co-proxamol. Stronger non-addictive analgesics include mephanamic acid (Ponstan), and buprenorphine (Temgesic). Some of these analgesics cause gastric irritation and should be taken with food; occasionally nausea is an unavoidable side effect which will respond to an antiemetic such as metoclopramide (Maxolon); some analgesics cause constipation.

3 Potentiate the effects of an analgesic by also giving a tranquillising preparation, e.g. chlorpromazine or diazepam.

4 Temporarily relieve the pain by a local injection.

i The distal part of a peripheral nerve can be destroyed by cryotherapy or injections of Depo-medrone, giving 3–6 months pain relief before the nerve regenerates; it is hoped that pain relief will be permanent, but if not, the treatment can be repeated. This treatment is particularly useful in the treatment of thoracic girdle pain, but does carry the risk of pneumothorax.

ii Depo-medrone can be injected outside the spinal theca (epidural injection) to relieve nerve root pain, and may be repeated.

5 Stimulate the painful area with a transcutaneous nerve stimulator. Two electrodes are placed approximately 15 cm apart over the painful area, the electrodes are attached to a small portable stimulator which has controls for intensity, duration and frequency of the impulses which the patient can control for himself when the pain is present.

6 Hypnosis and acupuncture have a useful part to play in the treatment of pain.

7 Relieve the pain with strong hypnotic and narcotic drugs, e.g. morphine, Brompton mixture (a syrup containing morphine and other additives, e.g. chlorpromazine), pethidine, dextromoramide (Palfium) and dipipanone co (Diconal). Oral administration is preferred, but if the need arises the drug will be given by injection; small continuous doses of the drug can be given throughout the 24 hours using an injection driver. A concurrent or alternative method of providing pain relief is by the administration of analgesic suppositories, e.g. oxycodone pectinate (Proladone). Diazepam suppositories or intramuscular injection are useful to assist relaxation and relieve depression.

8 Interrupt the pain pathways by making destructive lesions (Fig. 17.4). It is sometimes necessary to subject patients with intractable pain to some form of pain relieving operation. The success of certain surgical procedures in the relief of pain depends upon the duration and severity of the pain, the effectiveness of analgesia and whether the patient is excessively preoccupied with his pain. It is difficult to free a patient from pain when he has previously received ineffective analgesia for a long time, as a pain pattern will have become fixed in his brain. Operative procedures include:

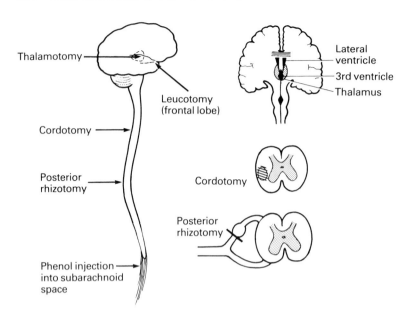

Fig. 17.4   Sites of surgical pain relieving procedures.

i Phenol injection into the subarachnoid space A phenol preparation is injected in the lumbar region to block the lumbosacral sensory nerves. This simple procedure is performed with great care as the phenol must not come into contact with the spinal cord, the lower sacral sensory nerves to the sphincters or the motor nerve roots, otherwise the patient will become paralysed and lose bladder control. Greât care must be taken to maintain the position recommended by the surgeon for the set period of time following the injection.

ii The insertion of a nerve stimulator Extradural electrodes are implanted against the posterior part of the spinal cord as the pain fibres enter through the posterior nerve root, ascend several segments and synapse in the substantia gelatinosa in the posterior horns of grey matter (see Fig. 17.1) The electrodes are implanted several segments higher than the pain level suggests, in the thoracic region for pain in the leg, and in the cervical region for arm and chest pain.

iii Posterior rhizotomy (sensory nerve root section) This operation is reserved almost exclusively for thoracic girdle pains; several sensory nerve roots must be severed to anaesthetise even a small well-defined area, as there is considerable overlap in function of adjacent sensory nerves. This operation is unsuitable when pain is very severe and widespread and will prove unsatisfactory in areas supplied by the brachial, lumbar and sacral plexuses as there is much reorganisation of nerve pathways and the extensive surgery necessary to guarantee complete loss of pain would also sacrifice the motor power of a limb.

iv Cordotomy The severe pain associated with cancer can only be abolished by dividing the pain pathways where they are all close together in the spinal cord. On entering the cord, pain fibres ascend for 2 to 3 segments (see Fig. 17.1) before crossing to the opposite side, then they travel to the thalamus in the spino-thalamic tract in the antero-lateral part of the cord; the operation of cordotomy interrupts these pathways high in the thoracic or cervical cord producing loss of pain and temperature appreciation in the opposite half of the body. A cordotomy at the first thoracic level would eradicate pain in the lower abdomen or leg, but for pain in the chest or upper abdomen it would be necessary to sever the tract at the first cervical level. These operations are most successful when the pain is unilateral; bilateral cordotomy is seldom performed as it may cause loss of bladder control, and in the cervical cord, temporary apnoea during sleep.

There are two ways in which cordotomy is performed.

(a) through a laminectomy to cut the spinothalamic tract which is located anterior to the dentate ligament. It is likely that the patient has undergone other major surgical procedures, is generally debilitated and therefore the risks are great.

(b) By coagulating the cord using an electrode guided by myelographic X-rays of the spine. This operation is performed under a local anaesthetic; the radio-opaque substance outlines the dentate ligament enabling the surgeon to locate the spino-thalamic tract which is destroyed by several short bursts of electrical current; great care is taken not to encroach upon the adjacent motor pathways. Between each coagulation, the surgeon assesses the extent of sensory loss in the opposite side of the body and the muscle power in the limbs on the side of the operation. The nurse must remember that postoperatively the patient will have also lost the ability to appreciate temperature sensation and great care should be taken to prevent burns; she should teach the patient how to care for the insensitive area and to be especially careful in testing the temperature of washing water, preferably using a thermometer.

For postoperative nursing care following spinal surgery see Chapter 12.

v Thalamotomy Stereotaxic thalamotomy attempts to interrupt the passage of pain impulses to the cortex where they pass through the thalamus; it is difficult to locate and destroy solely the pain fibres without causing other sensory loss and the effects are short-lived.

9   Change the patient's emotional response to pain. Leucotomy as a treatment for intractable pain is only performed as a last resort when pain due to an organic lesion such as carcinoma is so severe as to be unbearable in spite of treatment or, when a pain pattern (possibly originating in a past organic lesion, e.g. a wound) has become so indelibly impressed on the patient's brain that he is completely obsessed by it, allowing it to rule his life to the exclusion of all else. There are several types of operation which involve creating a small, precisely calculated destructive lesion in the frontal lobes. These either sever some of the fibres connecting the higher centres of emotion in the frontal lobes to other parts of the brain or destroy by the implantation of yttrium seeds, deliberately changing the patient's personality. There have been doubts about the ethics of performing such operations; it does not remove the pain, but changes the patient's emotional response allowing him to discuss it with bland indifference and may enable him to lead a more active life.

These apparently simple operations are not without possible complications and postoperatively the nurse should observe very carefully for signs of rising intracranial pressure due to haematoma or oedema. During the first 24 hours after operation there may be slight confusion, poor concentration, the patient may appear rather vague and there may be a flatness of emotional response; there may be occasional incontinence if the patient lacks the initiative to ask for bedpan or urinal. These symptoms, with the help of retraining, should recede or be overcome within a week of surgery. Lowering of consciousness and the presence of a hemiparesis are serious signs indicating possible intracranial complications and should be reported immediately to the doctor.

As soon as possible the patient must return to normal activities, getting up and dressed early in the day and attending to his personal hygiene regularly, as it is very easy for a patient who has had leucotomy to lapse into slovenly habits, a pattern which once established is difficult to break. The nurse may find that the patient aggressively refuses to get out of bed and she is fearful of enforcing her request in case she gets hurt; she must be firmly persuasive as these early patterns are so important to rehabilitation following leucotomy.

10   Hypophysectomy (see Chapter 7). The pain produced by tumours which are hormone dependent, mainly breast cancer, responds well to the removal of the pituitary gland (hypophysis). The gland can be totally or partially excised through a craniotomy or through the naso-pharynx (transphenoidal approach), destroyed by radiation or implantation of a radio-active substance, or the pituitary stalk may be cut. Diabetes insipidus may be a temporary problem postoperatively which will be helped by administration of desmopressin intranasally or by intramuscular injection.

Nursing care of patients in pain

A patient in pain is often unable to concentrate, is anxious, irritable, depressed and unable to eat or sleep. At home he may have borne his pain only by adhering to an almost obsessional routine and will resent any change when admitted to hospital.

On admission to hospital, to avoid disturbing the patient unnecessarily, most information should be obtained from the accompanying relative or friend. This should include the history of the patient's illness, nature and duration of pain and simple measures relating to position, posture, arrangement of pillows or clothing which bring relief, analgesics which are particularly effective and when they were last taken, and factors which aggravate pain. All this information should be rapidly communicated to each member of the nursing and domestic staff, who must be warned not to jolt the patient's bed, nor handle him roughly or become impatient if he is so absorbed with his pain that he does not immediately respond when addressed; they should also be asked to perform all their duties near the patient in a gentle, quiet manner.

Nurses may be able to influence and relieve pain by methods other than just 'giving a tablet':

i by allaying anxiety;

ii by attending to physical needs and comfort even before the patient needs to ask;

iii by providing a quiet sensitive atmosphere;

iv by encouraging relatives in the right approach and suggesting the best time to visit, length of stay and number of visitors that can be tolerated – the patient may find it an effort to talk to more than one person at a time and though he longs for peace and quiet will not like to ask his visitors to leave;

v by administering analgesia at the right time.

The patient who has been having regular analgesics must continue to receive them promptly or he will become agitated and lose confidence in the staff; he should be observed carefully throughout the day and night to assess pain and the effectiveness of analgesia. The nurse should never need to repeatedly ask 'Are you in pain?' but should notice pallor, inattention, restlessness or other signs of increasing discomfort and should promptly administer analgesics as prescribed, report their effectiveness and if the patient is receiving medication only 'when necessary', ensure that it is given when the pain starts and not when it has already reached an undesirable and uncontrollable intensity; mild analgesics may be surprisingly effective if they are given early with regularity. The doctor may wish analgesia to be temporarily withheld before adjusting dosage or introducing another drug; should this be necessary an explanation must be given to the patient.

Although the patient needs a quiet atmosphere and should be left undisturbed immediately after the administration of an analgesic or when the pain is at its worst, he must not feel deserted. The nurse should beware of looking gloomy or anxious and equally avoid heartiness of manner, but should uphold the patient by her presence and when she knows his pain is less severe and distracting, engage him in short periods of undemanding conversation.

The patient should be given an opportunity to discuss the cause of his pain with a doctor; patients sometimes jump to the wrong conclusions based upon 'old wives' tales' and fears engendered by 'well meaning' relatives and friends and their lack of knowledge of anatomy and physiology may lead to unnecessary acute anxiety. Proposed measures of treatment should be discussed every few days to ensure that the patient understands the overall plan, for example 'We would like to change the medicines you are having to try to find a better combination which does not make you so sleepy (nauseated or giddy) yet still relieves your pain. During the change-over the pain may not seem any better, it may even be a little worse for a day or two, possibly longer, try not to worry and bear with it, we shall find a way of helping you, but it will take time. When the pain is under control another doctor, who has had a great deal of experience in treating conditions like yours, will be seeing you to advise the next step in your treatment', or 'You will be able to go home and will be seen at the hospital regularly as an out-patient'.

Relatives should be discouraged from continual mention and enquiry about the patient's pain and adverse comment on his appearance. They should be kept informed in advance about the patient's treatment to prevent them continually pestering the patient for information, increasing his anxiety and they should also be warned that the patient may not be immediately pain-free and that treatment may take time.

Psychological pain
(psychogenic 'overlay' and 'hysterical' pain)

Nurses must be extremely careful to be impartial and objective when making observations and reports concerning any patient in pain; whether the pain is organic or psychogenic, the patient's behaviour is influenced by psychological factors and these may not be so obvious unless the patient is watched discreetly without her awareness. The cause of psychological illness may be revealed when there is a history suggesting previous nervous breakdown or obvious stress immediately preceding the present illness; the cause may only be revealed later during the course of conversation when the nurse has gained the patient's confidence.

The patient's behaviour may give clues which suggest the pain is of psychogenic origin.

i   Florid dramatisation of pain, the patient flinging herself on the bed, flouncing about loudly complaining and seeking attention.

ii   Her appearance belies her complaint, as she is neither pale, drawn, sweating nor does she neglect personal grooming, perhaps even applying make-up when no one is apparently watching; she may on the other hand deliberately refrain from improving her appearance in order to look wan and ill.

iii The patient's behaviour may differ according to whether she thinks someone is watching or not, when conscious of a nursing or medical audience he may writhe about in apparent pain, but when thinking herself unobserved may occupy herself in some normal activity or talk to other patients without any sign of discomfort. Facial expression and gait should be closely observed for inconsistencies.

iv There may be apparent loss of appetite yet no loss of weight or the patient may be eating normally, which suggests she is not in such severe pain as she would have everyone believe.

Inexperienced nurses should be very much aware that hysterical patients are skilled in the art of manipulating the staff, other patients and situations to suit their own ends. Nurses must be careful not to become over-involved with the affairs of such patients nor to be gullible in accepting every tale that is told of how the patient has been misjudged and maligned. On the other hand it is too easy to label these apparently tiresome patients 'hysterical' and overlook serious illness. Routine temperature, pulse, respiration and blood pressure recordings should be made without undue fuss and on occasions of 'collapse' sometimes it is necessary to inform a doctor who will observe the patient and possibly examine her in more detail; the inference given to the patient will be that the doctor just happened to come into the ward and not that he has been especially summoned. On no account should the patient be led to believe that the staff think her complaint 'of no consequence' or that they are harsh in their judgement. She must be treated kindly, but firmly encouraged to pursue normal activities for gradually increasing periods.

Patients whose pain is believed to be hysterical in origin or whose physical pain is aggravated by psychological causes may benefit from psychiatric treatment.

18

Demyelinating Diseases

The nerve fibres in the central nervous system are each covered by a fatty myelin sheath (see Fig. 2.1) which insulates the fibre and aids conduction of electrical impulses. There are several neurological conditions associated with patchy degeneration of the myelin sheaths and disordered conduction of nerve impulses. Though the myelin to some extent regenerates after each episode of demyelination, these areas gradually become sclerotic plaques. Demyelination is a feature of many neurological disorders, the best known being multiple sclerosis.

Multiple sclerosis

Multiple sclerosis (disseminated sclerosis) is one of the commonest diseases of the nervous system and in Great Britain affects 1 in 2000 of the population from all walks of life, women more often than men. The disease is not familial though occasionally two people in the same family are affected. It has been known for the onset to occur in the early teens, is commonest between the age of 20 and 40 and rarely occurs after the age of 60, in this latter instance it is possible that there have been previous unnoticed minor episodes. When the illness begins after the age of 35 its course is usually slowly progressive without remission.

The disease is characterised by scattered patches of demyelination in the central nervous system which occur at irregular intervals of time (disseminated in time and place). Areas of demyelination (Fig. 18.1) in the spinal cord, optic nerves, brain stem, cerebellum and subcortical regions of the cerebrum leave permanent sclerotic scars (plaques).

In spite of extensive research and some interesting observations about the worldwide distribution of the disease, as yet no single factor has been proved to cause multiple sclerosis, though theories have been advanced which suggest the disease may be caused by a virus or is an auto-immune response to a virus infection. There appear to be factors which consistently precede or aggravate the disease; upper respiratory tract infections,

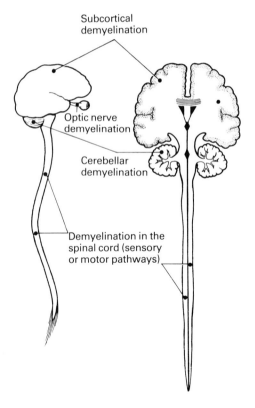

Subcortical demyelination

Optic nerve demyelination

Cerebellar demyelination

Demyelination in the spinal cord (sensory or motor pathways)

Fig. 18.1 Patchy distribution of demyelination in multiple sclerosis.

specific infectious diseases such as measles, fatigue and extremes of temperature. The disease occurs in temperate climates, particularly in the northern hemisphere; moving to tropical areas does not reduce the risk of its development, conversely moving from a tropical to a temperate climate puts a person at risk. All races living in a temperate climate are equally susceptible. The fluctuating nature of the disease has led to difficulties in trials of various forms of treatment and many patients have been exploited by the false claims of success of 'quack' medicine, when the 'cure' was probably a natural remission in the disease. The prognosis depends upon where the lesions are, their size and how rapidly one episode of demyelination follows another. In a greater number of patients than is often realised, the disease is relatively benign, with long remissions of up to 15 or 20 years; in others, there are frequent episodes for several years, then the disease arrests, leaving the patient only partially disabled. Sometimes there are repeated catastrophic relapses and in 2–5 years the patient becomes severely paralysed and helpless. The disabling effects of this disorder which occurs during the prime of life, its remitting and relapsing course and the fact that research has so far failed to discover the cause has led to many misconceptions about the disease, its treatment and prognosis, and perhaps an unnecessarily gloomy approach to the problems.

The onset of the illness may be acute or insidious and there are many different presenting symptoms, according to the site of demyelination. Retrobulbar neuritis (optic neuritis), often the first manifestation of multiple sclerosis, is caused by demyelination in one or both optic nerves; in this condition there is pain on movement of the eye or when pressure is applied to the eyeball, and mistiness of vision or blindness, the visual field defect is a central scotoma (see p. 15) and swelling of the optic disc (papillitis) is sometimes present. Optic neuritis may be very mild, lasting for a few days and only recalled on close questioning, or severe enough to render the patient blind for as long as three months; sight usually recovers. Sometimes a small scotoma persists, only obvious when the visual fields are plotted, and there is always permanent pallor of the temporal side of the affected optic disc. Retrobulbar neuritis may be accompanied by signs of demyelination in other parts of the nervous system, for example diplopia, unsteadiness of gait, limb weakness, abnormal

sensations of numbness or fleeting paraesthesiae. When the onset of multiple sclerosis is acute and severe, the patient is extremely ill and has vertigo, nystagmus, definite weakness or paralysis of one or more limbs, intention tremor and loss of position sense; there may be bladder disturbance.

The history of the illness and evidence of widespread scattered lesions in the central nervous system often establishes the diagnosis. During the first episode diagnosis is sometimes difficult if the symptoms and signs suggest one well defined lesion, for example in the spinal cord this could also be attributed to a spinal tumour; it is important that treatable lesions are always excluded. In some instances it is only the characteristic progression of the disease over a long period which confirms the initial tentative diagnosis of multiple sclerosis.

When the patient is first taken ill he is seen by his general practitioner who suspecting the possible diagnosis, refers him to a neurologist who sees him as an out-patient and usually recommends hospital admission for full assessment, investigation and treatment.

Admission to hospital

History and examination

When the patient is admitted to hospital a detailed history and thorough general and neurological examination is of the utmost importance to establish the diagnosis and assess the extent of neurological involvement. Direct questioning is often necessary to find out whether the patient has had other episodes of demyelination, as the patient may not appreciate the relevance of a short episode of blurred vision or difficulty with micturition. A general impression of the patient's personality, mood, intelligence and reaction to his illness and disabilities is soon gained during conversation; it is also helpful to know whether he suspects the nature of his illness. The patient's social background is important as there is always the possiblity that he will have a persisting or increasing disability:

i   Has he any dependants?
ii Is he regularly employed and what is his job?
iii How does he travel to work?
iv Does he live alone?
v   What type of accommodation does he have?
Relatives may be able to give helpful information

and must be interviewed if the patient has memory impairment or psychological disorder.

During examination scanning dysarthria (see p. 12) of cerebellar origin is often heard; in the early stages, it may pass unnoticed unless the observer listens very carefully.

Visual acuity may be impaired by retrobulbar neuritis. There may be diplopia, most commonly on lateral gaze, and difficulty in focusing when eye movements are disorganised by involvement of the IIIrd, IVth or VIth cranial nerves, due to disturbance in the upper part of the midbrain. Nystagmus is often present, a sign of cerebellar inco-ordination of eye movements most marked in the abducting eye.

The trigeminal nerve is sometimes affected resulting in facial sensory loss and there is sometimes bilateral trigeminal neuralgia (see p. 249). The VIIIth cranial nerve nucleus in the midbrain may be affected causing 'giddiness'.

Examination of the limbs usually reveals a mixture of signs indicating involvement of the pyramidal, cerebellar and sensory systems; symptoms of disturbance in one of these systems may appear first or predominate. The patient may have noticed that when he is tired he tends to stumble or drag one leg and it may be noticed that the toe of the shoe on the affected side is worn down more than the other. Signs may be asymmetrical, but though dysfunction appears to be only on one side, pathologically brisk reflexes on the other side indicate that the disease is bilateral; upper motor neurone signs are usually most marked in the legs. Intention tremor, a sign of cerebellar disturbance, is common especially in the later stages of the disease; the finger–nose test will demonstrate ataxia and tremor, which will be even more pronounced if there is also weakness and sensory loss. The patient's gait is unsteady and Romberg's sign is often positive. Unsteadiness may be due to several factors, cerebellar disturbance, weakness and sensory loss, especially loss of joint position sense.

Bladder control is affected in several ways, the most common symptoms are urgency and precipitancy of micturition which lead to incontinence of urine when facilities are not readily available. The 'spastic' bladder over-reacts to the presence of urine and often empties incompletely leading to stagnation of urine and infection which then increases the irritability of the bladder and leads to frequency and dysuria.

Investigations

The patient will not be subjected to unnecessary costly investigations when the diagnosis is obvious. When the diagnosis is uncertain, tests will include haemoglobin and white cell count, blood sedimentation rate, Wassermann and Kahn reaction, serum B_{12}, blood urea estimation and X-rays of the chest, skull and spine; a CAT scan will help to exclude other cerebral lesions.

There are two particular tests which though not diagnostic in themselves help to support a provisional diagnosis of multiple sclerosis made on clinical grounds.

1 A record of visually evoked potentials demonstrate the delayed passage of light stimulated impulses from the retina to the visual cortex (picked up by EEG electrodes over the occipital cortex) when patches of demyelination have affected the optic nerves.

2 Lumbar puncture. The CSF is sometimes abnormal during an active phase of the illness, the lymphocytes are increased to 50–80 per cu mm, the protein content is increased to 50–120 mg per cent and there is an abnormal Lange colloidal gold curve (see Chapter 24) of the paretic or sometimes luetic type in spite of a negative Wassermann reaction.

Magnetic resonance imaging will show patches of demyelination, but this expensive investigation will only be performed when in spite of other tests there is still doubt about the diagnosis.

Treatment

There is definite indication that during an acute phase of this illness, fatigue causes deterioration in the patient's condition; a period of complete bed rest is therefore recommended. There is no arbitrary period of rest, but it seems best for the patient to remain in bed until no new signs or symptoms have appeared for a day or two and existing ones have stopped getting worse. A course of oral prednisolone or intramuscular adrenocorticotrophic hormone (ACTH) is beneficial with each acute relapse and should be commenced at the earliest possible time, to halt the disease process and speed recovery; it is not curative and does not prevent another relapse. On the basis that vitamin B_{12} benefits the nervous system, monthly injections of this preparation are sometimes given and if nothing else, will benefit the patient psychologically.

When the acute phase of the illness is over, gradual mobilisation begins and, with physiotherapy and occupational therapy, the patient is encouraged to become as independent as possible. All forms of exercise will be given depending upon physical limitations, including training in coordination, balance and movement. The range of activities and periods of therapy are arranged according to the patient's exercise tolerance, activity must always stop before there are signs of fatigue. Nurses and therapists will become sensitive to when the patient needs a rest and when he can be encouraged to a little more effort.

When a diagnosis of multiple sclerosis is made, almost inevitably the staff feel dismayed and helpless, discussion of the illness is limited by fear of the patient's reaction to the devastating news that he has an incurable illness and the staff's feeling of inadequacy because they have no cure to offer. The patient will become anxious, suspicious and bewildered if he is not given sufficient information. The doctor should not be evasive or the patient, thinking that no diagnosis has been made, will seek other advice and may go from one doctor to another or to dubious sources of costly 'quack' medicine. The patient and his relatives must be given opportunities to ask the doctor questions; many doctors feel it is unwise to state a definite diagnosis of multiple sclerosis with all its unpleasant implications, after the first episode as it is insufficiently conclusive. The doctor can only advise and final decisions must rest with the patient, yet from past experience he can foresee some of the future problems likely to face the family; the worst feature of the disorder is its uncertainty. No one can say whether the patient will have a long remission or a paralysing relapse within the year. A young person needs to plan a career, too much sick leave will lead to dismissal, the individual may not recover sufficiently to continue his present employment or commute to work and it will be difficult for someone who is slow and clumsy and whose speech is indistinct to find employment. Is it fair to hold a fiancé(e) to promise of marriage when the future is uncertain

and parenthood might be a selfish additional burden, physically and financially? Many established marriages cannot take the strain of repeated ill health, unemployment, heavy financial stress (involving growing children, mortgage, help in the home and house maintenance) and the ultimate heavy nursing of someone who becomes increasingly paralysed and helpless. Those who are trapped in their own home by illness can so easily become so depressingly absorbed by the tedious details of their daily routine that they are no longer interesting companions and their depression may infect the whole family; it requires very strong family bonds to support and uplift such a situation.

It is inevitable that the patient will ask questions about his future, some of which cannot be answered. Most of the patient's supervision will rest with the general practitioner, who, knowing the patient and his family well, can avert some difficulties and solve others with the help of the social services. He will know when the patient and his family are ready to accept the full import of the illness and when to advise contact with the Multiple Sclerosis Society. Most patients will come to terms with their disability and the name of the disorder loses something of its sting as, with the passage of time, they become used to their way of life and familiar with their own pattern of disease.

It should be impressed upon the patient that if he cares sensibly for his general health he will run less risk of a relapse. Action Research into Multiple Sclerosis (ARMS) has recently published a diet (see Table 18.1) which, though it will not cure multiple sclerosis, is thought to be beneficial in keeping the patient in a stable condition. The research unit has made use of recent scientific work on nutrition in supporting the healthy functioning of the central nervous system. As bladder disturbance is a feature of multiple sclerosis the patient should be persuaded to adopt the habit of taking at least 2½ litres of fluid every day. He should avoid fattening foods and alcohol, should not 'burn the candle at both ends', never exercise to the point of exhaustion, avoid excesses of temperature (sunbathing, hot baths or becoming thoroughly wet and chilled) and avoid contact with common infections such as colds and influenza. He should be advised to contact his own doctor promptly if he feels unwell, develops any infectious illness or has a recurrence of symptoms and in any of these circumstances should go to bed immediately, never 'soldier on'.

Reasons for readmission to hospital

i   A further episode of demyelination
ii   A course of rehabilitation
iii Treatment of complications
iv   Social factors
v   Terminal care

Table 18.1   The ARMS recommended diet

1   Polyunsaturated margarine and vegetable oils instead of animal fats
2   Fish – three times a week
3   Liver – half a pound weekly
4   Lean meat – all traces of fat trimmed off
5   Cottage cheese, Dutch cheeses, Brie and Camembert
6   No more than two to three eggs weekly
7   Large portion of dark green vegetables daily
8   Fresh fruit daily
9   Salads with French dressing daily
10   Whole grain cereals and wholemeal bread
11   Plenty of skimmed milk and yoghurt
12   A reduction in all foods containing sugar

Nursing care

The patient may be admitted to hospital several times with this illness and it is helpful if he finds staff whom he knows, though to them it is distressing to see the patient becoming less able and more dependent, but this should not colour the nurse's approach and she should always be aiming to improve the quality and usefulness of the patient's life. The nursing care of a patient with multiple sclerosis is a real challenge as, in the absence of curative medicine, his well-being largely depends upon good nursing care through the prevention of complications (see Chapters 3 and 10). The patient is naturally extremely anxious about his condition; while he is forced to rest in bed every effort must be made to relieve him of worries associated with his home and family; the medical social worker should see the patient. The need for complete rest must be explained to the patient and his relatives; all physical and mental effort must be spared. Visiting should be restricted to close members of the family and the length of each visit should be limited. One of the patient's main worries concerns bladder control and, knowing how frequently and suddenly is the need to pass urine and not wanting to be a bother, the patient will fear accidents and wonder how to manage when confined to bed; nurses should always be willing and prompt with bedpan, urinal or commode to save the distress and embarrassment of incontinence. Care of the skin and bladder are two of the difficult and frequently discussed problems in relation to nursing patients who have multiple sclerosis. Throughout the illness, whether the patient is in hospital or at home, skin and bladder care, as described in Chapters 3 and 10, are important. There are problems associated with skin care: the patient may be immobile, overweight, have sensory impairment, incontinence and possible urinary infection. In the terminal stages of the illness the patient will have an indwelling catheter. Spasm of leg muscles and fixed flexion posture makes it difficult to position the patient, causes friction on knees and heels and difficulty in thorough cleansing of the genital area, a particular embarrassment during the menstrual period. All these problems will increase as the patient's condition deteriorates and their management needs careful consideration. It is not always possible to enforce bed rest for the sake of intact skin surfaces if the patient's happiness and independence is thereby forfeited, so a compromise must be achieved. Operative measures to correct flexion deformity or intrathecal injection of phenol in glycerine to relieve flexor spasm may indirectly assist in prevention of sores, though the latter sometimes increases the risk by further impairment of nerve supply to the tissues.

The most influential factors in the patient's well-being, irrespective of the progress of his illness, are his personality, his religious faith which carries him through difficult times, his determination to enjoy life, and whether he has intelligently caring relatives, friends and neighbours and lives in a lively community which recognises the disabled person's need for companionship.

Neuromyelitis optica (Devic's disease)

Neuromyelitis optica is a rare demyelinating disease which is characterised by the sudden onset of partial or complete blindness in both eyes due to demyelination of the optic nerves. There may be dense paralysis accompanied by severe pain in the back and limbs when demyelination attacks the spinal cord. Either optic or spinal symptoms appear first within a day or two of each other, or both may appear together. The disease may be rapidly fatal or the patient may make a complete recovery.

Rare diffuse demyelinating diseases

There is a group of very rare diseases in which severe demyelination starts in the occipital lobes of the cerebrum causing blindness and advances through the cerebral hemispheres causing mental deterioration and spastic paralysis; death occurs within a few months.

19

Epilepsy

Epilepsy is a symptom of disorder within the brain characterised by repeated stereotyped disturbances of consciousness, movement or sensation; it may be idiopathic (of unknown cause) or symptomatic of organic brain disease. An epileptic fit occurs when there are abnormal electrical discharges from the brain cells. These cells are highly sensitive to chemical changes and it is likely that this is in some part responsible for the disruption in the electrical rhythms which accompany an epileptic attack, but it is not understood why it occurs in certain individuals at particular times and intervals. Approximately 4 in every 1000 persons have some form of epilepsy and both sexes are equally affected. There is little evidence that epilepsy runs in families although it is possible for more than one member of a family to have fits, in which case it is usually because the family suffers from an hereditary disease which affects the brain; children of parents with idiopathic epilepsy are very unlikely to develop the disorder though if both parents are affected the risk is slightly greater.

It is known from birth that certain children with congenital abnormalities or whose birth has been abnormal are likely to develop epilepsy and it may also be anticipated if an infant has had brain infection, head injury or has had more than one febrile convulsion; these children will be seen regularly at out-patient clinics or by their general practitioner, and any suspicious attack will be immediately investigated. Older children who have been healthy and whose milestones have been normal may have attacks which pass unnoticed because they are momentary, are similar to childhood habits and tics or occur at night. The child may be taken to the family doctor because his school teachers are concerned about inattentiveness, learning difficulties, disruptive or inappropriate behaviour or because he has developed nocturnal enuresis. The first indication of epilepsy may be a sudden fit or 'blackout' which may happen anywhere, at home, school, work or in the street.

History and examination

When taking the history, after hearing about the patient's recent attack, the doctor will try to discover whether there have been any previous episodes which might suggest that the current attack is not an isolated event, but one of many, and possibly epilepsy. The doctor will ask about the patient's birth, childhood milestones, whether he has lived abroad and if there has been head injury or serious illness such as meningitis. Idiopathic epilepsy usually starts in childhood and the onset of attacks often coincides with the critical periods of life: starting school, puberty, leaving school or starting a career. In girls a fit is more likely in the days before menstruation when it is associated with premenstrual tension; fits may cease during pregnancy and recur after parturition. It is necessary to know of any family history of mental illness, hereditary disease, faints or fits. Throughout the examination the doctor assesses the patient's attitude to his attacks and the manner in which he describes them as it is important to differentiate between an epileptic fit and a 'blackout' due to hysteria or anxiety. A general and neurological examination (see Chapter 2) will either confirm idiopathic epilepsy, because there is a characteristic history, no demonstrable neurological abnormality and a typical electroencephalogram (EEG, see p. 28) or, will reveal signs of a symptomatic cause. A hint of a facial weakness or very slightly increased reflexes on one side of the body may suggest a brain lesion. Signs can be very slight, yet important, suggesting an event in infancy which caused brain damage, for example the only sign of an infantile cortico-thrombophlebitis may be one limb infinitesimally smaller than its opposite, only detectable by measurement. Other significant signs suggesting symptomatic epilepsy are mental retardation, vascular bruit, naevi, the large head and short neck of arrested hydrocephalus and

Arnold Chiari malformation and, in the fundi, hypertensive changes or papilloedema.

Discussion, management and advice

Only a few patients with epilepsy will need to be admitted to hospital, the majority will be kept under observation, seen by a neurologist at an outpatient clinic and have an EEG (Fig. 19.1); treatment with anticonvulsant drugs will be commenced. Very emphatic advice will be given about taking drugs; the patient must understand that these drugs will not cure epilepsy but will only reduce the incidence of fits. At no time should the patient discontinue or reduce the dosage even though he has been free from attacks for a long time, as missing a few doses may have very serious consequences. It is very easy to forget to take pills regularly and for this reason a system should be worked out so that the patient can check whether or not he has taken his medication (e.g. putting a full day's dose into a separate bottle). Repeat prescriptions should be obtained well in advance to avoid sudden last-minute panic and whenever the patient goes away he should take extra pills with him in case his return is unexpectedly delayed. A medi-

band should always be worn. Patients should be alert to the possibility of a dispensing error and should query any change in size or colour of their tablets. Relatives will be instructed about caring for the patient during a fit and the patient or relatives will be asked to keep a record of the description, frequency and duration of attacks, and also record menstrual periods. Witnessing a fit is distressing and the doctor will give a simple explanation of the nature of the disturbance, its transient effect on the brain and assure relatives that the cry preceding the grand mal attack is involuntary and not a sign of conscious distress and the patient does not suffer during a fit; the patient and his relatives need assurance that repeated attacks will not cause insanity and anticonvulsant drugs are not harmful. Some common-sense advice should be given about regular mealtimes, avoiding long periods of fast, regular hours of sleep, avoiding heights and dangerous machinery, swimming only when accompanied by a competent life-saver, and caution regarding the consumption of alcohol; otherwise the patient should lead a normal life. Laws that exist to protect society, in particular about driving a vehicle on the public highway must be strictly upheld. The patient will be seen at frequent intervals until his fits are under control; after 3 to 6 months another EEG recording will be made.

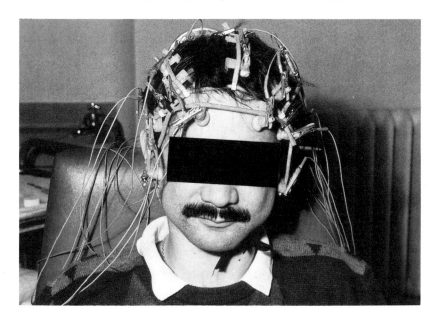

Fig. 19.1 Patient undergoing EEG.

Once the patient and his relatives have had time to get used to the idea of epilepsy, they will have many more questions to ask, will be more aware of the implications as they affect their family and the time will be right for expert medical advice.

The events in epilepsy are so unexpected, so dramatic and used to be so inexplicable, that there has always been a sense of mystery which has led to fear and superstition and, centuries ago was thought to be evidence of demon possession. Unfortunately for the person with epilepsy, who is nearly always physically and mentally quite normal, this leads to gross misunderstanding and can cause much frustration and unhappiness. No one should ever refer to a person with epilepsy as an 'epileptic', which seems to place him immediately outside normal society. Nurses have many opportunities to discuss and engender the right attitude towards epilepsy, when they meet the situation in the community, at outpatient clinics or in hospital. If the patient's relatives adopt these enlightened attitudes including an optimistic outlook and a sense of humour, they will influence a much wider circle of the general public and prevent some of the misconceptions and unfortunate situations which set up the familiar vicious circle of discontent, anxiety, more fits, more drugs and worse situation. The nurse must impress upon parents that their child should lead a normal life, taking part in the same activities as others of the same age with as few restrictions as possible. The child should be treated as a sensible individual and should be responsible for his drugs from as early an age as possible, setting a reliable pattern for the future. When a child is old enough to understand, he should be included in discussions with the doctor or he will feel resentful and suspicious and may become unco-operative, understandably feeling aggrieved that others are arranging his affairs behind his back; it is usually when things go wrong in family communication, that 'private' interviews are felt necessary. Parents should try to discipline all their children in the same consistent way and remember that at a very young age a child will learn to manipulate by using fits as an excuse to avoid any unwanted activity, even inducing an attack by holding his breath or by passing outstretched fingers rapidly across his eyes. There is sometimes difficulty in deciding whether disturbed behaviour is or is not a fit; some parents blame epilepsy for their child's unruly behaviour, others may not understand that such behaviour is the result of abnormal electrical discharges in the brain. The person with epilepsy should never feel he is being watched vigilantly for the occurrence of a fit. Parents have some difficult decisions to make, most parents are sensible and realise that their offspring must branch out on their own, but it must be difficult when they have the responsibility of a child with epilepsy, to know what degree of risk to take and if, at what age and how far, their son or daughter should be allowed to travel without an escort. Obviously parents will have greater peace of mind if the youngster is with a trusted friend, yet if they constantly express anxiety and hem him in with restrictions, that very aggravation will cause more fits.

A fit may be induced by certain visual (photic) and auditory stimuli: watching television, sunlight flickering through trees, lights at a discotheque, hearing a sudden loud noise, certain music or a droning voice giving a lecture. The patient and his relatives will become aware of and try to avoid the particular external influences which will always spark off a fit. Fits caused by the flicker of television can be avoided by viewing in a well-lit room at a good distance from the screen and by using remote control to switch on and off or adjust the set. The adverse effect of sudden flashes of light can be averted by pressing the palm of the hand firmly against one eye. In this light-provoked form of epilepsy the EEG is normal except during an attack.

The whole family are bound to be affected when one member has epilepsy; there are many restraints, anxieties and uncertainties. The anxiety of parents will reflect on the whole household, brothers and sisters may be jealous of extra attention and embarrassed when fits occur in front of their friends. The child with epilepsy may be teased by his contemporaries if he is incontinent, a change of clothing should be available and protective clothing worn if incontinence is a frequent occurrence. Travel can be a problem when there is no public transport nearby and a family will experience unexpected difficulties if the only driver develops epilepsy and loses his driving licence. The doctor will put the family in touch with the medical social worker who has all the information about special schools, assessment and training centres, employment prospects, holidays, life insurance and driving regulations. She will strongly advise them to contact the local branch of the British

Epilepsy Association where they will meet others with similar problems. Through lectures, discussion groups, films and literature, the family will gain information on every aspect of the disorder as well as enjoying the social activities in an atmosphere where they can really 'let their hair down' and it does not matter if the sufferer has a fit. It would be marvellous if everyone had this same understanding acceptance, but it will never be possible to create such a Utopian situation and everyone meets prejudice and problems in life, so someone with the additional hazard of epilepsy must be encouraged to develop a thick skin, branch out from any protected environment and learn to stand up for himself.

Parents may be faced with many environmental problems when they discover their child has epilepsy; they may live in a tenth floor flat, their garden back onto a river, and nearby roads may be heavy with traffic. If they have a choice and can move house, careful consideration should be given to the suitability of the proposed environment, the most ideal being in a locality near shops and schools where the child, known by many people, can go about freely; it will help the mother to know that there are others who are sharing the task of constant unobtrusive supervision. A bungalow may be safer for someone with severe epilepsy, failing that, all upstairs windows must be fitted with safety catches. Bathroom and lavatory doors should open outwards and have locks which, in an emergency, can be operated from outside; the patient should never have a bath unless there is someone in the home. Floor coverings should be soft, for severe head injuries can be sustained by falling on hard quarry tiles; children who have many grand mal fits must wear a protective helmet. A low bed is necessary and furniture should not have sharp corners and edges. Oil heaters should not be used as they may be knocked over, gas fires are dangerous as they do not always automatically ignite. All radiant bar and open fires should be surrounded by a sturdy fire guard, anchored on each side to the wall and set at a safe distance from the source of heat; not only may the person fall on a fire, but if he lies too near for a long period he may get badly scorched. Having taken all these precautions there will always be the unforeseen accident which must be handled with common sense and without reproach.

Schooling and employment

Most children suffering from epilepsy are educated in ordinary schools (about 90%), but a few mentally retarded, possibly also physically handicapped children who suffer from epilepsy need special schooling from the age of 5 years. A few who start normal schooling, but show learning difficulties and disturbed behaviour, will need to transfer to a special school, sometimes for a limited period of adjustment (18 months to 2 years). There must be close liaison between the parents, teachers, school doctor, educational psychologist and careers adviser and at no time should the student be pressured to reach academic levels beyond his abilities. Many finish school with very good examination results and may go on to university. A teenager will need guidance in choosing a suitable career to avoid disappointment, as some careers and professions are either unsuitable or are barred to someone with epilepsy. These youngsters, with the necessary qualifications for a particular job often have their application turned down and may have to accept a less skilled, poorer paid job. Job application forms always include questions about past medical history, a person is often turned down without interview if he is honest and declares his epilepsy or lives in fear of discovery and instant dismissal if he is dishonest. Failure to find employment leads to depression, more fits and even suicide. Though employers are supposed to employ a certain percentage of disabled persons, they would often rather take on someone with a severe physical handicap than someone who is unpredictable, may be an embarrassment and an accident liability; employers do not understand that there are different types of epilepsy and the disorder may be well controlled.

A person who suddenly develops epilepsy may be forced to give up a good job because he can no longer lawfully drive, his work would be too dangerous or because of the prejudiced attitude of his employer. It is difficult to find alternative employment; it may be helpful to be registered as a disabled person. The Disablement Resettlement Officer can recommend, and put in touch, a likely employer or he may suggest application for a government retraining course which will lead to better prospects of gaining suitable employment.

Admission to hospital

Admission to hospital is necessary for the following reasons.

1 To observe the patient and his attacks.
2 For special investigations of epilepsy of late onset and the exclusion of organic disease.
3 For stabilisation of drug therapy when this is not easily achieved as an outpatient.
4 For general review of the patient's life circumstances, education, career and employment.
5 For emergency treatment of status epilepticus.
6 For consideration of possible surgical treatment, e.g. temporal lobectomy.
7 For social reasons.

When the patient is admitted to hospital the accompanying relative should see the doctor to describe the patient's attacks. The incidence and frequency of attacks is important; when were the first and last attacks, how often do the attacks occur and have they changed in frequency or nature? The doctor will try to find out any relationship between the increase or decrease in the number of attacks and events in the patient's life. A clear and detailed account of one typical attack is essential and if there has been more than one type of fit, an account of each; it is helpful if a record of attacks has been kept. Entering hospital is a stressful situation and may even precipitate attacks; a relaxed but stable ward atmosphere is necessary to put everyone at ease, especially important when the patient is a child. It is helpful if the nurse is able to observe the interaction between the patient and his relatives and the behaviour of the relatives when the patient has an attack; relatives may panic, be over-anxious or smother the patient with unwanted attention to relieve their own anxiety. Patients who are already receiving regular anticonvulsant medication should be allowed to take their normal dosage when it is due, rather than wait to be seen by the admitting doctor, as it is unwise to delay medication. The nurse should be prepared from the time of admission to watch the patient unobtrusively, attentively and constantly, and record accurately on a specially designed chart every detail of all attacks.

Generalised epilepsy (involving the whole brain)

Petit mal

Petit mal attacks are a minor form of idiopathic epilepsy in which there are recurrent transient episodes of alteration in consciousness which appear in childhood and either disappear or are later replaced by major epileptic attacks. In an attack the child suddenly stops what he is doing (maybe breaking off in the middle of a sentence), looks pale, flutters his eyelids or blankly gazes into space and his hands may twitch; within seconds normal awareness returns, though sometimes there is momentary delay in picking up the train of thought or action. These attacks are sometimes so brief that they pass unnoticed, but when many occur in quick succession (100 or more a day) they interrupt the child's concentration and will result in learning difficulties at school and underachievement.

Grand mal

Grand mal attacks are a major form of idiopathic or symptomatic epilepsy and are seen when there is a generalised abnormal electrical discharge in the brain with loss of consciousness and a convulsion. A fit may be preceded by depression or tension for several hours and 60% of patients experience a warning (aura) before they lose consciousness. The aura lasts only a few seconds and may be an hallucination of smell, taste, vision or hearing, an emotion such as fear, inability to speak, a curious feeling in the epigastrium or other part of the body or an abnormal movement. The aura becomes familiar to the patient and may indicate the origin of the abnormal discharge in the brain. The tonic phase follows immediately or occurs suddenly without warning; contraction of the muscles of the chest, forcing air through closed vocal cords, may result in an involuntary cry as consciousness is lost, and the patient falls to the ground with all muscles in strong tonic spasm. The spasm is usually symmetrically distributed, but when it is not, the head, eyes or mouth may be drawn to one side; the arms are usually flexed and the legs extended with feet turned inwards. Temporary cessation of respirations and rapid metabolism of oxygen by the tonic muscles causes cyanosis. This tonic phase lasts about 30 seconds and passes into the clonic phase when the whole body jerks violently; there is frothing at the mouth and if the tongue is bitten, the froth is bloodstained; incontinence of urine is common. When the fit is nearing the end, intervals between muscular contractions become longer and finally the patient passes into a flaccid coma. During the clonic phase which lasts for a few minutes, and for a period afterwards, the pupils will be dilated and fixed to light, corneal reflexes and tendon jerks absent and plantar responses extensor. The period of unconsciousness lasts for up to half an hour, may be followed by a short period of automatism or, if undisturbed, the patient may sleep for several hours; on coming round he usually complains of headache, may be a little confused and does not recall the fit.

Frequent grand mal attacks can lead to brain damage through anoxia and repeated head injury; the latter may even lead to intracranial haematoma.

Minor epilepsy

There are other small epileptic events which are not, strictly speaking, petit mal though the interruption in consciousness without convulsion is similar. In these minor attacks which may be idiopathic or symptomatic only a small part of the brain is affected. There may be deviation of the eyes, twitching of the eyelids or other parts of the face, lolling or turning of the head and incontinence of urine. The duration of the fit is slightly longer than that of a petit mal attack and there may be a short period of confusion or odd behaviour (post-epileptic automatism) afterwards, the actions varying according to the part of the brain in which the attack arises. This type of fit may be seen when grand mal epilepsy is only partially controlled by anticonvulsant therapy.

Idiopathic epilepsy follows a recognisable progression:
i   petit mal for several years and then a major fit;
ii a major fit and then major and minor attacks at frequent intervals;
iii major attacks at infrequent intervals.
Approximately one third of those with idiopathic epilepsy have fits at any time during the twenty four hours; for the remainder the attacks occur only in the daytime, or always at night when they are usually associated with falling asleep or waking.

Focal epilepsy (involving part of the brain)

Focal epilepsy is seen when the electrical disturbance in the brain is confined to a specific area, the manifestations are as many as there are functions of the brain. Everyone has experienced the myoclonic jerk of a limb when falling asleep or the twitching of a muscle in the eyelid or corner of the mouth and these feelings are similar to those experienced by a patient with focal epilepsy, except that in epilepsy they are stronger and more persistent. The attack usually starts as a twitching in the parts of the body which have the greatest cortical representation (see Fig. 2.6), the thumb and index finger, corner of the mouth or the big toe. The fit may rapidly spread to adjacent parts of the body as the electrical disturbance spreads in the brain and may become generalised with loss of conscious-

ness. Sensory epilepsy, of which only the patient is aware, is less common and affects those parts which have greater representation in the sensory cortex. Focal epilepsy is often seen when there is localised brain disease; it is important to note which part of the body is first affected as this indicates the origin of the abnormal discharge and the site of the lesion.

Temporal lobe epilepsy (psychomotor epilepsy)

Though this is a focal epilepsy it is almost always idiopathic; to the observer there is often little to suggest epilepsy as many of the symptoms are sensory and behavioural and can easily be confused with psychiatric disorders. Epileptic attacks resulting from an abormal electrical discharge in one or both temporal lobes have curious features concerned with disordered perception and emotion and possibly complex motor disturbance; there may be sensory hallucinations of hearing, indescribable, usually unpleasant, smells and tastes, disordered appreciation of size and distance and unpleasant emotional experiences, for example unnatural feelings of intense fear, depression and depersonalisation. Déjà vu is a well known phenomenon associated with temporal lobe attacks when a person feels that he has lived through a particular experience before. During an attack the patient looks dazed and is unresponsive, but may continue apparently normal activities; following gustatory or olfactory auras chewing movements or smacking of the lips are sometimes seen (uncinate attacks which arise in the uncus of the temporal lobe). The patient sometimes runs off feeling the need to escape or following the directions of his auditory hallucinations, behaving abnormally and becoming very aggressive if thwarted. A momentary period of post-epileptic automatism is common, occasionally lasting for up to an hour; during this time the patient performs actions over which he has no control and later cannot recall, for example undressing in public, shop-lifting or even travelling many miles by car or public transport and 'coming to' in unfamiliar surroundings; he has almost superhuman strength, can lift very heavy objects or, if the need arises, fight off several people bigger than himself and could unknowingly commit a criminal offence. Each patient behaves differently and, in the way that he comes to recognise his aura, he will begin to recognise the results of his actions during the period of automatism. A temporal lobe attack may become a generalised convulsion.

Jacksonian epilepsy

This is a focal symptomatic epilepsy first described by Hughlings Jackson, a London physician, and its characteristic feature is that beginning in one part of the body, it marches on to affect other areas as the spread of electrical disturbance moves across the cortex from its original focus. It often begins with rhythmic twitching of the thumb and index finger of one hand, one corner of the mouth or in the big toe. The progression is then a natural sequence, for example finger to hand, wrist and arm; when there is severe clonic jerking of the whole of one side of the body a major fit becomes likely or the attack peters out. The patient may be fully conscious and frightened during the attack and the nurse must stay with him; in the early stage, if the part which is twitching is grasped firmly, the attack may pass off. There is sometimes residual weakness or paralysis (Todd's paralysis) on the affected side after an attack lasting from a few minutes to several hours.

Sensory epilepsy

When an abnormal electrical discharge occurs in the sensory cortex the patient feels an intermittent numbness or tingling in one part of the body; the spread resembles that of a Jacksonian attack and on reaching the motor cortex may lead to motor symptoms or a grand mal fit.

Epilepsia partialis continua (continuous epilepsy)

A focal lesion in the motor cortex occasionally leads to persistent clonic jerking of a small part of the body, usually flexion of the thumb or one or two fingers, which may persist for days or even months.

Observations during a fit

Observations should be written down immediately. It is possible for a fit to pass unnoticed, especially at night, but sore tongue, headache, damp clothing or bedding and the patient describing feelings in his limbs, similar to the after-effects of cramp, suggest that a fit has occurred.

1   Mode of onset:
i   What was the patient doing when the attack started?
ii   Was there any change in facial colour or expression?
iii Was there any alteration in state of consciousness or disturbed behaviour?
iv   Which part or parts of the body were first affected, were the head or eyes deviated to one side?
v   Did the patient fall to the ground?

2   How did the fit proceed?

3   How long did the attack last?

4   Mode of recovery.

5   Was there incontinence?

6   Was the tongue bitten during the attack?

7   Is there residual weakness of any part?

8   How long was it before the patient fully recovered?

When watching a patient during a fit the nurse must take note of every detail even if it seems irrelevant, as it may help the doctor decide the real nature of the attack and differentiate between epilepsy and the following:

(a) Syncope (faint) – the face is very pale and the patient slumps to the ground; the pulse is feeble and slow and the blood pressure is low.

(b) Anxiety attack – the circumstances leading to an attack may have obviously caused stress and tension; sighing may precede overbreathing, and the patient is flushed, complains of tingling in the arms and face and threshes wildly with his limbs.

(c) Hysterical fit – the attack usually occurs in the presence of onlookers and the patient rarely hurts himself as he falls; there is no tongue biting nor incontinence, the eyelids often flutter during 'unconsciousness' and an attempt to open the eyes is met with resistance, the pupils react to light and the plantar responses are flexor. These signs are in contrast to those seen during an epileptic fit, as are the wild threshing movements and noisy weeping during recovery.

Care of the patient during a fit

Most people have seen someone have a fit, but though 1 in 250 people suffer from epilepsy, it is extremely uncommon to come across this event in the street as most sufferers are well controlled by anticonvulsant medication and do not usually have an attack when they are concentrating on an activity; there are also those whose attacks only occur at night or on waking from sleep. Nonetheless fits can occur in situations which endanger the patient's life, for example on a crowded station platform or in a working situation near machinery or substances like grain or sawdust which can cause suffocation. Fits can also lead to other quite nasty accidents: bruising, lacerations, scalds and burns and a bitten tongue, a painful and common occur-

rence during a grand mal attack. During a fit the patient should be protected from injury, moved away from dangerous objects, prevented from falling, perhaps laid on the floor or steadied in his chair, until the fit passes; over-zealous physical restraint should be avoided as it may cause injury. Tight clothing should be loosened and if there is a denture this should be removed; it is unwise to force anything into the mouth once the jaws are tightly clenched, as this may break a tooth which can then be inhaled. A clear airway must be maintained and as soon as the clonic phase has passed the patient should be turned to the semiprone position with jaw pulled well forward to prevent the tongue obstructing the airway; this position must be maintained until the patient regains consciousness. Clothing and bedding must be changed with as little fuss as possible if the patient has been incontinent. The management of a patient during a temporal lobe attack or in a state of confusion or automatism following a fit is difficult; providing he is not harming himself or anyone else it is best to allow him freedom to wander accompanied until he regains full awareness. In hospital a nurse should accompany the patient to observe him and see that he comes to no harm and does not get lost in unfamiliar surroundings; she may also need to warn other people not to disturb him. It is unwise to restrain him as he may become extremely aggressive; without warning the nurse may suddenly be confronted with a terror-stricken patient whose disturbed brain misinterprets the motives of anyone who tries to restrain him (regardless of uniform or rank which he no longer recognises), and who feels the desperate need to escape. In this frightening situation men fight to survive and women struggle, scream and run away and this is exactly how the patient will behave. Confronting the patient, the nurse should speak to him calmly and with authority and try to gain his co-operation; this approach is sometimes surprisingly effective. Physical restraint and drugs such as diazepam or paraldehyde are occasionally necessary.

Status epilepticus

This dangerous condition, where fit succeeds fit without recovery of consciousness, may last for several hours; without treatment unconsciousness deepens and anoxia and hyperpyrexia cause irreparable brain damage, heart failure and death. The relatives must know of this risk, should contact the doctor if several fits occur in quick succession and should administer rectal diazepam which they keep stored for emergency use.

Those suffering from epilepsy risk status epilepticus if their medication is stopped suddenly, particularly if treatment is with barbiturates, or if their epilepsy is poorly controlled; nurses must notice and report to the doctor, any patient who has several fits within a few hours. Patients with frontal lobe lesions may develop status epilepticus with their first fit and those with subdural abscess are liable to almost uncontrollable status epilepticus. Every effort must be made to prevent the occurrence of this condition as it is difficult to control, can cause irreversible brain damage from hypoxia and may be fatal.

Prompt action is essential; the doctor must be notified immediately if a fit continues beyond the acceptable time or if, after a brief respite, it starts again. Arrangements are made for the patient to be nursed in the intensive therapy unit or 'specialled' on the ward by a trained nurse; resuscitation, suction and monitoring equipment must be avaiable and a continuous EEG record will be commenced. An intravenous infusion is set up to administer diazepam for the control of fits; intramuscular paraldehyde is a non-toxic drug which does not depress respiration and is still very useful for the treatment of status epilepticus in adults and especially in children. Should these medications fail to control fits it may become necessary to administer a muscle relaxant (tubocurarine) and maintain ventilation with a positive pressure ventilator to prevent anoxia and muscular exhaustion. It is usually necessary for a tracheostomy (using a cuffed tube) to be performed as endotracheal intubation is difficult. Anticonvulsant measures will be continued until the EEG shows that the fits are under control, then the patient's normal anticonvulsant drugs will be reintroduced, possibly in higher than usual doses or introducing or substituting another drug. The relatives must be notified that the patient is critically ill.

Care and observation of the patient is as for the unconscious patient using a ventilator – described in Chapter 3. Accurate records must be kept of each type of fit, their frequency and all drugs administered. Neurological assessment is of little value during the critical phase, as the patient's pupils will be dilated and fixed and stimulating his limbs is best avoided as it may trigger a fit. When status epilepticus is controlled the patient's level of consciousness should lighten; if it does not, the condition may be symptomatic of brain damage from anoxia or the underlying condition, for example tumour or subdural abscess. Nursing care should be given with as little disturbance as possible by using monitoring equipment for temperature, pulse and blood pressure and resisting the temptation to perform non-essential nursing duties, for example a blanket bath can wait until tomorrow. There will be an increase in body temperature due to continuous excessive muscular activity during the fits; hyperpyrexia is due to hypothalamic damage and measures should be taken to reduce the patient's temperature as soon as it starts to rise (see p. 88).

Identifying the cause and type of epilepsy

The diagnosis of epilepsy is made when other causes of paroxysmal disturbance of cerebral function have been excluded, the cause of epilepsy established or a characteristic abnormality is seen on an EEG; there then remains the question, is there a causal lesion and what treatment should be recommended?

Symptomatic epilepsy

Symptomatic epilepsy usually occurs in adult life and any patient who has his first fit after the age of 20 years should be investigated thoroughly in case he has a tumour or other treatable condition; in many patients no cause can be found.

Causes of symptomatic epilepsy

1 Local disease of the brain.
i Neoplasia
ii Head injuries – fits may occur following head injury, but a person subject to idiopathic epilepsy may sustain a head injury because he had a fit
iii Following supratentorial surgery
iv Congenital abnormalities
v Vascular disease
vi Infective disease
vii Degenerative disease
viii Parasitic infestation

2 General causes

i Metabolic and endocrine disease

ii Cardio-respiratory disorders which cause cerebral anoxia

iii Alcoholic intoxication

iv Barbiturate withdrawal

v Drugs and poisons

vi Fever

vii Toxaemia of pregnancy

Investigations

1 Electroencephalogram (EEG, see Chapter 2). Since 1929 when Hans Berger, a German physician, discovered a method of recording the brain's electrical activity, the subject of epilepsy has been better understood. It has been shown that attacks are related to abnormal electrical activity in the cortical cells possibly arising from the brain stem; an EEG is the most important investigation in the diagnosis of epilepsy. Certain sedative and tranquillising medications, which might disguise an abnormality in the record, will, on the instructions of the medical officer, be withheld before the EEG. When there is an abnormality it may be seen even when the patient is not having a fit; an abnormal electroencephalogram is sometimes found where there is no history of any kind of fit, and a normal recording can be found when fits are known to have occurred.

EEG telemetry

For many years after the discovery of electroencephalography arrangements were made to perform this test on a particular occasion in a specially adapted room or the record was taken in the ward. It was a matter of chance if the record coincided with the occurrence of a fit and sometimes measures were even taken to stimulate a fit by giving certain drugs, showing flickering lights or other stimulus. There were obvious limitations in the usefulness of this record which was taken under abnormal conditions and for a short period during daytime. Observation of the patient even in hospital could never be constant nor could the patient necessarily record every attack or remember the circumstances when an attack occurred, especially in the case of a child, confused or mentally retarded patient.

With the development of small, sophisticated electronic devices has come progress in electroencephalographic monitoring. Several methods are in use which enable the patient to be monitored for 24 hour periods while continuing normal activities in the ward or in some instances during prolonged periods at home, in school, at work, resting, sleeping, jogging or walking. The methods give a very accurate record with minimal artefact, pick up even very minor attacks which would otherwise be missed and in every instance there is absolute timing accuracy. Apparatus is light and convenient to wear, the miniature pre-amplifiers being easily hidden in the hair and the record box worn round the waist or hung on the shoulder. Replay can be interpreted quickly and records are helpful in diagnosis, differentiating between physical and psychological attacks and assessing the effect of different drugs.

The Oxford monitor using a cassette player records the EEG on the tape which can be transferred to paper. After 24 hours tapes, batteries and electrodes need changing.

Video telemetry using audio hi-fi 4-hour tapes can be used while the patient is in hospital. The screen is divided in two halves: one half shows the patient as he moves naturally about the ward pursuing normal activities and the other shows the EEG recording. When an attack occurs, either the patient, a relative or nurse, presses an alarm button. To review the record the doctor simply presses a key and the relevant section of telemetry can be scanned. Nurses are taught how to overcome small technical difficulties with either system of monitoring to prevent a hitch in the recording at night-time or during weekends.

A child suffering from petit mal can wear two hidden electrodes connected to a lapel badge which lights up or buzzes when an attack occurs. This is helpful at school, giving the teacher a guide to her expectations of the pupil's attention and consequent comprehension, and she can, if necessary, repeat an instruction.

2 Skull and chest X-rays

3 Computerised axial tomography

4 Cerebral angiography

5 Serological tests for syphilis

6 Psychometry to assess the patient's intellectual capacity

7 Psychiatric interviews

8 Other investigations to exclude systemic disorders which cause loss of consciousness or convulsions:

i   electrocardiography to exclude heart block

ii   blood sugar tests for diabetes and to exclude tumour of the islet cells of Langerhans

iii liver function tests

iv   renal function tests

v   X-rays of the muscles when cysticercosis is suspected

Treatment

The aims of treatment, once epilepsy is diagnosed, are to discover any treatable organic cause, control epileptic attacks with anticonvulsant medications and help the individual and his family to take life and its many problems in their stride. Although one wishes to convey the attitude that epilepsy is largely of 'nuisance value', the problems that it creates should not be minimised.

Anticonvulsant therapy will only be a successful form of treatment if the patient takes his prescribed drugs regularly; when someone is admitted to hospital because he is having more attacks the first thoughts are, is it because he has been negligent about taking his drugs or are there increased stresses in his life? Would another anticonvulsant drug or combination of anticonvulsant drugs suit him better or is there any underlying cause, organic or psychological, which has not been revealed? The period of late teens to early twenties is a time of upheaval with concern about adult responsibilities, breaking away from home, settling into employment, tangled love-life and marriage. What is on his mind? Admission to hospital is of mixed benefit and disadvantage; it is a time which is useful for investigations and interviews and here it is possible to get to know the patient and his relatives better than in a brief out-patient interview, but it is an artificial environment where the patient is removed from the sources of his normal tensions. In hospital it is possible to ensure that he takes his medications regularly, though he may deliberately hide them and induce more fits to prolong his stay in hospital and show the staff how really impossible life has become for him. Sometimes when the patient escapes from his tense home environment and is relieved of the ordinary day to day stresses and

anxieties, his fits temporarily cease. A week is not long enough to get to know and understand the patient's problems or observe the effect of a change of anticonvulsant and it is usual for the patient to be in hospital for 3 to 4 weeks. It would be a useless exercise to admit this healthy patient to hospital and allow him to spend the days idling on his bed, so a full programme of activities must be arranged with the help of the occupational therapist; these should include time spent at a rehabilitation centre, on escorted outings and weekends at home. Whenever the patient leaves the ward he must take medications with him, he will always be accompanied and whoever is with him on these occasions must see that he takes his medication when it is due and should be well acquainted with the variety of symptoms that occur with epilepsy and report any episodes accurately to the ward staff.

Anticonvulsant therapy

It has been found that certain drugs diminish or abolish the incidence of epileptic attacks; their action is partly sedative and partly one of protecting the cortical cells from the influence of abnormal electrical discharges. The principles of treatment with drugs are very important; the dosage is adjusted according to the patient's requirements, considering his weight, response to the drugs and the time of day when he usually has his attacks. The regime of drug treatment is carefully considered by the doctor and should then be continued for a reasonable period of time (6 to 8 weeks) before the situation is reviewed. Frequent chopping and changing of drugs and polypharmacy are avoided and the patient and his relatives must bear with this trial period. Satisfactory control may mean that it is preferable for the patient to have an occasional attack rather than have such heavy sedation that he cannot continue his normal life. Medications must be taken regularly at the appointed time, usually for the rest of the patient's life. When drugs are changed this is done gradually over a period of days, slowly withdrawing the original drug as the new is introduced. Sudden changes or withdrawal of drugs may lead to an increase in the number of attacks or even to status epilepticus and the patient must understand the very great risks involved in not taking the medication as prescribed. A relative will be responsible for the administration of drugs to a young child or to an adult if he cannot be responsible for them himself. Prophylactic anticonvulsant drugs may be prescribed for at least two years for certain patients who have sustained head injury, have had excision of a frontal space-occupying lesion (tumour or abscess) or who have had a postoperative fit. Treatment should not be discontinued unless the patient has been free of attacks and only then, gradually and with extreme caution under medical supervision.

In spite of extensive research there is no drug which completely controls all forms of epilepsy, suits every patient and has no side-effects. There are still many different drugs used in the treatment of epilepsy and if a patient is well controlled it would be unwise, in many instances, to experiment with a new drug, particularly if the patient has sucessfully completed the statutory 3 year period needed for a driving licence and is dependent upon driving a car for his livelihood (sufferers from epilepsy are permanently banned from driving heavy goods and public transport vehicles).

Sodium valproate (Epilim) is an effective drug, now widely used in all forms of epilepsy, with few side-effects and a less sedative action than other commonly used anticonvulsant drugs. Epilim may cause gastric irritation and should be taken after meals; it is absorbed very rapidly from the stomach and is excreted by the kidneys within 24 hours; it may give a false positive when testing urine for ketones and this should be considered in treating diabetes.

Phenobarbitone is a particularly useful drug for the control of grand mal epilepsy; it sometimes causes drowsiness and a sensitivity rash and can cause irritability and behaviour disorders in children.

Phenytoin sodium (Epanutin) is still one of the most used and effective of anticonvulsant drugs for the treatment of grand mal and temporal lobe epilepsy. Administration of large doses of phenytoin or prolonged use may cause slurred speech, ataxia and nystagmus; sensitivity rash, hirsutism and hyperplasia of the gums are fairly common. High doses of phenytoin sodium produce unpleasant side-effects and it is usual to give lower dosage combined with phenobarbitone which provides the sedative action that phenytoin lacks. It may be necessary to give phenytoin suspension to mentally retarded patients and children who have difficulty swallowing. Care must be taken to shake the bottle well as the drug does not stay in suspension and settles to the bottom of the bottle. *Primidone (Mysoline)* is sometimes used to control grand mal and temporal lobe epilepsy; it should never be used in conjunction with phenobarbitone as it is broken down by the body into more phenobarbitone.

Carbamazepine (Tegretol) is used for grand mal and temporal lobe epilepsy; the dosage is gradually introduced to a suitable level. Regular white cell counts are advised as leucopenia and aplastic anaemia have been reported with this drug.

Sulthiame (Ospolot) is effective in the treatment of temporal lobe epilepsy, but it may cause confusion, retardation, paraesthesiae and dyspnoea in the early days of treatment.

Diazepam (Valium). As it is so valuable for the treatment of status epilepticus it is not usually used in the routine treatment of epilepsy.

There are so many drugs used in the treatment of epilepsy that only a few are mentioned above. Alcohol enhances the effect of most of the anticonvulsant drugs and should be taken cautiously; patients will discover for themselves their safe tolerance level.

Drugs used in the treatment of petit mal
Epilim is the first choice of drug in the treatment of petit mal epilepsy as the drugs previously used, troxidone and others of the dione group and ethosuximide (Zarontin), caused blood dyscrasias and sometimes photophobia.

Pregnancy and anticonvulsant drugs
Research into the effect of drugs on foetal development has been difficult and most drugs are contraindicated in pregnancy especially during the first three months, including all anticonvulsants. There is a slightly higher incidence of foetal abnormality and stillbirths in women receiving anticonvulsant medication and this risk should be explained to them when they plan to have a child, but no woman with epilepsy should be denied motherhood. Some anticonvulsants are safer than others and when pregnancy is planned the patient should consult her doctor to discuss the suitability of her existing medication so that any necessary change can be made.

Surgical treatment

Anterior temporal lobectomy

Occasionally an EEG demonstrates a definite focus in the anterior part of one temporal lobe, and if the epilepsy cannot be controlled with drugs an anterior temporal lobectomy will be considered. The operation is less successful than the apparent cause and effect would suggest, but often brings about some improvement; unfortunately, once one temporal lobe has been partially removed the other which may have been dormant, sometimes becomes a focus for abnormal electrical discharges and the epilepsy persists. It is never possible for a patient to have bilateral anterior temporal lobectomy as it has been found to lead to profound behaviour disorders. During the operation the discharging focus is found by electrocorticography of the exposed brain; the surgeon then removes the focus destroying as little healthy brain tissue as possible, taking care not to encroach on the speech areas. Anticonvulsant drugs are continued indefinitely after this operation because of the risk of recurring epilepsy and the potential epileptic focus of scar tissue caused by an operation on the brain.

Hemispherectomy

This very rare procedure is performed if a child has severe grand mal epilepsy caused by an atrophied cerebral hemisphere. As the part of the brain removed is so abnormal and the child already hemiplegic, he can recover surprisingly well after this drastic operation and his epilepsy will be improved.

Long term management

Epilepsy is a life-long condition which changes with age and circumstances; anticonvulsant drug dosage is related to the patient's growth, age and type of attacks and needs to be reviewed from time to time. Unfortunately the only real indication that drugs need to be increased or changed is an increase in the number of the patient's fits. The patient must have regular medical supervision; the medical adviser needs wisdom and understanding and in the light of past experience can often foresee problems before they arise. For example knowing the family, he will know the worriers, the stoics, the martyrs and the flappers and will handle them accordingly; who after all is the normal patient or the normal family?

The general practitioner is able to put the patient in touch with the social worker and other departments of the District Health Authority as the need arises. He will also be called upon at various times for progress reports and to give his opinion about the patient's medical condition to school, prospective employer, vehicle licensing authority or to an insurance company; these occasions will be opportunities for him to keep in touch with his patient.

A very small number of individuals with severe epilepsy will continue to need a protected environment when they leave their special school; generally it is unfair to leave them to vegetate in their own home without gainful employment and where they are a burden to their family. There are Centres for Epilepsy (originally called 'colonies') where people can live in agreeable accommodation and work either for the benefit of their community or on contract work while receiving a salary commensurate with their job. Their social life, outings and holidays are arranged within the community aided by outside voluntary helpers. Though living away from home, they should keep in touch with their family.

Epilepsy is such a common neurological disorder from which anyone could suffer that it should be well understood; if the nurse could only put herself in the position of the patient she would have no difficulty in seeing his problems. He must be allowed to develop his full potential in spite of interrupted schooling, difficulty in finding employment, being barred from certain chosen professions and careers and not being able to drive or participate in some sporting activities; he must put his epilepsy behind him, lead a normal life and should not be denied the opportunities of marriage and parenthood.

Narcolepsy and cataplexy

Narcolepsy is a term used to describe a rare condition in which a person repeatedly falls asleep at inappropriate times without feeling tired or intending to do so; he can be roused as from sleep. The episodes may occur several times a day, are more common in the afternoon, after a meal or when the person is engaged in a monotonous occupation. Usually no cause can be found, but rarely the condition may be associated with a lesion in the region of the third ventricle. During an attack the EEG has a characteristic sleep rhythm with random slow waves, but at other times it is normal. Occasionally narcolepsy may be the only manifestation of an epileptic focus and there is a condition of recurring hallucinations associated with third ventricle and hypothalamic lesions.

Cataplexy is a condition sometimes associated with narcolepsy in which the patient, without loss of consciousness, loses all power of movement and posture; strong emotion and laughter lead to an episode when the person either feels weak and sags at the knees or falls limply to the ground with eyes closed usually recovering within a minute.

Amphetamine gives symptomatic relief for narcolepsy and cataplexy and may be given in spansule form; it should not be given late in the day or night-time sleep will be disturbed. A patient with either of these conditions should be treated sympathetically as, though the symptoms appear amusing in some circumstances, they are an embarrassment and an inconvenience; the patient must take care not to endanger himself or others. Attacks may continue indefinitely or inexplicably stop.

20

Extrapyramidal Disorders

There is a group of motor disorders which are the result of disturbance in the extrapyramidal system, a system responsible for maintaining normal muscle tone, posture and movement (see p. 21), which is closely linked with the pyramidal and cerebellar systems, and, through the thalamus, with incoming sensory information. The basal ganglia (Fig. 20.1), the nuclei of the extrapyramidal system, lie deep within the cerebral hemispheres and are grouped together on either side of the third ventricle surrounding the internal capsule and close to the brain stem. They are interconnected and exert an inhibitory action on each other, if one or more are damaged the others overact and it is not always possible to attribute a disorder to a particular structure. The ganglia from one cerebral hemisphere control the opposite side of the body and their fibres connect with the cerebellum and the lower motor neurones in the spinal cord.

There are many factors which influence the function of the basal ganglia:

1   Ischaemia, commonly caused by arteriosclerosis.
2   Degeneration which may be selective or associated with widespread cerebral atrophy.
3   Toxic substances
i   Drugs of the phenothiazine group especially in high doses, e.g. chlorpromazine and promazine.
ii   Copper, as in Wilson's disease; manganese and mercury ingested during industrial processes.
iii   Carbon monoxide.
4   The delayed effect of intracranial infection, notably encephalitis lethargica; there were several epidemics of this disease between 1916 and 1926.
5   Genetic factors – Huntington's chorea and Wilson's disease.
6   Intracranial tumours which directly compress the basal ganglia or cause compression by obstructing the ventricular system.

(a)

(b)

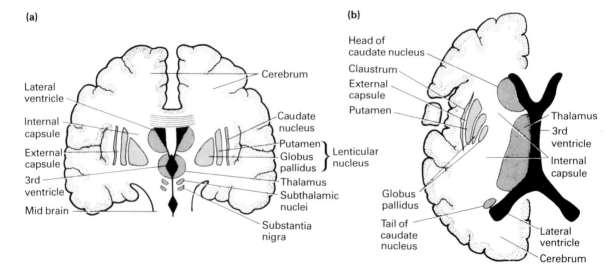

Fig. 20.1   The basal ganglia. (a) Coronal section of basal ganglia. (b) Horizontal section of basal ganglia.

Parkinson's syndrome

There is a group of symptoms often referred to as Parkinson's disease which is due to either an unknown cause, a sequel to encephalitis lethargica, associated with arteriosclerosis or induced by certain drugs. This syndrome, the commonest manifestation of basal ganglia disorder, was first described by James Parkinson, a London doctor, in 1817. He stated that the disease consisted of 'an involuntary tremulous motion, with lessened muscular power, in parts not in action and even when supported; with a propensity to bend the trunk forwards and to pass from a walking to a running pace, the senses and intellects being uninjured'. The clarity and accuracy of this description of idiopathic Parkinsonism (paralysis agitans) has not been surpassed. The cause of Parkinson's disease is now known to be degeneration of the substantia nigra, areas of grey cells in the cerebral peduncles, deep in the brain where the cerebrum joins the mid-brain. Paralysis agitans affects men more than women, usually occurring between the ages of 50 and 70 and having a slowly progressive disabling course, without shortening the normal life span. Post-encephalitic Parkinsonism appears at a younger age than arteriosclerotic Parkinsonism; in these two forms there are other symptoms not seen in paralysis agitans but there is the same progressive deterioration. Symptoms of Parkinsonism, induced by high doses of phenothiazine drugs for the treatment of mental illness (e.g. chlorpromazine), usually disappear when the drugs are withdrawn, though there is a danger of persistent involuntary movement.

The main features of Parkinson's disease are rigidity, difficulty in initiating and persisting in voluntary actions (bradykinesia) and tremor, which often affect the limbs on one side 2–3 years before the other. Rigidity causes gradual slowing up and loss of natural automatic movement (synergic movement, blinking or swinging the arms when walking); the coarse tremor is seen when the limbs are at rest, it disappears during voluntary movement and sleep. Complaints of cramp, aching muscles, a tendency to fall, difficulty in writing legibly are early symptoms which may not indicate the diagnosis as clearly as an obvious tremor. Though the rigidity and bradykinesia are the more disabling factors, it is usually the tremor which causes the patient most consternation and embarrassment. At first he and his immediate family may not notice subtle changes in his appearance, although the patient may subconsciously try to conceal a tremor by keeping his hand in his pocket; when he is seen by someone with knowledge of the disorder it may be obvious that the patient lacks facial expression, has an exceptionally quiet voice and difficulty in 'getting going', especially when getting up from a chair. Those whose occupation demands skills involving fine movement or clear speech (e.g., school teacher, dressmaker, precision engineer) will become aware of their disability early and will seek advice sooner than someone doing heavy manual work. The disease is often diagnosed by the general practitioner who himself prescribes treatment or refers the patient to a general physician or neurologist.

History and examination

The signs and symptoms of advanced Parkinson's disease are so characteristic that they are seen at a glance. The patient has a mask-like expression with unblinking stare, stooping posture with arms flexed close to the body, shuffling gait with small steps and a tendency to break into a run (festinating gait); his posture upsets his centre of gravity and he will either be suddenly propelled forwards or if he is off balance, start running backwards. There is commonly hesitation at the threshold of a doorway and difficulty in negotiating the way between obstacles even when there seems to be plenty of room. The patient has difficulty coming to a halt and when he stops, difficulty setting off again as though he were rooted to the ground; a deliberate effort of will is necessary to initiate all activities. When the affected hand is at rest a coarse rotational tremor with a pill rolling movement of the thumb and index finger is seen (Fig. 20.2); there may be an obvious tremor of the lower jaw and tongue and drooling of saliva. The patient's speech is quiet, monotonous, rapid, dysarthric and difficult to understand, though by leaning close with attentive concentration it is possible to 'tune in' and avoid letting relatives speak for the patient. Handwriting becomes very small, even illegible. An outward appearance of stupidity and dullness is

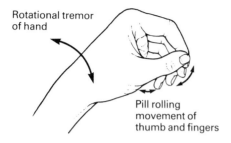

Rotational tremor of hand

Pill rolling movement of thumb and fingers

Fig. 20.2 Characteristic hand movements in Parkinson's disease.

misleading, as most patients with Parkinson's disease are mentally normal. The patient will be asked to give an account of his illness and will be closely questioned about his previous health.

1 Has he had an influenza-like illness in the past, with excessive sleepiness in the daytime and wakefulness at night (encephalitis lethargica); when did this illness occur? The symptoms of Parkinsonism caused by encephalitis lethargica develop 2–3 years after the illness.

2 Is there a history suggesting circulatory disorder?

3 Is the patient taking medication?

4 Has anyone else in the family had a similar disorder?

5 When did the first symptoms appear and what course has it followed?

6 What is his occupation and has he continued his usual employment or been forced by his disability to change his job or take early retirement?

7 Does the patient go out alone and manage his own shopping?

8 Is there any tendency to fall?

9 Has he any particular difficulties, e.g. in writing, doing up buttons, turning in bed or swallowing?

10 Does the patient require help with the activities of daily living and who is at home to help him?

11 Are his memory and concentration good?

12 Does he sleep well?

13 Has he received any previous treatment (physiotherapy or medication) for the disease?

14 Has there been personality change and is the patient emotionally labile or depressed?

(These questions are directed to the relatives in the patient's absence.)

A general and neurological examination is performed (see Chapter 2). The doctor and nurse, by their friendly approach, must try to allay the patient's natural anxiety about not being understood otherwise he will become agitated, making his speech less intelligible and affecting his ability to perform the physical tests of the examination. The patient's general health is usually good, his blood pressure normal but he is thin due to the constant muscular activity of tremor. The examination will reveal facial rigidity and tremor, jerky eye movements and tremor of closed eyelids; there is persistent involuntary blinking in response to repeated tapping of the centre of the forehead (a positive glabellar tap). There will be lead pipe (smooth) or cogwheel (jerky) rigidity in all limbs, worst in those first affected. Tremor affects the head, jaw, tongue and limbs and at a very advanced stage of the disease the whole patient may shake. All muscles are slightly weak and there is difficulty in performing repetitive or rapidly alternating movements (dysdiadochokinesis); reflex responses are usually normal.

In post-encephalitic Parkinsonism other symptoms are found: there is excessive salivation, the patient sweats profusely and has a greasy skin which may cause seborrhoea of the scalp; flexion deformities of the trunk and limbs may develop, most marked in the neck, hands and feet; the patient may lose his train of thought in the middle of a conversation (thought block) and there may be a history of oculogyric crises when the eyes have become fixed in an upward gaze for minutes or possibly hours (the pupils and iris almost disappear).

When Parkinson's disease is caused by arteriosclerosis there is evidence of widespread degeneration in the central nervous system (see Chapter 9) and the rigidity is much more marked. There is a very shuffling gait, memory loss, emotional lability and possibly incontinence; the reflexes of all limbs are increased, the plantar responses are extensor and a jaw jerk may be elicited.

Investigations

The diagnosis of Parkinson's disease is usually made on the clinical evidence, but certain routine tests are performed to make sure that the patient is in good general health, as the symtoms of Parkinsonism are aggravated by anaemia and chronic infection.

(a) A full blood count, sedimentation rate, blood urea and Wassermann and Kahn.

(b) Chest X-ray.

(c) Urinalysis and laboratory examination of urine for organisms.

(d) A CAT scan may be performed if there is any doubt about the cause of the disorder, e.g. Parkinsonian symptoms may accompany certain cerebral tumours.

(e) Psychometry will assess the patient's memory, concentration, grasp, intelligence and mood.

(f) A PET (positron emission tomograph scan will clearly demonstrate the substantia nigra.

Treatment

There is no curative treatment for Parkinson's disease; treatment began in Dr Parkinson's time with blood letting and intravenous injections of pure old oil of turpentine and continued with preparations from solanaceous plants, for example atropa belladonna (deadly nightshade) in about 1874, to extracts of belladonna and pure alkaloids of atropine and hyoscine and more recently to synthetic preparations. In the early 1970's there was a breakthrough in the treatment of Parkinson's disease due to the discovery that the cells of the basal ganglia which regulate extrapyramidal function are controlled by two balanced but opposing chemical systems: cholinergic and dopaminergic (Fig. 20.3). In Parkinson's disease for some unknown reason there is depletion of dopamine. Treatment is aimed at restoring the balance between these two chemical systems, preferably by replacing the one which is deficient, but dopamine does not penetrate the blood-brain barrier. A drug, levodopa, was found which could be converted into dopamine in the basal ganglia. Unfortunately levodopa is taken up by the liver, kidneys and intestine and unless it is administered in very large but toxic doses, insufficient reaches the basal ganglia. To inhibit the conversion of levodopa by these organs and free it for use in the basal ganglia, carbidopa was developed; Sinemet is a combination of levo-

dopa and carbidopa in the right proportions. This treatment has improved the outlook for those with Parkinsonism, enabling them to retain their mobility and independence for a longer period; 70–80% of sufferers are greatly helped as, though tremor persists, the most disabling features of the disorder, rigidity and bradykinesia, are improved. The results for some patients are astounding, releasing previously severely disabled housebound patients from their imprisonment and enabling them to resume normal activities. Even patients with quite severe symptoms are given a trial of levodopa as many benefit, though there are some whose basal ganglia are so damaged that the drug cannot be taken up or converted into dopamine.

The drug is introduced gradually over a period of three weeks until the patient is taking the recommended maximum dosage divided into 4 or 5 doses through the day, taken at times which best suit the individual's needs. There are unpleasant side-effects; gastric irritation with anorexia and nausea – the patient should be advised to take the tablets with food; postural hypotension is helped if the patient gets up slowly from the lying or sitting position, but hypotension may be so severe that the

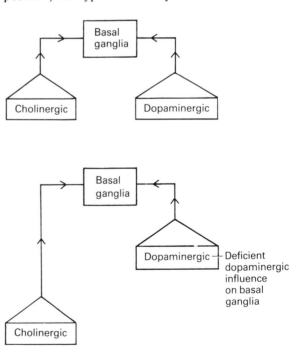

Fig. 20.3 Chemical influence on basal ganglia. **(a)** Normal, balanced influence. **(b)** Imbalance of chemical influence in Parkinson's disease.

drug has to be discontinued. Other side-effects include involuntary movements of face, neck and limbs, mental agitation, hallucinations and sexual overactivity.

There are a small number of patients who cannot tolerate levodopa at all or who can only take a low, less effective dosage; these patients are treated with anticholinergic drugs which dampen down the overactive cholinergic system allowing the existing, though deficient, dopaminergic system to be more effective. Anticholinergic therapy has been in use for many years and includes:

i   orphenadrine hydrochloride (Disipal)
ii   benzhexol hydrochloride (Artane)
iii procyclidine hydrochloride (Kemadrin)
iv   benztropine sulphonate (Cogentin)

The best dosage for the patient is often verging on toxicity and the side-effects of excessive dryness of the mouth, blurred vision and constipation are unpleasant, sudden withdrawal may cause a Parkinsonian crisis.

Medication must be taken for the rest of the patient's life; elderly patients are notoriously unreliable about taking their tablets regularly and they must be encouraged to devise a system to avoid missing a dose.

Stereotaxic surgery

For many years operations have been tried in an attempt to abolish the symptoms of Parkinson's disease; early operations were very hazardous and the results disappointing. In 1949 a stereo-encephalotome was developed which enabled the surgeon to reach a selected target deep within the brain with a guided probe passed through a burr hole. In basal ganglia disorders the target was the thalamus, part of which was coagulated by heat or destroyed by freezing. Stereotaxic surgery for the treatment of Parkinsonism has been superseded by levodopa therapy.

General management

Those with Parkinsonism are too inclined to sit at home all day and the less they do, the less they will want to do. It is most important that someone with this condition continues all normal activities and even when he has some slight illness, he should not lie about in bed for longer than absolutely necessary. A retired person should stick to a fairly rigid routine of getting up and dressed at a set time and going out each day, for example to buy the newspaper, visit the 'local', walk the dog. He should have regular meals and be encouraged to participate in outside social activities; there are day centres, social clubs for the over sixties and in some areas the Parkinson's Disease Association. A person who lives alone, unless he has good reason to go out, is likely to sit about, not eat properly and become depressed. Relatives must appreciate the need for the patient to keep as active as possible and should be discouraged from waiting on him hand and foot which is a natural inclination. They are emotionally involved with the patient and may smother him with kindness and help for, 'it is so difficult for him to do things and he is so slow if I let him do it himself'; the patient with Parkinson's disease often lacks drive and initiative. It must be remembered that his spouse may be equally elderly and any nursing duties will be a physical drain. A careful appraisal of home circumstances should be made as the introduction of a few simple devices may enable the patient to remain in his own home with his life-long partner, and prevent the loneliness and depression each will experience if the patient has to be admitted to hospital or nursing home. One tiresome aspect of the disease is the difficulty experienced in getting up from a chair, the patient is usually able to do so given time and the right equipment.

Occasionally a short burst of physiotherapy may be enough to put the patient back on his feet; this may be arranged as an out-patient visit to the physiotherapy department or be incorporated with occupational therapy in the programme of activities arranged by a hospital day centre. The social worker and occupational therapist will visit the patient's home and suggest ways and means of overcoming problems and arrange with the family a convenient time for the work to be done. Handrails are essential especially in the toilet and bathroom, raised or 'ejector type' toilet seats will help the patient to be independent with his personal toilet; a high-seated geriatric or rocking chair and a bed at chair height may be all that is needed to enable the patient to rise from chair or bed. Well meaning helpers, feeling the need to be in control of the situation and in a position to prevent a fall, prefer to take the patient's arm, but if the helper grabs the patient under an arm and hauls him to his feet, the patient may panic and be thrown off balance, his weight even toppling both of them to the ground; usually all that is needed is to offer the patient an arm.

Reasons for admission to hospital

1 To introduce a change in medication under close supervision especially if the patient has experienced side-effects.
2 For a complete review of medication including night sedation and treatment for depression, for active rehabilitation and attention to home circumstances.
3 To give the patient's relatives a rest.
4 For geriatric and terminal care.

Admission to hospital

The patient with Parkinson's disease, when admitted to hospital, may be moderately or severely disabled, he may have been sitting at home depressed, inactive and unable to take his pills, or may be emaciated, dehydrated, unable to speak coherently, with such complications as pneumonia or pressure sores. The nurse should always address the patient first, though she may be dependent upon the relatives for information; sometimes she may need to courteously dissuade the relatives from 'taking over' but she must be especially patient with elderly relatives who, having acted nurse-maid for so long, may appear unduly fussy, as to whether the patient 'wears a woolly vest or bed socks' and when he will require his 'laxative'.

Though a patient has Parkinson's disease, he is an individual who needs understanding; he bears stigmas that rob him of individuality, cause him embarrassment when he can no longer attend to his personal needs and cut him off from society because of his appearance and failure to communicate. Loss of the ability to speak coherently isolates the patient from intelligent discussion and even his relatives who can understand him better may have come to talk to him on a level that demands only brief answers. Not only is his communication limited through lack of speech, but he cannot give the normal smile of greeting and though he may be a humorous person his sense of humour cannot be expressed; this gives those he meets the wrong impression that he is 'an unfriendly misery who doesn't want to know them'. It is quite understandable too if the patients gets irritable when after repeating himself several times, and unable even to write down his wishes, the listener still does not understand. Shut into his inactive bodily shell, his active mind has nothing better to do than churn over his lost powers and worry about the future.

The patient will be seen and examined by the doctor; the nursing staff who are with the patient for much of the day will observe him unobtrusively and will report on his condition, whether he is quiet and withdrawn from social contact in the ward, how much stimulation and help he needs in normal activities, if he finds his way about the ward, is forgetful of recent events or is incontinent. The nursing staff should also notice if the patient's family visit him regularly and make a point of talking to patient and relatives together and in so doing, communicate a right attitude to disablement.

The mere change of environment for a housebound or elderly disabled person often brings a marked improvement in his spirits and general well-being, which becomes apparent after two to three days. At first, in unfamiliar surroundings with different routine and among strangers, tremor, gait and sleep rhythm may be worse than when the patient was at home; sometimes he shows a reverse pattern, maintaining a stoical front for a day or two and then suddenly releasing all his pent up anxieties revealing his depression. Anxiety, agitation and depression may cause a sudden deterioration. Any sudden deterioration is not due to the disease but to some other cause, even what may appear a relatively simple problem to nursing staff, for example constipation, may be a crisis to the patient of such magnitude that it robs him of his ability to walk.

Rehabilitation

The patient should be up and about and get dressed each day. He should be introduced to the occupational therapist and physiotherapist as soon as possible so that they can make a preliminary assessment of his difficulties and with the help and close co-operation of the nursing staff, take steps to overcome them. Everyone must know what the patient can do and the circumstances when help may be needed. Clothing needs to be light and warm using velcro fastenings whenever possible; sensible low solid-heeled shoes should always be worn for walking indoors and outdoors. The patient may have lost confidence in his ability to walk; he needs to be happy and relaxed in his new environment and have confidence in the staff to reap the most benefit from his treatment. The aims of physiotherapy are to correct posture and disturbance of balance, improve co-ordination and re-establish a sense of rhythm. The act of walking is no longer automatic and in order to correct it, a new pattern has to be taught in a drill-like manner which requires the patient's full concentration. Marching to music is beneficial, as are stepping lines and squares on the floor which encourage the patient to take longer steps in a set rhythm; should he suddenly start his small shuffling steps, he should be stopped and made to correct his balance before setting off again. Well-meaning by-standers, by coming to the patient's assistance or gazing at him anxiously, can disturb his balance and cause a fall, similarly, physical support and walking aids distract him from the natural rhythm of walking. Verbal encouragement on the other hand is very helpful, with reminders such as 'head up, look where you are going, left, right, left, right' etc. given from time to time, in a slightly jovial brisk manner. The patient may fall although this is not so often as would be expected from watching him; better to be active and fall than sit forever in a chair, feeling depressed and getting pressure sores and deformities. The nurse must not make too much fuss, but must ask the doctor to see the patient if he has had a fall; a precautionary X-ray may be ordered and, as a rule, as soon as it is known that no bones are broken, the patient must continue his usual exercise.

Physiotherapy is aimed at keeping the patient fully mobile and independent; intensive physiotherapy from time to time throughout the course of the disease will help to prevent the severe neck flexion and other deformities which could otherwise become untreatable features and cause many problems in terminal care.

Diet

The patient needs a well balanced diet with plenty of fresh fruit and vegetables; eating may be a slow and difficult process and though the patient should be encouraged to join others at mealtimes, if he is embarrassed having to use a spoon instead of a knife and fork, has excessive salivation or is dysphagic, his wish for privacy should be respected. Special feeding utensils may be necessary. A normal diet should be continued for as long as possible, soft diet only being introduced when the patient has dysphagia. It is often very difficult for the patient to eat or drink as he cannot close his mouth firmly or transfer food and drink from the front to the back of the mouth; though he can hold a cup, he cannot lift his arm and tilt his head back in order to drink and when fluid is poured into his mouth he may not be able to swallow because of his rigidity and posture.

Bladder and bowel care

When the patient with Parkinson's disease is admitted to hospital, circumstances have often led to an unsatisfactory fluid balance and disordered bladder function. A vicious circle is common, for example difficulty in taking fluids and in reaching the lavatory inevitably leads to fluid restriction, urinary stasis, infection, frequency, further fluid restriction, heavy urinary infection, sometimes incontinence and the patient becomes distraught and his Parkinsonian symptoms much worse. Some patients have difficulty in starting to pass urine, that same difficulty in initiation which occurs in other spheres of their activity, but it must be remembered that elderly men may have prostatic enlargement; there may be poor sphincter control or a spastic bladder. A urine specimen should be cultured, a high fluid intake encouraged, there should be easy access to the lavatory and the staff should adopt a calm unhurried attitude.

Severe constipation is a common problem because the patient is usually elderly, inactive, often depressed, may have difficulty taking a normal diet and adequate fluid and may be taking drugs which are constipating. Simple dietary measures (fresh fruit and vegetables, bran, prunes) may be all that is necessary, but should this fail, regular mild aperients should be given; if after 3–4 days, normal bowel activity has not been achieved, stronger aperients, suppositories or enemas must be used accordingly. A doctor may perform a rectal examination when there is spurious diarrhoea caused by impaction of faeces and to exclude rectal carcinoma.

Preparation for going home

Relatives take over the role of therapist when the patient returns home, so they must be encouraged to visit the patient regularly while he is in hospital, must be kept informed about his treatment and helped to understand the condition of Parkinson's disease and the importance of independence, activity, interests and optimistic encouragement. The period the patient spends in hospital should be no longer than is necessary to achieve the greatest possible improvement otherwise he may become dependent on the nursing staff, fearful of a change in routine and lose confidence, seeming reluctant to go home. Relatives suddenly finding themselves relieved of their burden of responsibil!ty may be reluctant to shoulder it again, however willingly they may have borne it for many years. Weekends at home are helpful in adjustment for both the patient and his relatives.

Terminal care

There is no curative treatment for Parkinson's disease and there is always deterioration due to degeneration of the basal ganglia and associated brain stem nuclei. The condition of some patients deteriorates rapidly to its fatal outcome over a period of 2–5 years while more commonly the disease slowly progresses for up to 20 years; death is usually due to general deterioration when the patient is bedridden, complicated by infection. These pathetically disabled patients demand all the skills that the nursing staff can muster; it is difficult to imagine the loneliness and isolation of such a helpless, stiff, incoherent, dribbling patient whose sense of hearing is preserved and whose mind is alert. Once there were many patients in this state, but with modern treatment the numbers have been reduced, as patients remain active for a longer period.

The patient must be nursed in a bright ward where he can see people coming and going, hear conversation and be drawn into it without needing to converse and hear familiar sounds like the comforting chink of tea cups. All nursing care should be anticipated; sedation will ensure a good night's sleep though changes of position must be continued and analgesia must be adequate to ensure comfort.

Heredofamilial or benign tremor

Heredofamilial tremor is a fairly common disorder which may be mistaken for Parkinson's disease; it starts in youth and is a fine bilateral intention tremor which mainly affects the hands, is not associated with rigidity, is made worse by emotional stress, relieved temporarily by alcohol and is probably to be found in at least one other member of the family. The tremor remains unchanged for many years with a tendency to increase towards old age. Treatment is only required if the patient is finding the tremor an acute embarrassment or it is leading to alcoholism; tranquillisers may be all that is necessary to calm the patient at times of stress and prevent him resorting to alcohol. Sterotaxic surgery though very successful in abolishing tremor is rarely necessary.

Chorea and athetosis

Huntington's chorea

In 1860 Dr Huntington of New York traced this rare hereditary disease through several generations to a family who emigrated from Bures in Suffolk to America on the Mayflower; in Britain 6000 families are affected and the disease is thought to originate from the same Suffolk family. This inherited disorder is carried by an autosomal dominant gene (passed to either sex and carried by only one parent) and is conveyed to half the sufferer's children; it is possible to determine by genetic tests which children will develop the disorder later. Sometimes the disease appears to develop spontaneously, but this may be due to premature death of a relative who would have developed the disease, or lack of information about the family history; some people are reluctant to disclose that there is or has ever been mental illness in their family.

The onset of the disorder is insidious; it affects both sexes equally, usually between the ages of 30–45 years; there is slowly progressive deterioration due to basal ganglia degeneration and the patient usually dies 10–15 years later. Symptoms of occasional facial grimacing, pursing and smacking of the lips and tongue are usually the first evidence of the disease. As in other basal ganglia disorders symptoms are increased by emotional stress and are less severe or absent during sleep. The family may notice that the patient is becoming unusually moody, irritable and fidgety. As the disease progresses, involuntary, jerky, grotesque movements affect the head, arms and then the legs. The patient learns to control these movements by trick methods to conceal them from onlookers, for example placing one finger on the cheek in a particular way to check abnormal head movements, or converting an involuntary movement into something purposeful, an abnormal arm gesture being used to push aside a strand of hair. Speech soon becomes dysarthric and increasingly difficult to understand and the flow of conversation is frequently interrupted by involuntary movements of the face, lips and tongue. When several years have elapsed the patient's symptoms will have become very severe with such wild excursions of the limbs and abnormality of posture (lower trunk thrown forwards and shoulders backwards) that walking or any task however simple would seem impossible, but surprisingly for some time the patient remains independent and manages incredibly well, and falls are far less common than one would expect. There is always progressive dementia, usually as a later symptom, but sometimes starting quite early in the course of the disease, which eventually leads to the necessity for institutional care.

Many patients who develop the disorder have watched close relatives through the course of their illness and will have anticipated early symptoms in themselves, even looking frequently in the mirror for the signs they are fearing. Their general practitioner, knowing the family history, may detect early signs when attending the patient for an unassociated illness, or the patient, suspecting the nature of her illness consults her doctor who will refer her for an out-patient appointment with a neurologist for confirmation of the diagnosis and to exclude other disorders.

The patient with early symptoms needs a great deal of understanding and help; explanations to relatives, friends and work associates will enable them to understand the difficulties and prevent the patient from being ridiculed; with this help they may be able to continue a near normal life for several years. The onset of mild dementia causes loss of confidence, anxiety and panic (see Chapter 9). A mild tranquilliser such as chlordiazepoxide may be prescribed which has the added benefit of calming abnormal choreiform movements; tetrabenazine may also be helpful. The patient may become depressed and housebound and there may be problems within the family when behaviour becomes difficult to live with, for example teenagers find their parents embarrassing or marriage breaks down. Parents, knowing the disease is passed on, will worry about their children; teenagers, those contemplating marriage and any sufferer likely to have children should receive genetic counselling as it can now be determined which person carries the disease. It is advisable that none of these carriers should have children, but this difficult decision will rest with the individual.

There will be financial hardship when the sufferer is a single person or breadwinner in the family and can no longer work, or a husband has to give up his job to care for his ailing wife. There will also be loss of companionship and normal social contacts outside the home especially when the patient is shy of talking because he cannot be understood and becomes almost mute; depression reduces conversation and increases the risk of suicide. Constant supervision becomes necessary when the patient's memory deteriorates, to safeguard him from gas and fire hazards and inadvertent or intentional drug overdosage. The healthy spouse should be relieved of some of the burden of responsibility; contact should be made with the community social worker who will arrange day centre care, voluntary visitors, meals-on-wheels and other assistance to enable the healthy partner to continue employment and outside activities for as long as possible; it is possible to arrange holidays for the disabled. The family should be introduced to 'Combat', the association for combating Huntington's chorea, who have 22 branches in Great Britain and who provide a family counselling service.

Medical advice

There is no curative treatment for this very disabling disorder. When the diagnosis is confirmed the patient and his relatives will need advice on how to cope with the various problems as they arise. Caring relatives and friends, marriage guidance counsellors, local church minister or priest, social worker, general practitioner, neurologist and psychiatrist all play an important part in supporting the patient and their family through a lengthy and difficult time, delaying for as long as possible the patient's permanent residence in hospital. Admission may be necessary for the following reasons.

1 Medical or surgical treatment of other conditions.
2 Treatment of injuries, burns or scalds, friction or pressure sores.
3 To relieve relatives of the patient's care for a limited time while they have a holiday.
4 For terminal care.

Admission to hospital is a stressful situation especially if the patient is not demented. He will be well aware of the impact of his grotesque appearance on strangers; nurses must contain their own reactions and give simple explanation to other patients and members of staff encouraging them to include the patient in conversation. The patient should be given the opportunity to be nursed in a single room where he will have privacy, but he must not be 'shut away' because of his appearance. While she is admitting the patient, the nurse should unobtrusively observe his capabilities, the severity and extent of involuntary movements and his mental state. She may tactfully enquire from relatives information relating to the patient's intellect, mood and behaviour; personality changes may have led to irritability and outbursts of aggression. Though a clearer assessment of intellectual ability may be gained by psychometry, nurses must

beware of assuming that a lowering of the patient's I.Q. represents an inability to appreciate their sad situation, though as time passes there will be a merciful blunting of this awareness.

Nursing care

It is essential to encourage complete independence for as long as possible; assistance is often more of a hindrance than a help and should only be given when absolutely necessary. There is very little the patient can do to alleviate boredom and he should be allowed to have his own radio and television, the company of frequent visitors if necessary out of hours, and for those who are permanently resident in hospital an opportunity for outings and weekends at home. Attractively served and interesting meals are one of the pleasures of the patient's life and should be according to his preferences; the patient expends much energy in constant muscular activity and his meals should have a high energy content (20 000 kJ) and be supplemented by a variety of nourishing drinks otherwise he will become very emaciated. Feeding is a difficult, messy and lengthy business and the patient may prefer to eat alone. Food should be cut into manageable sized pieces so that only a fork or spoon is necessary; if he is too afraid of making a mess or too little food is actually eaten the nurse will need to feed the patient. A stiff polythene drinking straw allows the patient to drink more easily with less spillage, but swallowing may be difficult.

Skin care and prevention of accidents
Really good general hygiene is very important; the nurse must notice when, due to physical or mental deterioration, the patient can no longer cope satisfactorily with personal hygiene, then she must be prepared to help with a daily bath. This will give her an opportunity to inspect the patient's skin for signs of dryness which needs treatment to prevent abrasion, crack or sore; the prevention of abrasions is essential as it is technically difficult to keep dressings in place and sores clean. Arachis oil keeps skin supple and zinc and castor oil cream soothes and heals sore areas. Night sedation may be necessary to ensure a good night's sleep; when asleep abnormal movements will be minimal but nonetheless it may be beneficial for the patient to lie on a sheepskin, and padded bedsides should

always be in position. Should the patient be confined to bed even for a short period of time he will be more prone to friction sores and the entire bed should be covered with sheepskin. All clothing and bedding should be of natural fibre as synthetic materials cause sweating and friction. Female patients find trousers more comfortable and less embarrassing for daytime wear as they do not ride up.

Although smoking is generally discouraged in hospital because of the known health risks, a patient with this disorder has so few pleasures that if he normally smokes he should be allowed to do so, but only with supervision as he may burn himself or set light to furnishings. Cigarettes and matches should be locked away and other patients and visitors must seek permission before giving the patient a cigarette.

As there is a risk of suicide, nurses must supervise the patient and ensure that tablets are swallowed.

Terminal care

When a patient can no longer be cared for in his own home, he will be admitted to a psychiatric hospital. A high standard of kind, caring nursing is necessary as, even for those who know the patient well, communication and anticipation of the patient's needs is difficult; the patient may become extremely distressed and het up over something as simple as wanting the light or television turned off.

Sydenham's chorea (St Vitus's dance)

Sydenham's chorea is the cerebral manifestation of infection by the organism streptococcus viridans which causes rheumatic fever; it affects girls more than boys between the ages of 5 and 15 years; it used to be a common disorder, but is now rare.

The parents first become aware that something is wrong when their child becomes clumsy and fidgety, jerky movements of the limbs and head soon develop which sometimes persist during sleep, the child is unable to sit still and becomes emotional and nervous. There may be quite marked weakness of the muscles, but there is never complete paralysis. Complete recovery is usual in 2–3 months, but occasionally abnormal movements may be per-petuated as a habit; in many instances the chorea recurs. An irregular and rapid pulse will indicate heart damage.

Treatment consists of complete rest in bed and sedatives will be prescribed to calm the child, dampen down abnormal movements and prevent strain on a possibly already damaged heart; rheumatic fever will be treated with antibiotics. Padded cot sides are necessary to prevent the patient falling out of bed and feeding utensils must be unbreakable. The child is often of above average intelligence and though a quiet atmosphere is necessary, every attempt must be made to prevent boredom; story telling or reading to the child are soothing yet entertaining. When choreiform movements have ceased and the pulse rate is normal, activities should be gradually increased and constructive toys and games used to help the child regain normal mobility. A suitable educational programme is desirable for the older child and will prevent excessive anxiety about lost schooling and forthcoming examinations. This condition occasionally occurs in pregnancy and is a rare complication of oral contraceptives.

Hemiballismus

This is a rare disorder of sudden onset affecting the limbs on one side of the body; continuous involuntary movements involve proximal muscles more than distal, are rapid, jerky and wild, only ceasing when the patient is asleep. The cause may be a small cerebrovascular accident affecting the basal ganglia. This condition is frightening to the patient, alarming to others and the patient may die of exhaustion unless the abnormal movements can be controlled.

Nursing care

The patient should be nursed in a quiet single room where he can be clearly seen from the nurses' station. Though there may be some clouding of consciousness the patient is sufficiently aware of the unpleasantness of his symptoms to need company and reassurance; the nurse must approach with confidence, and putting aside her natural response of shock, particularly when seeing the patient for the first time, must give prompt attention to his physical comfort, at the same time talking to him reassuringly. He will be embarrassed when, through no fault of his own, he strikes out at the nurse who is helping him or sends his food and drink flying from her hands.

The patient needs periods of rest and sedation will be prescribed; tetrabenazine is sometimes effective in controlling the abnormal movements of hemiballismus. All nursing care should be so arranged that the patient's rest intervals are not interrupted. Constant limb movements rapidly cause friction sores unless vulnerable areas are protected. No dogmatic statements can be made relating to skin care, but from the beginning observation of the patient's movements and which skin areas these are abusing must lead to their protection, with either orthopaedic felt (which should be left in place until it shows signs of wear and tear before being changed) or foam pads kept in place by crêpe bandages. Should any area become sore, for example the chest wall which is very difficult to protect, it should be treated with generous and frequent applications of zinc and castor oil cream. Eating and drinking are difficult and the patient will need to be fed; providing the nurse has patience, approaches the bed on his unaffected side, judges the right moment to put the food into the patient's mouth and praises him when he succeeds, adequate nourishment will be taken. Weight loss may occur as the violent continuous involuntary movements rapidly burn up calories.

Within a week to ten days the patient usually shows some improvement and it will be possible for him to sit out of bed, but a harness restraint will be necessary to prevent him throwing himself from his chair.

Stereotaxic thalamotomy may be an emergency procedure for very severe hemiballismus, or considered if disabling movements persist after several weeks.

Athetosis

Athetosis usually develops during childhood due to birth injury or asphyxia, but occasionally occurs at a later age; it may be unilateral or bilateral and associated with paralysis (cerebral palsy). The movements are slow, smooth, writhing and involuntary, affecting the arms more than the legs and distal more than proximal muscles. The movements are specific to the child, develop to their greatest severity during childhood, are increased by stress, lessen in intensity when the patient is lying

down and disappear during sleep. The cause of athetosis is obscure but it is associated with basal ganglia disturbance.

Infantile athetosis is first noticed at a few months old when the child develops abnormal movements and postures of his limbs; childhood milestones are delayed, walking is difficult and very ataxic and speech impossible to understand. When there is bilateral athetosis the muscles supplied by the cranial nerves are affected causing facial grimacing and tongue protrusion and withdrawal; when the muscles of swallowing are severely affected the child will be dysphagic. Many of these children are highly intelligent and become frustrated by their physical disability and their inability to communicate; sometimes there is mental subnormality.

Medical treatment is unsatisfactory; intensive physiotherapy and speech therapy is very beneficial and should involve the parents and other helpers as it must begin when the child is very young and be continued daily for many years. Much can be achieved by a painstaking loving family who devotedly encourage the child to develop his full physical and intellectual capacity. Residential care is sometimes needed if the family is emotionally, physically or financially unable to cope with the situation or the child's educational needs are not being met, but all ties with the family must be maintained through visits, weekends at home and holidays.

At a very early age the child will sense parents' embarrassment and notice strangers' reactions to his appearance. Communication and making a relationship with the child is difficult as, with the best will in the world, it is impossible to ignore facial grimacing, hold the child's gaze or know whether his concentration has been held, because he is constantly turning his head away and looking elsewhere; anxiety on both sides spoils communication and makes the child's writhings worse. A self-conscious child with unilateral athetosis will try to hide his abnormality by restraining the affected limb, even sitting on the hand. When such movements are really troublesome stereotaxic surgery for thermocoagulation, cryotherapy (ice destruction) or placement of electrical stimulators may reduce or abolish the movements, but there is a risk that the limb may be less useful. Surgery is not undertaken for purely cosmetic reasons for it is better to have imperfect function than a useless paralysed limb.

Spasmodic torticollis (wryneck)

Spasmodic torticollis is a slowly progressive condition in which tonic or clonic muscular spasm of the sternocleidomastoid muscles causes frequent repetitive lateral rotation of the head; occasionally the extensor muscles are affected causing head retraction with elevation of the eyes and eyebrows. Sometimes there are long periods free from spasm. The disorder is of the nerve supply and not within the muscles; it may be in the basal ganglia as it has been seen in association with encephalitis lethargica and other extrapyramidal syndromes, or in the peripheral nerve supply, as local causes such as cervical spondylosis with root pain cause muscle spasm. It may be precipitated by mental stress and conflict and often a combination of physical and psychological factors develop which make the disorder intractable. Although this is a unilateral disorder all muscles of the neck are involved, it is associated with pain which may be very severe and after some months muscle hypertrophy develops.

When the patient is first seen by a doctor a complete physical and neurological examination is necessary to exclude organic lesions and assess the patient's attitude to his disability. A firm but sympathetic approach is important and as this condition is very resistant to the limited treatments available, if the patient does not have confidence in his medical advisers, he will go from one doctor to another insisting that there must be a cure for his condition and becoming obsessed by his symptoms. Physiotherapy, various types of collar, surgical division of motor nerve roots and stereotaxic thalamotomy have all been tried without much success; tranquillisers and antidepressant drugs may help the patient's general well being. The patient should continue to lead as normal a life as possible and pursue some form of employment to divert his attention from his neck.

Wilson's disease (hepato-lenticular degeneration)

This is a rare inherited disorder carried by an autosomal recessive gene; it will affect children of either sex if both their parents are carriers of the disorder, whether or not the parents have any obvious clinical signs. The disorder is due to abnormal copper metabolism.

Normally copper ingested in certain foodstuffs in the diet is absorbed in small amounts through the gut, loosely bound to albumin, and carried to the liver where most of it is excreted in the bile; a small amount becomes firmly bound to globulin, forming caeruloplasmin in the blood (Fig. 20.4). In Wilson's disease excessive amounts of copper are absorbed through the gut, the bonding with globulin is defective (therefore the caeruloplasmin level is low) and copper is free; much of it is excreted in the urine, but a smaller damaging proportion is deposited in the liver, brain, kidney tubules and the membrane lining the posterior surface of the cornea (Descemet's membrane).

The biochemical abnormality is present from birth, but symptoms of the disease do not occur for several years; when they do they are either related to disorder of the liver or the brain. Liver symptoms which include recurrent episodes of jaundice, ascites, haematemesis, fulminating hepatic failure, chronic hepatitis or cirrhosis occur early, possibly even in childhood, and sometimes prove fatal before there are signs of cerebral involvement; cerebral signs are not usually seen until the early teens. The liver is always affected, but has often compensated in a remarkable way and there are no apparent symptoms.

The symptoms of cerebral disturbance arise when copper is deposited in the lenticular nucleus of the basal ganglia, the cerebral cortex and cerebellum causing degeneration and cavitation. The onset of the disorder is gradual and characterised by the development of tremor and rigidity similar to Parkinsonism, and sometimes there are choreo-athetoid movements. The patient develops a fixed smiling expression, his speech is very dysarthric, almost unintelligible, and there is excessive salivation and drooling. Degeneration of the cerebral cortex leads to dementia and the patient becomes irritable, childish and emotionally labile with progressive intellectual deterioration.

Early detection of Wilson's disease is vital so that treatment, which can be so successful, is commenced before there is permanent damage to major organs; for this reason when there is a known sufferer in a family, his children, his brothers and

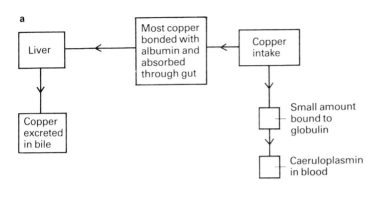

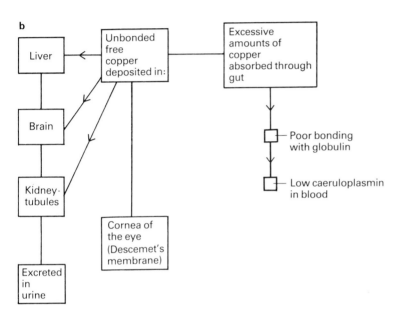

Fig. 20.4 Copper metabolism. **(a)** Normal absorption and excretion of copper. **(b)** Abnormal absorption and bonding of copper in Wilson's disease.

sisters and their children will be screened as they may have the disorder without any symptoms. Children with recurrent liver disorders are investigated for disturbance of copper metabolism and any child or young person with behaviour disorder will have a full neurological examination. Observant parents will consult their family doctor when they notice that their son or daughter has become ungainly, is less able to perform everyday tasks, speaks less distinctly, is falling behind with school work and is very unreasonable at home. Patients with suspected Wilson's disease will be referred to a

neurologist for thorough investigation and hospital admission is necessary for the patient to undergo certain biochemical tests, for assessment of his neurological condition, liver and renal function and to establish treatment.

On admission the patient will be examined in detail (see Chapter 2). The presence of a golden-brown ring of copper around the iris (Kayser-Fleischer ring) positively confirms the diagnosis of Wilson's disease; it may be clearly visible to the naked eye or detected using a corneal microscope and slit lamp.

Investigations

1   Tests related to copper metabolism
i   Serum copper estimation
ii   Caeruloplasmin estimation
iii   A 24-hour collection of urine for copper excretion – urine must be collected in a copper-free container

Low serum copper and caeruloplasmin estimations with a high urinary excretion of copper confirm the diagnosis.

2   Liver function tests
i   Blood tests
ii   Liver biopsy

3   Renal function tests
i   Urinalysis
ii   Serum uric acid
iii   Urinary aminoacids

4   Psychometry

These tests are of value in confirming Wilson's disease and in assessing the extent of liver, kidney and brain damage and will be repeated at intervals to assess the effectiveness of treatment.

Treatment

Without treatment Wilson's disease is fatal within a few years. The most effective drug is oral penicillamine, a chelating agent, which attracts copper from the liver, brain and kidneys and aids its excretion in the urine. This expensive drug is given in large doses 3–4 times a day before meals and continued for the rest of the patient's life; the dosage must be sufficient to correct and maintain the copper balance. The patient's neurological condition may deteriorate soon after treatment begins and sometimes a rash and raised temperature develop, there is often loss of the sense of taste and after several months many have proteinuria; fortunately these side-effects are usually self-limiting. Regular blood and urine tests should be performed throughout treatment to determine copper levels and detect any adverse changes in the blood picture caused by medication. There is usually a slow but steady improvement which continues for two years

or more and if treatment has begun early a good recovery can be expected. Symptoms which may persist for a long period in spite of prolonged treatment are excessive salivation, dribbling and emotional lability. If the brain has sustained irreversible damage the patient will be left with some permanent mental and physical disability.

Nursing care

Despite the availability of treatment, a few patients will have florid symptoms and will need expert nursing care if they are to survive (see Chapter 3); such a patient is very thin, debilitated, dysarthric, dysphagic, possibly dehydrated, prone to respiratory and other infections, to pressure sores, soreness in the hollows of the neck from dribbling, and may be losing large quantities of protein in his urine. The management of this very ill teenager, who would normally be eating and drinking heartily and who has much lost ground to make up, demands time and patience. Feeding is difficult because his attention wanders, his mouth hangs open, swallowing is poor, he is liable to cram too much food into his mouth in a childish manner and choke; suction apparatus should be at hand as the patient may have difficulty in expectoration. He may resent help, generally makes a great mess and it would be best for him to take his meals in a side ward where he has privacy and no one would know that his clothing has to be protected by a bib. It is important that his nutrition and hydration are adequate; a high protein low copper diet is necessary and a supplementary tube feed may be needed. The patient is unsteady on his feet and clumsy, is accident prone, should be supervised at all times and will probably need bedsides.

Even greater patience and understanding are necessary when the patient starts to improve, becomes physically more independent and shambles about the ward after the nurses, making a nuisance of himself. The day is long and can be boring to a young person with poor concentration and latent energy; he feels cooped up and restless, importunately seeks attention, is annoying to all with his loud talk, laughter and amorous slobbering advances. As the patient is so inarticulate, it is difficult for the staff and other patients to understand him; a system of communication must be established, all the while trying to improve speech and upgrade the level of conversation. Other patients, especially those with mutual interests and in the older age group, can exert a steadying influence on the patient's behaviour and keep him occupied; he may take correction better from other patients, whom he feels are on his side, than from a young nurse.

Recovery is never solely the result of administering tablets three or four times a day; there may be family problems to be solved by the medical social worker. All who have contact with the patient should understand the effects of the illness which gradually undermines health and causes emotional disturbance. This is a crucial time of life when the youngster is already experiencing the normal physical and emotional changes of adolescence, when schooling and examinations are vital to his career prospects and when it is so essential for him to make social contacts of his own age outside his home; unfortunately his objectionable appearance and childish demonstrative behaviour is a barrier which is likely to cause complete rejection.

Three months active residential rehabilitation is necessary for the severely disabled patient where a programme, planned to suit his needs covering physiotherapy, occupational therapy and speech therapy, aims to give him back his personal independence; weekends at home and outings give him confidence to face the outside world. At this stage full recovery will not have been reached and it is not possible to envisage how normal the patient will be in two years time nor how able he will be to train for a job which suits his talents and skills. In the meantime he may be able to keep himself occupied with unskilled employment, but whatever the situation this young person should not be allowed to idle away his time doing nothing; attendance at a day centre may help him pass this time until he is ready for assessment and training for suitable employment.

Kernicterus (haemolytic disease of the newborn)

Kernicterus is a disorder of the basal ganglia and auditory nuclei which occurs with neonatal jaundice especially in premature babies and those with Rhesus incompatability. Bilirubin released by haemolysis enters the circulation and as the immature baby is deprived of its maternal escape route through the placenta, bilirubin builds up in the blood to danger level and invades the nervous system. The baby has convulsions, loses consciousness, becomes rigid, adopts the opisthotonos position and may die. If the child survives, when he is several months old he will develop athetoid movements or spastic paralysis, will be deaf and mentally retarded. This disorder can be prevented by discovering Rhesus incompatability in parents, careful monitoring throughout pregnancy and early exchange transfusion, even *in utero*.

21

Disorders of the Labyrinth and Acoustic Nerve

Disorders of the labyrinth are usually treated by ear, nose and throat specialists, but as the symptoms are related to the nervous system and occasionally there may be some doubt about the diagnosis, the patient may be referred to a neurologist for special investigations.

Anatomy and physiology

The structures of the inner ear (Fig. 21.1) are situated within the petrous portion of the temporal bone. They consist of an intricate system of channels within the bone (bony labyrinth) containing membranous tubes (membranous labyrinth) of the same but smaller shape, which are attached to the bony walls by fibrous bands and surrounded and supported by a fluid, perilymph. The membranous labyrinth contains the fluid endolymph and in its walls are the fine nerve endings of the acoustic nerve.

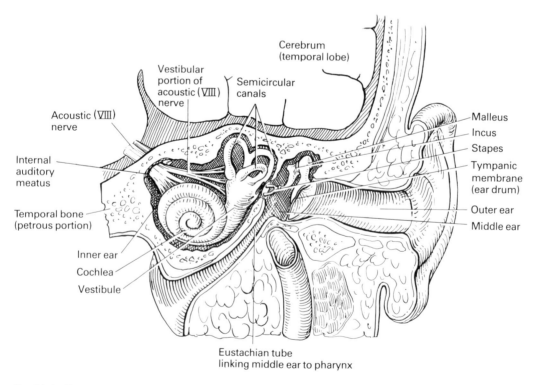

Fig. 21.1   The ear.

The bony labyrinth (Fig. 21.2) is divided into three connected parts, named according to their shape, the vestibule, cochlea and semicircular canals. Within the vestibule are two separate membranous sacs, the saccule which communicates with the cochlea and the utricle with the semicircular canals. Ducts from the saccule and utricle unite and enter the ductus endolymphaticus, a blind pouch which is on the surface of the temporal bone beneath the dura mater. The cochlea is the end organ of hearing; the vibrations of sound waves set the endolymph in motion stimulating the auditory nerve endings in the lining of the cochlea. Nerve impulses are transmitted by the acoustic nerve to the nucleus in the pons varolii and then by the auditory pathways to the temporal lobes of the cerebrum, each nerve relaying hearing to both temporal lobes. The three semicircular canals are at right angles to each other in different planes; information from the semicircular canals, utricle and saccule, about the position of the head, is picked up by the nerve endings of the vestibular portion of the acoustic nerve in the membranous lining and relayed via the brain stem to the cerebellum and, together with all the information coming in from the eyes, muscles and joints, is responsible for maintaining equilibrium.

Disorders which affect the labyrinth or the vestibular portion of the acoustic nerve produce vertigo which may be experienced in one of several ways: the surroundings may appear to rotate round the body, the body may appear to rotate or sway when the surroundings are apparently stationary (this movement may be within the body or the head) or the limbs especially the legs may feel spatially abnormal or unsteady. This true vertigo is not to be confused with the common symptoms of dizziness, giddiness or faintness. Everyone has experienced vertigo when, as a child, they spun round and round for fun and then tried to stand still; those who experience vertigo find it impossible to stand or sit and have to lie down and be very still or they will fall; they may vomit, are grossly ataxic and objects may appear to move to and fro in front of the eyes because of nystagmus; if the onset of vertigo is sudden the patient may momentarily lose consciousness. The first and subsequent attacks of vertigo can occur suddenly, without warning, in any circumstances and may endanger the patient or others; the patient may fall to the ground, sometimes from a height, have an attack while driving or, as a pedestrian, suddenly veer off course into the path of an oncoming vehicle. Wherever the attack occurs, unless it is very brief, the patient will need to lie down, remaining very still and quiet. The patient is usually treated by his general practitioner and even a severe attack will respond to medication, but patients are often referred to an otologist or neurologist to discover the cause of the disturbance, for special investigations to exclude

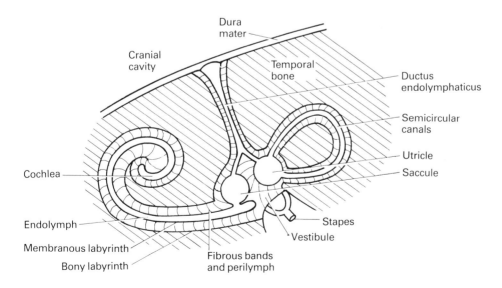

Fig. 21.2 Structures of the inner ear (only one semicircular canal shown for simplicity).

acoustic neuroma (see p. 114) and sometimes if vertigo is severe and recurrent, for consideration of surgery.

There are a variety of causes of vertigo: rapid unaccustomed external motion and visual stimuli (travel sickness), wax in the external auditory meatus, blockage of the Eustachian tube, infections of the middle ear, degenerative changes and inflammation of the labyrinth, damage to the vestibular portion of the acoustic nerve and sudden vascular changes in the brain stem and cerebellum (vertebro-basilar insufficiency; see p. 137). Certain drugs used in the treatment of pain, epilepsy, Parkinsonism and hypertension cause vertigo which will cease when the drug is stopped. Antibiotics such as streptomycin once used extensively in the treatment of tuberculosis, may cause permanent vestibular damage and even deafness.

Vestibular neuronitis occurs in small epidemics and is thought to be caused by a virus often following a respiratory infection; it is characterised by vertigo, vomiting and nystagmus, with no deafness. There is spontaneous recovery in about 3 weeks and the symptoms may be controlled by rest and by sedative and anti-emetic medication, for example prochlorperazine (Stemetil).

Benign positional vertigo may follow head injury or ear infections, but the cause is unknown. The patient experiences vertigo when bending down or moving his head slightly in certain directions. The condition resolves in time but it may take weeks or months; the patient learns to avoid movements which bring on the symptoms, but if these are very disabling they can be controlled by sedatives or prochlorperazine.

Meniere's disease

Meniere's disease is a disorder of the inner ear and acoustic nerve; the cause is obscure, but it is known that vasospasm contributes to dilatation, and an increase in the fluid pressure, of the endolymph system with progressive degeneration of the acoustic nerve endings. The onset of the disease can occur at any age from childhood onwards, but is usually in middle age; men are a little more often affected than women. The condition is usually bilateral, but worse in one ear than the other, it is characterised by tinnitus, increasing deafness and recurrent episodes of severe vertigo and vomiting. Tinnitus and deafness may be present for months or years before the onset of the more disabling symptom of vertigo which comes on suddenly and is of varying intensity and duration. The patient, pale and sweating, is so disturbed by rotation of his surroundings (less commonly rotation of himself) that if he is standing or walking he will stagger, veer sideways or possibly fall and may momentarily lose consciousness. The frequency, severity and duration of the episodes varies with each individual; they may occur at intervals of weeks, months or years and each may last from half a minute to many hours. Attacks are precipitated by certain movements of the head and may occur in circumstances which endanger the patient if he falls. Tinnitus and deafness are worse during an attack and vertigo subsides when the attack is over.

Examination

When the patient is examined during an acute attack it will be noticed that he looks pale, lies on one side and is resentful of interference wishing only to lie absolutely still in quiet surroundings; he may therefore be unco-operative should a doctor try to examine him. The only adverse signs to be elicited are rotary nystagmus which is most marked when the patient looks towards the affected side, and impairment of hearing in one or both ears. When the patient is examined between attacks, slight nystagmus may still be seen on looking to either side, but is most marked towards the affected ear. There will be unsteadiness when standing with eyes closed and difficulty in performing the heel to toe walking test. Nerve deafness will be demonstrated clinically by the Weber and Rinne tests (see Chapter 2).

Investigations

i   Skull X-rays are necessary to exclude acoustic nerve tumours which erode the internal auditory meatus.

ii Audiometry to accurately assess hearing in

each ear.

iii Caloric tests (see Chapter 2) which show that the labyrinth is unresponsive (canal paresis); as these tests give rise to unpleasant symptoms they are not performed in an acute phase of the disease.

Treatment

Medical treatment, which is usually satisfactory, is symptomatic and includes bed rest when symptoms are very severe, and sedative and anti-emetic drugs, prochlorperazine, perphenazine and dimenhydrinate. When vomiting is severe and persistent intramuscular prochlorperazine may be necessary. On the basis that the disorder is due to vasospasm, cinnarizine, a vasodilating drug is helpful and the antihistamine effect of betahistine dihydrochloride is also beneficial. A regular maintenance medication may prevent attacks. Patients with this condition are liable to become deaf in one ear over a period of time and, once they have lost their hearing, which may take years, many have no further attacks of vertigo.

When lengthy attacks of prostrating vertigo grossly disturb the patient's life, particularly if this interferes with his occupation, surgery is considered. Every effort is made to preserve hearing; operations include decompression of the labyrinth by sacculotomy, a shunt operation to drain endolymph from the saccule via the ductus endolymphaticus to the subarachnoid space, cervical sympathectomy to relieve vasospasm, and ultrasonic destruction of the vestibular labyrinth. Detailed surgery of the labyrinth is performed using a microscope. Total destruction of the labyrinth or section of the vestibular portion of the acoustic nerve are operations now rarely performed.

Nursing care of a patient with vertigo and loss of balance

When a patient has a severe attack of vertigo he will need to be helped to his bed, settled comfortably in quiet surroundings and given anti-emetic sedative drugs as prescribed. While he is intensely vertiginous and nauseated nurses must be very patient and gentle, encouraging him to take regular small amounts of fluid as he may be very reluctant to drink, helping him with oral hygiene to prevent his tongue from becoming furred and as his symptoms subside, persuading him to take a light nourishing diet and resume all normal activities. Patients who have experienced severe vertigo are understandably apprehensive and afraid to move, physiotherapy will help posture and balance and prevent unnecessary invalidism; similar rehabilitation is necessary after surgery. While the patient is subject to attacks of vertigo he should not drive and it will help his confidence to be accompanied when out in the street.

22

Motor Neurone Disease

Motor neurone disease is a widespread degenerative disorder of the upper and lower motor neurones causing severe muscular wasting and paralysis. The cause of the disease is unknown and there is no sensory nerve involvement; it affects men more than women, usually occurring between the ages of 50 and 70 years and has occasionally been noticed to follow a severe injury, electric shock, viral infection, contact with a toxic substance, or the patient recalls that another member of the family had a similar disorder; these associations may be purely coincidental.

The onset of motor neurone disease is insidious, it may pass unnoticed or be attributed to old age; when the patient's occupation requires skillful hand movement, slight disability may prompt him to seek early treatment. The first symptoms vary according to which part of the nervous system is affected; there is generally rapid deterioration and death occurs from 2 to 4 years after the onset.

Symptoms and signs

1 Lower motor neurone symptoms and signs

i *Weakness* This usually starts in the hands, one hand as much as a year before the other, but occasionally in the shoulder muscles or in the bulbar muscles of the throat and tongue (bulbar palsy). It is flaccid and spreads to involve the entire musculature including the muscles of respiration.

ii *Wasting* Muscles which are weakened by lower motor neurone degeneration lose their tone and rapidly become wasted; this usually starts in the small muscles of the hands and spreads to other muscles. Wasting affects the circular muscle around the mouth (orbicularis oris), making it difficult for the patient to purse his lips or whistle, and later the circular muscles around the eyes (orbicularis opticae), other facial muscles and the tongue which appears shrunken and wrinkled. The face takes on a characteristic flattened, somewhat sad expression. The loss of subcutaneous fat and dysphagia (see below) increases the overall emaciation.

iii *Cramp-like pains* in the limbs.

iv The *reflexes* are usually increased as rarely is the weakness of purely lower motor neurone origin.

v *Fasciculation* is a sign of motor neurone degeneration. It consists of a fine twitching of a bundle of muscle fibres or a group of muscles and is seen as a superficial rippling under the skin; the patient may have noticed this twitching which is a prominent feature of motor neurone disease. Fasciculation may not be obvious at first but can be elicited by tapping the muscles or shortening them by passive movement of the limb. It is commonly found in the muscles of the chest and shoulders even though there is no weakness or wasting, may be evident in the tongue and widespread throughout the body – an indication of the advancement of the disease.

vi *Dysarthria* The speech becomes slow, slurred, quiet and nasal due to weakness of the muscles of articulation, the vocal chords and the palate, particularly affecting the enunciation of consonants; when these muscles become completely paralysed speech is impossible.

vii *Dysphagia* Swallowing progressively deteriorates as the bulbar muscles become more paralysed and food will regurgitate through the nose; the patient will choke, inhaling food and liquid.

2 Upper motor neurone symptoms and signs

i *Weakness* Spastic weakness is most apparent in the legs, increases the weakness in the arms, affects the bulbar muscles of the throat and tongue (pseudobulbar palsy) and the muscles of the trunk.

ii Reflexes The leg reflexes are increased and the plantar responses are extensor; reflexes are usually brisk in the arms, even when wasting suggests lower motor neurone disturbance. The jaw jerk, palatal and pharyngeal reflexes are all exaggerated and reflex coughing and sneezing can be readily provoked.

iii Dysarthria The muscles of articulation are weak and spastic.

iv Dysphagia The muscles of swallowing are spastic.

v Emotional control When there is advanced pseudobulbar palsy the patient finds it difficult to control his emotional reactions and may laugh or cry uncontrollably; this may be quite unrelated to his true feelings.

vi Sphincter control There may be slight precipitancy or hesitancy of micturition.

History and examination

When the patient has severe dysarthria it may be kinder and easier to gain as much information as possible about the history of the illness from his relatives, asking the patient to fill in those details of which the relatives are uncertain. The doctor will need details of how the illness started, its duration and how rapidly it has progressed; he will need to know the patient's occupation, whether he has been able to continue in full time employment and any difficulties he has met in his work or recreation. Should the patient be severely disabled details will be required of how much assistance the patient needs to look after himself and walk.

A full general examination will be performed by the doctor who will check the patient's general health, condition of his heart and lungs paying particular attention to his respiratory capacity. This will be followed by a complete neurological examination when an assessment is made of mental and emotional state, posture, facial expression and extent of paralysis, muscle wasting, fasciculation and reflex changes. He will pay particular attention to the patient's speech and will examine the throat and tongue assessing the extent of cranial nerve involvement and will enquire whether the patient has difficulty swallowing or has had episodes of choking.

Investigations

The diagnosis is usually clear from the patient's history and examination but there are several disorders which commonly affect the same age group of people causing similar signs and symptoms and may confuse the diagnosis. Investigations may be necessary to exclude malignant disease, cervical spondylosis, respiratory and cerebro-vascular disease; they will also reveal general disorders which if treated will improve the patient's physical abilities.

i Blood tests – haemoglobin estimation, full blood count, blood sedimentation rate, blood urea and Wassermann and Kahn reaction

ii Chest X-rays

iii Cervical spine X-rays

iv A complete ear, nose and throat examination including laryngoscopy and pharyngoscopy will be necessary for those patients suffering from dysphagia and dysarthria

v Electromyography and muscle biopsy to exclude primary muscle disorders

Treatment

There is no specific treatment for this disorder because its cause is still unknown. The patient's general health should be maintained and he should be encouraged to continue suitable light employment for as long as possible; fatigue and exposure to cold should be avoided. The patient and his relatives will need advice and many problems can be averted and panic prevented if there is intelligent anticipation and close co-operation between the hospital, general practitioner, medical social worker and district nurse.

The patient has often fairly advanced disease before he sees his general practitioner as he may have experienced no disabling symptoms for the first 6 to 12 months. The general practitioner, suspecting the purely neurological nature of the disorder and its poor prognosis, requiring specialised care in the final stages, will refer the patient to a neurologist.

Admission to hospital

Detailed examination and investigation is necessary to exclude other disorders and confirm the diagnosis. It is useful for the medical team to get to know the patient, his response to illness and his general condition and disabilities. The neurologist will discuss the illness and its prognosis with the patient's relatives, answer their questions and when the patient is discharged from hospital will give advice concerning:

i   walking and other aids and adaptations which will assist the patient's mobility in his home and prevent falls;
ii employment or other activities;
iii diet;
iv particular indications for contacting the family doctor.

Other reasons for admission to hospital are respiratory infection, assessment of dysphagia and introduction of tube feeding, to give relatives a holiday, the patient a change of scene, provide an opportunity for physiotherapy, speech therapy and give encouragement to boost the patient's morale. Ideally during the final stages of the illness the patient will be nursed at home even though he requires a 24-hour nursing service, but sometimes hospital admission is necessary.

Nursing care

A patient with motor neurone disease has a distressing, progressive disorder which after only a year or two changes an able-bodied, healthy individual into an alert, severely paralysed, skeleton-like wraith who can only mumble inarticulately, constantly drools, who cannot take food without spluttering and choking or has to be fed through an indwelling tube. It is almost impossible to imagine the patient's distress and the intensity of hopelessness felt must vary from one individual to another. As there is no treatment for this disorder there must be times when the patient notices his deterioration and lack of definite treatment or medication. Those caring for the patient inevitably feel compassionate but helpless, yet the patient still turns to them with pleading eyes for help and support. Though the situation is so hopeless there is much that can be done to alleviate the patient's anxiety, prevent mental anguish and the intense feeling of isolation which occurs when he becomes unable to communicate. The patient needs spiritual and physical comfort; this comfort is often given in the unspoken, sympathetic understanding shown by nurses when they anticipate his needs before ever he has struggled to utter a whispered inarticulate request.

When the patient arrives in hospital he is often agitated and apprehensive, frightened of what the doctor's examination and investigations will reveal and if he has been nursed at home, afraid that the nurses will not understand his speech or realise the particular care he needs. An experienced nurse will gain much useful information from a few minutes conversation with the patient and his relatives; this will be conveyed to other members of the medical team. Her discerning observations will reveal the patient's abilities, special difficulties in mobility, his attitude to disability and how his relatives react. The nurse's obvious interest and concern will itself relieve anxiety and form a basis of understanding with the patient and his relatives which will be invaluable for future admissions to hospital when the patient is no longer able to communicate and is completely helpless. Nurses should always be very attentive to small points mentioned by relatives regarding the patient, his preferences and normal daily routine. As soon as possible patient and relatives should be given some idea of aims of treatment and expected duration of hospital care.

Some thought should be given to the position of the patient's bed in the ward, especially when he is very disabled and inarticulate; he will feel less cut off if he is near the nurses' station, has a good view of the ward, is able to look out of a window and can see the ward clock. A bed cradle must be carefully placed so that it does not obscure the patient's view and lead to difficulty in attracting a nurse's attention. Suction apparatus should be available at the bedside and nurses should always be particularly alert to the possibility of the patient choking (not only at mealtimes, but at any time as the result of inhalation of saliva or during an uncontrolled episode of laughing or crying), as the patient has not the power to cough strongly and there will not be the normal explosive choking noise.

The patient should be introduced to other patients in the ward and it should be obvious from the nurse's example that, though the patient's speech and expression may suggest mental deficiency, he is mentally normal. While he is able the patient should be up and dressed each day but activities should avoid excessive fatigue. The patient's morale will be helped by the niceties of life, a daily bath with the use of good quality soap and talcum powder, with general grooming, manicure and pedicure, application of a lady's make-up, hairdressing and shaving; the daily routine needs to be adaptable as the patient may have less energy on some days than others. When the patient's neck muscles are weak care should be taken to support his head during any procedure particularly when helping him in and out of bed, brushing his hair or cleaning his teeth; should his head flop suddenly it is not only painful, but will give him the feeling he is being throttled; he will be embarrassed if lifted in a way which allows his saliva to dribble on the nurse's uniform.

A patient who has difficulty swallowing usually finds a soft diet of a porridge-like consistency easier to manage than solids or fluids. The patient should be encouraged to feed himself, he should be sitting comfortably and the use of the right type of bowl and perhaps a teaspoon instead of a soup or dessert spoon may allow him to take more nourishment and prevent distressing spills and choking; each patient should be asked his preference in these details. The patient may need help towards the end of a meal when he is exhausted by his efforts to feed himself. When feeding a patient the nurse should always sit down and appear unhurried; the patient will find swallowing easier at the start of the day or after a period of rest. A careful record of fluid intake and output should be recorded; it may be necessary to give supplementary fluids by intragastric tube once or twice a day.

When there is difficulty swallowing and coughing the patient may become 'chesty'; a 4-hourly record of the patient's temperature, pulse and respiratory rate will reveal an infection not otherwise obvious. The patient with poor respiratory capacity cannot breathe deeply, cough or expectorate and apart from alteration in the vital signs, the only other indications of chest infection are deterioration in general condition, drowsiness, pallor or flushing and slight cyanosis. The patient needs careful observation throughout the 24 hours as he may be unable to attract attention when he is silently choking. Through her knowledge of the patient and alert observation the nurse will know when suction is necessary; the only indication being a look of agitation and intense fear.

During this illness most patients will spend more time at home than in hospital and there may be a period of a year to eighteen months after the first diagnostic period in hospital before the patient needs readmission; then the pattern of admissions is likely to be two or three weeks in hospital periodically until the possible need for terminal care. During the early stages of the illness the patient should be encouraged to remain as independent as possible and his relatives must be warned not to be oversolicitous, making an invalid of him sooner than necessary. A home visit by the occupational therapist will reveal hazards likely to cause falls and adaptations necessary to increase the patient's safety and enable him to be less reliant on others (see p. 366 for Disabled Living Foundation). The patient should wear suitable well-fitting shoes, floors should have a non-slip surface and rugs and mats removed; his bed may need to be moved downstairs, handrails fitted where necessary and a non-slip mat used in the bath. Arrangements must be made and equipment obtained speedily or the patient, with short expectancy of life, will derive little benefit.

The general practitioner will arrange to see the patient at regular intervals; should the patient develop a respiratory infection, a productive cough, difficulty in swallowing or episodes of choking the doctor must be notified immediately. A district nurse will visit the patient frequently if he has no close relatives or when he becomes severely disabled. The social services department will put the family in touch with voluntary helpers, medical loans department of the British Red Cross, taped book facilities or other necessary services.

Terminal care

It is a mixed benefit when, for the final stages of his illness, the patient returns to the ward where he has become well known; he and the staff will be only too aware of the change in his condition. The patient will feel he has let the nurses down because he has not responded to previous care, though he rarely seems to harbour bitterness about his illness, the staff feel helpless; even so it is a comfort to the patient to know those who care for him and they will better understand the patient and his relatives. Deterioration must be met with practical assistance and good humour; though the patient may be unable to talk or find it a great effort to do so, nurses should continue to talk of topics which may interest him according to their previous knowledge, rather than with gloomy face dwell on nursing procedure and his state of health. Only discerning observation will tell the nurse when the patient would welcome a little idle chatter or when he would rather turn inwards on himself and just watch ward activities because it is too much effort to concentrate; noise can be very aggravating if it cannot be escaped. The days may seem interminable especially at first when mealtimes are no longer a social event and pleasure, and until a routine has been established. Short spells of reading, being read to, listening to the radio and cassette recordings or watching television may help to pass the time and finally it is probably a comfort just to know there are staff and other people close by, even if all are going about their own concerns, something the isolation of a single room does not provide. Visits from relatives or friends should be frequent but not too long and kept to one or two visitors at a time. Inability to communicate and especially to call for help at times of emergency are common experiences in nightmares and the sensation of choking is always terrifying; how very sensitive nurses must be to help the patient who is daily in these situations.

In the early stages of dysarthria, speech therapy may be of value in improving breathing control. At all times the patient has to make a great effort to produce any utterance and it is therefore important to tune in and try to understand what he says at the first attempt; he may be unable to lift his head to look at the person to whom he is speaking so the nurse or visitor should sit down. The patient should not feel hurried fearing that the nurse may rush away; the nurse should give him her undivided attention, watch his lip movements or if this is hindering her comprehension just try listening without looking. When only part of the sentence is heard the nurse should repeat that which she has understood so that the patient need not repeat everything; the nurse should only ask questions which require a 'yes' or 'no' answer. Whichever member of the staff is best able to understand the patient should be used as interpreter to save unnecessary distress. Often it is a nurse or ward orderly who is constantly with the patient who can help 'speak' to the doctor or other visitor on his behalf; she should be aware that strangers visiting the patient will have difficulty understanding him and be available should they need assistance. It is unforgivable for a nurse to rush away from the patient when she knows he is trying to tell her something.

The patient's mouth is liable to become extremely dirty and the tongue coated because of muscle inactivity, residual food particles collecting in the mouth and dehydration caused by dysphagia; supplementary tube feeds will be necessary and a full regime of tube feeding may eventually be required. Frequent mouth care will be important to improve the patient's comfort and help prevent chest infection and other complications; the lips and corners of the mouth should be lubricated with petroleum jelly to prevent cracking and the soreness arising from the constant dribble of saliva.

These emaciated patients will be more comfortable nursed on a sheepskin with their heels protected by sheepskin bootees or on a ripple bed.

Relatives will need a great deal of support from the nursing staff during this anxious time, but if they and the staff have already developed a good relationship and understanding they can together help the patient to a peaceful dignified death.

23

Myasthenia Gravis

Myasthenia gravis (grave muscle tiredness) is a rare disorder in which a chemical disturbance at the neuromuscular junction causes muscle weakness, which is worse after exercise and improved by rest; there is no sensory nerve involvement and no muscle wasting until the late stages of the illness. It usually affects young women more than men, occurring between the ages of the late teens and forty years, but on rare occasions occurs in infancy, childhood or old age. The older patients are more often men and the course of the illness is then more chronic. The cause of the disease is unknown, but is thought to be an autoimmune process affecting the neuromuscular junction caused by antibodies produced initially by the thymus gland.

Anatomy and physiology

Normal muscular activity (see Chapter 28) is dependent upon a continuous process of chemical interactions, each muscular contraction and relaxation lasting about a thousandth of a second. Motor impulses which stimulate skeletal muscle to contract are conceived in the motor cortex of the brain, pass through the spinal cord and along the peripheral nerves to the nerve endings where a chemical, acetylcholine, is released; this attaches itself to the acteylcholine receptors in the motor end plate (a special sensitive area in each muscle), the muscle then contracts; an enzyme, cholinesterase, circulating in the blood, immediately cancels the effect of acetylcholine and the muscle relaxes (Fig. 23.1).

Symptoms

The effect of acetylcholine deprivation is extreme muscle fatigue and paralysis, mainly affecting those muscles which are in constant use, the focusing muscles of the eyes, those of the upper eyelids, the muscles of facial expression and mastication. The muscles of the shoulders and upper arms are more severely affected than other parts of the trunk and limbs and the respiratory muscles are affected

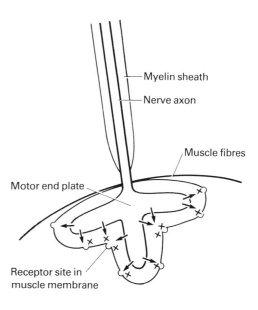

Myelin sheath

Nerve axon

Muscle fibres

Motor end plate

Receptor site in muscle membrane

↓ Acetylcholine released from motor end plate (stimulates muscle contraction)

× Cholinesterase released from muscle (cancels muscle contraction)

Fig. 23.1 Chemical interaction at neuromuscular junction.

in more advanced disease. In the less common bulbar form the fatigued muscles of the throat make swallowing difficult and cause regurgitation through the nose.

The course of myasthenia gravis is very variable and unpredictable; in some patients the disorder is limited to the ocular muscles, in others the whole body is affected. The onset of the disease is gradual with fluctuating physical ability, better in the morning than the evening, with improvement following a rest, and greater strength some days than others. There may be spells when the young person feels quite normal. The fatiguability of muscles is most clearly seen in repetitive activities which starting normally, become slower and weaker and, in spite of mental effort, fade out completely. After a rest, with renewed muscle power, the activity can be resumed, but soon fades out again. More severe episodes of weakness may occur for no obvious reason or coincide with emotional stress or prolonged physical effort, mild respiratory infection, certain drugs, surgical procedures under anaesthesia or pregnancy. The disease may only mildly limit the patient's activities for many years or, within a few months lead to severe irreversible paralysis and dependence upon a mechanical ventilator; very occasionally there is complete remission.

Fatigue is a common complaint during adolescence, it can be a sign of serious ill-health, but is more often the result of rapid growth and development and sometimes an excuse to avoid unwanted activities, some young people may be said by their parents to have been 'born tired'. The early signs of myasthenia gravis may be falsely attributed to the effects of adjusting to adult life, examinations, starting a career, emotional disturbances, girl/boy relationships or domestic stress. A young person who limits her activities because of exhaustion may be regarded as psychologically disturbed; parents and friends may badger her and even her own doctor may be unable to find a cause for her listlessness, leaving the patient with feelings of anxiety, inadequacy, frustration, depression and rejection, when she is no longer able to take part in the energetic activities of her contemporaries. She may be embarrassed, wanting to retreat into isolation when symptoms alter her facial appearance. Finally when the true nature of the disorder is suspected, the general practitioner will arrange for the patient to see a neurologist; a few patients may experience such severe symptoms at the outset that

they will need urgent admission to hospital. When a diagnosis of myasthenia gravis is made, though the disorder may mean physical limitation and the outlook is uncertain, the patient will often experience a sense of relief to be given some definite guidance after a long period of unexplained ill-health.

Reasons for admission to hospital

i   For careful examination and investigation when there has been some doubt about the diagnosis, and for introduction of drug therapy

ii   For adjustment of drugs, e.g. when there is systemic infection, pregnancy or if the disorder is poorly controlled

iii   For thymectomy

iv   For a course of steroid therapy

v   When the patient's condition is deteriorating in spite of treatment

vi   When the patient has collapsed in either a myasthenic or cholinergic crisis (see p. 307)

vii   If the patient is to undergo anaesthesia or surgery

viii   For long term care of the severely disabled patient who may be dependent on a ventilator

History and examination

The patient, usually quite a young woman, gives a history of becoming easily and excessively fatigued; she may complain of double vision especially when tired at the end of the day, drooping of the eyelids, fading of her voice almost to a whisper during prolonged conversation and difficulty in finishing a meal when chewing becomes an effort or attempts to swallow give rise to choking and regurgitation. All the symptoms are less severe after rest and worse at the end of the day.

On examination (see Chapter 2) the patient, often of slim build, appears debilitated and lifeless. Ptosis, which may be so severe that it obscures the patient's vision, is often more marked on one side than the other. In order to see, the patient holds her head in a characteristic backward tilted position giving a false appearance of haughtiness; weak facial muscles cause lack of facial expression and a smile is like a sneer. When the muscles supporting the jaw are so weak that the mouth hangs open, the patient finds it necessary to prop up her jaw with her hand. Mildly affected patients appear normal if seen after a rest and then only the doctor's testing will induce symptoms. During history taking it may be noticed that, having started quite strongly, the patient's voice becomes a whisper. The doctor can verify this observation by asking the patient to count to 50; this test may also demonstrate breathlessness caused by fatigue of the respiratory muscles. When ptosis is not immediately obvious the doctor asks the patient to gaze at the ceiling for a minute or so without tilting her head; the eyelids may then begin to droop very slightly causing narrowing of the palpebral fissure. There may be an obvious squint, but sometimes in spite of the patient's complaint of double vision, no visible weakness of the ocular muscles can be found even when eye movements are tested carefully. Movements of the face, jaw and neck are tested, the patient may be unable to tighten facial muscles, close her mouth or resist attempts to move her head; the power of limbs and trunk are also tested, to demonstrate the fatiguability of muscles the patient is asked to perform repetitive actions. The doctor examines the patient's chest and observes the movement of the chest wall, notes the rate, depth and character of respirations and tests the patient's ability to cough. Should there be any suspicion of weakness of the intercostal muscles or diaphragm he will measure the ventilatory capacity using a spirometer, and if there is any reduction will arrange for the test to be performed daily at a regular time each day and with the same time relationship to the patient's medication. When the medical staff are aware that the patient is developing respiratory failure, it is far better, with the patient's co-operation, to electively use a ventilator to avert a crisis. A full general examination is necessary as symptoms similar to those of myasthenia gravis sometimes accompany thyrotoxicosis and carcinoma.

Investigations

1   Tensilon test   A useful test to confirm the diagnosis of myasthenia gravis is the administration of 10 mg of intravenous edrophonium chloride (Tensilon), an anticholinesterase drug with a rapid brief action lasting about 5 minutes.

There may be immediate severe reactions to this drug including nausea, vomiting, increased salivation and abdominal cramp, and the antidote, 0.6 mg of atropine sulphate should be drawn up ready for injection. Observing the patient carefully the doctor injects 2 mg of edrophonium chloride; if, within 30 seconds, there is no adverse reaction, the remaining 8 mg is given. Myasthenia gravis will be confirmed by dramatic short-lasting relief from symptoms, but someone who is not myasthenic will experience twitching of the facial muscles.

2   Blood tests
(a)   Routine blood tests will ascertain the patient's general health and exclude anaemia
(b)   Examination for antibodies
(c)   Tests to exclude collagen diseases which are sometimes associated with myasthenic symptoms

3   Chest X-ray   A necessary investigation to exclude respiratory infection and carcinoma, and certain views may show the shadow of a thymic tumour.

4   Estimation of **ventilatory capacity**.

5   Sputum specimen to search for organisms and malignant cells.

6   A **radioactive iodine test** is necessary for those patients who show signs of thyrotoxicosis.

7   Electromyography   This is a delicate test of nerve conduction and muscle function and will help the doctor to locate the disturbance when the results of the Tensilon test are uncertain or when myasthenic symptoms accompany carcinoma.

8   A **body scan**.

Treatment

When the diagnosis of myasthenia gravis has been confirmed the patient will be given some simple advice about physical exertion. She should organise her daily routine so that periods of activity alternate with rest and even though she is feeling quite well, should conserve her energy whenever possible by using mechanical aids (electric mixer, toothbrush and free-standing hair-dryer, etc.) and should never be tempted to exert herself to the point of exhaustion nor take part in competitive sport. Extremes of temperature, sunbathing, hot baths or exposure to very cold weather, should be avoided.

Without treatment the patient may survive as an invalid, her very existence threatened by even a common cold; treatment with drugs greatly improves the patient's quality of life, for though not curative, they lessen muscle fatiguability. The two most commonly used drugs in the treatment of myasthenia gravis are neostigmine bromide (Prostigmin) and the longer-lasting but slower acting pyridostigmine bromide (Mestinon). These act by inhibiting the neutralising action of cholinesterase; they are used with caution in patients suffering from bronchial asthma as overdosage causes an increase in bronchial secretions. Pyridostigmine bromide is the drug most suitable to carry the patient through the night as it has a long-lasting effect, the quicker acting neostigmine bromide being more effective during the daytime as it can be taken to coincide with periods of increased activity. Neostigmine bromide is more rapidly excreted and there is less risk of toxicity, but patients prefer pyridostigmine as it is less inclined to cause diarrhoea. These drugs can be given intravenously if the patient is dysphagic and pre- and post-operatively. Intestinal disturbance, diarrhoea and abdominal colic are common effects of the administration of anticholinesterase drugs, but can be greatly reduced if tablets are taken with food, and diarrhoea further controlled by propantheline or codeine phosphate. The level of anticholinesterase medication is possibly on the brink of toxicity and should the patient experience abdominal cramp, diarrhoea, nausea, vomiting or increased salivation, the early warning signs of drug excess, she must contact her doctor without delay. When myasthenia gravis is accompanied by other auto-immune conditions, rheumatoid arthritis, diabetes mellitus or thyrotoxicosis, treatment of these disorders usually brings about an improvement in myasthenic symptoms.

The disease and its drug therapy must be clearly and simply outlined to the patient without causing unnecessary alarm, the booklet *The Myasthenia Gravis Companion*, produced by the Muscular Dystrophy Group of Great Britain, is helpful. When the patient starts medication and while dosage is being adjusted, she will be seen frequently by the neurologist and given guidelines on drug dosage and information about side-effects. The patient must be warned to resist the dangerous temptation of taking extra tablets to eradicate all residual symptoms, tiredness at the end of the day is to be expected and to increase the dosage will not necessarily reduce the symptoms, but may make them very much worse or lead to complete collapse. Certain medications in common use will aggravate the symptoms of myasthenia and the patient's condition must always be outlined to anyone who gives them treatment.

The relationship between the thymus gland and myasthenia gravis has been suspected for a very long time. The thymus gland is normally partly responsible for the development of maturity and for antibody formation in childhood; the gland, which lies behind the sternum in the thoracic cavity, enlarges during childhood, begins to atrophy after puberty and by old age remains as only a very small remnant. In myasthenia gravis, microscopical examination of thymus tissue always reveals some abnormality; the gland is sometimes enlarged (thymic hyperplasia) and 15% of patients have a benign thymoma. At one time thymectomy was performed if there was a thymoma, the gland was enlarged, or if the patient had not responded to medical treatment or was gravely ill. The operation had such grave risks that it was only performed as a last resort and the results of surgery appeared inconclusive. It is thought that myasthenia gravis is an autoimmune disease, the thymus gland producing lymphocytes, which produce antibodies that destroy the receptor sites for acetylcholine; therefore, the sooner the thymus gland is removed the more dramatic the recovery, but some patients improve within a few weeks while others not at all. Only a lengthy study has shown that the benefits of this operation may be delayed for several years; a study of 100 patients treated in this way showed a 50% improvement after 2 years, but when 5 years had elapsed 90% had greatly improved and many seemed completely cured.

Thymectomy remains a risky operation and should only be performed in a unit which has intensive care facilities and staff who are used to caring for patients with myasthenia gravis. The risks are those of giving a general anaesthetic to a patient with poor respiratory excursion and general muscular weakness; the operation involves opening the thoracic cavity by splitting and retracting the sternum to expose the soft vascular gland which lies close to the trachea and major blood vessels of the heart. A course of radiotherapy will be given before surgery for the removal of thymic tumour. The best results following thymectomy are seen in young women who have had the disorder for no longer than 3 years; thymectomy does not relieve the symptoms of the purely ocular form of myasthenia gravis.

Another treatment, plasma exchange, removes harmful antibodies from the circulation and it is hoped will speed recovery following surgery.

On the basis that myasthenia gravis is an auto-immune disease steroid therapy has been given, but is usually withheld until after thymectomy. Effective treatment requires high dosage, but this may cause a severe exacerbation of myasthenic symptoms, possibly necessitating the urgent use of a positive pressure ventilator, therefore steroid treatment is given in hospital; if treatment is introduced gradually and given on alternate days complete collapse can be avoided. It is thought that steroid therapy exerts its beneficial effects at the neuromuscular junction, but it is not known exactly how. Improvement is sometimes seen during the course of treatment, but may be delayed.

Complications

Comparatively minor illness, for example respiratory and urinary infection, can be serious and necessitate hospital admission for someone with myasthenia gravis, when their myasthenic symptoms worsen and do not respond to normal or increased anticholinesterase drug dosage. When the infection has been treated by rest and antibiotics, myasthenic symptoms will recede and the patient can resume her normal regime of anticholinesterase medication.

When the condition of a patient with myasthenia gravis continuously deteriorates in spite of treatment, the dosage of neostigmine or pyridostigmine is likely to have been increased to the limit of the patient's drug tolerance. Any further worsening in the patient's condition is difficult to treat and it becomes uncertain whether deterioration is due to exacerbation of myasthenia gravis (myasthenic crisis) or the result of overdosage by the cumulative effects of the longer acting anticholinesterase drugs (cholinergic crisis). The patient may have collapsed suddenly and in this crisis situation, on the brink of respiratory failure, equipment must be ready to assist respiration. Unless the events preceding the crisis are witnessed by the staff or other responsible person, it is not possible to determine the nature of the crisis without performing a Tensilon test. The signs of cholinergic crisis are:

i   diarrhoea, nausea and vomiting;
ii   muscular cramp and fasciculation;
iii increased salivation;
iv profuse sweating and pallor;
v   small pupils;
vi increased bronchial secretions;
vii muscle and respiratory paralysis.

The symptoms of a myasthenic crisis are:
i   dysphagia;
ii   muscle paralysis and respiratory failure.

All medication will be withdrawn for a few days until the patient's system is cleared of all drugs; this drastic measure will not be a threat to life providing that respirations are maintained. During this period the patient's condition may surprisingly improve, but on the other hand the patient may become completely paralysed and dependent on the ventilator. After a few days medication can be gradually re-introduced.

For nursing care of a patient using a ventilator see Chapter 3.
For care of a paralysed patient see Chapter 10.

There has been extensive research into the physiological process at the neuromuscular junction and the effect of various forms of treatment on the symptoms of myasthenia gravis and the course of the disorder. Early diagnosis and thymectomy can leave the patient symptom-free eventually, but anticholinesterase drugs still have a part to play and plasma exchange is a possibility. Still there are patients who have an idiosyncratic reaction to drugs, those whose condition is complicated by other serious medical disorders and those whose condition steadily deteriorates in spite of treatment. Myasthenia gravis may still be so gradual in onset that it passes unrecognised, or advance so rapidly to paralysis that planned treatment is impossible and the patient only survives the crisis through skilled nursing and medical care and a combination of all available forms of treatment. The outlook with myasthenia gravis is improving yearly, but because it is so individual and unpredictable, and threatens the patient's power to breathe, swallow and cough, careful observation must never be relaxed.

Nursing care

Although most patients with myasthenia gravis are treated as outpatients, the condition is always potentially dangerous and it may become necessary to admit the patient to a hospital equipped to give emergency resuscitation at a second's notice. Skilled nursing and observation are essential as the myasthenic patient with failing muscles cannot call for help and may quietly die from asphyxia or respiratory failure.

Communication with the patient may be one of the most difficult problems as the patient's voice may fade to an inaudible nasal whisper and written communication is equally difficult; nurses must be quick on the uptake and listen very attentively to the patient's first request as repetition may be impossible (see Chapter 22).

Nutrition and elimination

Small meals at frequent intervals supplemented with milk or high calorie drinks will be more easily taken without fatigue and the patient may prefer a soft diet which needs little chewing; ice cream and cold fluids improve swallowing. A liquidised normal diet will provide the best balance of nutritional requirements and can include fibre. Crushed pills are more easily swallowed and if taken with food or a milk drink prevent gastric irritation; neostigmine should be given at least an hour before a meal and a rest before meals can be helpful. The patient, conscious of her difficulty and messiness when eating will prefer to eat apart from other patients; malnutrition is a risk as the patient may give up the struggle part way through a meal, fearing choking and the unpleasantness and embarrassment of nasal regurgitation. The patient will be watched carefully during mealtimes as suction may be necessary. Patients with periodic dysphagia may need supplementary intragastric feeding but patients with persistent severe dysphagia or those requiring mechanical ventilation will need a full regime of tube feeds.

The drugs used to treat myasthenia gravis often cause diarrhoea and codeine phosphate, prescribed to overcome this problem, may be taken too liberally causing constipation; reduction of codeine phosphate may be all that is necessary, but should an aperient be needed, only very mild medication such as Lactulose should be given. **An enema should NEVER be administered as the patient may collapse, be severely shocked, and even die.**

Visual disturbances

Diplopia is a most unpleasant and disabling symptom which can be relieved by the use of an eye shield, worn alternately on each eye to prevent the suppression of vision in one eye. Ptosis, a feature of myasthenia gravis, is embarrassing and inconvenient and when severe can prevent the patient from seeing. Lundie loops fitted to a pair of spectacles raise the eyelids by gently pressing them upwards above each eyeball (Fig. 23.2); the device can be retracted during periods of improved muscle power.

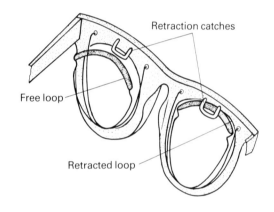

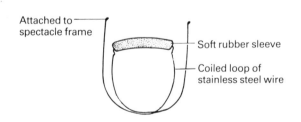

Fig. 23.2 Lundie loops. Redrawn from *The Myasthenia Gravis Companion*, by kind permission of R.G.N. Lundie and the publishers, The Muscular Dystrophy Group of Great Britain and the British Association of Myasthenics.

Outlook

Recent advances in treatment and greater understanding of myasthenia gravis allow many sufferers to lead a relatively normal life. The patient will have to take tablets several times a day, possibly for the rest of her life and try to avoid contact with colds or influenza; she should wear a Medic alert necklace or bracelet and should always carry a supply of tablets with her (see p. 265). The patient is herself more acutely aware of how well she feels than any observer, and only she will know when to rest and when to take medication. When she understands her disease with its fluctuating course she will herself become responsible for minor adjustments in medication; should a mild infection develop a slight increase in drugs is necessary, on the contrary early signs of drug overdosage suggest a necessary reduction of medication; should the illness or drug side-effects be severe or persist for more than a day or two the patient must contact her doctor immediately. Toxic effects from drugs may be a good sign and indicate that the condition of myasthenia gravis is improving and that the patient needs less medication.

Relatives need to fully understand the patient's illness and should avoid fussing and making unnecessary reference to the illness or treating her like an invalid. Schooling and advanced education should continue and transport to and from college will prevent the fatigue of walking or cycling; teachers must understand the fluctuating nature of the disorder and the need for curtailment of energetic activities. Employment should continue if it does not involve too much physical effort, sometimes a change of job is necessary.

It is not possible to foretell the effect of pregnancy and childbirth, but if the patient is quite severely disabled it might be wise to delay having a family for a year or two. Antenatal care will be extra carefully monitored and, although the delivery may be uncomplicated, the baby may show myasthenic symptoms at birth (weak cry, inadequate respirations, poor sucking and weak limb movements), probably because of the transference of antibodies through the placenta. The condition though serious, responds to treatment with anticholinesterase drugs and will resolve completely within a few weeks. Breast feeding is contraindicated as anticholinesterase drugs are secreted in breast milk.

Myasthenia gravis remains a serious unpredictable illness, but in spite of set backs any patient with this disorder can now feel optimistic about the future.

24

Neurosyphilis

Syphilis, one of the venereal diseases, is a chronic infection caused by the spirochaete, *Treponema pallidum*, which is transmitted from one person to another during sexual intercourse. Should the primary infection remain untreated, in 10% of persons the disease invades the central nervous system, men being more often affected than women. Whereas neurosyphilis was once the commonest disease of the nervous system, it is at present very uncommon. It is all important that the general public, particularly teenagers, are well informed about syphilis; they must know of the early symptoms of painless ulcers and discharge from the genital tract and how the disease is transmitted from person to person and from generation to generation (an infected mother can pass it to her unborn child). They must know how and where to seek treatment and the importance of completing a course of penicillin injections, however painful they may be; if they do not have the recommended course of treatment or have only a few injections they run a very grave risk of syphilitic invasion of the nervous system which causes insanity or paralysis or both. It is essential that expectant mothers attend ante-natal clinics for their blood to be tested for syphilis; should the result be positive, treatment can be given to prevent the foetus from being harmed.

Syphilis was once a very common disease in this country; there was no cure, but various treatments were tried including injections of arsenical compounds, bismuth and mercury. At the turn of this century and until recent times, mental hospitals had complete wards full of demented patients suffering from general paralysis of the insane, one of the forms of neurosyphilis, and in those days anyone with knowledge of the disease could easily notice in a crowd, one or two young people with the obvious stigmas of congenital syphilis. The discovery that high fever improved the symptoms of syphilitic infection of the brain led to the once favoured use of malarial treatment. This unpleasant treatment, which gives the patient malaria and allows him to suffer controlled hyperpyrexia for several days before anti-malarial drugs are given, destroyed the spirochaete, but could not undo the damage already sustained by the nervous system. The advent of penicillin and its success in the treatment of syphilis dramatically reduced the incidence of neurosyphilis and probably gave a false sense of security; because of current attitudes to sexual relationships and contraception, society has become more promiscuous and there has been a reported increase in syphilis, the results of which are yet to be seen.

There is a stigma attached to the name 'syphilis'; it is a disease that is still talked of secretively and with some shame because of its mode of transmission and implications of promiscuity or unfaithfulness; this disease is one of the very real reasons against promiscuity as venereal diseases are easily spread and contacts are difficult to trace.

The spirochaete has an affinity for certain parts of the central nervous system, but the signs and symptoms of neurosyphilis are as varied as the parts of the nervous system affected. At first the disease may be symptomless, then there may be evidence of disturbance in the meningo-vascular system or of the cells and fibres of the brain and spinal cord.

Although three main types of neurosyphilis are described, there is in reality much overlapping of the disorders and all three may appear in the same patient.

Meningo-vascular syphilis

Meningo-vascular syphilis affects the walls and surrounding tissue of the blood vessels within the meninges of the brain and spinal cord narrowing their lumen, causing ischaemia and possibly leading to thrombosis and necrosis. The symptoms typically appear within a few months to 5 years of the initial infection, but can appear in any subsequent period in the patient's life. Symptoms include:

Those caused by general infection of the central nervous system
(a) headache
(b) mental disturbance
(c) papilloedema
(d) convulsions

Those caused by meningitis at the base of the brain
(e) optic atrophy

(f) reflex paralysis of the muscles of the iris causing unreactive pupils (Argyll Robertson pupils, see p. 312)
(g) other cranial nerve palsies

Those caused by disturbance of sensory nerve pathways of the spinal cord
(h) loss of deep and superficial sensation, particularly in the lower part of the body with loss of sphincter control and incontinence of urine and faeces

Unless the patient receives treatment he will lapse into unconsciousness and die. A localised syphilitic lesion may cause hemiplegia or cranial nerve palsy; the oculomotor (IIIrd cranial) nerve is particularly susceptible and neurosyphilis is a possible cause of a painless IIIrd nerve palsy without other adverse neurological signs.

Tabes dorsalis

As tabes dorsalis implies, the signs and symptoms of this disorder are mainly due to degeneration of the dorsal (posterior) part of the spinal cord (Fig. 24.1). The area involved includes:
i   nerve pathways of joint position and vibration sensation;
ii posterior horns of nerve cells in the spinal cord;
iii sensory nerve roots entering the spinal cord.
The myelin sheaths of the nerve fibres degenerate with subsequent loss of nerve conduction; the presence of Argyll Robertson pupils suggests the disorder is widespread in the nervous system and not confined to the spinal cord.

   The onset of tabes dorsalis is slow and progressive, the patient often giving no history of previous syphilitic infection which may have occurred as many as 5 to 20 years before. The condition may be asymptomatic and found only during routine examination; symptoms may appear unrelated to disorder of the nervous system until the patient is carefully examined. When the patient is first interviewed he may complain of characteristic stabbing pains ('lightning pains') in the legs lasting only a

few seconds, occurring repeatedly in the same spot, though they may flit from area to area in the same limb, thought by the patient to be caused by rheumatism. Pain may occur in other parts of the body, particularly in the chest and abdomen where it is felt as a constricting band sometimes referred to as 'girdle pain'. Other distressing symptoms may be 'pins and needles' in the legs and numbness of the feet with its unnatural feeling of walking on cotton wool. Incontinence of urine or faeces occur (see pp. 179 and 180) when, through loss of sensation, the patient is unaware of a full bladder or loaded rectum; the bladder often empties incompletely. There may be very slight unsteadiness of gait particularly on turning due to loss of joint position sense and absence of incoming sensory impulses which provide information relating to posture and movement (spino-cerebellar tracts); it is worse if the patient tries to walk in the dark or shuts his eyes (as when washing his face) because he can neither feel nor see the position of his body in relation to his surroundings. When the patient's ataxia increases, he develops a characteristic gait walking with his feet wide apart to steady himself, lifting them high

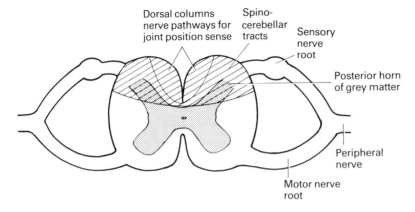

Fig. 24.1 Area of spinal cord degeneration in tabes dorsalis.

and stamping them down heavily because he is unsure where they are in relation to the floor; this gait contributes to the damaged joints which occur in this condition, the knee joint being particularly susceptible. The patient feels no pain even after repeated injury, an effusion and swelling develops and the joint becomes unstable (Charcot's joint). Pads of hard skin resembling corns develop on the soles of the feet; these, particularly if the patient tampers with them, may become painless ulcers with sinuses extending into the bone. Tabetic crisis, an uncommon event in any of its forms, is often characterised by bouts of epigastric pain accompanied by vomiting; these episodes which last for a few hours or days may lead to unnecessary emergency laparotomy. Other crises affect the larynx, bladder or bowel.

Signs and symptoms

The patient is usually pallid, of slim build and normal mentality. There may be slight bilateral ptosis with compensatory wrinkling of the forehead caused by constant efforts to lift the eyelids and open the eyes more widely; the iris is often a muddy indefinite colour. There are other cranial nerve signs:

(a) primary optic atrophy with impairment of visual acuity;

(b) Argyll Robertson pupils which are irregular in outline, unequal, small, do not react to light, but react to accommodation;

(c) diplopia, if there is poor counterbalance of the eye muscles;

(d) anosmia;

(e) deafness;

(f) laryngeal paralysis;

(g) impairment of sensation on the face, particularly affecting a small butterfly-shaped area including the nose and extending across the cheeks.

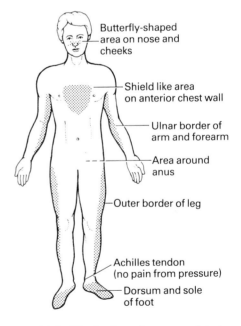

Fig. 24.2 Distribution of sensory disturbance in tabes dorsalis.

Examination will reveal bilateral signs affecting the legs more than the arms. Muscle tone is decreased; reflexes, particularly those of the legs are diminished or absent as the reflex arc is broken; abdominal reflexes are often brisk and the plantar responses flexor. Joint position sense is affected (see p. 24) and a positive Romberg's sign will be found. There is no weakness or wasting because the motor nerve pathways are intact.

Disturbance of sensation is patchy but characteristic (Fig. 24.2), affecting the nose area (see above), a central shield-like area on the anterior chest wall, the inner aspect of the arms and outer border of the legs, the feet and a small area surrounding the anus. Pressure on the normally pain-sensitive Achilles tendon causes no response and there is a generally delayed response to any form of pain.

Treatment with a course of penicillin will halt the disease process and prevent further deterioration; without treatment this disorder usually arrests spontaneously but the patient's disability is by then quite severe.

General paralysis of the insane

General paralysis of the insane occurs 15 to 20 years after the primary infection when the spirochaete invades the brain tissue, especially that of the anterior two-thirds of the cerebrum, causing chronic encephalitis with degeneration of the frontal and parietal lobes.

Signs and symptoms

1 Mental changes are related to frontal lobe disorder
i Impairment of memory for recent events
ii Poor concentration
iii Dementia which may be either
(a) simple dementia with dysphasia, dyspraxia and general slowing of the mental processes or
(b) grandiose dementia (less common) when the patient has delusions of grandeur, is euphoric, boastful and identifies himself as crowned head of a country or other famous person, confabulating in an exaggerated manner

2 Physical changes are related to disorder of the frontal and parietal lobes and other parts of the brain

i Generalised epileptic fits
ii Signs of pyramidal tract disturbance
(a) increased muscle tone, pathologically brisk reflexes and extensor plantar responses
(b) pseudobulbar dysarthria (slow slurred speech) due to spasticity of the muscles of articulation
iii Tremor of the lips and tongue and sometimes also of the limbs
iv Argyll Robertson pupils
v Optic atrophy

In the early stages of the illness, personality changes pass unnoticed, then workmates and relatives begin to notice that the patient's standard of work and personal care have deteriorated; he himself shows no insight into his condition and often exhibits a vacant facial expression or fatuous smile, though he may on the contrary be irritable and morose. As the dementia worsens he will become careless about his appearance, oblivious of his unkempt state and may squander money which he can ill afford; urinary and faecal incontinence may develop. Later, physical abnormalities and progressive weight loss occur and movement of the limbs becomes weak, tremulous and ataxic. Finally the patient will become completely demented, bedridden and will die from intercurrent infection.

Congenital neurosyphilis

An infant may be affected by transplacental spread or by direct contact with a syphilitic chancre during birth. Mortality is high; the foetus may be stillborn and macerated with evidence of miliary gummata. A baby born to a mother with syphilis should be isolated from other babies to prevent cross infection, as discharge from the eyes and nose is highly infectious; antibiotic treatment will be commenced promptly to prevent infective destruction of the nasal septum. Mildly affected children show certain stigmas; the face is characteristically wizened with flattened nasal bridge, there is deafness and the incisor teeth are peg-shaped (Hutchinson's teeth). There may be no evidence that the baby is affected at birth, but he may later develop:

(a) syphilitic meningitis followed by hydrocephalus;

(b) cerebrovascular lesions which lead to thrombosis;

(c) juvenile tabes dorsalis;

(d) general paralysis of the insane at 12 to 15 years of age.

Admission to hospital of a patient with neurosyphilis

Admission to hospital is necessary to confirm the diagnosis by investigation, to treat complications, to rehabilitate or to provide a protected environment for the mentally sick patient who cannot be cared for at home. A careful history is taken and the patient examined (see Chapter 2). Patients are often reluctant to reveal that they have had past treatment for syphilis; a history of a course of injections or a lumbar puncture may be significant.

Investigations

The most important investigation is the blood Wassermann reaction which is a routine test for every patient with neurological disorder of any kind. Blood Wassermann reaction is sometimes positive in other conditions and not always so in neurosyphilis and for this reason CSF analysis is often necessary. Neurosyphilis may be discovered accidentally during the course of investigation for some other disorder. In the presence of neurosyphilis the white cells in the CSF (lymphocytes) are increased, the protein level raised, Lange colloidal gold curve abnormal and CSF Wassermann reaction is positive (Table 24.1 and Fig. 24.3). There were always some negative Wassermann reactions in both blood and CSF, but since the more general use of penicillin this is a more likely occurrence and other tests have been developed, for example treponema immobilisation and flourescent antibody tests. Other investigations are sometimes necessary for differential diagnosis; these may include any of the special investigations discussed in Chapter 2. It is important to realise that during the long natural course of neurosyphilis the patient may develop another neurological disorder and symptoms may be due to either condition, for example a patient with tabes dorsalis and a prolapsed intervertebral disc may have retention of urine; a myelogram may be necessary to determine the cause.

Treatment

The importance of penicillin injections in the treatment of primary syphilitic infection has already been mentioned. When, during the investigation of neurological disorder, active disease is found, the spirochaete must be abolished by treatment with a full course of penicillin by intramuscular injection 1 mega unit daily for 3 weeks. To ensure that the disease is no longer active, CSF analysis is usually repeated after a period of 3 months and an annual blood test for 5 years is sometimes recommended. The CSF white cell count and protein level should return to normal though the Lange curve and

Table 24.1   Investigations for neurosyphilis

Type of neurosyphilis	Blood	CSF			
	WR	Cells	Protein	WR	Lange
Meningo-vascular	+ve in 60–70% of patients	Increased 20–100/cu.mm lymphocytes	0.05–0.1%	+ve in 90–100% of patients	1355421000 or 5542210000
Tabes dorsalis	+ve in blood alone; 5% +ve in blood and CSF; 65% −ve in blood and CSF; 20%	Increased 20–70/cu.mm lymphocytes	0.05–0.1%	+ve in CSF alone; 10% +ve in blood and CSF; 65% −ve in blood and CSF; 20%	1344310000
General paralysis of the insane	+ve in 90–100%	Increased 20–100/cu.mm lymphocytes	0.05–0.1%	+ve in 100%	5554311000 or 5555555444

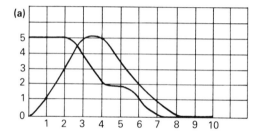

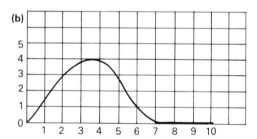

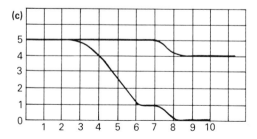

Fig. 24.3   Lange colloidal gold curves. **(a)** Lange curve in Meningovascular syphilis. **(b)** Lange curve in tabes dorsalis. **(c)** Lange curve in general paralysis of the insane.

Wassermann reaction may remain abnormal. The development of additional neurological symptoms at any time is an indication for further CSF analysis. It should be understood that penicillin treatment is curative for primary syphilis, but only arrests neurosyphilis, and those parts of the nervous system already destroyed by the disease will not recover.

Herxheimer reaction
Herxheimer reaction is an extremely rare occurence when, during the course of penicillin treatment, an exacerbation of symptoms with pyrexia occur. The reaction is thought to be due to the toxins released during mass destruction of spirochaetes; there may be serious consequences if the patient has cardio-vascular disease.

Lightning pains (see p. 311)
Analgesics are generally ineffective for the treatment of lightning pains.

Nursing care

This is a difficult subject to discuss as the patient presents such diverse signs and symptoms, with every degree of disability from slight ataxia to the complete dependence of a demented bedridden patient; it is more easily considered if each patient is assessed and the aims of treatment and rehabilitation are planned to suit each individual.

Many nurses are concerned about the possibility

of contracting syphilis when nursing patients suffering from neurosyphilis; they should be reassured that no barrier nursing precautions are necessary during this tertiary stage of the disease. There is sometimes a tendency for nursing staff to be prejudiced, because of the manner of transmission of the disease and long established ideas on morality; such feelings must never influence the patient's care, however depraved his demented habits in the late stages of the illness.

All patients with neurosyphilis should be encouraged to be as active and independent as possible; the patient with tabes dorsalis should not be confined to bed unless absolutely necessary as constant use and practice in walking are essential to compensate for loss of proprioception. Epilepsy is commonly a symptom of meningo-vascular and general paralytic forms of neurosyphilis; the nurse should carefully but unobtrusively observe her patient to make certain that, in the event of a fit no injury is sustained; low beds may prevent serious injury. It is equally important that the patient with general paralysis of the insane should continue normal routines, getting up and dressed each day and being encouraged to take an interest in his appearance and personal hygiene.

In every instance the nurse should only help the patient with those matters which he cannot do for himself; the patient with poor vision will need more supervision than others to ensure that he does not fall. A bright attractive environment and cheerful understanding nurses will help to prevent the demented patient from sinking further into his apathy. Patients with delusions of grandeur should not be contradicted or they may become aggressive, ways and means should be found to deter any unacceptable behaviour; tranquillising drugs are sometimes prescribed which calm the patient's response and though he may continue to speak of his delusional ideas he will less readily act upon them. Every effort should be made to maintain the patient's nutrition and general health.

Care of the skin and painless ulcers of the feet

All patients should take a daily bath. The patient with tabes dorsalis should be taught to take particular care of his skin, to dry his feet carefully and apply a good foot powder. He should be told the importance of wearing comfortable easy fitting shoes with a solid based heel; these will not only prevent the development of corns and abrasions on his feet, but will also enable him to walk more steadily. While he is in hospital and when he goes home, his skin should be inspected daily and he should be advised to seek medical advice if at any time he gets a sore which is slow to heal, even though the sore is painless. Painless ulcers of the feet should be relieved of pressure and when not walking about, the patient should sit with his feet elevated; a swab should be taken for culture of organisms and the sore cleaned with a de-sloughing solution (Aserbine) twice daily and covered with a sterile dressing. A superficial sore can be treated with Aserbine cream, but should the ulcer have any depth, a wick of ribbon gauze soaked in Aserbine solution should be inserted; the appropriate antibiotic will be prescribed. An X-ray of the foot is necessary as there may be bony involvement.

Charcot's joints

The basis of treatment is to prevent further damage to the joints; supporting bandages should be used to prevent hyperextension, and nurses and physiotherapists should teach the patient to walk as correctly as possible using a walking aid if necessary.

Care of the bladder

1   A high fluid intake should be encouraged and a fluid balance record maintained.

2   A clean specimen of urine should be sent to the laboratory for analysis and urinary infection will be treated with antibiotics.

3   The bladder should be palpated after the patient has passed urine to assess residual urine; when the bladder is emptying incompletely the patient will be persuaded to pass urine at 2-hourly intervals even if he has no sensation of bladder fullness and taught to use manual compression during micturition.

4   Catheterisation is used only to relieve retention or to assess the amount of residual urine. When retention has been relieved by catheterisation it is sometimes possible to establish bladder training as described in **3** above.

Physiotherapy

All patients with neurosyphilis benefit from a programme of exercises to strengthen muscles, improve co-ordination and correct posture and gait; this is especially beneficial to the patient suffering from tabes dorsalis.

Occupational therapy

The occupational therapist will assess how independent the patient can be in daily living and his mental and physical capacity for work. She will also concentrate on helping the patient to pursue activities which practise exercises taught by the physiotherapist to strengthen and co-ordinate movement.

Social factors

The patient's family should be seen by their doctor and their blood should be tested in case they have contracted syphilis. This is a situation which calls for tact and discretion on the part of the medical and nursing staff; relatives may be distressed and critical of the patient and need help and support in adopting a reasonable attitude.

25

Peripheral Nerve Disorders

The body is supplied to its furthest extremity with a complex network of peripheral nerves (including the cranial nerves) which convey sensation to the spinal cord and brain stem and thence to the brain, and provide the returning motor nerve pathways to initate movement (see Chapter 10 and p. 13).

Anatomy and physiology

In foetal life the spinal cord fills the entire length of the vertebral canal and the spinal nerve roots run in a horizontal direction. As the vertebral column elongates in infancy the spinal cord is drawn upwards and the roots assume an increasingly oblique and downward direction toward their exit foramina. There are 31 pairs of peripheral nerves (see Fig. 10.8), arising from the spinal cord, which contain both sensory and motor nerve fibres. Those in the cervical region supply the arms, neck and upper thorax; the thoracic nerves supply the remaining part of the thorax and the upper abdomen and the lumbar and sacral nerves (the cauda equina) supply the lower trunk and legs. The cervical, lumbar and sacral nerves are organised into plexuses and re-emerge from these as major nerve roots (Fig. 25.1). The peripheral nerves leave the spinal cord in pairs (one on each side), puncture the meningeal sac enclosing the cord and pass out through the foramina of the spinal column. They are joined by branches of the autonomic nervous system (see Chapter 2) and extend to the areas of skin, muscle and joint which they supply (see Fig. 10.9). There is considerable overlap of function between adjacent peripheral nerves and damage to a single nerve root as it emerges from the spinal column may produce little, if any, obvious weakness or sensory loss, as the nerve roots are then reorganised in the plexus. On the contrary, damage to a nerve near the periphery will give very obvious sensory or motor disturbance.

The efficiency of each nerve is dependent upon the health of the nerve cells in the spinal cord or

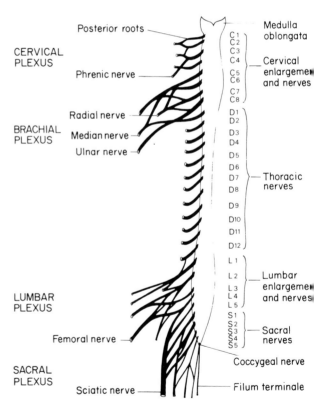

Fig. 25.1 Organisation of peripheral nerves into plexuses and major nerve trunks.

sensory root ganglion. Any deficiency or toxicity affecting the cells, deprivation of essential vitamins or poisoning by infection or chemicals will render them inefficient and cause symptoms and signs which start in the fingers and toes and creep towards the spinal cord, as it is the extremities of the nerves which are affected first. Each nerve fibre is protected by a covering of myelin which insulates the fibre and aids conduction of nerve impulses; it is then encased in a tube of neurilemmal cells which nourish and maintain the myelin (see Fig. 2.1). Destruction of the myelin causes haphazard conduction or loss of nerve impulses; as long as the myelin sheath remains intact the nerve cell is capable of stimulating the damaged fibre to regrow though this process is extremely slow and may be incomplete.

Some nerves, because they lie near the surface of the skin or are closely related to bones and joints, are liable to injury; congenital anomalies may also place nerves in a more vulnerable position. Nerves may be damaged by tearing, wrenching, crushing or they may be completely severed; they may be compressed by scar tissue, tumour or external mechanical factors such as pressure from splints or crutches. Peripheral nerve injuries and disorders are more likely to occur at birth, during wartime when gunshot wounds are common or in old age when falls and fractures are likely, arthritic joints (especially in the neck) compress nerves, and general illnesses cause nerves to function less efficiently. Occupational factors are complex and individual; any patient who complains of a peripheral nerve disturbance not associated with direct injury should be closely questioned about his daily activities. Work or leisure pursuits may involve repeated lifting of heavy weights, constant pressure, or repetitive actions which hammer, jar or vibrate a nerve. An individual may become more susceptible to nerve damage owing to increase or loss of weight, a change in his general health, or because of his particular posture, build or age, be more susceptible to nerve damage than another person in the same job.

When a nerve is damaged the part of the body innervated by that nerve will be affected, the severity of symptoms depending upon the extent and site of damage and ranging from tingling or mild weakness to complete numbness and paralysis.

Aims of treatment

1   To relieve pressure upon the nerve by
    (a)   advising the patient to avoid the aggravating cause,
    (b)   advising him to adopt a better posture,
    (c)   surgical decompression.

2   To rest the affected part if necessary by the use of slings or splints.

3   To improve physical fitness and general health while natural repair and recovery takes place, by giving adequate diet, supplementary vitamins and physiotherapy.

4   To search for metabolic and genetic disorders, sources of infection or a latent carcinoma causing peripheral neuropathy.

5   To anastomose a severed nerve as soon as possible – the full extent of recovery will take at least 18 months.

While the patient is disabled he will rest more contentedly if anxieties regarding finance, future employment and family are allayed – contact will be made with the medical social worker.

Brachial plexus disorders

The brachial plexus is a network of nerves in the lower neck just above the first rib; it is formed by the 5th, 6th, 7th and 8th cervical nerves and the 1st thoracic nerve which enter the plexus, divide, reorganise and emerge to form three main nerve roots: the median, ulnar and radial nerves (Fig. 25.2). In some individuals the brachial plexus is at a slightly higher level and includes the 4th cervical nerve, in other individuals it is lower taking in the 2nd thoracic nerve. The brachial plexus may be involved in head, neck, shoulder and arm injuries.

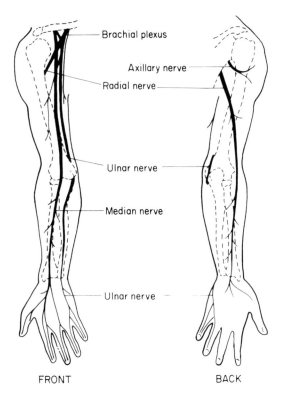

FRONT   BACK

Fig. 25.2   Brachial plexus, median, ulnar and radial nerves.

Upper brachial plexus injury

Forcible stretching of the neck by opening up the angle between the head and shoulder sometimes leads to damage of the 5th and 6th cervical nerve branches to the plexus. This may be a birth injury (Erb's paralysis) or the result of a fall; the muscles which move the shoulder and supinate the forearm become paralysed and the affected arm hangs limply with the elbow extended and the forearm pronated. Treatment is by splinting the arm with the shoulder abducted allowing freedom of movement at the elbow; recovery may be complete, but there is sometimes residual weakness.

Lower brachial plexus injury

Sudden traction on the outstretched arm may tear the 1st thoracic nerve causing weakness and loss of sensation in the small muscles of the hand which become wasted and develop into a 'claw-hand'. There is no specific treatment except rest and analgesia.

Cervical rib and costo-clavicular syndromes

Congenital anomalies, more common in women, frequently involve the bony structure of the opening at the top of the thoracic cage and may affect the nerves and blood vessels which supply the arm. Variations in position of the brachial plexus may also be present; higher placement may be associated with an extra, poorly formed rib, usually on the right side, sometimes bilateral, or the relationship between the brachial plexus and the scalene muscles (beneath the trapezius muscles in the neck) may be abnormal. These anomalies are aggravated by carrying heavy shopping bags.

Symptoms

The patient's usual complaint is of pain in the ulnar border of the hand and the distal half of the forearm possibly associated with numbness and tingling. The patient may have noticed that the circulation of one or both hands is poor and find that raising the arm above the head brings relief from pain and discomfort. Symptoms usually develop gradually, they may only occur at night after lying down for some time or be related to carrying something heavy.

Examination

There may be local tenderness or deformity in the neck (evidence of a cervical rib) and pressure on this area may cause pain or tingling, referred to the ulnar border of the hand and forearm, or disappearance of the radial pulse. There may be obvious circulatory impairment in the fingers with blanching, cyanosis or rarely gangrene; the radial pulse may be feeble or absent in the affected arm. Weakness and wasting of the small muscles of the hand and change in sensitivity (hyperalgesia or analgesia) may be demonstrated in an area on the ulnar side of the hand and distal part of the forearm. It may be noticed that the patient has a slight ptosis on the affected side, a small pupil which reacts to light and there may be absence of the normal sweating response on the same side of the face (Horner's syndrome, see p. 17). This is caused by the unopposed action of the parasympathetic nerves when the sympathetic nerve supply is damaged. The sympathetic nerve supply to the eye is from the 8th cervical and 1st and 2nd thoracic nerves which enter the sympathetic nerve trunk and pass into the skull with the internal carotid artery.

Investigations

X-rays of the thoracic outlet will reveal the presence of an extra pair of ribs (cervical); even though a cervical rib is seen on X-ray it may co-exist asymptomatically with other disorders, for example carcinoma at the apex of a lung or syringo-myelia; in the latter, congenital abnormalities of the cervical spine may be seen. Electromyography will be performed to exclude lesions of the ulnar and median nerves and motor neurone disease.

Treatment

The surgical excision of a cervical rib is a simple operation; it is usually more successful if the symptoms have not existed for too long. Other operations will be devised according to the cause of nerve and blood vessel compression. Postoperatively a course of physiotherapy will strengthen the muscles of the shoulder girdle and when there is no major structural abnormality, rest and shoulder girdle exercises are the only form of treatment.

Carpal tunnel syndrome

This is a condition in which the median nerve becomes compressed as it passes through the carpal tunnel (Fig. 25.3). The tunnel, at the wrist, is formed by a rigid band of tissue (flexor reti-naculum) overlying the carpal bones through which the median nerve and some flexor tendons pass completely filling the space in the channel. Any condition which further narrows the tunnel, swelling of the synovial sheaths of the tendons or swelling of the nerve, leads to nerve compression causing symptoms of pain and disordered sensation. The compressed nerve will become oedematous, and unless pressure is relieved it will, over a period of time, slowly degenerate and fibrose.

Carpal tunnel syndrome most frequently affects middle-aged women and may be associated with fluid retention and aggravating repetitive occupations such as vigorous scrubbing which cause pressure upon the nerve. It may also occur during pregnancy, when fluid retention is probably the most important factor, or occasionally in a young person when it may be associated with a particular activity, for example riding a motor-cycle or ski-ing, or relate to the person's occupation. Other influencing factors are fractures or arthritic changes at the wrist, rheumatoid arthritis, myxoedema or acromegaly. The condition is usually bilateral though it may be noticed on one side months before the other.

Symptoms

The first symptoms are of pain and tingling in the thumb, index and middle finger and the radial side of the ring finger (Fig. 25.3). Symptoms are particularly troublesome at night and on waking in the morning; patients often describe how they hold their arm over the edge of the bed to try to obtain relief. The patient may complain of numbness of the finger-tips and difficulty in picking up and manipulating small objects; medical advice is usually sought before there is any noticeable weakness of the hand.

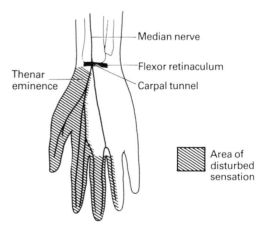

Fig. 25.3 Palmar surface of the hand showing site of compression in carpal tunnel syndrome and distribution of sensory disturbance.

History and examination

The patient usually gives a clear history of the complaint. The doctor may enquire about possible contributing factors (wrist injuries, recent weight gain and occupation), he will also look for evidence of rheumatoid arthritis, myxoedema and acromegaly. On examination there may be obvious wasting of the thenar eminence. Sensation and power will then be tested and will show characteristic impairment of sensation in the distribution of the median nerve supply to the finger-tips and weakness in moving the thumb across the palm of the hand. When the patient has no symptoms at the time of the examination these can sometimes be induced by pressure or percussion over the median nerve on the front of the wrist. Electromyography to assess nerve conduction is performed if there is any doubt about the diagnosis.

Treatment

When carpal tunnel syndrome occurs during pregnancy, treatment is usually unnecessary as the condition resolves after delivery. Medical treatment affords only temporary relief, diuretics may

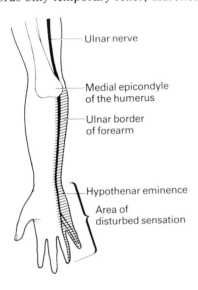

Fig. 25.4   Distribution of weakness, wasting and sensory disturbance in ulnar nerve lesions.

be prescribed when fluid retention is thought to be a factor and splints may be used at night to keep the wrist immobilised in a neutral position. The operation of carpal tunnel decompression in which the flexor retinaculum is divided to relieve pressure on the median nerve is a very successful form of treatment. There is usually full recovery of sensation and power within 6 months to 1 year.

Ulnar nerve palsy

The ulnar nerve (Fig. 25.4) is often injured and compressed at the elbow in association with fractures, arthritic changes, neuroma or ganglion formation, but may be injured in the palm.

History and symptoms

The patient notices changes in the appearance of his hand before complaining of alteration in sensation.

Examination

The ring and little finger are weak and held in a semi-flexed position; there will be evidence of wasting of the small muscles in the interosseus spaces of the hand, the hypothenar eminence, those muscles of the thenar eminence which are supplied by the ulnar nerve and the muscles of the ulnar side of the forearm. Loss of sensation will be found in the little finger and along the ulnar border of the hand. When the deep branch of the ulnar nerve is damaged by prolonged pressure upon the ulnar side of the palm there is only weakness and wasting of the interosseus muscles and the adductor muscles of the thumb.

Investigations and treatment

Electromyography will establish the level of the lesion. The nerve may in some instances be transplanted to the front of the internal condyle of the humerus to relieve chronic nerve irritation and injury at the elbow.

Labels on figure:
- Ulnar nerve
- Medial epicondyle of the humerus
- Ulnar border of forearm
- Hypothenar eminence
- Area of disturbed sensation

Radial nerve palsy

The radial nerve (see Fig. 25.2) is particularly susceptible to injury. It may be compressed in the axilla through the use of crutches or compressed where it winds round the humerus, when the arm of an intoxicated person hangs over the edge of a chair or if the arm of the anaesthetised patient is allowed to hang over the edge of the operating table. Penetrating wounds and fractures of the humerus may also cause radial nerve injury.

The symptoms depend upon the level at which the nerve is injured, if this is in or above the axilla there will be paralysis and wasting of all the muscles it supplies. When pressure occurs where the nerve winds round the humerus it is usually only the muscles below the elbow which are affected; features of this injury are wrist and finger drop due to paralysis of the extensor muscles of the wrist and hand.

Treatment

A splint is necessary to maintain the wrist in a position of extension without rigidly fixing the fingers, as they must be free for exercise.

Injuries of the long thoracic nerve

The long thoracic nerve is a combination of nerve roots from cervicals 5, 6 and 7 and may be injured as the result of a sudden blow on the shoulder or as the result of pressure from constantly carrying heavy weights on the shoulder, for example sacks of coal. The patient will find difficulty in thrusting his arm forward and in raising it above his head, as the serratus anterior muscle which normally holds the scapula against the chest wall is weak or paralysed allowing winging of the scapula. The weak muscle must be rested, but should it not recover, an operation will be performed to transplant the sterno-costal portion of the pectoralis muscle from the arm to the inferior angle of the scapula.

The lumbar and sacral plexuses

The lumbar and sacral nerve roots, after leaving the spinal cord, unite and divide in the lumbar and sacral nerve plexuses and re-emerge to form the main nerve roots to the legs (Fig. 25.5).

Disturbance of the lateral cutaneous nerve of the thigh (meralgia paraesthetica)

The lateral cutaneous nerve enters the thigh under Poupart's ligament to supply the antero-lateral aspect of the thigh. The nerve is sometimes constricted by fibrous tissue as it leaves the pelvis or enters the thigh muscles. The patient is usually a middle-aged overweight man; the condition may affect a woman in the third or fouth month of pregnancy or it may be due to prolapse of the intervertebral disc between the 3rd and 4th lumbar vertebrae. As the nerve is entirely sensory the symptoms are pain and numbness down the outer side of the thigh.

Treatment

The condition usually recovers spontaneously after a few months; mild analgesics may be helpful and the patient will be advised to lose weight. Surgical decompression or section of the nerve will only be necessary if the patient finds the persistent pain unbearable.

Disturbance of the femoral nerve

The femoral nerve arising from the lumbar plexus passes beneath the psoas muscle close to the pelvis and hip joint on its way to the anterior muscles of the thigh and knee. The nerve roots may be compressed by the less common prolapsed intervertebral disc between the 3rd and 4th lumbar vertebrae. The nerve itself may be damaged in association with dislocation of the hip, fractures of the pelvis or femur, or compressed by a psoas abscess or pelvic tumour.

Symptoms

The patient will complain of pain and tingling or numbness in the front of the thigh, that his leg sometimes gives way as he is walking, he has difficulty lifting and straightening the leg and in climbing stairs.

Examination

On examination there may be obvious wasting of the quadriceps muscles, sensory loss in the distribution of the femoral nerve (the front and inner

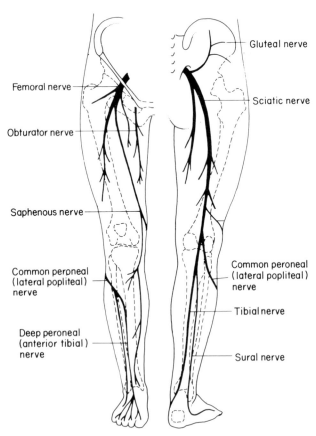

Femoral nerve

Obturator nerve

Saphenous nerve

Common peroneal (lateral popliteal) nerve

Deep peroneal (anterior tibial) nerve

Gluteal nerve

Sciatic nerve

Common peroneal (lateral popliteal) nerve

Tibial nerve

Sural nerve

Fig. 25.5 Distribution of nerve supply to the leg.

aspects of the thigh) and weakness of the muscles which flex the hip and extend the knee, the knee reflex may be absent.

Treatment

The condition will resolve when the cause of the disturbance is treated.

Disorders of the sciatic nerve

The 4th and 5th lumbar and 1st, 2nd and 3rd sacral peripheral nerves enter the sacral plexus, are rearranged and emerge as the sciatic nerve (see Figs 25.1 and 25.5). This important nerve trunk passes through the great sciatic notch close to the acetabulum, down the back of the thigh and divides to become the common peroneal and tibial nerves. The common peroneal (lateral popliteal) nerve passes round the outer side of the knee and down the shin as the deep peroneal (anterior tibial) nerve to the foot, and the tibial nerve passes down the back of the leg to the foot. These nerves supply sensation and power to the back of the thigh and most of the leg and foot except for the small area of the inner leg and foot supplied by the saphenous nerve, a branch of the femoral nerve.

The commonest cause of sciatica is a lumbar disc protrusion (see p. 214) compressing one or more nerve roots before they enter the plexus; the nerve may also be damaged by fractures of the pelvis or femur, gunshot wounds of the buttock and thigh or the compression of pelvic tumours. Great care is necessary when giving intramuscular injections into the buttock (see Fig. 25.5) as an injection incorrectly positioned may enter the sciatic nerve.

Symptoms and signs

The sciatic nerve is rarely completely destroyed. The onset of symptoms suggesting involvement of the sciatic nerve may be sudden, following fracture or gunshot injuries, but more commonly they develop gradually. The patient will complain of pain extending down the back of the thigh, the side of the leg and into the toes. He will find difficulty in walking as the leg becomes weak and flaccid and foot-drop may cause him to trip unless he consciously lifts his leg as he takes each step; the weak leg may suddenly give way and cause a fall. There is evidence of muscle wasting at the back of the thigh and in the leg, and an area of diminished sensation in the same distribution. Sweating is absent in the leg due to interruption of the autonomic nerve supply and the skin below the knee will be dry; considerable thickening of the skin of the toes and sole of the foot occurs. The circulation in the lower leg is poor and the foot swollen and discoloured, ulceration is likely in the insensitive areas. The ankle and plantar responses are diminished or absent, but the knee reflex is present as it is supplied by the femoral nerve.

Treatment

The aims of treatment are to locate and relieve pressure upon the nerve, to provide physiotherapy to strengthen weakened muscles, and support the paralysed limb by the use of a caliper and toe spring. Insensitive areas of skin should be inspected daily for signs of redness or abrasion as prompt treatment will avoid ulceration; the dry skin should be oiled and callouses carefully removed by a chiro-

podist. Swelling of the foot and ankle can be reduced by wearing an elastic stocking or supportive bandage to assist venous return and by periods of exercise alternating with periods of rest with the foot raised.

The common peroneal nerve

Injuries to the knee, in particular fractures of the upper end of the fibula, or a tight bandage applied to the knee may damage the common peroneal nerve as it winds round the outside of the knee joint. Symptoms of disturbance may arise spontaneously in healthy persons, or may occur as the result of pressure during sleep, especially in the elderly who also suffer from arteriosclerosis or diabetes mellitus (see p. 329). The first symptom is usually of pain down the outside of the leg which is present for two or three days and is followed by the sudden onset of weakness of the lateral and anterior muscles of the leg. There is foot-drop and sensory loss in the outer part of the leg and upper surface of the foot and later some wasting of the paralysed muscles. Recovery is slow and usually incomplete; the weak foot is supported by the use of a toe-spring and caliper during the day and by a supportive boot at night.

Bell's palsy

The onset of Bell's palsy is usually rapid. After some pain behind the ear, the patient wakes in the morning to find his face paralysed on one side; sometimes this paralysis develops more slowly over a period of 24 to 36 hours. The paralysis can be very severe involving the forehead as well as the rest of the face, the lower eyelid will not close, tears run from the eye and the mouth sags at the corner. The pain in the side of the head, behind the ear or in the neck on the affected side, rapidly disappears; there is increased sensitivity to sound in the affected ear and the sense of taste is often diminished.

The cause of this catastrophic event, which may affect anyone between the ages of 20 to 60 years, is inflammation of the facial (VIIth cranial) nerve; this peripheral nerve to the face contains mainly motor fibres supplying power to one half of the face with a small sensory branch which transmits taste from the anterior two-thirds of the tongue and

the soft palate. The cause of inflammation is unknown though a virus or autoimmune reaction may be responsible; sometimes the disorder occurs in association with herpes zoster. The rapid onset of such a disfiguring condition will undoubtedly cause much anxiety as it may be several hours before the patient sees his doctor and is given assurance that the condition will get better; the patient may fear he has had a 'stroke'.

Complete recovery is usual without treatment. The forehead and eye recover first and within 3 to 6 weeks paralysis totally disappears. In some instances recovery will take much longer (from 3 months to 1 year) and may be incomplete. During recovery there may be some disorganisation of the nerve pathways as the nerve fibres regrow, for example the patient may find when he smiles that he also involuntarily winks or that when he eats, tears pour down his cheek.

Until the use of steroids there was no effective treatment for Bell's palsy. The chances of complete recovery are increased if treatment with steroids is commenced during the first 4 hours before paralysis is complete, and total paralysis may also be averted. Prednisolone is given orally in high doses for 5 days and then tailed off gradually. Mild analgesics may be necessary for a few days. During the period when the eyelid is paralysed the eye must be protected to prevent inflammation and ulceration (see p. 57); a lateral tarsorrhaphy may be required until the eye closes normally, usually within a few weeks.

Polyneuropathy

Polyneuropathy (sickness of many nerves) sometimes inaccurately called polyneuritis, is a term used to describe simultaneous disturbance of the function of many peripheral nerves. It leads to symmetrical muscular weakness and wasting usually accompanied by sensory disturbance which starts in the distal parts of the extremities and may also involve the cranial nerves. The disorder is acute or chronic and may be part of a generalised illness, the brain or other major organs also being involved. There are two ways in which the nerves are affected.

(a) the disorder may be in the nerve cell body and its axon and result in the nerve dying back from its extremity

(b) the neurilemmal cells of the insulating cover of the nerves may be affected and lead to demyelination.

There may be a combination of these processes or some unknown factor.

Known causes of polyneuropathy

1 Metabolic disorders
i Nutritional
(a) Alcoholism causing malabsorption and deficient intake of vitamin B_1
(b) Beriberi – dietary deficiency of vitamin B_1
(c) Subacute combined degeneration of the cord – malabsorption or lack of vitamin B_{12}
ii Endocrine disturbances especially diabetes, but also myxoedema, acromegaly and more rarely, thyrotoxicosis.
iii Poisons
Prolonged and repeated contact with heavy metals such as lead, mercury, copper and gold and other organic compounds used during industrial processes (triorthocresylphosphate, acrylamide and disulphiram).
iv Drugs
Prolonged treatment with isoniazid (by causing vitamin B_6 deficiency), vincristine used in the treatment of malignant disease, sulphonamides, nitrofurantoin and rarely phenytoin.
v Porphyria, a genetically determined metabolic disorder in which there are episodes of haemoglobin breakdown; these are often precipitated by administration of barbiturates, alcohol and other drugs, and cause intermittent attacks of intestinal colic and constipation, or confusion associated with peripheral nerve disorders. Excessive excretion of porphyrins in the urine and faeces will be found during an acute attack and characteristically the urine, a normal colour when it is passed, later becomes darkish red.
vi Uraemia

2 Infection
Polyneuropathy is associated with certain infections more usually as the indirect effect of toxins rather than a direct effect of bacteria or viruses.
i Direct infection may be from the viruses of mumps and herpes zoster or the leprosy bacillus.
ii Indirect infection may follow glandular fever, infective hepatitis or diphtheria.
iii Following an injection of tetanus serum or an inoculation.

3 Vascular disorders
The effect upon the nervous system is usually the result of ischaemia but there may be other additional factors in such disorders as diabetes mellitus where metabolism is also disturbed.

4 Generalised disorders

Carcinoma, sarcoidosis and polyarteritis nodosa in which there are abnormalities in the metabolism of serum proteins.

5 Genetic disorders

These include peroneal muscular atrophy (see Chapter 29).

Often the cause of polyneuropathy remains undiscovered.

History

The history will vary according to the cause of the neuropathy; in some cases the symptoms are rapid in onset, in others gradual. The first symptoms are usually tingling, 'pins and needles' and numbness affecting the extremities of all four limbs, firstly in the feet, later the hands and then spreading up the limbs in a symmetrical way (glove and stocking distribution, Fig. 25.6) over a varying length of time. There may be considerable pain and tenderness of the calf muscles and night-time cramp. The patient complains of weakness and unsteadiness when walking, difficulty in fine movements such as fastening buttons, and mentions that when he is handling familiar objects they 'feel different'.

The doctor will observe the patient carefully for signs of contributory illness, will assess his mental state, note his general appearance and state of nutrition, look for oedema, abnormal pigmentation of the skin and tremors. He will ask searching questions to find out if the patient has symptoms of diabetes mellitus, has been in the habit of taking alcohol regularly (particularly spirits and wines) is taking drugs, or if his occupation is likely to have brought him into contact with a toxic substance. He will enquire about the patient's appetite, diet, digestion and whether he has had a recent illness.

Examination

A full general examination may reveal signs of early heart failure, enlargement of the liver, palpable carcinoma or evidence of respiratory disorder.

Neurological examination will reveal a flaccid

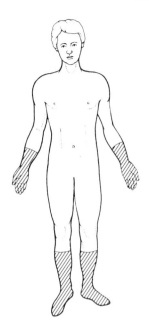

Fig. 25.6 Glove and stocking distribution of sensory loss in polyneuropathy.

lower motor neurone weakness affecting the legs more than the arms, there will also be ataxia due to loss of postural sensibility, loss of all forms of sensation, diminished or absent tendon reflexes and the plantar response may be flexor or unobtainable. There may be wasting of muscles. The skin of the hands and feet is often shiny and oedematous. There is a characteristic high-stepping stomping gait due to foot-drop and loss of sensation in the feet. The patient often experiences a delayed sensation of severe pain when pressure has been applied to the calf muscles or the plantar reflexes have been tested.

Investigations

The many causes of polyneuropathy often necessitate lengthy and detailed investigation, and yet the cause may remain obscure. All non-essential medications will be withdrawn and no treatment begun until investigations have been completed.

1 Routine chest X-rays will be scrutinised for evidence of a neoplasm

2 Blood tests will include
i full blood count, haemoglobin and blood sedimentation rate
ii blood urea
iii fasting blood sugar
iv serum proteins
v vitamin B_{12} estimation
vi viral studies
vii liver function tests
3 Urine tests
i routine ward tests
ii urinary examination for excreted drugs or metallic substances
iii urinary porphyrins
4 Glucose tolerance test
5 Pyruvate tolerance test (see p. 332)
6 Diagnex blue test
7 Histamine test meal
8 Examination of faeces for
i occult blood
ii porphyrins
iii fats
9 Lumbar puncture
10 Electrophysiological tests
11 Nerve biopsy

Many factors influence the incidence of neuropathy. In certain countries vitamin deficiency diseases are common due to acute shortage of food supplies, local dietary habits or lack of understanding of food values. Alcoholic neuropathy is likely to be more common in those countries where spirits and home brewed wines are drunk to excess. Controlled drug trials help to prevent the marketing of drugs with harmful side effects and factory controls and legislation influence the health of industrial workers, but regular inspection is necessary to prevent slovenly standards and malpractice from creeping in. Immunisation programmes have eliminated many diseases which were once prevalent and led to polyneuropathy, but inoculation itself is sometimes thought to be a cause; diseases which cause neuropathy are still common in certain parts of the world.

Acute post-infective polyneuritis (Guillain-Barré syndrome)

This can be a very severe illness affecting young to middle-aged people which may cause rapid deterioration in the patient's condition and even death, but if excellent medical and nursing care is given the patient may make an astonishing recovery despite several weeks of complete paralysis and inability to swallow, or breathe without mechanical aid.

The illness often begins with a mild upper respiratory infection, fever, headache and general malaise followed within 24 hours by numbness and loss of power in the legs. Rapidly ascending paralysis involves the trunk and upper limbs, the shoulder and pelvic girdles being as severely affected as the extremities; the cranial nerves may also be involved. Despite extensive paralysis the respiratory muscles may be spared, but each patient must be carefully observed for signs of impending respiratory failure and difficulty in swallowing as inhalation of saliva or vomit must be avoided; prompt tracheal intubation, tracheostomy and mechanical ventilation may become necessary.

Nursing care

Good nursing care is vital if the patient is to escape the many complications which can retard recovery or leave the patient unnecessarily disabled (see Chapter 10). During the acute phase of the illness a full regime of chest care must be given with the assistance of the physiotherapist who will also give passive exercises and advice about the use of splints. An intravenous infusion will be necessary if the patient is very ill or has difficulty swallowing and, after a day or two, if dysphagia persists, will be replaced by intragastric feeding. Retention of urine is common in the early stages of this illness and will necessitate catheterisation; a self-retaining catheter on open drainage will be necessary until the patient's condition improves. The patient will need reassurance and, fortunately, this can be confidently given, as the more acutely this illness begins the more rapid the recovery; the whole course of the illness usually takes a period of 3 to 6 months. Nurses need to be very watchful as sometimes a patient shows signs of slight recovery and then relapses to the point of having respiratory and swallowing difficulties. It is important that the patient should at no time be over-fatigued by excessively enthusiastic physiotherapy and rehabilitation, too much too soon may cause a relapse. Occasionally permanent disability remains, particularly some loss of sensation in the hands and feet.

Alcoholic polyneuropathy

This is a chronic painful neuropathy caused by vitamin B_1 deficiency arising from the increasing intake of alcohol, the toxic effect of the alcohol itself, gastritis and the exclusion of normal diet. The condition will resolve if the patient can be persuaded to refrain from alcohol soon enough, take nourishing meals and is given a multi-vitamin preparation.

Diabetic polyneuropathy

This form of neuropathy usually leads to increasing weakness and sensory loss in the legs accompanied by severe burning pain in the lower part of the legs. Isolated cranial or other peripheral nerve palsies may be the only symptoms, probably the result of small vascular incidents. Distal trophic lesions of skin and joints occur because of the combined effects of neuropathy and poor circulation. Occasionally there is marked wasting and pain affecting only the thigh muscles (diabetic amyotrophy). Diabetic polyneuropathy may affect the autonomic nervous system when disturbance of bowel function and impotence become distressing symptoms; there may be postural hypotension from pooling of blood in the legs resulting in attacks of syncope. Patients suffering from diabetes mellitus are more susceptible to carpal tunnel syndrome and to nerve root pain associated with cervical and lumbar spondylosis. Polyneuropathy does not develop purely because a patient has severe diabetes mellitus, it may accompany mild diabetes, though better control of the diabetes does improve the symptoms of polyneuropathy.

Carcinomatous neuropathy

A patient who has carcinoma may develop polyneuropathy and it is particularly associated with carcinoma of the bronchus; the lesion itself may be asymptomatic or very small and difficult to detect on X-ray or body scan. As the carcinoma enlarges the symptoms of polyneuropathy increase; they usually resolve once the tumour is treated. The symptoms affecting the limbs may be sensory, motor or a combination of both; there may also be cerebellar degeneration, polymyositis or myopathy (see Chapter 28). Symptoms may be similar to myasthenia gravis, motor neurone disease, encephalomyelitis or metabolic disturbance (hyper-

calcaemia or abnormal secretion of anti-diuretic hormone).

Diphtherial polyneuropathy

Diphtheria is now almost unheard of in the developed countries due to mass immunisation of children, but in countries where immunisation is not practised, the disease is quite common and often fatal.

The toxins of diphtheria have an affinity for the peripheral nerves and when the disease affects the nervous system the first signs, which are usually those causing paralysis of the palate and external ocular muscles, are seen during the second week of the illness. The patient's voice develops a nasal tone, fluid tends to be regurgitated through the nose and there is difficulty in focusing the eyes. These symptoms persist for 10 to 20 days, then rapidly resolve. A few patients with diphtheria develop widespread polyneuropathy which very occasionally leads to paralysis of the diaphragm and respiratory muscles necessitating the use of a mechanical ventilator. When diphtheria is complicated by involvement of the central nervous system, complete recovery usually takes 6 months.

Treatment and nursing care of patients with polyneuropathy

Treatment will depend on the cause of neuropathy. Rest is important in the initial stages of acute severe illness especially if tachycardia suggests cardiac involvement, as sudden syncope and death have been known to occur. Any patient who has an ascending paralysis must be observed at all times for signs of impending respiratory failure and difficulty in swallowing; over-fatigue must be avoided to prevent a relapse. A patient with chronic neuropathy must keep active and follow their normal routines or they run the risk of becoming helpless and bedridden. Every patient will need reassurance and encouragement during what may be a long frightening illness or involve almost daily lengthy investigations necessitating overnight fasting, no breakfast and late lunch. The patient's general health must be maintained by a well-balanced diet and vitamin B supplements (see Chapter 26). When the patient is known to have gastritis or faulty absorption, vitamins must be given by injection.

Those who have been accustomed to taking excessive alcohol will suffer withdrawal symptoms and as, during investigations, tranquillising drugs are contraindicated, care will be taken that the patient receives supportive psychotherapy during his period in hospital and following discharge home. The patient should be carefully observed to ensure that he does not secretly obtain alcohol; the co-operation of relatives will be necessary and the patient and relatives can be encouraged to contact the Alcoholics Anonymous organisations. A patient with any form of neuropathy may have anxiety, depression, pain or insomnia, but care will always be taken in prescribing medication for someone with neuropathy as it may increase the symptoms, further confuse the diagnosis or lead to addiction. Lack of medication is an additional hardship for the patient and there is unfortunately little relief obtainable for those with painful neuritis apart from general measures to improve the neuropathy and the passage of time. When the patient is suffering from neuropathy due to poison-ing with heavy metals, penicillamine is given (see Chapter 27).

Steroid therapy is specifically used in the treatment of acute post-infective polyneuritis; there appears to be evidence that the illness is less severe and recovery more rapid if cortico-steroids are administered, though there is some risk of accelerating respiratory infection.

Nurses may be able to pass on helpful information to the doctor when, during conversation with the patient or his relatives, relevant details of the patient's way of life, activities, hobbies or habitual medicines are revealed. The patient may need encouragement to take a healthy diet, avoid factors which have caused the neuropathy and follow the advice and treatment recommended by the doctor.

An intensive course of rehabilitation is always necessary (see Chapters 3 and 10); there may be some residual disability, but some patients will recover completely. Close co-operation is necessary with social welfare and public health authorities.

26

Deficiency Disorders

A healthy individual – man, woman, child or infant – needs a diet which provides protein, fats and carbohydrates in the correct balance, calories in proportion to energy expended, minerals, calcium, potassium, magnesium, sodium, iron and vitamins (Fig. 26.1). Caloric requirements vary according to age, activities and climate. Nutrition is dependent on agriculture, economic factors, education, racial and religious habits and taboos; there are places where the inhabitants suffer from malnutrition though food is available, they may for instance be forbidden to eat meat or fear the consequences of eating unfamiliar foods which are regarded as poisonous and whose food value is not appreciated. In certain remote parts of the world the inhabitants barely scrape a living, the soil is poor, drought and lack of irrigation prevent growth of crops and there is no easy route for supplies by road and rail; the inhabitants suffer from severe malnutrition and many die of starvation. Medical advisers are powerless to improve their patients' health though they clearly see the cause of ill-health and the results of particular deficiencies. Government and administrators can assist in road building, distribution of supplies, provision of machinery and by teaching methods of irrigation and cultivation. Education is a continuously important factor or facilities may be misused. Health centres are necessary with emphasis on ante-natal and post-natal care, infant welfare and care of the sick and aged. Other parts of the world are rich in money and provisions yet deficiency disorders still occur, particularly among the very young, pregnant and nursing mothers, the ignorant, the aged and infirm, those with dietary fads and the mentally ill (those with anorexia nervosa, endogenous depression, chronic alcoholism and dementia). There may be not only inadequate intake of essential food, minerals and vitamins, but also defective absorption and utilisation when there are stomach, intestinal and liver disorders. Certain medications similarly affect absorption, for example antibiotics destroy the flora and bacteria of the gut which normally assist in the metabolism of folic and nicotinic acids and riboflavin, anticonvulsants (phenytoin sodium, primidone and phenobarbitone) cause deficiency of folic acid, isoniazid (an anti-tuberculous drug) destroys vitamin B_6, and regular doses of liquid paraffin coat the bowel. Alcohol taken habitually in excess, not only acts as a gastric irritant, but may be consumed in preference to normal food.

One of the essential factors in maintaining normal healthy function of the nervous system is the presence in the diet of certain organic substances, vitamins. Those necessary are in the vitamin B complex and include thiamine (B_1), nicotinic acid, riboflavin (B_2), folic acid, cyanocobalamin (B_{12}) and pyridoxine (B_6). These substances are unrelated, but often found in the same foods; yeast, the husk and germ of wheat, egg yolk and liver. Smaller amounts are found in milk, green vegetables, potatoes, tomatoes and meat. Glucose,

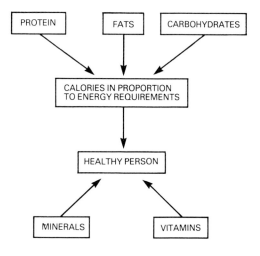

Fig. 26.1 Dietary needs of a healthy person.

calcium, potassium, magnesium, sodium and iron are also essential to the nervous system. Although a deficiency disorder may appear to suggest lack of one particular vitamin or mineral, it is rarely limited to one factor and the patient is often generally debilitated and undernourished.

Deficiency of vitamin B₁

Conditions which can result from a deficiency of vitamin B₁
i Beriberi
   (a) 'wet' (cardiovascular) beriberi
   (b) 'dry' beriberi
ii Wernicke's encephalopathy

Beriberi occurs chiefly among rice eating nations whose diet of 'polished' rice has lost vitamin B₁. The condition is rare in temperate climates for though much refined white flour is used, a varied diet supplies the vitamin in other foods. The symptoms of beriberi occur however when gastro-intestinal disease, vomiting during pregnancy or alcoholism cause defective absorption of vitamin B₁. Lack of this vitamin causes imperfect growth in children, loss of appetite, defective metabolism of carbohydrates and loss of normal peristalsis; in the nervous system it causes polyneuropathy and encephalopathy.

'Dry' beriberi

This may be acute or insidious in onset. The patient is usually undernourished and has had a diet deficient in the entire vitamin B complex for a long period; underfeeding and protein deficiency are thought to play a part in the disorder. On examination a bilateral symmetrical peripheral neuropathy will be noticed involving the motor and sensory nerves causing weakness, muscle wasting and loss of tendon reflexes (lower motor neurone) and impairment of all forms of sensation.

Investigations
See Chapter 25

Pyruvate tolerance test

The patient is fasted and then takes a measured amount of glucose by mouth; intravenous blood is then taken at intervals. Normal pyruvic acid level is 0.5–1 mg per 100 ml; disturbance of carbohydrate metabolism in vitamin B₁ deficiency leads to a raised pyruvic acid level.

Treatment

The most important feature of treatment is an adequate well-balanced diet and the importance of this should be explained to the patient who may not at first relish unfamiliar foods. Diet must be supplemented by foods rich in vitamin B₁, yeast, wheat germ and liver extract and intramuscular Parentrovite may be administered to correct overall vitamin deficiency caused by undernourishment. Physiotherapy is important to maintain and restore muscle power and prevent deformities. An acute polyneuropathy responds to treatment more rapidly and fully than one of slower onset. The patient should be persuaded not to return to previous dietary habits when he is discharged from hospital; this can be most difficult to prevent in some sections of society who have very rigid eating habits.

'Wet' (cardiovascular) beriberi

This is a distinct form of beriberi and though it does not affect the nervous system, must be mentioned here as it occasionally occurs with the 'dry' form and carries the risk of sudden heart failure. The symptoms are entirely due to disordered carbohydrate metabolism and lack of thiamine (vitamin B₁); there may also be evidence of deficiency of protein, iron, vitamin A, nicotinic acid and ribo-flavin. Patients with this form of beriberi have suffered from incorrect nutrition with lack of thiamine, but are not necessarily undernourished and appear obese due to oedema and excessive carbohydrate intake.

Treatment

Emergency treatment is necessary when signs of impending heart failure are present. The patient will require hospital treatment, complete bed rest and administration of thiamine hydrochloride 30 mg daily which is at first given by intramuscular injection. Following these injections the patient must be observed carefully for anaphylactic shock; oral thiamine hydrochloride, the safer form of treatment will be instituted as soon as possible. The effect of thiamine is dramatic, it rapidly reduces the heart to normal size and function and this produces a sudden diuresis. The patient's general condition must then be treated and a full programme of physical and social rehabilitation completed.

Wernicke's encephalopathy

This condition, a serious and infrequent result of vitamin B_1 deficiency, leads to areas of congestion and small haemorrhages in the medial aspect of the thalamus and hippocampus and in the hypothalamus and grey matter of the upper part of the brain stem. The condition, with its early signs of difficulty in concentration and disturbed sleep, may have passed unnoticed until the patient suddenly becomes noisy, confused, disorientated, deluded and unco-operative. Untreated the patient will lapse into unconsciousness.

On examination, in addition to the patient's abnormal mental condition, there will be signs of cranial nerve involvement, loss of pupil reaction, weakness or paralysis of all the eye muscles and nystagmus; there may be evidence of polyneuropathy. Examination may be difficult or impossible if the patient is so confused that he is unable to co-operate.

Vitamin B₁₂ (cyanocobalamin) deficiency

Vitamin B_{12} is contained in certain foods, especially meat and liver, and its absorption and utilisation are dependent upon the secretion of intrinsic factor by the lining of the stomach. Vitamin B_{12} and the intrinsic factor are stored in the liver and are used by the bone marrow along with other vitamins, proteins and chemicals in the manufacture of red blood cells. One of these chemicals, folic acid, may be deficient in the diet or destroyed by prolonged treatment with anticonvulsant or barbiturate drugs; this causes megaloblastic anaemia and may lead to neurological symptoms as found in subacute combined degeneration of the cord. Vitamin B_{12} is also necessary to maintain the health of nerve tissue.

Two factors affect the absorption of vitamin B_{12}

i Lack of secretion of intrinsic factor which may follow total gastrectomy or is more commonly due to atrophy of the gastric mucosal glands in later life, the result of a genetic tendency.

ii Insufficient vitamin B_{12} in the diet; this sometimes happens in strict vegetarianism.

Effects of vitamin B₁₂ deficiency

(a) Pernicious anaemia
(b) Peripheral neuropathy
(c) Spinal cord degeneration
(d) Encephalopathy – manifest by mental irritability, confusion and convulsions
(e) There may be a combination of (a) – (d).

The first results of vitamin B_{12} deficiency may either be shown by the central nervous system or the bone marrow or the two systems may be affected almost simultaneously. The severity of the anaemia in no way predicts involvement of the nervous system, as a very mild anaemia may be closely followed by a progressive neurological disorder and a severe anaemia by no neurological involvement.

Pernicious anaemia

In this condition there are fewer than normal red

blood cells in the circulation and some of these are large and immature. Anaemia caused by vitamin B$_{12}$ deficiency is corrected by injections of cyanocobalamin (Cytamen).

Subacute combined degeneration of the cord

The spinal cord seems to bear the brunt of the effect of vitamin B$_{12}$ deficiency, hence the misleading name given to this disorder which frequently also involves the peripheral nerves and sometimes the cerebral hemispheres and brain stem. Demyelinating degeneration occurs mainly in the posterior sensory pathways and the lateral motor pathways throughout the length of the spinal cord (Fig. 26.2), causing poor conduction of nerve impulses; later the nerve fibres die because they have lost their protective nourishing coverings.

Subacute degeneration of the cord has become more rare since vitamin B$_{12}$ has been used in the treatment of pernicious anaemia; however, when it occurs it usually affects either sex over the age of 50 years.

History

There may be a family history of pernicious anaemia and the patient may already be receiving treatment for the condition; he may feel tired and lifeless, breathless on exertion, have ankle swelling, a sore tongue (glossitis) and suffer from indigestion. Additional recent symptoms are unpleasant sensations of tingling and 'pins and needles' (paraesthesiae) starting in the toes and creeping up the legs with similar feelings in the fingers and hands. Other abnormal sensations may be described as a feeling of wetness and coldness of the legs and 'walking on cotton wool'. The patient may complain that his legs are tired, he is unsteady on his feet and tends to trip; his hands may also be clumsy. Relatives may have noticed that the patient has become forgetful, irritable and sometimes slightly confused.

Examination

There may be a yellowish tinge to the skin and other signs of anaemia. The signs in the nervous system will vary considerably from patient to patient depending on the extent to which the spinal cord or the peripheral nerves are affected, for example predominant peripheral nerve involvement leads to a flaccid paraparesis whereas a mainly spinal cord degeneration produces a spastic weakness. One particular feature of vitamin B$_{12}$ deficiency neuropathy is the intensely painful nature of the paraesthesiae and the tenderness of the legs. There may be optic atrophy.

Investigations

1　Full blood count
2　Blood vitamin B$_{12}$ estimation
3　Serum folate estimation (folic acid)

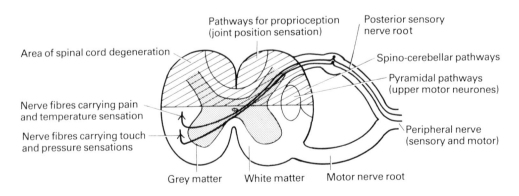

Fig. 26.2 Distribution of spinal cord degeneration in subacute combined degeneration of the cord.

4 Diagnex blue test and histamine test meal to diagnose achlorhydria, as without hydrochloric acid there can be no intrinsic factor
5 Radioactive vitamin B_{12} estimation

A very small number of patients with signs of dementia may be suffering from undiagnosed vitamin B_{12} deficiency; to prevent these few who have a treatable condition from being permanently detained in an institution, it is important that in every instance of dementia a full blood count and vitamin B_{12} estimation are performed.

Treatment

Treatment with injections of cyanocobalamin will produce a marked improvement in the patient's condition. Intramuscular injections are given every other day during the first week, then weekly, and after several months a maintenance dose is given every 3 to 4 weeks for the rest of the patient's life. Regular haematological analysis and a periodic neurological examination are essential.

The earlier the patient's disorder is discovered the more complete will be the cure. Those who suffer from pernicious anaemia or any form of vitamin B_{12} deficiency always need careful neurological examination as, though the blood count may have returned to normal, a considerably higher dosage of cyanocobalamin is advisable if the nervous system shows any signs attributable to vitamin B_{12} deficiency. The patient who has adequate treatment for pernicious anaemia may never develop signs related to the nervous system. All patients with subacute combined degeneration of the cord treated with cyanocobalamin will show some improvement as peripheral nerves slowly regenerate and there is recovery of myelin, but there is no regeneration of nerve tissue in the spinal cord once it is totally destroyed and some patients will be left with loss of joint position sense (proprioception) and signs of mild spastic paraparesis; the patient will probably notice these disabilities more with increasing age.

Nursing care

(See Chapter 10)

All vitamin deficiency disorders need prompt diagnosis and effective treatment to prevent irreversible damage to the nervous system. Many deficiencies pass unnoticed until they become quite severe and chronic. Old people living alone do not bother to eat a well-balanced diet, there is no pleasure in solitary mealtimes and their appetite diminishes, until a cup of tea and a biscuit often replace a meal. Mental deterioration caused by old age is aggravated by dietary deficiency and more florid signs of confusion develop. Alcoholic addiction is often a secret concealed by the individual and his or her family. Community health workers need to be very observant and play an important part in the aftercare of patients who have been treated for malnutrition and deficiency disorders.

27

Poisoning

Since earliest time the effects of poisons on the nervous system have been observed and recorded. It was noticed that after eating certain plants, berries and fungi or being attacked by creatures which protect themselves with deadly venom or poison, a person would become very ill with delirium, paralysis, convulsions or loss of consciousness and soon die. Early man, observing the effects of these natural poisons, used them to make poisoned darts and arrows with which he caught his prey and killed his opponent in battle. Through the centuries men and women have been murdered simply and speedily by the addition of a small quantity of poison to food or drink. In an attempt to ward off poisonous 'evil' spirits, amulets were worn and these early people believed in the magic power of particular stones; witch doctors, sorcerers and others mixed antidote potions for a variety of ills, some of which were as lethal as the poisons they were intended to treat. For many centuries 'doctors' tried to help the sick, but their remedies were primitive, often 'hit and miss' and very costly.

During the last century science has advanced so rapidly, to such a depth of understanding, that poisons can be measured in parts per trillion and it is known that a miniscule amount of poison, only two-tenths of a milligram, can kill a man weighing 500 million times more. Scientific advances have led to more accurate diagnosis and effective treatment; antidotes have been found to many poisons and toxins, but some are so rapidly fatal that it would be a miracle if the antidote were at hand in time. Knowledge of the effect of certain drugs upon the nervous system has been put to good use in the development of local and general anaesthesia, in the control of pain, insomnia and epilepsy and in the treatment of psychiatric illness, but on the other hand useful drugs are abused and poisonous substances are sometimes used by the individual experimentally for 'kicks', to heighten perception, as a means of escape from reality or in the extreme to destroy life. Young children are in danger because they grow up in an environment where pills and medicines are freely taken, advertised on television and kept in every home, and in the countryside there are many poisonous plants, berries and fungi.

There are certain communities in the world, who though free of industrial contamination are poisoned by the effects of natural phenomena; in many parts of the world there is little variety in the diet which is sometimes limited by choice, availability or failed harvest to one or two foodstuffs which may contain natural poisons or toxins, for example casava, insufficiently cooked, contains cyanide, fish may be contaminated with mercury, and lathyrus, an Indian pulse, sometimes the only crop to survive a drought, contains a toxin. Nearly every community in a search for pleasure and as a means of escape from the monotony of their lives, have discovered the stimulating and pleasantly relaxing effects of alcohol and drugs and their use has become a socially acceptable feature of life leading to addiction and chronic poisoning. The complexity of modern civilisation and industrialisation has increased the risk of chronic accidental poisoning by chemicals. For generations man has polluted his environment, at first in ignorance and now, though he has begun to understand the dangers, is unable to check the process, being in the grip of huge multi-national companies, high finance, politics and the energy crisis. Chemical fertilisers and weedkillers are widely used to make the land more productive, industrial wastes are dumped onto the land and into streams and rivers, contaminating plants, animal life and water supplies. Radioactive materials are used in a variety of ways and though they are handled with care and stored in protective containers, their waste products are always a problem for disposal and there may be accidental leaks. Pollutants in the air settle on the land, and the seas have become a dumping ground for sewage, oil, detergents and many other chemicals which eventually reach man in the air he breathes and in his food and drink. Unknowingly or uncaringly man bombards himself with a variety of chemicals as preservatives, flavouring and colouring in foodstuffs, he fills his lungs with cigarette smoke, swallows medicines for every ache, pain or minor ailment and to escape from a seemingly meaningless life in a hostile world, may resort to drugs and alcohol. Every year throughout the world poisoning accounts for thousands of deaths, especially in the under fives and the 14–25 age group.

A poison is any substance which destroys life or impairs health. Poisoning may be accidental or intentional, acute or chronic, the poison entering the body (Fig. 27.1) through the lungs (inhaled), gastrointestinal tract (ingested) or skin (absorbed, injected or trapped in wounds). The effects depend upon whether the poison or gas has an affinity for protein, blood or nerve tissue. The blood-brain-barrier prevents some water soluble poisons from leaving the blood stream and entering the nervous system, but many other poisons, once they have reached the circulation, affect the function of the nervous system despite the efforts of the liver and kidneys to rid the body of all unwanted substances.

Poisons and gases affect the nervous system (Fig. 27.2) by:

i   depriving the nerve cells of a constant supply of oxygen

    (a)   disturbing cell metabolism and prevent-

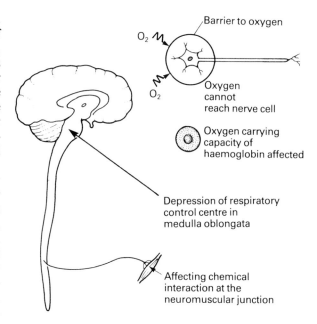

Fig. 27.2 Effects on the nervous system of poisonous substances.

ing the uptake of oxygen from the blood; cyanide has this effect

    (b)   affecting the oxygen-carrying property of haemoglobin; oxygen is displaced by the poisonous carbon monoxide gas which is three times more readily taken up by haemoglobin

ii   depressing the function of the respiratory control centre in the medulla oblongata thereby slowing the respirations, e.g. the action of morphine.

iii   affecting chemical interactions at the neuro-muscular junction by

    (a)   preventing the release of acetylcholine; this is the toxic effect of botulism

    (b)   blocking the uptake of acetylcholine by the muscle; this is the action of tubocurarine which, within minutes of entering the body, paralyses all muscular activity including respirations.

In Great Britain natural gas has replaced town gas, poisonous snakes are few and industrial and agricultural legislation has done much to eliminate poisoning despite the dangerous chemicals used, but accidents still happen.

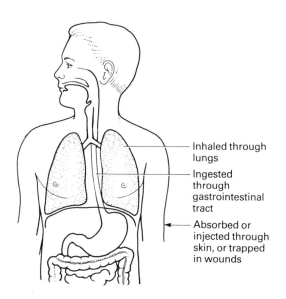

Fig. 27.1 Mode of entry of poisons into the body.

Inhaled through lungs

Ingested through gastrointestinal tract

Absorbed or injected through skin, or trapped in wounds

Poisons

1 Drugs
i hypnotics and narcotics
ii anti-depressants
iii stimulants
iv tranquillisers
v hallucinogenics
vi analgesics
vii any drug to which the patient is allergic

Many potentially poisonous drugs are prescribed by medical practitioners for a variety of conditions, especially for the treatment of anxiety and depression. A depressed person is more likely to take an overdose as an act of self-poisoning or suicide, and as the drugs most readily available are his or her own tranquillisers or anti-depressants, these are most commonly used, sometimes taken with alcohol or as a mixture of drugs which may be antagonistic to each other. An overdose of any drug will cause poisoning and will affect the nervous system, those which are addictive are most often abused. The elderly are forgetful and sometimes take more than the prescribed dose and hoarded drugs can be sampled by children.

2 Alcohol – alcohol dependence is very common and alcohol intensifies the effect of drugs.

3 Gases – in particular carbon monoxide from town gas, car exhaust fumes and the incomplete combustion of faulty camping stoves. The level of carbon monoxide is highest near the ground and children run the greatest risk.

4 Inhalants – glue, butane gas and solvents, e.g. paint strippers and dry cleaning fluids.

5 Metals – lead, copper, mercury and manganese which usually cause chronic poisoning.

6 Inoculations – especially the whooping cough (pertussis) vaccine which occasionally causes an encephalopathy with mental retardation.

7 The effect of general disease which disturbs the normal blood chemistry, e.g. diabetes mellitus, liver failure and uraemia which cause toxic confusional states.

8 Subsistence on certain foods which contain toxins and poisons.

9 Bacterial toxins, e.g. tetanus and botulism.

10 Snake venom.

The severity of poisoning depends upon the strength of the poisonous substance, the person's tolerance to a drug, the number of poisonous substances involved, the amount entering the body, whether the poison directly enters the blood stream, which tissues or organs are involved and the age and health of the individual.

Acute poisoning

As members of the general public, nurses should help to educate others and practise correct procedures designed to prevent accidental poisoning; there should be good publicity about the risks incurred by children. It is possible to impress upon very young children that medicines and other products are dangerous and will make them very ill; nonetheless inquisitive children do not always heed warnings and all medicine bottles must have child-proof lids, medicines should be carefully labelled, stored in a locked cupboard (never in household containers) and all household cleaning fluids, cosmetics and alcohol kept out of reach. A hearing aid battery, a seemingly small and harmless item, can rapidly act as a corrosive if swallowed by a small child; early surgery is the only course of action. Educational programmes in schools should include talks and films on the dangers of experimenting with drugs, inhalants, alcohol and cigarettes, to prevent youngsters from embarking on the downward road which leads to drug dependence and early death. All adults should know the emergency measures to take in the event of accidental or intentional poisoning; the conscious person should be made to vomit (unless he has swallowed petroleum products or caustic and corrosive substances), by putting a finger or spoon handle into the throat or administering strong salt water. The patient who has inhaled gas or noxious fumes must be moved to fresh air. Medical aid should be sought urgently, but if a doctor is not immediately available the victim should be rushed by car or ambulance to the nearest casualty department taking with them all empty containers found beside the victim. It is helpful if a third person can telephone the casualty department to give information in advance concerning the nature of the incident. Some poisonings are within the scope of treatment by the general practitioner who can give activated charcoal which absorbs the poisonous contents of the stomach, or the emetic, syrup of ipecacuanha. Many patients are treated by their doctor and remain at home, cared for and upheld by their relatives and friends.

As the incidence of acute poisoning in adults and children has increased, the possibility of 'overdose' is always considered when the cause of unconsciousness is not immediately obvious. The life of the patient often depends on prompt emergency resuscitative treatment which should not be delayed by attempts to identify the poison. Overdosage of sedative and hypnotic drugs depress the respiratory centre and inhaled noxious gases lead to respiratory crises. A clear airway must be maintained, dentures removed, the patient carefully positioned (see Fig. 3.6) and secretions and vomit aspirated from the throat. An endotracheal tube may be necessary and should the patient fail to breathe spontaneously after a short period of simple artificial respiration, a mechanical ventilator will be needed; this is the only way to ensure that respirations are adequate (see p. 50) and the brain is not deprived of essential oxygen.

Caution should be exercised in the administration of oxygen and when possible the percentage of oxygen and the rate of flow should be prescribed by the doctor; too high a percentage given to patients with chronic lung disease reduces the stimulus which carbon dioxide normally exerts on the respiratory centre. An assessment should be made of the respiratory capacity, a minute volume of 4 litres per minute is adequate; blood gases will also be estimated. When unconsciousness has been caused by severe poisoning the vasomotor centre in the medulla is usually disturbed, gravely affecting the patient's cardiovascular system; the heart becomes a less efficient pump, the blood vessels dilate, venous blood pools in the extremities, the excess fluid gathers in the tissues and there is poor venous return to the heart. The blood volume is diminished, systolic blood pressure is low and the patient is very shocked; he is not dehydrated and intravenous fluids are given with great care to avoid overloading the circulation, further embarrassing the heart and increasing the likelihood of pulmonary oedema. A simple measure to assist venous return to the heart is to raise the foot of the bed or trolley. Cardiac and venous pressure monitoring guide the doctor in his plan of treatment, especially regarding fluid replacement; there are instances when large volumes of intravenous fluids are necessary to quickly restore a normal blood volume, crystalloid solutions and plasma expanders (e.g. haemaccel) may be infused. When the blood volume has been corrected the use of isoprenaline, dopamine or dobutamine may be beneficial.

History and examination

While these emergency measures are undertaken, the person who accompanies the patient to hospital (relative, friend or police officer) should be interviewed by an experienced member of the medical or nursing staff; there must be close co-operation with the police force who are often involved in these circumstances. Parents or close relatives are likely to be panic stricken, often guiltily blaming themselves. Panic is very infectious, but everyone must remain calm for accurate details to be obtained. The following facts should be elicited:

1   The story of the poisoning and/or the circumstances in which the person was found; the victim may be a child and it may not be clear what was taken or whether more than one substance was sampled. Empty containers will be examined to identify the contents.

2   Details of the patient's household, social circumstances and domestic relationships. Important factors include parental fights and separation, legal wrangles over children, unemployment, drug addiction and alcoholism.

3   The patient's state of physical and psychological health before the incident and whether he has been receiving treatment. A few patients exhibit a sudden, severe idiosyncratic reaction to a commonly prescribed medication, e.g. chlorpromazine, or an ordinary food substance, e.g. milk.

4   The nature of employment – the person may have been subjected to sprays or fumes in an enclosed area.

The cause of poisoning in many young children at the exploratory age of 18–36 months when everything goes into the mouth, is often lack of parental supervision and availablity of poisonous drugs which look like sweets. The child's mother may be very busy and harassed by several young children or pre-occupied by a family crisis; she herself may be ill and receiving treatment for anxiety or depression, or be a drug addict and carelessly leave medicines lying about. Young to middle-aged women who become lonely, depressed or have tangled love affairs may take an overdose as a plea for help in an insoluble and intolerable situation (parasuicidal act), not as a deliberate suicide attempt; the patient may make several half-hearted attempts on her life, sometimes in ignorance mixing drugs with alcohol. 'Down and out' drug and alcohol dependent persons are repeatedly seen in casualty departments when they want a 'fix' or a bed for the night where they manipulate the staff to get what they want; it is not always clear whether they are genuinely ill or their odd behaviour is due to inebriation or head injury sustained in a fall (see Chapter 5). Many of those dependent on alcohol and drugs become very depressed and make serious attempts to end their lives. It is a difficult task for the casualty officer to sift malingerers from the genuinely ill who, not showing obvious symptoms at the time, may later develop neurological complications or require the help of a psychiatrist.

A detailed general and neurological examination is necessary (see Chapter 2). An assessment of the patient's conscious level will be made as soon as he reaches hospital and compared with previous assessments made by police, ambulance personnel and others. The nurse will continue frequent regular observations paying particular attention to the rate and character of respirations and level of consciousness. If the patient is unconscious his response to painful stimulus is a more reliable guide to his condition than the pupillary response which

has been influenced by drugs or other medical factors; pupils are constricted by morphine or the drugs used in the treatment for glaucoma and dilated by belladonna and excesses of anti-depressant drugs. There may be clues to the nature of the toxic agent:

i   Barbiturate burns (also caused by tricyclic anti-depressants and carbon monoxide) – areas of erythema often surmounted by a blister are most commonly found where two skin surfaces have pressed together.

ii   A particular smell associated with a poison, e.g. alcohol, bitter almonds (cyanide) or pear drops (nail varnish remover).

iii   Pink discolouration of the skin and mucous membranes suggesting carbon monoxide or cyanide poisoning.

iv   Pin point pupils, depressed respirations and vomiting indicative of poisoning by morphine and allied substances.

v   Vomiting and a very slow irregular pulse associated with excesses of digoxin.

vi   Overbreathing, flushing, sweating and tachycardia suggestive of salicylate poisoning.

vii   The cyanosis of methaemoglobinaemia associated with overdosage of codeine and phenacetin preparations.

viii   Local signs of burning on lips and mouth suggesting ingestion of caustic and corrosive substances.

ix   Characteristic signs of diabetic or insulin coma.

Doctors and staff of accident and emergency departments know the treatment of common poisons, have reference books and charts including one giving information on drugs which are antagonistic to each other, and have access to a 24-hour Poisons Information Service in major cities where they can gain information about a specific rare or new poison and its treatment.

Forensic tests and treatment

Since 1940 the number of poisons available has risen dramatically from as few as 60 to many thousands, even to a possible 250 000. To identify an offending poison would seem impossible, but usually there are clues to its nature and location in the body; an empty bottle may be lying beside the unconscious person or in the other extreme it may be known that the victim was a possible assassination target because of his political affiliations or the nature of his job. To search for poisons in the living victim, specimens of body fluids are collected in metal-free containers, carefully labelled and analysed in the laboratory as soon as possible.

i   Blood – at least 10 ml.

ii   Urine – at least 20 ml; catheterisation may be necessary.

iii   The entire stomach aspirate.

iv   The entire fluid from a stomach washout. A stomach washout, which may prevent further absorption of the poison, should only be performed on the recommendation of the doctor and his decision depends upon:

(a)   the substance ingested

(b)   the patient's level of consciousness

(c)   the length of time since the poison was ingested

Stomach washout is of value especially if the drug has been taken within the previous 4 hours; this time is extended to 12 hours for a tricyclic antidepressant and up to 24 hours for salicylates, as they cause pyloric spasm and the drug is retained in the stomach for longer.

A cuffed endotracheal tube protects the patient from inhalation of regurgitated fluids. When corrosive substances, caustics, paraffin oil and petroleum products have been ingested, intubation is never performed as the risk of regurgitation and inhalation during the procedure is too great and even a small amount of these substances in the lungs will cause pneumonia. When the patient is gravely ill from a massive overdose and delay has allowed large quantities of poison to be absorbed into the blood stream, other measures are employed to hasten elimination. These include diuresis, peritoneal dialysis, haemodialysis and haemodetoxification. During any of these forms of treatment the patient's blood chemistry and fluid balance must be carefully monitored.

When a victim is brought in to hospital already dead, specimens of organs are subjected to forensic testing; there are very sophisticated methods of detecting minute amounts of poison, including neutron activation and the radio immune technique.

Nursing care

The assessment of conscious level at frequent regular intervals throughout the 24 hours must continue until the patient has been fully conscious and alert for several hours. At first fluctuation can be expected and any deterioration must be promptly reported. Patients often show signs of self-neglect and there should be an early and thorough inspection of the skin and pressure areas for sores, abscesses, blisters, infected injection sites or reddened areas caused by pressure; a 2-hourly change of position is necessary avoiding any damaged skin area. Hypothermia is a common complication; a low-scale rectal thermometer must be used as the patient's temperature may be below 30°C. Except when there is severe hypothermia, active rewarming is unnecessary, but further heat loss should be prevented by keeping the patient warmly covered, especially during examination, using a foil space blanket.

Recovery period

When the patient regains consciousness he may be restless, confused and disorientated for hours, days or even months. Careful observation and nursing care are always necessary and the following should be noted and reported.

1   The patient's mood. He is often quiet, withdrawn and depressed and given the opportunity may make another attempt to end his life. On the contrary he may be tearful and filled with remorse. Nurses and medical staff must show a friendly and uncritical attitude and be prepared to listen if the patient wants to talk.

2   Withdrawal fits (see Chapter 19).

3   Abnormalities of response, behaviour or movement which suggest transient or permanent brain damage; aggressive behaviour and restless agitation are very common and blunting of awareness and signs of basal ganglia disturbance sometimes occur.

4 Pyrexia. Mild pyrexia is to be expected, but simple causes of pyrexia (deep vein thrombosis, urinary and respiratory infections) should be excluded.

5 Irregularities of the pulse.

6 Peripheral nerve palsies (see Chapter 25). The commonest of these are ulnar, radial and lateral popliteal nerve palsies due to prolonged pressure on these superficial nerves. Recovery is spon-taneous, but may be incomplete and physiotherapy will be given to prevent contracture deformities.

In every instance of attempted suicide, the patient should be persuaded to see a psychiatrist while he is in hospital; should the patient try to discharge himself while he is still mentally disturbed it may be necessary to sedate him and arrange for transfer to a psychiatric hospital for compulsory detention under the Mental Welfare Act.

Chronic poisoning

Regular repeated ingestion, inhalation or skin absorption of poisonous substances results in chronic poisoning and without treatment leads to tissue damage, especially of the liver, kidneys and nervous system. The true cause of headache, lethargy and loss of appetite, the early symptoms of poisoning, is often unsuspected and even more florid symptoms may be wrongly attributed to other diseases. The hazards of chronic poisoning are unseen; the victim is often unaware that his polluted environment is endangering health, does not realise for example that acid substances leach poisons from cooking utensils and preserving crocks, and when harmful habits are perpetuated, it is often done in ignorance of the consequences and in secret. Poisoning may affect an individual, a family, a group of workers or a whole community; everyone exposed to the risk of poisoning must be screened and if necessary treated, even though they have no symptoms, for it is important for an early diagnosis to be made and treatment begun before there is permanent mental and physical damage. Attempts are being made to exclude toxic substances from industrial processes and manufactured goods. When there has been a breach of the factory safety regulations an enquiry will be held; sometimes the patient is involved in a prolonged legal wrangle for compensation which may delay his recovery. Alcoholism (see Chapters 5, 9, 25 and 26) and drug addiction are also forms of chronic poisoning.

Lead poisoning

Lead is found in the air, the soil and in water supplies, but is an element unnecessary to the human body in even the smallest quantity. Everyone takes in a certain amount of lead each day, but there are important safety limits for children and adults (Lead in Food Regulation, 1961) controlling permitted lead levels in drinking water, baby foods and all consumer products. City dwellers are subjected to higher lead levels than those living in the countryside because there is a greater volume of traffic giving off lead laden exhaust fumes. Young children living near busy road intersections are particularly vulnerable because they live and play in an atmosphere of heavy pollution where even the household dust contains lead; children naturally play on the dusty floor and suck their fingers and toys. Though the use of lead in toy manufacture is now prohibited, it must be remembered that old lead toys are a risk. There are still many old houses with lead pipes and water tanks, and woodwork with several layers of lead-based paint beneath a superficial covering of less harmful modern paint. Other people at risk of lead poisoning are those who work in or live near a lead processing plant, plumbers, painters and those engaged in the manufacture of products containing lead; lead is still found in paints, cosmetics, batteries and astringent lotions.

Lead poisoning is rare and is usually a chronic illness due to repeated intake of small amounts of lead over a long period; as little as a fingernail-sized flake of lead paint eaten daily by an infant is sufficient to cause severe lead poisoning in as short a time as a month. The cause of lead poisoning is sometimes bizarre, for example a child daily tasting her mother's hair dye, or an artist licking his paintbrushes.

Lead is mainly absorbed through the small intestine and lungs, is readily taken up by plasma and red blood cells and is excreted in sweat and urine. Organic lead is rapidly absorbed through the skin into the soft tissues, especially those of the kidneys and liver and after a longer period reaches the bones, hair and teeth. Lead crosses the placental barrier and can reach a baby through the mother's milk. The smaller the individual the greater the effect of a small amount of lead.

History and examination
See Chapter 2

All persons suffering from suspected lead poisoning or who have unexplained or unusual symptoms not attributable to any other condition will be admitted to hospital for thorough examination and investigation. Taking a very careful medical history the doctor will try to establish from the patient and his relatives when the patient was last physically and mentally in good health and when he first started feeling 'off colour'. Enquiries will be made of a child's parents whether early milestones were normal, when development came to a standstill and how and when other symptoms occurred and progressed. The locality in which the patient lives and works, his past and present occupations, leisure pursuits and curious habits are all very relevant.

The first symptoms of chronic lead poisoning are anorexia, constipation, headache and sometimes vomiting; a condition of 'lead colic' causes severe abdominal pain. There is always a mild degree of anaemia associated with lead poisoning. As the disease progresses the patient becomes tremulous and has poor co-ordination, he may either develop peripheral neuropathy (see Chapter 25) which selectively affects the motor fibres causing weakness of the extensor muscles of the hands with wrist drop (the feet are rarely affected), or lead encephalopathy with irritability, hypersensitivity and mental dullness; pregnancy may end in abortion due to tonic contraction of the uterus. Unless the patient is removed from exposure to lead contamination and receives treatment his condition will deteriorate. Signs of severe poisoning include visual disturbance, persistent vomiting, ataxia, delirium, epileptic fits and coma.

The most pertinent observation during the examination which confirms the diagnosis is the discovery of a black or blue 'lead line' on the gums at the base of the teeth, a line which unfortunately is not present if the patient is edentulous.

Investigations

1   Blood tests
i   Haemoglobin, full blood count and sedimentation rate
ii   Wassermann reaction
iii   Lead levels
iv   Liver function tests
2   Urine tests
i   Routine ward tests
ii   Laboratory analysis including a 24-hour collection of urine for estimation of lead content
3   X-rays of wrist, knee and ankle joints
4   Electrophysiological testing of nerve conduction
5   Electroencephalography
6   Psychometry – an initial test may be necessary to give an accurate assessment of the patient's mental state and ability, and later tests will help to assess improvement after treatment and assist the choice of suitable employment.

Treatment

Chelating agents will be given to rid the body of lead deposits; for diagnosis and rapid excretion when the poisoning is severe, sodium calcium edetate is given for a short while and for long term treatment penicillamine is used (for side-effects see p. 292). Treatment must continue for some time after urinalysis returns to normal and anaemia must be corrected. The patient must be removed from exposure to the poison. An extensive search may be necessary in the home with the help of the Public Health authorities; the water supply and preparations in regular use will be analysed.

Mercurial poisoning

Mercury is a naturally occurring substance found in the soil and water; everyone takes a small amount in their daily diet, but it is not necessary to the body. Elemental mercury, as found in thermometers, if swallowed causes little harm, for it is poorly absorbed and some can remain in the body without causing toxic effects. In contrast mercurial vapour and compounds are highly toxic even in small amounts and methyl mercury has a particular attraction for the nervous system and is slow to be excreted. Mercury crosses the placental barrier and affects the foetus. A careful watch is kept on contamination of foodstuffs and there are regulations relating to the use of mercury; it is still used in disinfectants, parasiticides, fungicides, as a seed dressing, for preservation of eye drops and injection solutions, in dental fillings, hair dye and in industry. Certain teething powders, infant dusting powders and ointments that contained mercury have been withdrawn from sale and mercury is no longer used in purgatives and diuretics. In spite of regulations there have been episodes where large numbers of people have been affected by contaminated fish, or bread sprinkled with seed previously treated with organic mercurial seed dressing.

Mercurial poisoning is very rare; chronic poisoning occurs from:

i   The regular inhalation of small amounts of mercurial vapour, e.g. from industrial processes or in a dentist's surgery.
ii The absorption of mercurial compounds through the skin, e.g. when a hairdresser regularly handles hair dye without wearing gloves. It is unwise to handle any substance containing mercury, but should some splash on to the skin it must be washed off thoroughly with soap and water.
iii The ingestion of poorly soluble mercurial salts.

History and examination
See lead poisoning

The effects of mercurial poisoning involve all parts of the nervous system especially the cerebellum and pons varolii and damage may be permanent. Symptoms include tremor, excessive salivation, motor and sensory disturbance sometimes including disturbance of vision and hearing, irritability, emotional lability, mental deterioration, ataxia, dysarthria, chorea, athetosis and myoclonus; an unusual effect is a neuromuscular disorder similar to myasthenia gravis (see Chapter 23). Anaemia is

common and liver and kidney damage occur. In severe poisoning there is loosening of the teeth and a blue line on the gums.

Investigations

Investigations to detect mercury are similar to those used in the investigation of lead poisoning.

Treatment

The patient should be removed from the source of poisoning and elimination of mercury will be hastened by the use of penicillamine; anaemia will be treated.

Manganese poisoning

The body needs a small amount of manganese (2–3 mg) daily. Poisoning is the result of inhalation of manganese dust from industrial processes. It causes respiratory irritation and secondary infection, dermatitis, liver enlargement, headache, sleep disturbance, irritability and progressive basal ganglia disturbance similar to Parkinsonism. Treatment is with sodium calcium edetate and the symptoms of Parkinsonism may be relieved by levodopa and anti-cholinergic preparations.

Nursing care of patients suffering from metal poisoning
See also Chapters 9 and 25

When a patient with chronic metal poisoning is admitted to hospital, his condition may be the result of slow deterioration which has taken place over many months or years. A middle-aged man may appear aged beyond his years, mentally slow, tremulous and unsteady in gait. His relatives may have paid little attention to the change, but the nurse who has not known the patient before will immediately notice his mental dulling, lack of initiative, neglect of personal hygiene and general apathy. It is important for an accurate written report to be made as a base-line for future assessments and a comment from relatives on the patient's previous personality traits is also useful. The patient should be encouraged from the beginning to be as independent and active as possible. Detailed daily written observations of his physical condition, spontaneous activities, sociability, mood and sleep rhythm will be helpful information for the doctor during what may be a very slow, almost imperceptible recovery. Children should be detained in hospital for as short a time as possible as they will benefit most by their home environment and will be seen frequently in the out-patient department.

Rehabilitation
See also Chapters 3 and 10

A full programme of rehabilitation will include occupational therapy and physiotherapy; there may be some residual damage in the nervous system and re-education and change of employment may be necessary. The medical social worker will be in close contact with the family throughout the patient's illness, giving advice about financial matters and rehousing; later she will act as a liaison with the community social worker, council departments and employers.

Careful follow up is necessary to ensure that treatment is continued as prescribed without ill effects and that the patient is no longer exposed to the poisonous substances; blood tests will be performed regularly to ascertain the blood metal levels and to check that the patient is not anaemic.

Tetanus

Tetanus is a condition caused by the infection of a wound by *Clostridium tetani* bacteria; being anaerobic these bacteria thrive in deep wounds, in the presence of a foreign body, or when there is sepsis or necrotic tissue. The tetanus bacillus is found in the faeces of many animals, especially horses and sheep, and is therefore in the soil and on the road; it forms spores which lie dormant for many years. When the bacteria enter a wound they cause infection and release toxins which enter the peripheral nerves and track into the central nervous system.

This is a very serious illness, but nowadays the population is protected; most children are immunised against tetanus during infancy and receive booster injections of tetanus toxoid at 5 years of age and again before leaving school. Should a person so protected sustain an injury, a further dose of tetanus toxoid is given which gives life-long immunity. Anyone who has not had this final injection or someone who has never been given protection and who sustains a potentially dangerous injury, will be given an injection of human antitetanus immunoglobulin for immediate protection and tetanus toxoid for future immunity.

The incubation period for tetanus is usually 7–8 days; the first symptoms the patient notices are difficulty in opening his mouth ('lockjaw' or trismus) due to spasm of the masseter muscles, headache, stiff neck, dysphagia, back pain and cramp-like stiffness in the legs due to muscle spasm. The patient's face develops a fixed expression, his forehead is wrinkled, eyes sunken and half closed, and mouth pulled into a sardonic smile (risus sardonicus). Head retraction develops, the back is arched, legs rigid and extended and the abdomen becomes board-like. Superimposed upon this rigid state are very painful paroxysmal muscle spasms which are precipitated by unexpected external stimuli such as noise, touch or sudden movement and may be so forceful as to cause fractures. Spasms of the diaphragm, laryngeal and intercostal muscles will cause choking episodes which, though not truly hydrophobic, may be provoked by attempts to drink; the spasms may be prolonged and cause asphyxiation. When the autonomic nervous system is affected the patient sweats excessively, has a rapid irregular pulse and a fluctuating blood pressure; his temperature is variable, and hyperpyrexia a serious symptom.

Although the toxin itself does not cause permanent brain damage, death may result from exhaustion caused by continual paroxysmal muscle spasms, asphyxia due to laryngeal spasm or inhalation pneumonia; however ill the patient, he does not lose consciousness unless death is imminent.

Treatment will commence immediately the diagnosis is made. A dose of intravenous antitetanus immunoglobulin is given to prevent further absorption of toxins from the wound; benzylpenicillin will also be administered to destroy the *Clostridium tetani* bacteria. Sedatives and antispasmodic drugs (diazepam) will be administered to keep the patient calm and reduce muscle spasm. Intravenous feeding will be necessary if the patient is dysphagic or when severe muscle spasms make it impossible for him to take enough fluid. Spasms may be so severe that muscle paralysing agents (tubocurarine) become necessary and respiration must be maintained by a positive pressure ventilator via a tracheostomy.

Nursing care
See also Chapter 3

The patient will be 'specialled' in a single, quiet, darkened room; notices will be posted at strategic places in the ward, requesting 'Quiet please'. Equipment must be ready to give suction and artificial ventilation. A smooth sequence of nursing care will prevent the patient being unnecessarily disturbed and stimulated; any lengthy nursing procedure must be given at an interval after the administration of sedative and muscle relaxant drugs, when the patient is most relaxed. Quiet explanation of all procedures is always necessary as the patient will remain fully conscious.

This is still a very serious illness and the prognosis is poor, but if the patient can be kept alive without complications while the tetanus toxin is naturally eliminated from the body, the chances of survival are improved.

Botulism

Botulism is an extremely rare notifiable disease; it is a very acute form of food poisoning, often rapidly fatal, caused by eating improperly processed bottled or canned foods infected by *Clostridium botulinum* bacteria which thrive in alkaline anaerobic conditions and give off a highly poisonous toxin. The bacteria are destroyed by boiling, but the spores are only destroyed at a higher temperature. Inspection and regulations controlling the commercial preparation of bottled and canned foods prevent the incidence of botulism except in very rare instances. Housewives must use correct procedures for bottling foods and appreciate the risks of using the contents of bent, punctured and 'blown' cans.

There are rare incidences of botulism poisoning a single person or a small number of people who have eaten contaminated food. The poisoning affects the central nervous system more than the gastrointestinal tract and symptoms include general weakness, dizziness, headache, ocular, pharyngeal or other cranial nerve palsies, vomiting and sometimes diarrhoea. In some instances the patient's condition deteriorates so rapidly with the occurrence of convulsions, coma and respiratory failure that the victim dies before anyone is aware that he is ill. On the other hand the patient may be rushed to hospital suffering from very severe food poisoning with characteristic signs and symptoms which differ from any other form of food poisoning. The contents of the patient's stomach are aspirated and saved for analysis, a stomach washout is performed and an intravenous injection of botulinum antitoxin is given. Respiratory failure is usual and a tracheostomy and artificial ventilation using a positive pressure ventilator are necessary (see p. 51). Skilled nursing and medical care are essential to keep the patient alive and free from complications while the body rids itself of the poisonous toxins; even so, few patients survive.

When the source of poisoning is discovered, the Public Health Authority and the Department of Health take appropriate steps to ensure that no other member of the public is poisoned; this may result in the withdrawal of a particular batch of food and a public warning about goods already retailed.

28

Muscle Disorders (Myopathy)

Anatomy and physiology

A muscle is composed of many elongated cells called fibres, some large, others small, interlaced with connective tissue and bound together into bundles. Many of these bundles bound together form a muscle; the whole muscle is enveloped in connective tissue called fascia which tapers at each end into a tough, inelastic flexible tendon continuous with the periosteum. Muscle tissue has some important characteristics; it is capable of receiving and responding to an electrical stimulus by contraction, and its elasticity allows it to be stretched and to spring back into shape. To remain healthy and function satisfactorily the muscle must have:

1   an adequate blood supply containing nutrients in the right proportion;
2   an intact nerve supply
   (a)   sensory fibres which convey impulses to the brain
   (b)   motor fibres which convey impulses from the brain to the muscle;
3   a balance between the chemical, acetylcholine, and the enzyme, cholinesterase, at the neuromuscular junction;
4   a balance between certain chemicals, in particular, sodium and potassium, and enzymes concerned with normal muscle metabolism; this is not yet fully understood though in certain muscle disorders variations have been observed; and
5   the muscle must be used.

Sometimes, at any time from infancy to old age, muscles become weak and wasted; this may be an inherited disorder, the effects of disease, malnutrition, or due to normal ageing processes. The conditions are usually chronic and progressive.

Muscular dystrophy

There is a group of fairly uncommon hereditary disorders of unknown cause which are characterised by progressive unrelenting degeneration of certain groups of muscles, without involvement of the nervous system. Weakness and wasting of these muscles affects both sides of the body, skeletal deformities develop (scoliosis, lordosis and winging of the scapulae) and fibrosis and shortening of the atrophied muscles cause painful contractures. In some instances the 'muscle' increases in size due to useless deposits of fat (pseudohypertrophy). Ultimately the degeneration of muscle will interrupt the reflex arc and tendon reflexes will be lost. Though several apparently clearly defined forms of muscular dystrophy are described there may be considerable overlap, especially in the adult forms; some begin earlier or later than usual and do not advance at the expected rate. One or more members of a family may be affected and there may be a history of the disorder in previous generations. In general, the earlier the child is affected the more rapid the deterioration and the poorer the prognosis. The diagnosis is usually obvious from the family history and examination of the patient; electromyography, muscle biopsy, blood and urine tests may be helpful if the diagnosis is uncertain. No specific treatment has yet proved effective. These disorders are very distressing; the pathetic physical disablement and in some instances actual facial disfigurement of a young child of normally bright disposition and intellect, the curtailment of life expectancy and important genetic implications, give a sense of urgency to research programmes which, though assisted by modern laboratory techniques, are still hampered by limited financial support. Known sufferers of the disorder and members of their family should be referred to a Genetic Counselling Centre for advice regarding family planning; by estimating the serum creatine phosphokinase, it is sometimes possible to discover subjects who are carrying the disorder even though there is no clinical evidence of the disease.

Pseudohypertrophic muscular dystrophy (Duchenne type)

This is the most common form of muscular dystrophy and usually affects young boys, is rapidly progressive and runs its full course within 15 years. The condition is transmitted by the mother who is a carrier, though she herself shows no signs of the disease. The main feature of this disorder is a characteristic change in the muscles; the muscle fibres atrophy, connective tissue increases and fat deposits occur. The affected muscles, those of the calves, buttocks, front of the thighs and some of the muscles of the shoulders and back, appear more bulky (pseudohypertrophic) and firmer to the touch than normal, but despite their highly developed appearance they are very weak. Other muscles of the chest and back are wasted without pseudohypertrophic changes; the face and hands are unaffected.

The disorder is usually first noticed when the child, at about 5 years of age, begins to walk in an ungainly way, tends to stumble, cannot run without falling and when he falls finds difficulty in getting up from the ground; before this he may have appeared normal and achieved normal milestones of development though some children have never walked normally. On examination the child may look deceptively sturdy as he stands with his trunk thrown back and large shoulder and calf muscles (Fig. 28.1), the term 'infant Hercules' has sometimes been used to describe this appearance. Winging of the scapulae, due to weakness of the serratus anterior muscles, and lumbar lordosis will be obvious. One feature of movement always observed in association with this disorder is the child's method of getting up from the ground; he

first rolls onto his hands and knees and then pushes himself upright by walking his hands up his legs; this method is necessary because of weakness of the extensor muscles of the spine and knees. Within a few years these children usually lose their ability to walk and, becoming increasingly helpless, resort to a wheelchair existence. They often become overweight as the result of inactivity, and kyphoscoliosis makes it difficult for them to sit, comfortably supported, in a wheelchair; unless there are restraining straps the child may very easily fall out of the chair, particularly when going down steep slopes. Children with this disorder rarely live beyond the age of 20 years and usually die as the result of intercurrent respiratory infection.

Limb girdle muscular dystrophy

This type of dystrophy occurring during adolescence or in early adult life affects boys slightly more often than girls. The disorder is caused by a recessive gene which can transmit the tendency without actually producing the disease; this is passed to successive generations. When two people

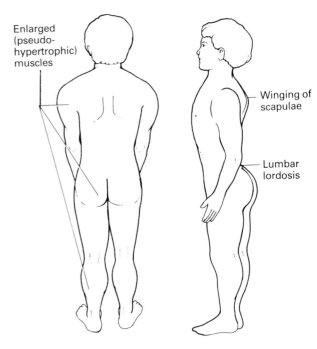

Enlarged (pseudo-hypertrophic) muscles

Winging of scapulae

Lumbar lordosis

Fig. 28.1 Child with pseudohypertrophic muscular dystrophy.

with this abnormal gene have children, though neither of them may suffer from the dystrophy, 1 in 4 of their offspring will develop the condition.

Symptoms of weakness and wasting first develop in the muscles of the shoulder girdle making it difficult to raise the arms, or in the muscles of the pelvic girdle causing difficulty climbing stairs or rising from a sitting position. The symptoms are slowly progressive and may be confined to one group of muscles for many years. Many with this disorder lead a relatively normal working life within the limits of their disability, but for some, the disease advances more rapidly and by middle age they are quite severely handicapped.

Facio-scapulo-humeral dystrophy (Landouzy-Dejerine)

This is the rarest and usually most benign form of muscular dystrophy and can affect both sexes though more commonly it affects boys. The facial and shoulder girdle muscles slowly and progressively become weak and wasted; many years later there may be involvement of the legs. The disorder is passed on directly by the affected individual to half of their children of either sex. The onset is usually during adolescence or early adulthood and the first complaint is of difficulty in raising the arms above the head. The muscles of the face are not always involved, but when they are, the bilateral facial weakness gives a flat expressionless appearance, the eyelids close incompletely, the lips are thick and pouting due to pseudohypertrophy, the patient is unable to whistle and he has a leering smile. The youngster appears exceptionally thin with obvious wasting of the upper arms and winging of the scapulae; when the lower limbs become involved, bilateral foot-drop develops and the patient tends to trip, when he is usually unable to save himself because of muscular weakness, and invariably falls flat on his face causing disfiguring bruises and abrasions. The disorder progresses slowly, the patient continuing to walk after a fashion, though with increasing difficulty especially when going upstairs, getting on and off buses and on uneven ground. There comes a time when appliances (toe springs, calipers and spinal supports) become necessary to enable the patient to walk and maintain his posture though they add to the difficulty of getting dressed.

Ocular muscular dystrophy

This is a rare slowly progressive condition in which there is bilateral ptosis and weakness of all the muscles which move the eyes. In some patients there may also be other weak muscles but the disorder is relatively benign.

Distal muscular dystrophy

This disorder is very rare indeed; it affects the small muscles of the hands and feet giving them a claw-like appearance; it then gradually spreads to involve the lower muscles of the legs and forearms. There is often no family history, but in some families it is passed on by an affected person to half of their children of either sex.

Care and management of patients with muscular dystrophy

There is no effective treatment or cure for muscular dystrophy; handicapped children or adults can lead a fuller life than was at one time possible, because of present knowledge of the importance of remaining active and involved in life and the availability of helpful social services. Nothing can alter parental distress when they are first told the diagnosis and prognosis for a child with muscular dystrophy. During any child's first year parents are watchful and half anticipate some slight abnormality or delay in development, but when that time has passed they assume they have a normal healthy child. It comes therefore as a great shock when they notice deterioration in their child's agility and are told that he has an inherited disorder which will cause progressive disability and gives a short life expectancy; there may be the additional distress of finding that other younger children in the family also have early signs of the disorder. Most parents will come to terms with the situation, but a few continue to harbour resentment and some may never accept that their child has an incurable disease. As soon as the diagnosis has been made both parents should be fully informed about the illness and its expected course. Confidence in their medical adviser is essential or parents may continually waste energy, time and money seeking a cure, and their attitude of restless discontent will distress the child. Parents may be burdened with guilt when they know they have been responsible for passing the disorder to their child; when both parents have carried the abnormal gene, guilt is shared, but they may be self-reproachful and heartbroken as they consider the child's future. The parents may not at first realise the burden they will have to bear as the disability relentlessly increases, the child needing continual encouragement, help, support and finally full nursing care, day and night; this burden falls mainly on the mother though indirectly it affects each member of the family. Each family will respond in a different way to crises; some have neither the financial nor psychological reserves to call upon. In some instances the situation is made even worse when the father and breadwinner is also disabled; this will add to the mother's burden, as she cannot call upon her husband to help with the many tasks involved in maintaining the house and garden, or do anything which involves lifting or climbing steps or ladders; in his efforts to be helpful the husband may take unnecessary risks.

A child affected by muscular dystrophy is at an age when he will be keenly aware of what is going on and parents and others will need to control and hide their feelings of distress very rapidly and remember that a child's hearing is very acute. Fortunately, small children are generally adaptable and find fun and interest more easily than adults; adolescents are more likely to ask questions and feel depressed about their condition. Every parent is responsible for their child's attitude to life, self-reliance and mature development. It cannot be easy for parents to treat and discipline a disabled child as they would a normal one, but over-protection and indulgence will do the handicapped child nothing but harm; what he needs more than anything, is as normal a life as can possibly be created and the love and security of a happy home.

The growing child must retain his independence for as long as possible and this includes the freedom to take decisions and discuss plans regarding education, outings, holidays and recreational pursuits. He may be able to enjoy some rather unexpected outdoor and indoor activities for a time; there has been great interest recently in sports

for the disabled including swimming, sailing, horse-riding, archery, fencing and table tennis. It will give a young person greater contentment of mind if he has at least experienced the pleasure of these activities, and later, when he can no longer take an active part he will still be able to follow them with interest. The child also needs to cultivate more sedentary interests; he can be encouraged to read, collect stamps or coins, or have pen friends – interests he will be able to continue in the late stages of the illness when he is severely disabled. Disabled children also enjoy belonging to such organisations as the Guides or Scouts, and friends made in these companies will be even more valuable when the youngster is completely helpless.

Education
(see pp. 183 and 201)

Many children with the less severe forms of muscular dystrophy will be able to attend a normal school, but those who use a wheelchair will attend a special school for the handicapped, as a day pupil, weekly or full-time boarder, depending what suits the family best. It may be hard for parents to accept that their child will be better off away from home and they may think they are shirking their responsibilities, but the disabled child is sometimes happier among others with similar disabilities and will find school interesting and the days fully occupied. Parents, brothers and sisters can arrange weekend outings or welcome the youngster home for weekends and holidays when, as the mother is not so tired and harassed as she would be were she giving full time care, the time can be a particularly happy reunion. In a few instances arrangements are made for the child to be educated at home, but this provides no change of scene or company.

Finance and facilities
(see p. 194)

Families are sometimes ill-informed and reluctant to claim their rightful financial assistance; the father may be disabled, possibly in poorly paid employment or unemployed, and if the mother is caring for a handicapped child or other young children at home, she will find it impossible to go out to work. A car is essential for someone who has difficulty walking and can no longer board and alight from public transport; the family may need to run two cars or a large car to accommodate one or more wheelchairs, which means high petrol consumption. Rising costs may limit family travel especially when there are so many other extra calls on a family's limited income; mobility allowances are available, but the busy, tired mother may not make the effort to visit the local Department of Health and Social Security nor feel like answering endless questions and filling in forms to put in a claim, unless she is encouraged to do so. The community occupational therapist and social worker should visit the home to assess the entire situation, to see whether it will be necessary for the family to be rehoused in ground floor accommodation, or whether adaptations can be made to the existing premises. Grab rails and ramps may be fitted, a telephone, electric wheelchair, 'hospital' bed or hoist may be necessary; a stair lift may be required (in this case some of the cost is borne by the family or a charitable organisation). Voluntary organisations may be helpful too in supplying such items as a television set or night storage heaters; an inactive person always feels the cold and the room temperature needs to be higher than in a normal household; less additional heating will be required at night if a continental quilt is used. Other expenses are incurred when clothing has to be adapted to suit an individual's needs (velcro fastenings simplify dressing and going to the toilet) and shoes are soon worn out. Clothing damaged by falls may need to be replaced; a businessman could not possibly go to work with patched trousers.

It is only possible to achieve a smoothly run household if considerable thought is given to the planning of each day. Each person's interest and well-being must be studied, neither parent should be overburdened, those who are handicapped never cast on one side, lonely and unoccupied, nor over-protected and indulged, nor must the normal child be sacrificed for the sake of the disabled. There should be no hesitation in accepting and requesting help from Social Services, voluntary organisations, relatives, friends and neighbours as it is very important that the mother should not become exhausted to the point of collapse. When heavy day and night nursing is necessary this is even more important, it is particularly difficult to find someone willing to sit with a severely disabled teenager or take on night care.

Parents should be introduced to the Muscular Dystrophy Association where they will be given the opportunity to meet and discuss their problems with others who have had similar experiences, and to take part in the varied social activities arranged by its members.

It is essential for both parents and children to go out, but even minor shopping expeditions can prove difficult unless there is a great deal of advance planning. Car parking facilities for the disabled are not always available, few places are without steps and stairs and toilets are often inaccessible; unless there are separate toilets for the disabled it is impossible to help a disabled person of the opposite sex, for example a mother may not be able to help her teenage son.

Home nursing care

The care of children and young people with a progressive degenerating disorder is inevitably time consuming as these children are rarely admitted to hospital; it is the mother who needs to be prepared for the many problems before they arise. Independence should be encouraged; difficult as it may be for a mother to stand idly by, watching her child struggle to complete a fairly simple task, if she realises the many years of nursing care ahead she will not make an invalid of her child too soon.

Diet is important from the outset. A healthy child who is constantly 'on the go' uses an immense amount of energy, but as the child with dystrophy becomes gradually less active his diet must change or he will slowly and imperceptibly gain weight (see p. 181). Constipation may be a problem and may lead to incontinence of urine.

Mealtimes may become a 'messy business', but independence in feeding should be encouraged. A high table allows food to be placed on a level with the child's mouth enabling him to feed himself with little effort. When the muscles of the neck and lower jaw are weak, the sufferer usually props up his floppy head and lax jaw with his hand.

Physiotherapy should begin early to prevent contractures. Parents may learn the techniques from the physiotherapist and find it simpler and more beneficial to give the daily treatment themselves at home to avoid the difficult, time-consuming excursions to hospital; periodic check up at the physiotherapy department is advisable. Even with the most diligent care it may be impossible to avoid contractures, in particular those affecting the legs; surgical transplantation of tendons may be helpful. The child may need a spinal support. The physiotherapist will also teach the mother the techniques of postural drainage, 'clapping' and shaking (see p. 50); common colds are often followed by chest infection and as the child's respiratory muscles and cough are weak he will find difficulty in expectoration. Falls are commonplace; once the disabled person finds it difficult getting up from the ground he cannot be left unattended nor allowed out on his own. When helping someone up from the ground, not knowing how much assistance is necessary, an inexperienced helper may 'let go' before the disabled individual has regained his balance; nurses should appreciate that such a past experience may be the cause of apparently unnecessary agitation and lack of trust in the nursing staff.

Hospital care

Hospital admission, though the patient may be severely disabled, is rare. Reasons for admission include surgical treatment for contractures, severe chest infection, other general illness unassociated with muscular dystrophy and, if the patient is severely disabled, when those upon whom he is dependent are ill and unable to care for him. Nurses should appreciate that the patient's family obviously know the details of his care better than they do, and must always be prepared to listen to their suggestions.

Polymyositis

Polymyositis is a widespread inflammatory disease allied to the collagen diseases which cause destruction of muscle fibres and inflammation of connective and subcutaneous tissues and blood vessels. The disease is rare, affecting men and women equally, usually between the ages of 30 to 60 years. In most instances no cause can be found, but the disease is sometimes associated with carcinoma, especially of the bronchus. There is much variation in the onset, progression and prognosis of polymyositis, ranging from an acute and rapidly progressive illness, to one which is chronic and slowly progressive over many years with remissions, regression and occasionally spontaneous arrest.

Symptoms

In acute polymyositis the muscles become swollen, tender and weak and there is oedema of the subcutaneous tissues and skin. There may also be obvious skin lesions, erythema, pigmentation and telangiectasis; the term dermatomyositis is usually applied in this instance. The proximal muscles are first affected, then other muscles waste and become weak, leading to complete paralysis. The tendon reflexes are lost when there is little remaining muscle with the power to contract. The patient is feverish and a blood count will show an increase in polymorphonuclear leucocytes.

Analgesics will be given for pain. Steroid therapy is the only specific treatment for polymyositis and since its use the prognosis for young patients with the acute form of the disease has greatly improved; oedema and inflammation soon subside and the true extent of muscle wasting will then be apparent.

The patient with chronic polymyositis does not feel generally ill, but tires easily; all his muscles including those of the face, throat and neck are weak, wasted and readily fatigued. Complete recovery is unlikely even when the disease has arrested spontaneously, but there may be some slight improvement with the regeneration of partially damaged muscle fibres.

Examination and investigations

1 A full physical and neurological examination
2 Blood tests
   (a) A full blood count will show evidence of inflammatory disease
   (b) An ESR – this will be raised according to

the degree of active muscle inflammation and destruction

3 Urinalysis – a more accurate assessment of muscle damage can be made by measuring the levels of muscle enzymes, e.g. creatinine kinase

Occasionally the diagnosis may be difficult and, to differentiate this from other diseases with similar symptoms, (motor neurone disease, thyrotoxic and carcinomatous neuropathies and muscular dystrophies) the following tests are necessary

4 Electromyography
5 Muscle biopsy

Nursing care

The patient suffering from acute polymyositis must have complete rest in bed during the acute phase; thereafter he will be mobilised and rehabilitated within the limits of his disability. Severe paralysis may mean a wheelchair life, adaptations to his home, possible change of employment and all aids for independence (see p. 181). The care of a patient with chronic polymyositis must be adapted to his gradually worsening condition, retaining his independence as far as possible. (For care of the chronically disabled see Chapter 18.)

29

Inherited and Familial Neuromuscular Disorders

There are a few, rare, inherited and familial disorders which develop during infancy, childhood or adolescence, for which there is no curative treatment and which progress slowly over a period of many years. The latent tendency to develop a particular disorder is passed from one generation to the next by a recessive or dominant gene; genetic counselling is important for members of these families. Several members of the same family may be found to suffer from a particular disorder; even when it appears to miss a generation, apparently healthy members of the family may have single associated features especially cataract, scoliosis or pes cavus. The cerebellum, brain stem, spinal cord and optic nerves may be simultaneously or individually affected and degeneration gives rise to ataxia, dysarthria, nystagmus, intention tremor, loss of postural sense and muscular weakness. On examination, optic atrophy may be discovered, but complete blindness is unusual; the heart may be affected.

Friedreich's ataxia

The name of this familial disorder is somewhat misleading as ataxia, though the first, is not the only symptom. An ataxic gait is noticed, usually between the ages of 5 and 15 years; on examination at this stage, the only other abnormalities are scoliosis and pes cavus. The disorder progresses very slowly; several years later movement of the arms becomes ataxic and the hands become wasted, dysarthria, nystagmus, intention tremor and paraparesis also develop. Sensory changes are variable, but postural sensation is often diminished. The plantar reflexes are extensor and firstly the ankle and then the knee reflexes are lost; the sphincters are not affected. Fibrotic changes sometimes enlarge the heart muscle causing cardiac dysrhythmias, heart block and eventual death from heart failure.

There is no effective treatment for Friedreich's ataxia, but occasionally the disorder arrests spontaneously before the patient is so severely disabled that he becomes entirely dependent upon others.

Peroneal muscular atrophy (Charcot-Marie-Tooth disease)

This disorder is more widespread in the nervous system than the name implies. The degenerative process mainly affects the branches of the common peroneal nerves (see p. 325) which supply the legs and feet, but also involves the posterior columns of the spinal cord, the cortico-spinal (motor) pathways and the anterior horn cells (see Figs 10.13 and 10.15). This is a very slowly progressive disorder which may arrest at any time; many members of a family may be affected, some obviously, but others apparently unaffected have mildly deformed feet suggesting that the disease arrested before any disabling symptoms arose. The first symptoms are noticed in the early teens, when a claw-like foot-drop and high stepping gait develop as the result of progressive weakness and wasting of the muscles of the feet. Gradually, wasting spreads up the legs to the mid-thighs and then involves the hands and forearms; sensory loss involves the feet, legs and hands and all reflexes are lost. The patient learns to live with the disablement which in no way shortens life expectancy.

Nursing care

Patients who suffer from these rare conditions spend only a limited time in hospital, but they and their families need compassionate care and support as the prospect for the young person is usually of increasing disability. These patients are seen by a neurologist at an out-patient department, a diagnosis is made and they and their parents are given advice. This initial examination, correct diagnosis and interview are important as they will dispel doubts and uncertainty and prevent the family seeking other opinions, endless examinations and investigations which focus attention on the disorder. The child should be treated as normally as possible with a little extra attention to safety measures, prevention of falls, use of fire guards and care in the kitchen to avoid burns and scalds caused by weakness or inco-ordination. Treatment which involves resting in bed is harmful as the patient will readily lose mobility. Education will depend upon the facilities available in the district and will need to be adapted to the child's mental and physical abilities. A secure happy home environment is a great benefit and normal social contacts should be encouraged; a youngster will be self-conscious of his ungainly way of walking or of wearing heavy surgical boots, supports or calipers.

There may be difficulty finding suitable employment on leaving school despite the advice of the disablement resettlement officer (DRO), but at all times it is important that useful, creative and preferably gainful employment should fill regular hours of the day, preferably in an environment away from home. Parents are often anxious for the future when, due to their advancing age, they will become less able to help and nurse a disabled person; adequate provision for the young chronic sick is essential.

An understanding general practitioner will know a disabled child and his family and put them in touch with social services according to their needs and will realise the implications of such ordinary illnesses as influenza, especially if the patient already has an abnormal heart. When there are problems at home he will arrange for the patient's admission to hospital for assessment, physiotherapy and occupational therapy to ensure that the patient is as mobile and independent as possible and to allow those looking after him to take an annual holiday, or the disabled person may be accommodated in a holiday residence for the disabled.

Dystrophia myotonica

This is a rare disorder combining muscular dystrophy and myotonia mainly occurring in the male members of certain families. It may appear to skip several generations, but cataract, a feature of the disorder, is found with greater frequency and at a younger age in apparently unaffected members of these families. The first symptoms are usually noticed between 20 and 30 years, when the patient complains of weakness, difficulty in swallowing and difficulty in releasing his grasp (myotonia) when shaking hands or holding on to a handrail.

Examination

The patient speaks with a nasal intonation, may be mentally normal or, more often, a little dull or noticeably of subnormal mentality. His face is usually rather expressionless, with smooth brow, premature frontal baldness, drooping eyelids, flattened cheeks, sagging jaw and a long thin wasted neck with wasted or absent sternocleidomastoid muscles (Fig. 29.1) and the patient's head

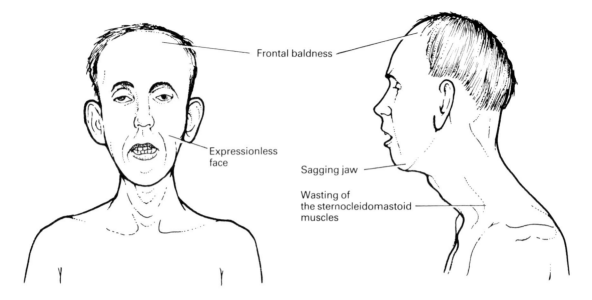

Fig. 29.1 Patient with dystrophia myotonica.

adopts a forward protruding position. There may be gradually increasing weakness and wasting of the muscles of the shoulder girdle, forearms, hands and most of the muscles of the legs; tendon reflexes are absent in the wasted muscles. Symptoms of myotonia, which are increased by fatigue, emotion or cold, are most noticeable in the flexor muscles of the fingers, the facial, masticatory and leg muscles; most tiresome to the patient is difficulty in relaxing his grasp, which persists beyond voluntary effort. Percussion of the tongue and the thenar muscle of the hand can demonstrate this muscle abnormality, as a weal or dimple is produced which only gradually disappears. The patient's heart will be carefully examined as it may be affected and heart block is a possibility. The patient may complain of impotence or amenorrhoea due to atrophy of the testes or ovaries.

Investigations

1 Electrophysiological tests show a characteristic record in the presence of myotonia.

2 Electrocardiography will be necessary if there is any suspicion of heart disease.

3 Intelligence quotient tests will assist placement in suitable employment.

Treatment

There is no specific medical treatment except to achieve some relief of myotonia by the administration of procaine amide. Anaesthesia can endanger the patient's life and should be avoided if possible. The patient can usually lead a fairly normal life within the limit of his mental capabilities and should be encouraged to pursue a useful occupation however simple the task. Those with dystrophia myotonica rarely live beyond early middle age.

Myotonia congenita (Thomsen's disease)

This is a very rare hereditary muscle disorder of childhood, characterised by prolonged contraction and delayed relaxation of muscles after voluntary movement. It causes a considerable handicap as the child is prevented from freely changing his posture.

Family periodic paralysis

This rare familial disorder which renders the patient paralysed, particularly on waking in the morning, is thought to be due to an abnormal level of potassium in the muscles, either too much or too little, or to a lack of sodium. Treatment consists of giving oral potassium or sodium chloride when those levels are too low for diuretics to excrete excessive potassium.

The 'floppy' infant

Infantile muscular weakness may be caused by:

1 Progressive spinal muscular atrophy This familial disorder is due to progressive lower motor neurone degeneration which causes weakness and wasting of muscles. Affected infants are normal at birth but after a few months weakness and wasting begin in the muscles of the back, spread to the shoulder and pelvic girdles and eventually involve the entire body. The infant usually dies within a few months to one year.

2 Benign congenital hypotonia In this condition the muscles are extremely weak and the baby very floppy from birth (like a rag doll). There may be slow improvement enabling the child eventually to sit up and walk. Musculo-skeletal deformities and mental retardation are usual.

3 Congenital myopathy This sometimes familial condition may be present at birth or reveal itself soon after. The proximal limb muscles are small, weak and hypotonic. Some children may slowly improve until they are able to sit up, perhaps to walk, but may deteriorate again. Other members of the same family may develop myopathy later in life.

A muscle biopsy is usually performed to differentiate between these three forms of myopathy.

Appendix

The neurological centre

Patients with disorders of the nervous system often have such major disturbance of consciousness, mental state, speech, hearing and movement that their recovery demands very special nursing skills; the selection and training of all grades of staff and the situation and design of hospital and equipment are important factors for effective treatment and rehabilitation.

A hospital or unit for nervous diseases usually has a large catchment area and patients and relatives will be forced to travel some distance for out-patient appointments and visiting; some have cars, but for those who have not, a regular reliable public transport service is essential. All patients value visiting times, and relatives should always be able to stay with critically ill patients. For those who are semiconscious or have difficulty in communication there are also important therapeutic reasons for regular visiting, as the patient needs to be stimulated to awareness by well-recognised voices and talk of familiar things and needs to learn how to communicate with his family in spite of slurred or disordered speech. During rehabilitation relatives must learn how and to what extent they can lend assistance and will help to maintain the morale of a long stay patient. Relatives must also be available when the patient is unable to give the doctor information. A few relatives will need to stay overnight at the hospital and separate accommodation near the ward will include a bedroom, comfortable sitting room with books and periodicals, television viewing room and facilities for making a cup of tea or coffee, though the comfort given by a thoughtful nurse personally bringing a cup of tea to distressed relatives should never be underestimated; a canteen service will provide main meals. The hospital may have a list of local residents who provide more long term accommodation at an acceptable cost. A public telephone kiosk will keep relatives in touch with home and enable them to pass on information about the patient's condition to family and friends.

Ideally, the neurological centre is part of a large general hospital, as consultants from all fields of medicine, surgery and psychiatry will be needed from time to time, yet it is essential that it is a self-contained unit with its own operating theatre, X-ray department, intensive therapy unit and facilities for rehabilitation. There will be departments for physiotherapy (with a hydrotherapy pool), occupational therapy, speech therapy, accommodation for the medical social worker, an outpatient department and a pharmacy nearby. Facilities for audiometric testing (a sound-proofed room), ophthalmological examination, electro-encephalography and electro-myography are necessary. A chapel should be available for the use of patients, relatives and staff and for services conducted by the chaplain.

The ward units of the neurological centre are ideally sited on the ground floor to give disabled patients access to an open veranda or garden, and for speed of evacuation in case of fire. Fire exits must be kept clear, extinguishing equipment regularly maintained and day and night staff must be familiar with fire drill and attend regular practices. Each room or annexe must have an emergency bell by which patients and staff can summon help.

In the authors' opinion each ward should accommodate no more than 20 patients otherwise the nurse in charge cannot be expected to know each patient, his close relatives and their home circumstances, her nursing and domestic staff, remember the patient's past medical history, present illness and current neurological assessment, results of tests and treatment and be able to communicate all this information to medical, nursing and ancillary staff, not to mention dealing with other ward matters. Less than 15 patients may not provide sufficient variation for teaching purposes nor stimulate the nurses' interest.

The layout of the ward with its ancillary rooms is important; the nurses' station with telephone extension is in the acute area containing beds for 6–8 seriously ill patients. A treatment room in which all dressings and sterile treatments are performed will lead off from the acute area; the room will be large enough to accommodate the patient in his bed, the nurse's treatment trolley and space for at least three people to work comfortably. When a treatment is in progress a notice on the door will prohibit admission; this area must never be a main 'thoroughfare', racks for storage of sterile supplies being replenished from outside. Throughout the unit every possible care is taken to prevent infection, so serious in the central nervous system. Adequate storage space for drugs and lotions, a locked drug trolley and a storage area for emergency resuscitation equipment will be nearby; a nurse must check this equipment at the beginning of each shift. The dirty utility room (sluice) will be distant from the treatment room but near the patient areas.

The remaining beds can be arranged in bays (2–4 per bay) so that the patients will enjoy a certain degree of seclusion while still under the nurses' observation, bathrooms, toilets, lounge-dining room and television room so situated that there is no need for these patients to pass through the acute area; two single rooms will be available for isolation, quiet and privacy. It should be possible to see into side rooms easily and reinforced half-glazed doors and walls are essential. For some very severely disturbed noisy patients there is no better alternative than a room with padded walls and floor; this may be a converted side ward with detachable rubber covered foam sections attached to the walls and door and a thick fitted mattress on the floor. To prevent injury lighting and other wall fittings must be at a high level and there can be no other fittings in this room.

The ward kitchen, a large linen cupboard and storage for disposable supplies with a recess for a clean linen trolley should be near the patient areas to save unnecessary footsteps. Plenty of storage space must be provided for large items of equipment (bed cradles, walking frames and aids, 'monkey pole' hoists, electric fans, ripple bed motors, hair drier on stand, etc.) and standing space for wheelchairs. Other ancillary rooms and offices are necessary for doctors, ward sister, examination of patients and interviewing of relatives and a teaching room for the clinical nurse teacher. The ward receptionist will be accommodated in a bay close to the main ward entrance in a quiet area where she can take accurate details of names, addresses and telephone numbers; as her job is mainly clerical she will be supplied with a desk and comfortable chairs for herself, the patient and relatives.

Automatic reinforced, glazed main ward doors will facilitate entry of trolley-borne patients and equipment, and automatic entrance doors into the bathroom, toilet and sluice area will ensure that these doors are always shut when not in use to prevent unpleasant smells from pervading the ward and to limit noise nuisance. All doorways should be wide enough for the passage of wheelchairs and the bathroom doorway for entrance of a hoist. Safety catches are essential on all windows to safeguard confused or suicidal patients, and windows low enough for a seated person to look out at the scene. The ward must be bright, but blinds are necessary to prevent glare and excessive heat from the sun and for night-time use. Both natural and artificial lighting must be adequate as observation of the patient's colour is important and slight changes will not be noticed in a dim light, nor will early warning signs of pressure sores or small cracks in the skin. An even temperature (16–18°C) and ventilation without draughts will help keep patients comfortable, prevent cross infection and pressure sores, assist in controlling body temperature of patients with hypothalamic disturbance, expel the odour from incontinent patients and keep the staff alert and fit. All flooring even when wet should be a non-slip matt finish as a high gloss surface is a psychological barrier to walking; some areas can be carpeted.

Beds should have easily applied reliable brakes, a simple device for raising or lowering the head or foot and for adjusting the height. Nurses must raise the bed to prevent unnecessary strain when lifting and turning the patient or making the bed, but at other times it is advisable to have the bed at a low level for a restless patient or at a height suitable for the disabled person to get in and out easily. A detachable bed head is essential and a firm base will be necessary to facilitate cardiac massage and for treatment of spinal conditions. Each bed needs fittings to support an intravenous infusion stand (which can be stored when not in use in a recess in the bed), for inserting a 'monkey pole' hoist, overhead mirror or padded bedsides. It is necessary to have a comfortable, heavyweight, waterproof foam mattress which does not slip about when the bed is made and is weighty enough to keep bedding firmly tucked under. A waterbed, ripple beds and a sectional mattress for prevention and treatment of pressure sores will be available from a central store. More sophisticated beds such as a low air loss bed system for totally immobile patients can be rented from the manufacturers or purchased by an Area Health Authority. Piped oxygen supply, suction and an electric point are necessary at each bed space and there should also be a wall mounted sphygmomanometer, clinical thermometer, and a plastic coated wire basket for tissues, disposable gloves and suction catheters.

In the acute area several electric points are needed at each bed space for use with the following equipment:

electric fan
electric blanket
ripple bed
portable X-ray machine
artificial ventilator
cardiac and other monitoring equipment

Each patient needs a bedside locker which, in the medical and rehabilitation wards will include a small hanging wardrobe; a cantilever table is useful for those having meals in bed or when sitting in an armchair. An angle-poise lamp is necessary over each bed with a dimmer switch for use at night-time. In the acute area there must be enough space around each bed to manoeuvre trolleys and bulky equipment (Fig. A.1); a ventilator, cardiac monitoring equipment and portable X-ray machine may all be in use simultaneously and the space must also comfortably accommodate several doctors, nurses and technicians.

Three bathrooms are necessary, two of which should be very large with a central bath allowing easy access for nurses on either side and for the use of a hoist. Also required are a toilet and low level washbasin. The third smaller bathroom is for the use of more able patients. Useful additions to the bathing area are a separate shower room with thermostatically controlled shower and in a female ward, a bidet, and washbasin with shower attachment for hair washing. Each fairly shallow bath with a textured non-slip base will be fitted with handrails on each side and with an easily reached hand-operated plunger mechanism for the plug. An overhead hand hold, which can be hooked out

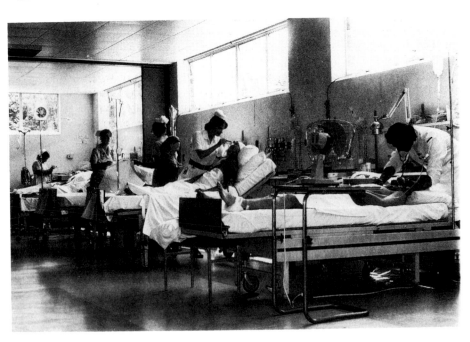

Fig. A.1   Intensive therapy unit.

of the way when not in use, will help the patient pull himself up out of the bath. A bell pull must always be within the patient's reach or for a nurse to summon extra help and there should be hooks for hanging clean clothes and a container of disposable bath mats in each bathroom. At least two other toilets with handrails are necessary, both with doors opening outward (in case the patient collapses), one large enough to accommodate a wheelchair and an attendant and having its own washbasin. Lavatories are often too low for the elderly and disabled and even though there are handrails, a raised lavatory seat may be necessary; a frame round the lavatory will give security when the patient has loss of balance. Several washbasins in curtained alcoves with a variety of lever or foot-operated taps and plugs will suit a variety of disablements. A vanity area with a formica topped shelf, mirror, good lighting and a shaving point is useful. Mirrors are necessary over each washbasin and throughout the ward in strategic places, full-length mirrors will help patients with posture and balance and to get into the swing of walking; an uncluttered walking area is essential.

Most patients, even those who are incontinent, will feel more comfortable wearing their own clothing rather than hospital garments. There are many appliances and waterproofed garments to protect clothing but patients may be messy eaters, may vomit or be incontinent and an automatic washing machine and tumble-drier are necessary items of equipment.

There are many models of commode on the market, some are unsuitable for disabled patients. A suitable commode must be lightweight and easily mobile and have:

a comfortable, commodious toilet seat;

a receptacle (this can be disposable) which can be removed while the patient is still seated, to enable the nurse to clean the patient; a sanichair is suitable for those patients who can be wheeled to the lavatory;

a comfortable padded chair wide enough to seat a large patient comfortably; and

reliable brakes on all four wheels.

A variety of good quality, lightweight comfortable, washable chairs are needed to suit all shapes and sizes. When seated the patient should be well back in the chair with 5–8 cm between the front edge of the seat and the knees, with feet comfortably planted on the floor; there should be no rail between the front legs of the chair to enable the patient to put his feet back as he gets up from the sitting position. Chairs of different height and seat depth will be available for selection to suit individual patients' needs; wing armchairs give support to the back and head without extra cushions; chairs with castors must also have brakes. Dining chairs must be comfortable, washable and well-designed. Several well supporting high-backed wheelchairs will be necessary for ward use and must incorporate removable arms and hinged foot rests; they must be lightweight, compact, fold away for storage, smooth running and have good brakes. Patients who become dependent on a wheelchair must have one made to individual specifications, the chair will need regular servicing.

Electric wall clocks with clear dials and automatic calendars are essential to keep the patient orientated in time. A selection of interesting colourful pictures on the walls can be supplied by the picture library of the British Red Cross Society and colourful curtaining will brighten the ward environment.

A children's ward must be bright and attractively decorated with wall murals and patterned floor tiling. Several mother-and-child rooms, a school room, a play room with a variety of constructive toys and a television, and a quiet play area are necessary. There are many safety aspects which should always be considered in any children's ward – fixed low windows, reinforced glass for all interior glazing, and the ward needs to open onto a safe fenced garden. Electric points must be out of reach of inquisitive children and fitted with safety covers, plastic disposable bags and draw sheets stored well away from the reach of children and waterproof pillowcases stitched on to the pillows. The safety aspect of toys is important and all toys must be washable. Large foam play blocks allow freedom of play with safety for mentally subnormal, physically disabled, disturbed and hyperactive children of all ages. Baby bouncers and walkers may be useful, but used with discretion for only short periods.

The rehabilitation centre

One of the most important developments of recent times is the rehabilitation centre for patients with disorders of the nervous system. A centre is costly to equip and staff, but money can be saved in the long run when many patients are so successfully rehabilitated that they are able to resume their normal lives; others become sufficiently independent to relinquish their dependence on community services and chronic invalidism is prevented. The rehabilitation unit is a separate community of about 45 in-patients and an equal number of out-patients attending daily. Patients are carefully selected ranging in age from 18–55 years although there may be exceptions outside this age bracket (there are special paediatric and geriatric rehabilitation centres); a team comprising the medical officer in charge, a psychologist, physiotherapist and occupational therapist are responsible for assessment and selection of patients. The atmosphere in the centre is one of self-help achieved by the encouragement of staff and other patients. A disciplined individual programme is designed to increase the patient's self-confidence and sense of responsibility, improve memory and concentration and take him step by step through the stages of rehabilitation; there is always a certain amount of helpful competition amongst patients of like disability. Patients come from all walks of life, have many different personalities and have suffered a variety of disorders affecting the brain and spinal cord. There may be a clash of personalities and some patients who have suffered brain damage are outspoken, ill-mannered and unco-operative and care is necessary in arranging shared-room accommodation. Irresponsible youngsters need controlling guidance with regard to their consumption of alcohol when they start excursions into the nearby town as part of their rehabilitation programme, because they do not appreciate the effects of combining alcohol with drugs nor their greater susceptibility to intoxication due to brain damage.

Sleeping accommodation is furnished in a homely style with adjustable divan beds, each room being shared by 2–4 persons; a small ward is necessary for those patients who still require some nursing care. Other accommodation includes sitting rooms and a cafeteria dining room; walking frames with a built-in tray enable the patient to carry his own food.

The rehabilitation day is a full one and demands stamina, the patient rising, dressing, having breakfast and being ready for 'work' by 0930 hours. Apart from coffee and lunch breaks and a short rest after lunch, one activity follows another until 1700 hours and there may be entertainments and social activities in the evening.

The day's activities are divided between the physiotherapy and occupational therapy departments, patients working in groups in the gymnasium yet each exercise or activity adapted to suit the individual, the hard work of exercising against springs and weights being contrasted with more light hearted, but nonetheless useful team games. Some individual physiotherapy treatment sessions will be given including passive exercises, manipulation to correct deformity, heat treatments and electrical stimulation of nerves. Certain patients will be selected for hydrotherapy, small groups being treated at one time. Speech therapy will be given individually or in small groups; this will include the use of picture/word matching sets and games, and learning to read and write. In therapeutic workshops patients' ability, skills and potential for employment are assessed and developed (Fig. A.2); some suitable occupations include typing, printing, metal and woodwork, and machine sewing. Each occupation not only uses the patient's present powers, but also strengthens weak muscles and increases work tolerance; some patients are deliberately given a task which involves standing, even though they are so weak at first that they require a supporting harness.

Some patients recover completely, but many remain paralysed and must be taught to manage in spite of their disability, using alternative methods or gadgets to do everyday tasks. The therapy kitchen, bathroom and laundry are fitted with every imaginable gadget and modification to enable the patient, with guidance, to select the items most suited to his needs and practise using them before going home. The kitchen is a high risk area in any home and for the patient who is unsteady on his feet, has to operate everything with one hand or work from a wheelchair the risk is increased; reduced visual acuity, loss of the sense of smell, insensitivity to pain and weak unsteady

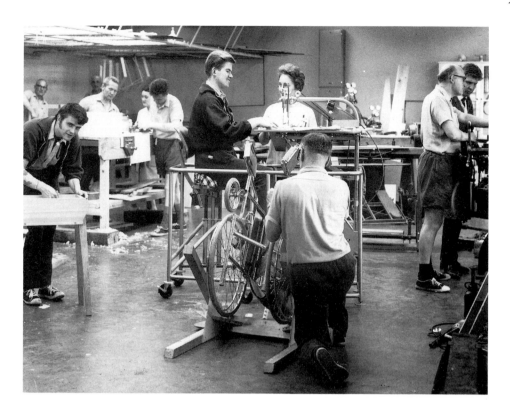

Fig. A.2 Therapeutic workshop in the rehabilitation centre.

hands all add to the dangers of handling heavy pans of boiling water, hot oil and the use of gas and electrical appliances.

Gardening and greenhouse work are useful occupations and tools and gardens can be adapted for the disabled, with long handled implements and raised wall beds. These activities can be mentally relaxing and are very suitable for those who have lost their power of speech; patients can be usefully employed in the hospital gardens.

The next stage is for the patient to venture into the outside world with all the anxiety, embarrassment, lack of confidence and fear of what other people may think and say, especially when he is severely disfigured or has a speech impediment. Patients in a wheelchair or obviously disabled receive more help and understanding than those who are just slow and find difficulty calculating or handling money and who become more agitated,

tense and fumbly when they sense impatience and intolerance from a queue of people waiting behind them at the cash desk; they are naturally reluctant to repeat the experience. In preparation for going out and about patients need practise getting on and off public transport; the platform section of a bus can be set up in the occupational therapy department. The patient will be accompanied on his first excursion by a member of staff, then by another patient and finally will venture out alone. Some patients will be dependent upon their own car for transport. Cars can be amazingly well adapted to suit even severely disabled patients, who need to learn new ways of handling the controls; this can be learned on a simulator and then practised on their own vehicle. When he goes shopping the patient must be able to unload his wheelchair from the car and get into it, then reload it again.

Nursing staff

Neurological and neurosurgical wards need a high staff/patient ratio, as nurses will be needed for 'specialling' seriously ill patients, escorting patients to X-ray for special investigations and accompanying patients to the lavatory and, if necessary, staying with them. Many patients need total nursing care and it is always necessary to have two nurses, sometimes as many as four, to lift a patient. Incontinent patients require frequent attention and may even need to be bathed more than once a day. Senior staff need to be well qualified and trained in the specialty, should be physically fit, emotionally stable, good leaders, able to organise, delegate, teach and inspire all their staff with enthusiasm. They must be cool-headed in emergency and have a good sense of humour. They will be subjected to mental and physical fatigue, to the tensions that arise when medical and nursing staff are anxious about acutely ill patients whose lives are in the balance, to the strain of imparting bad news, meeting distressed relatives and the constant emotional strain of supporting chronically ill patients and their families. All nurses should wear name badges with their rank and qualification, be equipped with a watch with a clear dial and central second hand, a narrow beam torch, red and blue pens and a pair of sharp scissors.

Reliable domestic staff will relieve the senior nursing staff of an added burden of constant domestic supervision. Ward hostesses are invaluable in answering the telephone, receiving new patients and relatives, listing property and performing other clerical tasks as directed.

The ward sister and senior nurses should be aware of all the community services available and if in doubt should contact the medical social worker. They are also responsible for co-ordinating voluntary workers who help with speech therapy, visit the lonely, read to patients and write letters; for arranging appointments with chiropodist, hairdresser, dentist, optician, hearing aid centre and making all the arrangements for the patient's homegoing, including notifying relatives, arranging transport, contacting the district nurse and passing on all the details of the patient's care, arranging meals-on-wheels and home help, outpatient appointments and, should there be any cancellations, making sure that the appropriate department is notified to avoid wasting the time and resources of these hard pressed services.

Glossary

Agnosia Inability to recognise familiar objects
  Visual agnosia Failure to visually recognise objects
  Auditory agnosia Failure to recognise sounds
  Tactile agnosia Failure to recognise objects solely by touch
Akinesia Absence of voluntary movement
Anarthria Inability to speak through failure to articulate words
Anosmia Loss of the sense of smell
Aphasia Loss of the ability to understand or express oneself using speech (language)
Aphonia Loss of voice
Apraxia Inability to perform a purposive movement in spite of understanding its nature and, in the absence of paralysis, sensory loss or ataxia
Astereognosis Inability to recognise familiar objects by touch
Ataxia Inability to co-ordinate muscular movement
Athetosis Slow, writhing, purposeless movements of the limbs

Bruit Swishing noise heard over a blood vessel

CSF Cerebrospinal fluid
Chemosis Oedema of the conjunctiva
Choreiform Jerky, irregular, semi-purposeful, non-repetitive movements of limbs, trunk or head
Clonus Rapidly alternating contraction and relaxation of muscle following sudden stretch stimulation
Confabulation Relating of facts which bear no relation to truth to compensate for failing memory

Decerebrate Without cerebral control
Diplopia Double vision
Dysarthria Difficulty with articulation of words
Dyscalculia Difficulty with mathematical calculation
Dysdiadochokinesis Inability to perform alternating movements with speed and regularity
Dysgraphia Difficulty of expression by the written word in the absence of paralysis
Dyslexia Inability to recognise the written symbols that make up words (word blindness)
Dysphagia Difficulty in swallowing
Dysphasia Difficulty in expressing or understanding speech (language)

Echolalia Automatic repetition of words in a parrot-like way
Emotional lability Difficulty with controlling emotional responses. Easily moved to tears with pleasant experiences
Euphoria Sense of well-being, not always with foundation

Fasciculation Involuntary twitching of muscle bundles or groups of muscles
Flaccid Floppy, limp

Hallucinations A false perception of objects (visual) or sounds (auditory) which have no basis in reality
Hemianaesthesia Loss of sensation on one side of the body
Hemianopia Loss of one half of the field of vision
  Homonymous hemianopia Loss of vision to the same side in both eyes
  Bitemporal hemianopia Loss of the temporal field of vision in each eye
Hemiparesis Weakness of the muscles of one side of the body
Hemiplegia Paralysis of one side of the body
Hyperaesthesia Increased sensitivity to touch
Hyperalgesia Increased awareness of pain

Intention tremor Tremor, mainly of the hand, which increases as it nears its intended objective
Intrathecal Within the meninges (theca)
Ipsilateral On the same side as

Mutism Complete loss of speech which is neither aphasia nor anarthria
Myoclonus Clonic contraction of muscles

Neuralgia Pain in the distribution of a peripheral nerve
Nystagmus Ataxia of gaze, involuntary, rapid movements of the eyeballs which may be horizontal, vertical or rotary

Opisthotonus Extreme arching of the spine with head retraction

Paraesthesia Disordered sensation. Feelings of

prickling, crawling, 'pins and needles', heat and cold

Paraparesis Weakness of legs and lower trunk

Paraplegia Paralysis of legs and lower trunk

Perseveration Involuntary repetition of words or actions

Photophobia Dislike of light

Proprioception Joint position sense

Proptosis Protruding eyeball

Ptosis Drooping of the upper eyelid

Quadriparesis Weakness of all four limbs and trunk

Quadriplegia Paralysis of all four limbs and trunk

Spastic Increased muscle tone

Theca The coverings of the brain and spinal cord (meninges)

Tinnitus Noises in the ear

Titubation Fine, rhythmical, involuntary tremor of the head

Vertigo Dizziness

Xanthochromic Yellow coloured

Bibliography

Brain, L. (1985). *Clinical Neurology*. Oxford Medical Publications, Oxford.

Brooks, N. (ed.) (1984). *Closed Head Injury: Psychological, Social and Family Consequences*. Oxford University Press, Oxford.

Carr, J. and Shepherd, R. (1979). *Early Care of the Stroke Patient: A Positive Approach*. Heinemann Medical Books, London.

College of Speech Therapists (1973). *Without Words: A Guide for Nursing and Medical Staff on Speech and Language Problems*. (A leaflet obtainable for a small fee from The College of Speech Therapists, London.)

Disabled Living Foundation, 380 Harrow Road, London W9 2HU. The Aids Centre will send on request literature concerning the many aids that will help a disabled person towards independence.

Guyton, A.C. (1984). *Physiology of the Human Body*. Holt-Saunders, London.

Guyton, A.C. (1986). *Textbook of Medical Physiology*. W.B. Saunders, USA.

Matthews, W.B. (1985). *Multiple Sclerosis: The Facts*. Oxford University Press, Oxford.

Nathan, P. (1983). *The Nervous System*. Oxford University Press, Oxford.

Netter, F.H. (Ed.) (1985). *Nervous System, Part 1 – Anatomy and Physiology*. Vol. 1 of *CIBA Collection of Medical Illustrations*. CIBA Pharmaceutical Co., USA.

Saunders, C. and Baines, M. (1983). *Living with Dying: Management of Terminal Disease*. Oxford Medical Publications, Oxford.

Williams, M. (1979). *Brain Damage, Behaviour and the Mind*. John Wiley & Sons, Chichester.

Winwood, R.S. and Smith, L.J. (1985). *Sear's Anatomy and Physiology*, 6th edition. Edward Arnold, London.

Index

abdominal reflex   23
abscesses
  cerebral   93
  intracerebral   102
  intracranial   103-5
  spinal   227-8
acetylcholine deprivation   303
acidophilic cells   116
acoustic nerve disorders, *see* labyrinth and acoustic nerve disorders
acoustic neuroma   114
ACTH   260-1
acupuncture   253
acute poisoning   338-42
  emergency measures   339
  forensic tests   340-1
  history and examination   339-40
  treatment and care   341-2
acute post-infective polyneuritis (Guillain-Barré syndrome)   328
acyclovir   106
adhesions in meningitis   102
airway, maintenance of   40-2, 50-1
alcoholic poisoning   338
alcoholic polyneuropathy   329
anarthria   12
anencephaly   70
aneurysms
  anterior communicating artery   133
  'berry'   133
  micotic   134
  middle cerebral artery   133
  posterior communicating   134
  subarachnoid haemorrhage   132-4
angiography   29-31, 131
angiomata   81, 114, 118, 205
  migraine   248
  subarachnoid haemorrhage   134-5
ankylosing spondylitis   241-2
anosmia   85, 117
anticonvulsant therapy   274-5
antihistamine   249
antitetanus immunoglobulin   346
aphasia   11, 44, 129, 146
apraxia   12
arachnoiditis   227
Argyll Robertson pupil   17, 311, 312, 313
Arnold Chiari malformation   70, 77, 265
arterial spasm   30, 128
articulation disorders   12, 302, 308
Aserbine   316
assessment of patient
  general   42-3
  neurological   43-4
ataxia
  in brain stem and cerebellar disorders   129
  in encephalitis   105
  in multiple sclerosis   260
  after post-fossa craniectomy   122

in tabes dorsalis   311
  see also Friedreich's ataxia
atherosclerosis, cerebral   137-9, 147
athetosis   289, 293
atropine sulphate   305
audiometry   296-7
aura
  in epilepsy   268
  in migraine   247

Babinski response (plantar reflex)   23
back pain, *see* spinal injury
bacteria causing intracranial infection   97
barrier nursing   110, 225
basophilic cells   116
Battle's sign   86
bed rest, complete
  for chronic spinal disorders   218-20
  for multiple sclerosis   260
  for polymyositis   353
  for subarachnoid haemorrhage   94
  for Sydenham's chorea   288
behaviour   10
Bell's palsy   325-6
benzhexol hydrochloride (Artane)   282
benztropine sulphonate (Cogentin)   282
benzylpenicillin   346
beriberi   332-3
betahistine dihydrochloride   297
birth injuries   96
bladder problems
  in multiple sclerosis   260, 261
  in neurosyphilis   316
  in unconsciousness   60-1
blood tests   25
blood vessels, tumours of   114
botulism   346
bowels, problems of
  in brain disorders   146
  in paralysis   180-1
  in unconsciousness   61
brachial neuropathy   239
brachial plexus disorders   319-23
brain
  death, diagnosis of brain   67-8
  degenerative disorders of   151-60
  displacement of   37-8
  see also dementia
brain tissue tumours   112-13
Brompton mixture   253
bronchopneumonia   49
Brown-Séquard's syndrome   169
  brucellosis   97
bruit   13, 118
buprenorphine (Temgesic)   253

Cafergot (engotamine tartrate and caffeine)   249

caloric tests 35, 297
canal paresis 35
carbamazepine 231, 250, 252, 275
carcinomatous neuropathy 329
carpal tunnel syndrome 321-2
CAT (computerised axial tomogram) 26
    in encephalitis 106
    in head injuries 89, 90, 92
    in infantile hydrocephalus 73
    in intracerebral abscess 104
    in intracranial tumours 118
    in intracranial vascular disorders 131
    in multiple sclerosis 260
    in tubercular meningitis 101
cataplexy 277
catheterisation 61
    in paralysis 179-80
cerebellar system 21-2, 260
cerebellar tumours 78
cerebral haemorrhage 127-8
cerebral ischaemia 128, 137-9
    emboli 138
    thrombosis 138
cerebral oedema 48, 89
cerebrospinal fever ('spotted fever'), *see* meningitis, meningococcal
cerebrospinal fluid (CSF), *see* CSF
cerebrovascular accident
    care in 140-7
    causes of 127-8
    cerebral ischaemia 137-9
    cranial haemorrhage 131-7
    history and examination 128-9
    investigations 130-1
    mobilisation following 147-8
    rehabilitation following 148-50
cervical disc lesion 221-2
cervical myelopathy 239
cervical rib and costo-clavicular syndrome 320
cervical spondylosis 238-41
    brachial neuropathy 239
    cervical myelopathy 239
    reasons for admission 240
    treatment 239-40
cervical sympathectomy 297
Charcot-Marie-Tooth disease 354
Charcot's joint 312, 316
chemosis 44
chemotherapy, cytotoxic 119, 122-3
Cheyne-Stokes respirations 48, 85, 90
chlordiazepoxide 286
chlorpromazine 253
cholesteatoma 80, 98
chordoma 80-1
chorea 285-9
    see also Huntington's chorea
choroid plexus papilloma 113
chromophobe cells, tumours of 116
chronic poisoning 342-5
    lead 342-3
    manganese 344
    mercury 343-4
    nursing care 344-5
cinnarizine 297
cisternal myelogram 34
'clapping' 49, 50
Cloward's operation 241
codeine phosphate 89, 308
colloid cyst 113
colloidal gold curve 314
communication disorders, spoken, *see* aphasia, articulation, dysphasia, phonation

communication disorders, written 12
compensation neurosis 95
confused patient, management of 61-2, 88
congenital cranial disorders 69-81
congenital dislocation of hip 196
congenital neurosyphilis 314
congenital spinal disorders 185-205
    see also diastematomyelia, spina bifida, spinal angioma, syringomyelia
congenital tumours 80-1
consciousness, levels of 36-68
    after angiography 30
    in cerebrovascular accident 129
    in ventriculography 31-2
    see also unconsciousness
consent for procedures
    radiological 29-35
    unconscious, for the 65
continuous epilepsy 270
contractures 3, 55, 56, 177-8
contre-coup injury 84
copper metabolism
    serum copper estimation 292
    in Wilson's disease 290-1
co-proxamol 253
cordotomy 254-5
corneal abrasion 58
corneal reflex 18, 23
corneal smear in rabies 109
corneal ulceration 38
cortical atrophy 94
corticothrombophlebitis 102
coxsackie virus 98
cranial disorders, congenital 69-81
cranial haemorrhage 131-7
    intracerebral 131-2
    subarachnoid 132-7
cranial nerve palsy 42, 79, 102, 105, 311
cranial nerves 13-21
cranial nerves, tumours of 114
cranial surgery
    craniectomy 121-2
    cranioplasty 93
    craniotomy 120-1, 136-7
craniopharyngioma 80
craniostenosis 81
craniotomy 120-1, 136-7
Creutzfeld-Jakob disease 154
cryoblock 250
cryotherapy 253, 289
CSF (cerebrospinal fluid), description of 33
Cushing's syndrome 116
cyanocobalamin 333, 335

deafness 18
death 66-8
deficiency disorders 331-5
degenerative disorders 151-60, 238-242
dehydration 60, 95
dementia 152-60
    arteriosclerotic 153
    care of 155-60
    causes of 152
    deficiency disorders 335
    general paralysis of insane 313
    history and examination 154-5
    Huntington's chorea 286
    investigations 155
    pre-senile 154
    senile 153-4
    signs and symptoms 153
demyelinating disease 258-63

Depomedrone 253
dermoid cysts 80, 98
Devic's disease 263
dexamethasone 48, 89, 119, 139, 211
dextromoramide (Palfium) 253
diabetes insipidus
    following head injury 95
diabetic polyneuropathy 329
Diagnex blue test 335
diastematomyelia 205
diazepam 253, 272, 275, 346
Diconal (dipipanone co.) 253
diffuse demyelinating diseases 263
di-hydrocodeine 253
dimenhydrinate 297
diphtherial polyneuropathy 329
dipipanone co. (Diconal) 253
diplopia 17, 100, 260, 308, 312
discriminative sensations 24
Disipal (orphenadrine hydrochloride) 282
disorders of the spine, *see* spinal disorders
disturbances of sensation and power 162-184
dopamine in Parkinson's disease 281
dysarthria 12, 21
    in brain stem and cerebellar disorders 129
    in Huntington's chorea 286
    in motor neurone disease 298-9
    in multiple sclerosis 260
dysphagia 20, 21, 49
    in cranial nerve damage 85
    in motor neurone disease 298-9
    after posterior fossa craniectomy 122
    in tetanus 345
dysphasia 11-12, 117, 119
dyspnoea 30
dystrophia myotonica 355-6

echoencephalogram (ultrasound) 27
    infantile hydrocephalus 73
echolalia 154
echo virus 98
edrophonium chloride (Tensilor) 305
electroencephalogram (EEG) 28-9
    epilepsy 106, 264
    telemetry 273
electromyography 305, 321
emergency equipment for the unconscious 39
encephalitis 98, 99, 105-7
    herpes simplex 106
    inclusion body 98, 107
    investigations 106
    lethargica 98, 106-7
    meningoencephalitis 105
    nursing of 106
    treatment 106
encephalocele 70
encephalomyelitis 99-100, 105
    caused by herpes zoster 229
    caused by toxoplasmosis 98
    see also rabies
endocrine disorder
    in cerebral tumour 118-20
    in hydrocephalus 79
endocrine glands, tumours of 114-16
ependymoma 113, 234
epilepsy 94, 264-77
    admission 268
    care during fit 271-2
    causes of 272-3
    in encephalitis 105
    focal 118, 269-70

continuous 270
    Jacksonian 270
    psychomotor 269-70
    sensory 270
generalised 93, 118, 268-9
    grand mal 268-9
    minor 269
    petit mal 268
in general paralysis of the insane 313
in head injury 88
history and examination 264-5
investigations 273-4
management 265-7
observations 270
status epilepticus 271-2
treatment 274-6
ergotamine tartrate 249
examination of patient
    central nervous system 8-25
    see also under particular disorder
exophthalmos 15
external ventricular drainage 49, 79-80
extradural haematoma 89-90
extrapyramidal diseases 278-93
extrapyramidal system 21
eye care
    in head injuries 88
    in unconsciousness 57-8
eye movements 17-18

family periodic paralysis 356
fasciculation 22, 23, 298
fat emboli 94
fatigue, excessive 260, 304
femoral nerve disturbance 323-4
festinating gait 279
finger/nose test 22, 35
first aid in head injury 86
'floppy' infant 357
fluid balance chart 95
foil space blanket 341
foraminotomy 220
fortification spectra 247
fractures
    at birth 96
    and CSF leak 92-3
    of skull 25
    of spine 210-11
Friedreich's ataxia 354
fundus of eye 16
fungal infections 98, 110

gag reflex 20
Gasserian ganglion block 251, 252
general paralysis of the insane 313
glandular fever (infectious mononucleosis) 98
glioma 234
grand mal 268-9
Guillain-Barré syndrome 328

haemangioblastoma 114
haemangioma 233
haematomata
    in head injury 89-92
        extradural 89-90
        infantile subdural 96
        intracerebral 92
        subdural 90-92
    injection site 30
haemorrhage
    cerebral 127-8

cranial 131–7
    intramedullary 237
    subarachnoid 30, 94, 132–7, 236
hallucinations 10
headache 47, 79, 105, 118, 129
    atypical facial pain 252
    causes of 245–7
    in meningo-vascular syphilis 311
    migraine 247–9
    neuralgia 249–52
    temporal arteritis 252–3
    see also intracranial pressure and tetanus
head injury 82–96
    admission 86–7
    anatomy related to 83–6
    birth injury 96
    brain stem 85
    care of 87–9
    causes of 82
    complications of 89–95
    contre-coup 84
    cranial nerve damage 85
    examination and investigation 87
    first aid 86
    prevention of 82–3
    shearing lacerations 85
heel/shin test 23
helminths (worms) 98
hemianopia 15
hemiballismus 288–9
hemiparesis 91
hemispherectomy 276
hepato-lenticular degeneration (Wilson's disease) 290–3
heredofamilial or benign tremor 285
herpes
    simplex 98, 100, 106
    zoster 98, 229–31
Herxheimer reaction 315
histamine test meal 335
Holmes Adie syndrome 17
Horner's syndrome 17, 320
humidifier, mechanical 52, 53
Huntington's chorea 278, 285–8
Hutchinson's teeth 314
hydrocephalus 71–80
    as complication of
        meningitis 102
        spina bifida 195
        subarachnoid haemorrhage 137
    infantile 72–7
    later childhood 77–80
hydrocortisone
    in meningitis 102
    post-craniotomy 120
hydronephrosis in spina bifida 195–6
hydrophobia in rabies 108, 110
hygiene, *see* oral, pressure sores, care of, and skin, care of
hyperalgesia 320
hyperpyrexia 88
hypnosis 253
hypophysectomy 255
    see also craniotomy and intracranial tumours
hypopyrexia 88
hypothermia 341
'hysterical' pain 256–7

infantile hydrocephalus 72–7
infantile subdural haematoma 96
infections, *see* fungal, intracranial, parasitic intracranial and spinal
inherited and familial neuromuscular disorders 354–7
intelligence on examination 11

intracerebral haematoma 92
intracranial abscess 103–5
intracranial infection 97–110
    anatomy related to 4–7, 36–8
    infecting organisms 97–9
    routes of entry 98–9
intracranial pressure, raised
    in craniostenosis 81
    in head injuries 88
    in hydrocephalus 79
    implications of rising 1, 8, 13, 16, 47
    in meningitis 102
    methods of reducing 48–9
    in subarachnoid haemorrhage 132
    in tumours 117–18, 119
    after ventriculography 32
intracranial tumours 111–23
    anatomical and functional localisation 111–16
    growth of 117–18
    history and examination 118
    investigations 118
    nursing care 119–22
    signs and symptoms of 116–18
    treatment 119
intracranial vascular disorders 124–50
    see also cerebrovascular accident
intragastric feeding
    in myasthenia gravis 308
    in posterior fossa craniectomy 122
    in the unconscious 59–60
intramedullary haemorrhage 237
'iron lung', *see* ventilator
irrigation of eye 58
ischaemia, cerebral 104, 128, 137–9
    see also consciousness, levels of

Jacksonian epilepsy 270
jaw reflex 18, 23, 299
joint position sense (proprioception) 24

Kayser-Fleischer ring 291
Kemadrin (procyclidine hydrochloride) 282
keratitis 58
kernicterus (haemolytic disease of the newborn) 152, 293
Kernig's sign 93
    in epilepsy 106
    in meningitis 100
    in subarachnoid haemorrhage 132
Korsakow's syndrome 154

labyrinth and acoustic nerve disorders 18, 294–7
    anatomy and physiology of 294–6
    examination and investigation 296–7
    Menière's disease 296
    treatment and care 297
labyrinthine function, tests of 297
Lactulose 308
laminectomy 220–2
Lange colloidal gold curve 314–15
laryngeal obstruction 52
laryngeal paralysis 312
leucotomy 255
levodopa 281–2
light touch 24
lightning pains 311, 315
limb size in examination 23
lobectomy, anterior temporal 276
'lockjaw' (trismus) 345
long thoracic nerve injuries 323
lower brachial plexus injury 320
lumbago, *see* spinal injury, chronic

lumbar and sacral plexus disorders 323–5
lumbar myelogram 34
lumbar puncture 32–3
  in acute aseptic meningitis 102
  in cerebrovascular disorders 130
  in encephalitis 106
  in multiple sclerosis 260
  in pyogenic meningitis 100–1
  in rabies 109
  in spinal disorders 175–6, 218, 237
  in tubercular meningitis 101
Lundie loops 308

magnetic resonance imaging (MRI) 26–7, 260
malarial parasites 98
Mannitol 44, 48, 89
Mantoux test 101
Maxolon (metoclopramide) 123, 253
mechanical ventilator, *see* ventilator
medulloblastoma 113
melanoma 118
memory on examination 10–11
Menière's disease 35, 296
meninges, tumours of
  meningioma 13, 111–12, 233
meningitis
  aseptic (acute non-pyogenic) 102–3
  basal 77
  in head injury 93
  meningococcal 99–100
  meningo-vascular syphilis 311
  pyogenic 97–103
  tuberculous 97–103
meningocele 186
meningo-vascular neurosyphilis 311
mental state of patient 10–11, 44, 47
  see also dementia
mephanamic acid (Ponstan) 253
meralgia paraesthetica 323
Mestinon (pyridostigmine bromide) 306
metabolic disorders in head injury 94–5
metastases, carcinomatous in brain 112–13
metoclopramide (Maxolon) 123, 253
metrizamide 35
microencephaly 70
migraine 247–9
migrainous neuralgia 249
Migril 249
motor neurone disease 298–302
  admission and care 300–1
  history and examination 299
  investigations 299
  symptoms and signs 298
  terminal care 301–2
  treatment 299
motor neurones, lesions of 24
motor system 21–4
mouth, care of, *see* oral hygiene
MRI (magnetic resonance imaging) 26–7, 260
multiple sclerosis 258–62
  diet 262
  history and examination 259–60
  investigations 260
  nursing care 262
  treatment 260–2
muscle wasting 22, 23
  in motor neurone disease 298
  in muscular dystrophy 347
  in myasthenia gravis 303
muscular disorders (myopathy) 347–52

muscular dystrophy 347–52
myasthenia gravis 303–9
myelitis, spinal 224–5
myelocele 188–9
myelography 218
  cisternal 34
  lumbar 34
myelo-meningocele 186
myopathy (muscular disorders) 347–52
myotonia congenita (Thomsen's disease) 356
Mysoline (primidone) 275

narcolepsy 276
nerve stimulator
  insertion of 254
  transcutaneous 253
nerves, tumours of 114
nervous tissue, anatomy of 4–7
neurofibromatosis 118
neurological centre 358–61
neurological examination 13–25
neuromuscular disorders, inherited and familial, *see* Charcot-Marie-
    Tooth disease, dystrophia myotonica, family periodic para-
    lysis, 'floppy' infant, Friedreich's ataxia and myotonia
    congenita
neuromyelitis optica (Devic's disease) 263
neurosyphilis 310–17
  admission 314–15
  care of 315–16
  congenital 314
  general paralysis of insane 313
  infecting organisms 97
  meningo-vascular 311
  tabes dorsalis 311–13
Norton Scale 54
nursing care
  of the paralysed 171–81
  of the unconscious 39–60
  see also under names of disorders
nursing staff, neurological 364
nystagmus 18, 35, 46, 105
  in brain stem and cerebellar disorders 129
  in labyrinth and acoustic nerve disorders 295–6
  in multiple sclerosis 260

occupational therapy
  in multiple sclerosis 261
  in neurosyphilis 317
  in spina bifida 200
  in syringomyelia 204
oedema, cerebral 89
ophthalmoscopy 16
opisthotonos 42, 100, 109, 293
optic nerve ghoma 114
oral hygiene 56–7
orientation 10
orphenadrine hydrochloride 282
Ospolot (sulthiamine) 275
osteoma 98
otorrhoea 93
overhydration 60, 95
oxycodone pectinate (Proladone) 253
oxygen administration 50

Paget's disease 242
pain 244–57
  anatomy and physiology related to 245
  causes of 245–7
  nursing care of 255–6
  pathways of 246
  psychological 256–7

pain-relieving drugs   253
Palfium (dextromoramide)   253
papilloedema   16
    in cerebrovascular accident   129
    in hydrocephalus   79
    in meningitis   100
    in meningo-vascular syphilis   311
    in suspected cerebral tumour   118
paracetamol   253
paraesthesiae
    in deficiency disorders   334
    in rabies   108
    in tabes dorsalis   311
paralysed patient, care of   171-81
paralysis
    family periodic   356
    poliomyelitis   225
parasitic intracranial infections   98
Parentrovite   332
Parkinson's syndrome   279-85
    admission   283
    diet   284
    history and examination   10, 279-80
    investigations   280-1
    management of   282, 284
    rehabilitation   283-4
    terminal care   285
Parkinsonian symptoms in encephalitis   107
parotitis   57
penicillamine   330
penicillin
    in neurosyphilis   313, 314-15
    see also benzylpenicillin
peri-anal reflex   23
peripheral nerve blocking (cryoblock)   250
peripheral nerve disorders
    anatomy and physiology of   318-19
    see also Bell's palsy, brachial plexus disorders, lumbar and sacral
        plexus disorders, and polyneuropathy
pernicious anaemia   333-4
perphenazine   297
PET (positron emission tomograph)   281
pethidine   253
petit mal   268
phenobarbitone   275, 331
phenol injection   254
phenytoin sodium (Epanutin)   231, 250, 252, 275, 331
phonation disorders   12
physiotherapy
    in cerebrovascular accident   141-5, 149
    in cervical spondylosis   240
    in Guillain-Barré syndrome   328
    in multiple sclerosis   261
    in muscular dystrophy   351
    in neurosyphilis   317
    in paralysis   178
    in Parkinson's disease   282
    in poliomyelitis   227
    in sciatica   325
    in spina bifida   194-5
    in spinal injury   212, 217
    in syringomyelia   204
plantar reflex (Babinski's response)   23
    in epilepsy   106
pneumothorax after angiography   31
poisoning   336-46
    acute   338-42
    botulism   346
    chronic   342-5
    tetanus   345-6
poisons and drugs causing unconsciousness   39

poliomyelitis
    care of   226
    observation of   226
    stages of disease   225-6
    ventilator in   226-7
    virus of   98, 169
polymyositis   352-3
polyneuropathy   326-30
Ponstan (mephanamic acid)   253
positioning of patient
    in cerebrovascular accident   141-5
    in chronic spinal disorder   216
    in lumbar puncture   32
    in paralysis   176-7
    in poliomyelitis   226
    in spina bifida   193
    after spinal surgery   220-1
posterior fossa exploration   251
posterior rhizotomy   254
post-herpetic neuralgia   231
Pott's disease   228-9
power, disturbances of   162-84
prednisolone (oral cortisone)   230, 260
pregnancy in the unconscious   61
pressure and friction sores   54-6
    in paralysis   175-7
    in spina bifida   199
pressure sensation   25
primidone (Mysoline)   275
prochlorperazine   297
procyclidine hydrochloride (Kemadrin)   282
Proladone (oxycodone pectinate)   253
proprioception (joint position sense)   24
proptosis   15, 44, 118
Prostigmin   306
protozoa in intracranial infections   98
psychomotor epilepsy   269-70
ptosis   16, 17, 44, 91, 304, 320
pupil abnormalities, see Argyll Robertson, Holmes Adie and Horner's
pyramidal system   6, 8, 21
    in general paralysis of insane   313
    in multiple sclerosis   260
pyrexia   88
    in head injury   93
    in meningitis   100-3
pyridostigmine bromide (Mestinon)   306
pyruvate tolerance test   332

Queckenstedt's test   33, 101, 102

rabies   107-10
radiculography   35, 218
radiotherapy
    in intracranial tumours   119, 122-3
    in Paget's disease   242
    in spinal neoplasm   235
    see also intracranial pressure, raised
Rathke's pouch, tumour of   80
rebound phenomenon   23
Recklinghausen's disease, von   114
reflex arc   5, 313
reflexes
    abdominal   23
    corneal   18, 23
    cutaneous   23
    gag   20
    jaw   18, 23, 299
    peri-anal   23
    plantar   23, 106
    tendon   23
rehabilitation

in cerebrovascular accident   148–50
in disturbances of sensation and power   181–4
in head injury   95
in poliomyelitis   227
in polyneuritis   328
in spinal injury   212
in unconsciousness   62–6
rehabilitation centre   362–3
relatives, interviews with   64–6, 123
renal failure in paralysis   178–80
repetitive movements, tests for ability in   22–3
respiratory problems
in bronchopneumonia   49
Cheyne-Stokes   48, 85, 90
failure   51–2
in head injury   90, 92
obstruction   50–1
in posterior fossa craniectomy   122
in rabies   109
stridor   42
retrobulbar neuritis   15, 259
Rheomacrodex (dextran)   135
rhinorrhoea CSF   93
Rinne's test   19–20, 296
risus sardonicus   345
Romberg's test   23, 24, 35
in multiple sclerosis   260
in tabes dorsalis   313

sacculotomy   297
sacral plexus, disorders   323–5
St Vitus's dance (Sydenham's chorea)   288
scalp and skull tumours   111
sciatica, *see* sciatic nerve disorders and spinal injury, chronic
sciatic nerve disorders   324
scotoma, central   15
sensation disturbances   162–84
sensory epilepsy   270
sensory inattention   24
septicaemia, acute   100
shearing lacerations in head injury   85
'shingles', *see*, herpes zoster, skin, care of
in Huntington's chorea   287
in neurosyphilis   316
in paralysis   176–7
in poisoning   341
in radiotherapy   123
in the unconscious   53–5
'sleeping sickness' (trypanosomiasis)   98
sodium valporate (Epilim)   275
spasmodic torticollis (wryneck)   290
speech centre   7, 11–12, 44
speech therapy
in cerebrovascular accident   141–2
in intracerebral haemorrhage   132
in motor neurone disease   302
spina bifida   185–202
admission to specialist hospital   190–1
complications
congenital hip dislocation   196
hydrocephalus   195
hydronephrosis   195–6
talipes equinovarus   196
family involvement   193
further care   196–202
medical and surgical management   189–90
medical social worker   193–4
meningocele   186
myelocele   188
myelo-meningocele   186
occulta   185

physiotherapy   194–5
spinal abscess   227–8
spinal angioma   205
spinal cord compression   1, 175, 211
spinal degenerative disorders   238–42
spinal disorders   161–242
admission of   171–4
anatomy and physiology of   162–9
care of   175–81
congenital   185–205
degenerative   238–42
infection in   223–31
injury in   206–22
investigation of   174–5
neoplasm   232–5
observation of   173–4
rehabilitation of   181–4
vascular   236–7
spinal fusion   220
spinal infection   223–31
spinal injury
acute   206–12
chronic   213–22
spinal neoplasm   232–5
spinal vascular disorders   236–7
spirochaete organisms   97
Spitz-Holter valve   74–6
spondylolisthesis   242
'spotted fever'   99–100
squint (strabismus)   17, 44, 85, 305
status epilepticus   271–2
stereognosis   25, 117
stereotaxic surgery   282, 289
steroids
in ankylosing spondylitis   241
in Bell's palsy   326
in cerebral oedema   89
in encephalitis   106
in Paget's disease   242
in polyneuritis   330
in temporal arteritis   253
Stokes-Adams attack   46
stomatitis   57
strabismus   17, 44, 85, 305
'stroke', *see* cerebrovascular accident
Sturge Weber syndrome   81, 135
subacute combined degeneration of cord   334–5
subarachnoid haemorrhage   30, 94, 236
see also aneurysms
subdural haematoma   90–2
subdural hygroma   92
suction technique   41–2
contraindication   93
in motor neurone disease   300–1
in posterior fossa craniectomy   122
in tetanus   346
suithiame (Ospolot)   275
swallowing mechanism   20
Sydenham's chorea   288
syphilis, *see* neurosyphilis
syringomyelia   169, 202–4
syringo-myelocele   188

tabes dorsalis   311–13, 316
talipes equinovarus   196
taping of eyelids   57
tarsorraphy   58
Tegretol (carbamazepine)   231, 250, 252, 275
teichopsia   247
telemetry   273
Temgesic (buprenorphone)   253

temporal arteritis   252-3
Tensilon test   305
tentorium cerebelli, tumours above and below   117
teratoma   80
tetanus   345-6
tetrabenazine   286
thalamotomy, stereotaxic   255
Thomsen's disease (myotonia congenita)   356
thymectomy   306-7
thymus gland   303, 306
thyroid replacement therapy   120
tic douloureux   249-52
tinnitus   19, 296
Torkildsen's operation   78, 119
torulosis   98
toxoplasmosis   98
tracheostomy   52-3, 272
traction of spine   219
tranexamic acid (Cyklokapron)   135-6
trigeminal neuralgia (tic douloureux)   249-52
trigeminal thermocoagulation   251-2
trismus ('lockjaw')   345
trypanosomiasis ('sleeping sickness')   98
tuberculoma   102
tuberculosis of spine (Pott's disease)   228-9
tubocurarine   51
tumours, congenital   80-1
    see also cerebellar and intracranial
two-point discrimination   24-5

ultrasound   27
unconsciousness
    anatomy related to   36-8
    causes of   38-9
    nursing care   40-68
unconscious patient, care of
    continuing   42-68
    deterioration in conscious level   47-8
    feeding of   58-60
    general assessment   42-6
    hygiene and care of skin   53-5
    immediate   39-42
    levels of consciousness   43-4
    vital functions   46-7
unishunt, *see* ventriculo-peritoneal shunt
urinary retention   61, 328
urinary tract infection in paralysis   178-80
urinary tract management
    in spina bifida   200
    in spinal disorders   179-80, 211-12

Valium (diazepam)   253, 272, 275, 346
vascular disorders *see* intracerebral, intracranial and spinal
ventilator   48, 51, 87
    in myasthenia gravis   307
    in poliomyelitis   226-7
    in status epilepticus   272
    in tetanus   346
ventricular system   70-1
ventricular tap
    external drainage   49, 79-80
    in infantile hydrocephalus   73-4
ventricular tumours   113-14
ventriculo-artrial shunt   76
ventriculography   31-2
ventriculo-peritoneal shunt   74-6
    in infantile hydrocephalus   118-19
    in spina bifida   199
vertigo   9, 18, 19, 20, 295-7
vestibular function   20
vibration sense   24
viruses causing intracranial infection   97-8
visual acuity   15, 260, 312
visual field examination   15
visual pathways   14, 15-16
vital functions
    in head injury   88
    in the unconscious   46-7
vitamins
    B_1 329, 332
    B_2 331
    B_6 331
    B_{12} 261, 333
    K   96

wasting, muscle   22, 23
    in motor neurone disease   298
    in muscular dystrophy   347
    in myasthenia gravis   303
Weber's test   19, 296
Weil's disease   97
Wernicke's encephalopathy   332, 333
Wilson's disease (hepato-lenticular degeneration)   290-3

xanthochromia in CSF   130
    see also lumbar puncture

yttrium seeds implantation   255